D0216855

Physical Dimensions of Aging

SECOND EDITION

Waneen W. Spirduso, EdD
The University of Texas, Austin

Karen L. Francis, PhD
University of San Francisco

Priscilla G. MacRae, PhD
Pepperdine University

**HUMAN
KINETICS**

Library of Congress Cataloging-in-Publication Data

Spirduso, Waneen Wyrick.
    Physical dimensions of aging / Waneen W. Spirduso, Karen L. Francis, Priscilla G. MacRae.--2nd ed.
        p. ; cm.
    Includes bibliographical references and index.
    ISBN 0-7360-3315-7 (hard cover)
1. Aging--Physiological aspects.
    [DNLM: 1. Aging--physiology. 2. Aging--psychology. WT 104 S759p 2005] I. Francis, Karen L., 1961- II. MacRae, Priscilla G., 1955- III. Title

QP86.S65 2005
612.6'7--dc22   2004016531

ISBN-10: 0-7360-3315-7
ISBN-13: 978-0-7360-3315-2

Copyright © 2005 by Waneen W. Spirduso, Karen L. Francis, and Priscilla G. MacRae
Copyright 1995 by Waneen W. Spirduso

All rights reserved. Except for use in a review, the reproduction or utilization of this work in any form or by any electronic, mechanical, or other means, now known or hereafter invented, including xerography, photocopying, and recording, and in any information storage and retrieval system, is forbidden without the written permission of the publisher.

The Web addresses cited in this text were current as of October 14, 2004, unless otherwise noted.

Acquisitions Editor: Judy Patterson Wright, PhD; **Developmental Editor:** Renee Thomas Pyrtel; **Assistant Editor:** Ann M. Augspurger; **Copyeditor:** Julie Anderson; **Proofreader:** Sarah Wiseman; **Indexer:** Betty Frizzéll; **Permission Manager:** Dalene Reeder; **Graphic Designer:** Nancy Rasmus; **Graphic Artist:** Kathleen Boudreau-Fuoss; **Photo Manager:** Kareema McLendon; **Cover Designer:** Keith Blomberg; **Photographer (cover):** Robert Baumgardner; **Photos (interior):** Human Kinetics except where otherwise noted; **Art Managers:** Kelly Hendren and Kareema McLendon; **Illustrator:** Mic Greenberg; **Printer:** Edwards Brothers

On the cover: Constance (Connie) Douglas Reeves, at 101 years. Story on page 44.

Printed in the United States of America   10

The paper in this book is certified under a sustainable forestry program.

Human Kinetics
Web site: www.HumanKinetics.com

United States: Human Kinetics, P.O. Box 5076, Champaign, IL 61825-5076
800-747-4457
email: humank@hkusa.com

Canada: Human Kinetics, 475 Devonshire Road Unit 100, Windsor, ON N8Y 2L5
800-465-7301 (in Canada only)
email: info@hkcanada.com

Europe: Human Kinetics, 107 Bradford Road, Stanningley, Leeds LS28 6 AT, United Kingdom
+44 (0) 113 255 5665
email: hk@hkeurope.com

Australia: Human Kinetics, 57A Price Avenue, Lower Mitcham, South Australia 5062
08 8372 0999
e-mail: info@hkaustralia.com

New Zealand: Human Kinetics, P.O. Box 80, Torrens Park, South Australia 5062
0800 222 062
e-mail: info@hknewzealand.com

To those who make it possible for us
to teach, research, write books,
and be happy doing it . . . .

Craig Spirduso

Holden, Micala, Manali MacRae, and

Bear, Karen's best friend, biggest fan,
and most ardent supporter.

Contents

Part III Motor Coordination, Motor Control, and Skill

Part IV Physical–Psychosocial Relationships

Preface

One of the certainties of life is that every day everyone grows older. A time comes in each of our lives when this fact becomes personally relevant. The time is different for everyone, and the awareness may be sudden or subtle, but at some age each of us understands for the first time that we are not immortal. For many people this revelation is precipitated by a physical experience—a father's unexpected loss to his son in a short race, sore muscles following softball at the company picnic, the first time you wonder if you can climb all the steps to the top of the monument on vacation. Of all human dimensions, the physical is usually the first to convince us that no one is an exception to the rule—we all are aging. Not only does the physical dimension provide us with clues to this effect, but it becomes a constraining factor in what we can do, and if we live long enough, physical aging begins to define our quality of life. Because physical function is central to most of our activities, our physical efficiency permeates all aspects of our life. Physical aging affects us cognitively, psychologically, socially, and spiritually.

The focus of the second edition of this book has not changed from that of the first edition. This book discusses how people age physically and how this aging affects other dimensions of life. It will be of interest to anyone who is personally experiencing signs of aging, which includes almost everyone over the age of 40. Primarily, however, *Physical Dimensions of Aging* is written for upper level undergraduate and graduate students planning to be professionals or researchers who work with adults and the elderly, in such areas as counseling psychology, gerontology, health promotion, medicine, psychiatry, nursing, occupational therapy, pharmacy, physical fitness, physical therapy, and social work. Because the book is research based, it provides a resource for researchers who study physical aging in these professions and in disciplines such as biomechanics, exercise physiology, and psychology. We have integrated findings on physical aging from more than 100 different journals in myriad fields, creating interdisciplinary coverage of the topic.

So much has changed about what we know about physical aging since the first edition was published in 1995 that very little of the first edition remains. Although the scope of the first edition was daunting, our scientific community has been so productive over this 10-year period that it was impossible for one person to edit this book. Fortunately, two outstanding former students of the author (Spirduso) agreed to assist in the massive task of editing this book. Our initial dismay at how much we would have to revise eventually merged into gratification that we know so much more about the physical aging process now.

What is different about this second edition? Chapter 13, Job Performance, was eliminated because this topic has grown so large and complex that it requires a book on its own. Chapter 10, Health, Exercise, and Emotional Function, and chapter 11, Health, Fitness, and Well-Being, were merged into one chapter in the second edition, chapter 10, titled Health-Related Quality of Life. The organization of most chapters has been updated. In this edition, we have tried to focus even more on what students and working professionals need to know about physical aging to conduct clinical research or to work with clients and patients. Consequently, we have focused less on explaining the measurement techniques and research design of studies and more on the outcomes of the studies and their implications for everyday living. The book now has a structural organization more conducive to learning. It includes objectives for each chapter; key points that students should remember above all else in the chapter; sidebars of capsule research studies; testimonials, vignettes, and other tidbits that tie the research information to the real world; and review questions to assist students in synthesizing the information and remembering it. We have added a glossary of key terms at the end of the book and a short list of suggested readings at the end of each chapter for those who want to pursue the topic in more detail. For the most part, we have tried to include in this list interesting review articles with good graphics from magazines such as *Scientific American* and *American Scientist*.

As in the first edition, we have worked hard to write this book in an integrated and cohesive manner, so that as many times as possible in a chapter we refer to related information in other chapters. We also maintained the original goal of emphasizing the strong role that good health habits and physical exercise play in modifying functional age and in determining the quality of life of older adults.

The book concludes with a section on physically elite older adults, because the capabilities that result from their consistent and hard efforts are wonderfully inspiring to us all. With so much negative news about physical ability and aging, analyses of the great athletic performances of some of our septuagenarians and octogenarians, as well as the incredible physical feats of older mountain climbers, rock climbers, and long-distance swimmers, raise the bar for all of us. Most people underestimate the physical abilities and potential of older adults. At a time in their lives when so many people are telling older adults that they can't, we as professionals at least should be telling them that they can.

Acknowledgments

Gerontology is an extremely comprehensive and complex field of study. Physical, psychological, social, and environmental systems interact so that it is extremely difficult to identify causal relationships. We have presented the information that we think is relevant and is valid as fairly as we can, but there are only three of us, and no one is an expert on every subject. Thus, we are indebted to several people for reading manuscripts and for helping us "get it right." We are grateful to the following people for reading chapters and giving us advice: Hiro Tanaka, Jan and Terry Todd, and Roger Farrar, The University of Texas; Jim Martin, University of Idaho; Marialice Kern, San Francisco State University; and Ken Fink, Pepperdine University.

It may not take "a village to write a book," but it certainly takes a lot of assistance. We are so grateful to Sandy Graham (U. Texas) for all of her help on technical matters, content, coordination of the authors, and commonsense advice as well as work on the book. She was able to view it as both a student and an experienced health professional, and her contributions are greatly appreciated. Also, thanks to Mina Rathbun and Patty Cauffman (U. Texas), Linda Platas and Rian Tierman (San Francisco State University); and Leslie Branch, Andrea Docherty, and Kami Teal (Pepperdine University) who provided excellent technical support and solved administrative problems that made the book a reality.

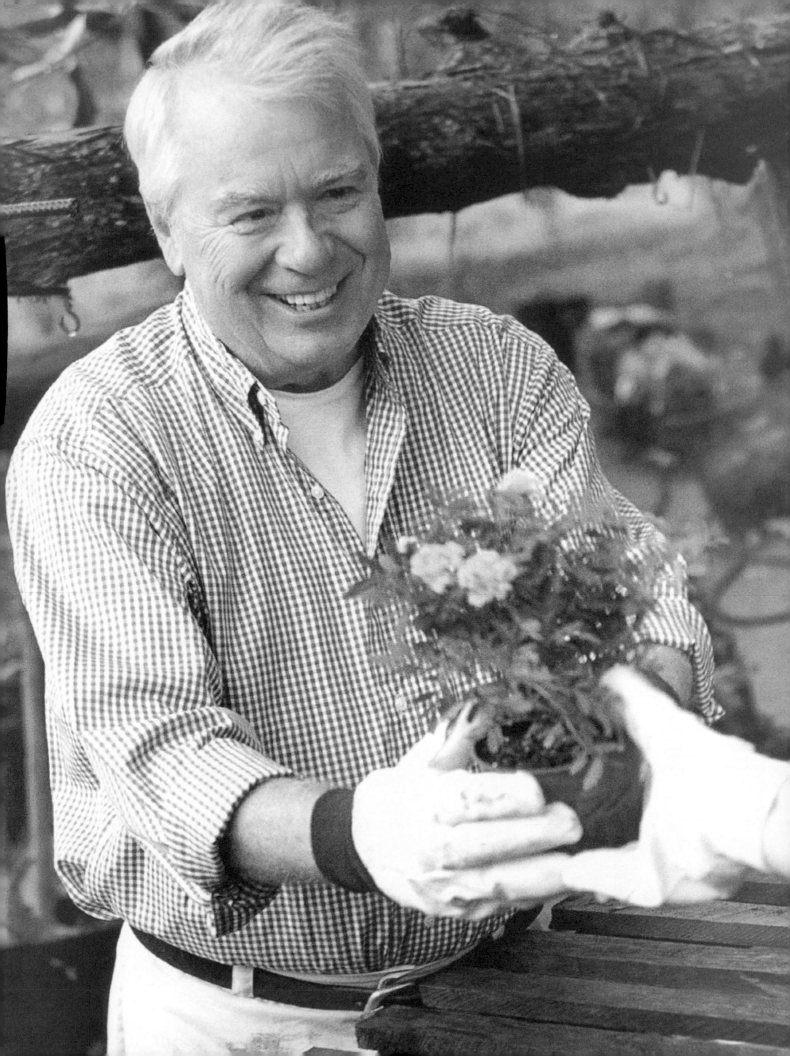

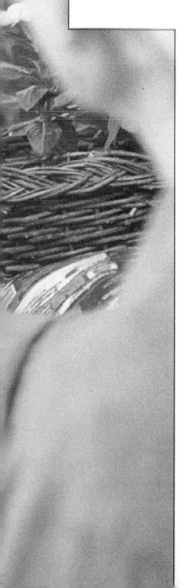

PART I

An Introduction to Aging

Quantity and Quality of Life

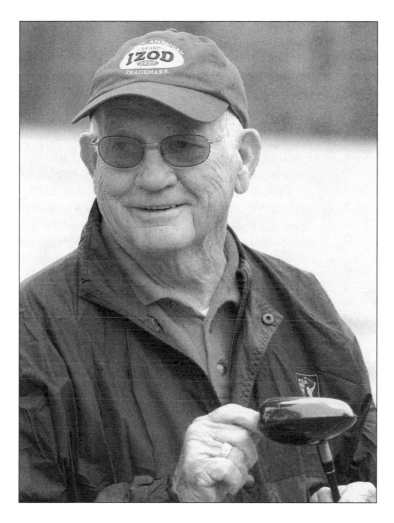

The objectives of this chapter are

- to describe aging and how it is measured,
- to examine the issues involved in trying to delay the aging process,
- to show how physical aging affects the quality of life of all individuals, and
- to introduce the theories that are currently used to explain aging.

Aging is an experience that every human being shares but no one fully understands. Many throughout human history have pondered the same questions about aging: What is aging? What is its nature? Why do living organisms age? Can aging be stopped or slowed?

Although all people age, they do so in different ways and at different rates. Some people live longer and have a higher quality of life than others. The basis of gerontology is the study of these differences, their causes, and the factors that amplify or attenuate them. The length of time that people live, or quantity of life, is easily measured. Statistical survival curves have been developed to describe the life spans of many species, and from these, predictions can be made about the quantity of life and the rate of aging. But scholars and scientists want to understand the fundamental processes and causes of aging so that the quantity of life for humans can be maximized. The results of their studies of basic mechanisms have provided the basis for several theories of aging.

Not only is understanding the fundamental processes of aging essential to determining what causes aging, but it is also necessary if interventions are to be developed that can postpone or stop the aging process. The goal of applied health and social scientists is to change the shape of the human survival curve so that most individuals can live long lives, and several controllable factors, such as food restriction and nutrition, general activity level, and physical activity, have some promise in fulfilling that goal. Most people would agree that long life without health and physical mobility is undesirable, yet many people live their terminal years in a state of **morbidity**, or complete physical dependence and poor health. A substantial thrust in recent research has thus been to determine whether the occurrence and duration of morbidity in the population can be compressed. Discussions of extending the life span are always entangled with issues of quality of life.

This chapter introduces some of the fundamental questions and basic terminology of gerontology. What is aging? How is it described? What causes it? Can the aging process be slowed? And how is the quantity of life related to the quality of life?

What Is Aging?

On the simplest level, physical age seems easy to define. It is the chronological time something has existed or the number of elapsed standard time units between birth and a date of observation. On this level, age and time are synonymous. On another level, however, the physical dimension and meaning of time depend totally on the biological, psychological, and social significance attached to time; for that reason the concept of time has been the subject of philosophical debate for centuries. Because time and chronological aging can be viewed as synonymous, it is impossible to divorce aging from the passage of time. Yet biological processes that occur in youth are thought of as developmental, whereas time-related changes that lead to disability and dysfunction are thought of as adult aging, or senescence. When does this change in definition occur? Does aging begin in all body cells simultaneously or in different systems at different times? When does aging start? As complex as these issues are, rational discussion requires some agreement on definitions among professionals.

In this text, the term *aging* refers to a process or group of processes occurring in living organisms that with the passage of time lead to a loss of adaptability, functional impairment, and eventually death. These processes are distinct from daily or seasonal biological rhythms and any other temporary change. It is particularly important to distinguish aging effects from **secular effects**, which are environmental effects that influence all people who live within an identified period. For example, during the late 1970s and early 1980s, serum cholesterol levels decreased over 7-year intervals in all age groups studied in the Baltimore Longitudinal Study of Aging (BLSA). The dietary cholesterol and fiber of these subjects also changed. Attributing the decrease in cholesterol to aging would be an inaccurate conclusion. Much more probable is that many of the BLSA subjects, as well as countless numbers of young adults, changed their diets as a result of heavy media advertising regarding the benefits of low-fat and high-fiber diets.

Aging is a logical extension of the physiological processes of growth and development, beginning with birth and ending with death. The emphasis of this text is on the latter portion of this continuum of life span growth and development.

Aging occurs with the relentless march of time, but relatively few people actually die of old age. Most die because the body loses the capacity to withstand physical or environmental stressors. Through youth, bodies have reserve physiological capacities and system redundancies that enable them to adapt to physical challenges or insults, such as exposure to viruses or to extreme heat and cold. Accompanying aging, however, is a loss in reserve capacity and redundancy, which reduces the ability to adapt quickly and effectively. For example, a young adult might be able to dodge an oncoming automobile on a hot summer day and avoid being struck. An older person, however, who has suffered cumulative losses in peripheral vision, hearing, muscular strength, reaction time, and heat adaptation, might marshal his or her resources just a step too late and be hit by the car.

Although physical age differences are apparent, the physiological effects of aging are hardly visible between a 20-year-old and a 70-year-old when the two are sitting quietly in chairs. But these differences are more noticeable when they rise and walk across the room, and the differences are striking if an alarm sounds and the two must leave the room as quickly as possible. The age differences will be even more dramatic if the older person has had frequent sicknesses and accidents, has one or more chronic diseases, and has chronically insulted his or her body (e.g., by smoking or using drugs). Losses in vision, hearing, and strength, for example, are primary aging, and the accelerated aging that occurs as a result of disease or environmental factors is secondary aging.

> *Aging* refers to a process or group of processes occurring in living organisms that with the passage of time lead to a loss of adaptability, functional impairment, and eventually death.

Primary and Secondary Aging

Aging processes are different from the process of aging. Aging processes represent universal changes with age within a species or population that are independent of disease or environmental influence (Hershey, 1984). The onset of puberty in children and menopause in women, for example, are age-related changes that are not disease-dependent. The process of aging refers to clinical symptoms (the syndrome of aging) and includes the effects of environment and disease. Busse (1969) described aging processes as primary aging and the process of aging (which includes the interaction of aging processes with disease and environmental influences) as secondary aging. Although the causes of primary and secondary aging are distinct, they do not act independently. Rather, they strongly interact with each other. Disease and environmental stress can accelerate basic aging processes, and aging processes increase one's vulnerability to disease and environmental stress.

> *Aging processes* (primary aging) are universal age-related changes within a species that are independent of disease or environmental influence.
>
> The *process of aging* (secondary aging) refers to clinical symptoms (the syndrome of aging) and includes the effects of environment and disease.

Rate of Aging

The rate of aging is the change in function of organs and systems per unit of time. In normal aging, these deleterious changes roughly follow a linear senescence over the life span. It had been thought that the rate of aging was roughly exponential after age 40; that is, mortality intensity would double following equal periods of time after a person reached 40 years of age. But the aging rate is different in men and women (Ekonomov et al., 1989). The rate at which males age slows monotonically with time, whereas females age at a slower rate between 45 to 60 years of age than they do between 70 to 80 years of age. Disease and accident can change the rate of deterioration, and thus of aging, in a system, but although many researchers have tried, only two interventions, caloric restriction and genetic manipulation, have been shown to change the rate of aging positively by increasing the life span. Caloric restriction is a very robust intervention, seen in most studies of rodents, other small animals, and primates, but genetic manipulation has been shown only in *C. elgans,* a species of nematode (Johnson, 1990).

How Is Aging Described?

The simplest way to describe aging is to categorize it. Age categories are divisions of chronological age, such as those shown in table 1.1, that are used for purposes of discussion and clarification in gerontology. These divisions seem straightforward, but a major problem in gerontology research has been that age categories have not been standardized across the field of gerontology. Some professionals describe a 55-year-old as old, whereas others call the same-aged person middle aged. Within the gerontology literature, 20 different terms have been used to describe middle-aged or old adults (Crandall, 1991). Reviewing several research studies will show that subjects ranging in age from 35 to 100 years have been labeled "old." This is an unfortunate state of affairs, because to interpret the results of research studies in which old are compared with young, it is important to know what *old* means. (For purposes of discussion, the age categories shown in table 1.1 will be used in this text; the term *older* or *old* refers to persons older than those in the middle-aged adult category, i.e., > 65 years of age). The "young-old" category, comprising those between 65 and 74, is a relatively new division by which gerontologists acknowledge the growing number of older Americans who, by virtue of their active lifestyles, have continued behaving as young and middle-aged people well into the ages that were once described as old. George

Table 1.1 Age Categories

Description	Age (years)	Decade
Infant	0-2	1st
Child	3-12	1st-2nd
Adolescent	13-17	2nd
Young adult	18-24	2nd-3rd
Adult	25-44	3rd-5th
Middle-aged adult	45-64	5th-7th
Young-old	65-74	7th-8th
Old	75-84	8th-9th
Old-Old	85-99	9th-10th
Oldest-old	100+	11th

Bush, Sr., the 41st president of the United States, sky-dived from an airplane on his 73rd birthday, 50 years after his aircraft was shot down in World War II. He is an excellent example of a member of the young-old age category. Most young-old can maintain their jobs and productivity if they choose to do so.

Another important point shown in table 1.1 is that the first decade of life includes children from birth to age 9, the second decade includes individuals from 10 to 19, and so on. Thus, if someone describes individuals as being in their sixth decade, they are chronologically between 50 and 59. Yet another way to describe older adults is as sexagenarians (60-69), septuagenarians (70-79), octogenarians (80-89), nonagenarians (90-99), and centenarians (100+).

All individuals in an age category may be loosely described as cohorts, that is, people who are more likely to experience common environmental conditions and events, such as wars, environmental disasters, or economic booms or downturns. Birth cohorts include all people who have the same year of birth and who are compared from the same fixed time origin. Although all individuals have very different personalities and experiences, persons who were beginning their career during World War II and who also lived through the Great Depression, for example, collectively share some attitudes and behaviors that are different than those of young adults who began their careers in the post-Vietnam era. The radically different life events that shaped different cohorts play a substantial role in shaping their behaviors, so that what might be interpreted as an aging effect in one cohort could be in reality an effect of a specific

environmental event experienced by one cohort but not by the other. Physical and social environments that differ in health risks and medical care affect the **life expectancy** of a cohort.

The most highly publicized cohort in American society includes individuals born between 1946 and 1960, the baby boomers. This cohort is the largest in the United States. After World War II, babies were born at a faster rate in this country than in any other period of time. Consequently, one out of three people in our society is a baby boomer. The sheer size of this cohort has influenced every aspect of our society—schools, housing, marketing, job availability—and continues to do so as this cohort ages. Indeed, one reason that gerontology and issues of aging are attracting so much attention today is that the baby boomers are now at midlife and are requiring more and more health care. Many are predicting that when the baby boomers reach retirement age, if health insurance, medical disability, and retirement policies are not radically changed, the health care system will completely collapse under the weight of the needs of this large cohort of society.

Human Survival Curve

Another way to describe the aging of various species is to develop a survival curve, depicting the percentage of a population that survives at each age throughout the life span of the entire population. Survival curves for any species are important to describe changes and shifts in populations as well as to understand the factors that influence these changes. Some sample life spans determined from the survival curves of several species are shown ordered by length in figure 1.1. Note that although humans have a relatively long life span compared with many other species, humans are certainly not the longest lived species. In the human species, each person has a specific life span, ranging from perhaps only a few minutes to more than 100 years. Several aspects of the human survival curve are shown in figure 1.2. The percent of persons surviving out of 100,000 is shown on the vertical axis for each age group.

Since the mid-19th century, the life expectancy of the U.S. population at birth has nearly doubled from 40 to 75.9 years. The longer the life expectancy of each new cohort, the greater the percentage of the total population represented by the older cohort and the older the population as a whole. In 1995, the Census Bureau reported that the life expectancy of the U.S. population was 75.9. The Census Bureau's low, middle, and high projections for life expectancy in 2050 are 74.8, 82.0, and 89.4.

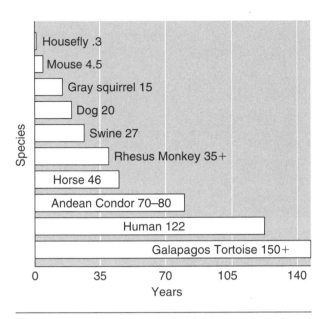

Figure 1.1 Maximum recorded life spans for selected mammals, birds, reptiles, amphibians, and fish.

Data from Arking (1998)

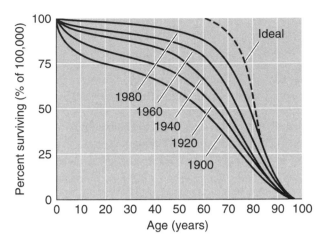

Figure 1.2 Cumulative survival curves for both genders. The increasing life expectancy for each cohort (1920, 1940, 1960, and 1980) reveals that the survival curves are becoming more rectangular. One goal of medical science is to find ways to reduce accidents and eliminate disease, thus rectangularizing the human survival curve so that most individuals can expect to live the average biological life span for humans.

Adapted, by permission, from J.F. Fries and L.M. Crapo, 1981, *Vitality and aging* (New York: Freeman), 7.

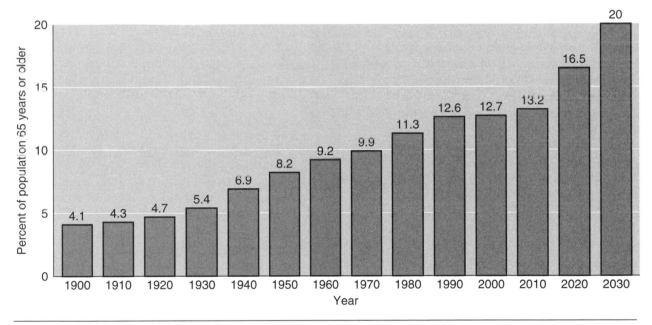

Figure 1.3 Percent of U.S. population aged 65 years or older.

Data from Older Americans 2000 (2000): Administration on Aging. www.aoa.gov/agingstats/chartbook2000.

From 1995 to 2010, the 85+ population is expected to increase 56%, compared with approximately 13% for the population between 65 and 84. It is estimated that by 2030, 20% of our population will be 65 years or older (figure 1.3; Older Americans, 2000). Today, 3.4 million people are older than 85. It is projected that in 2050, 21.5 million, or seven times more, will be 85 or older. The fastest growing age category is the centenarians, those more than 100 years old. It is estimated that 72,000 Americans are more than 100 years old, and projections are that 131,000 centenarians will be living in this country by the year 2010 (Krach & Velkoff, 1999). Those now living are predominantly female and white, approximately half

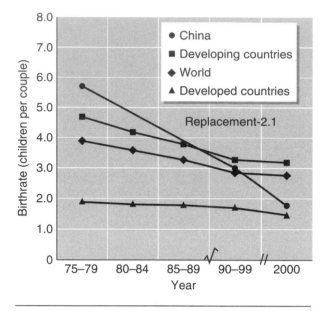

Figure 1.4 The birthrate is plummeting in many countries, but especially in the developing countries. The birthrate considered necessary for the replacement of the human species is 2.1. The world birthrate is still well above that number, but many developed countries have fallen below it, so that the average for developed countries has been below the replacement rate since 1975.

Data from Department of Family and Community Services (2001).

live in homes rather than institutions, most have very low incomes, and more than 75% are native-born Americans.

The "graying" of the population is not limited to the United States: It is a global phenomenon. Most of the increases in life expectancy in the early part of this century were attributable to declining rates in neonatal, infant, and maternal mortality. But today, increases in the median age of populations are being fueled by dramatic improvements in public health, medical treatment of chronic diseases, and lowered birth rates. In the United States, fertility rates have dropped from 2.48 to 2.06 in less than 30 years, and Canada's fertility rate has decreased to less than half, from 3.90 to 1.66. Spain's fertility rate was the lowest in the world at 1.15 when the data shown in figure

1.4 were obtained. The combination of millions of people growing older and a plummeting birth rate in all developing countries is dramatically changing the demographic profile of the world (Holden, 1996).

Maximum Life Span Potential

The **maximum life span** potential is the survival potential of members of a population. The members of a species who live the longest provide an operational definition of the maximum life span for that population. As of 2000, the oldest verified age for a human was that of Jeanne Louise Calment, who lived to be 122. Some demographers believed that, in the absence of some genetic or medical technological breakthrough, 115 to 120 years would be the maximum human life span potential (Rothenberg et al., 1991). Obviously they underestimated the human life span potential!

Average Life Span

The **average life span** is the average age by which all but a very small percentage of the members of a population are deceased. Most gerontologists agree that the average biological limit to human life is approximately 85 years, because only about 12% of the population exceeds that age. Figure 1.5 shows the distribution of age at death in the hypothetical situation where no premature death occurs from accident or disease (Fries, 1980). This suggests a genetically endowed limit to life even for a member of a population free of all exogenous risk factors. Indeed, the life span of humans has not changed much since the beginning of recorded history. The 90th Psalm in the Bible declares a human's natural life span to be three-score years and ten, or 70 years, which is not radically different from present values.

Life Expectancy

Life expectancy is the average number of years of life remaining for a population of individuals, all of the same age, usually expressed from birth as

An Aging World

The phenomenon of an extended life expectancy for millions of people is not limited to the United States. The median age of almost all developing countries is increasing rapidly. At the same time, as is true in the United States, the birth rate is declining. Women are having fewer children than they used to, and thus the average age of persons in developing countries is increasing. The combination of people living to extraordinary ages and a decreasing birth rate means that for the first time in recorded history, in several countries people are not replacing themselves. See the figure on the next page.

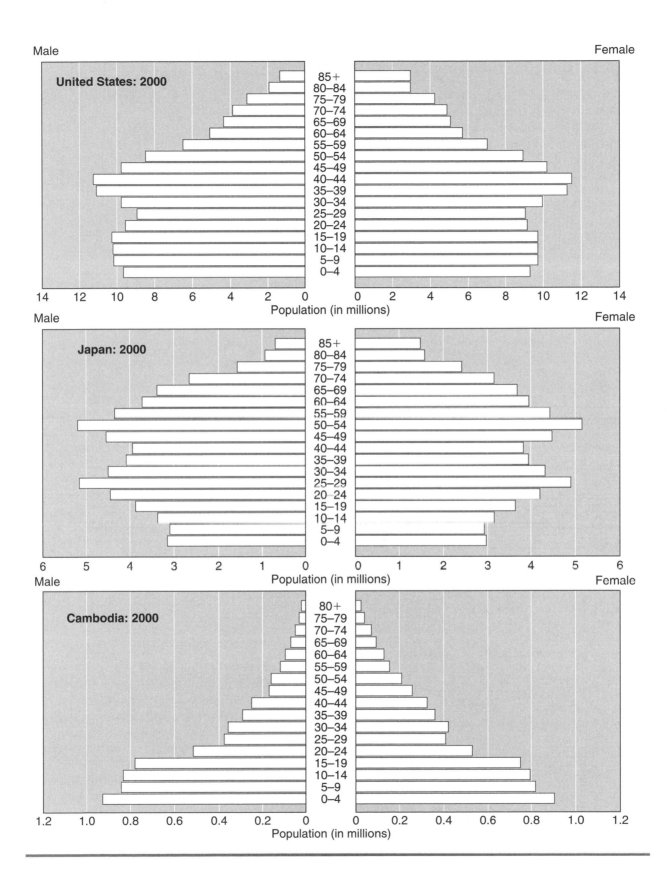

An Extraordinarily Long Life

Jeanne Calment lived until very near her death in a house that was in a prime location in Paris. An amusing story is told about an ambitious real estate broker who sought to buy her house when she was in her 80s. She refused, and so thinking that he had put something over on her, he agreed to a contract in which she sold the house to him, received the money, but was allowed to live in the house until her death. He surely anticipated that, given her advanced age, he would have the house in just a few years. Approximately 30 years later, she was still in her house, and the real estate agent was dead.

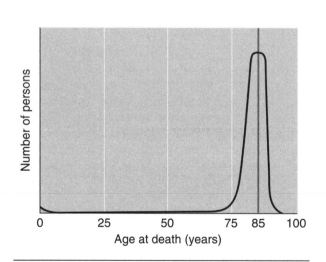

Figure 1.5 Mortality rate according to age in the absence of premature death. If the survival curve were completely rectangularized, that is, everyone died of old age and no one died prematurely (because of accidents, war, or disaster), almost all natural deaths would occur at about 85 ± 10 years of age, which is the average human life span.

Adapted, by permission, from J.F. Fries, 1980, "Aging, Natural Death, and the Compression of Morbidity" *New England Journal of Medicine* 303: 134.

Table 1.2 Life Expectancy in 1996 for Selected Countries

	Men	Women
Japan	76	83
Canada	76	83
Australia	76	83
France	74	82
Sweden	76	82
Israel	76	81
Spain	74	81
New Zealand	74	80
Cuba	75	80
United States	73	79
Mexico	70	77
Poland	68	76
Russia	57	70
Egypt	60	63
Kenya	56	56
Morocco	68	72
South Africa	57	62
Cambodia	48	51
Zambia	36	36

Note: Data from World Health Organization, Census Bureau.

the average number of years of life that newborns might expect to live. Life expectancy is different for males and females. For those born in 1946 (leading edge of the baby boomers) in the United States, the life expectancy is 73 for males and 79 for females. That is, the largest number of deaths in this group occurs at these ages. Although life expectancy is usually thought of as length of life from birth, the life expectancy of 50-year-olds can also be calculated. In this case, life expectancy is defined as the average

number of years of life remaining. In contrast to the average life span, life expectancy for both genders increased significantly throughout most of the 20th century in most countries. Life expectancy is different for people of different ages, cohorts, genders, and ethnic backgrounds. It is also greatly different in various geographic locations (table 1.2). However, of all the biological, social, and cultural differences in life expectancies, one of the most striking is that of gender.

In recent years, gains in life expectancy have been achieved by reducing mortality attributable to cardiovascular disease. Thus, deaths from infectious diseases have been replaced by deaths from chronic degenerative diseases. It is estimated that the life expectancy of males at age 30 could be increased by more than 15

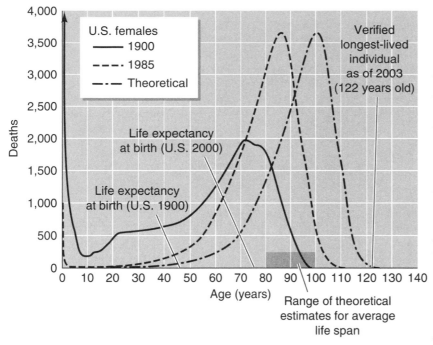

Figure 1.6 Observed and theoretical distribution of deaths of females in the United States, 1900 and 1985.

Reprinted, by permission, from S.J. Olshansky, B.A. Carnes, and C. Cassel, "In search of Methuselah: Estimating the upper limits to human longevity," *Science* 250: 635.

cancer (which causes about one fifth of all deaths in the United States) and heart disease. Olshansky and colleagues (1990) have been studying this issue for some time. It is comparatively easy to increase life expectancy in countries where it is low, but as life expectancy approaches the 80s, increasing life expectancy is more and more difficult and requires that huge decreases in mortality rates occur. For example, even eliminating all forms of cancer would increase life expectancy at birth by only 3.17 years for females and 3.2 years for males. To make large increases in life expectancy by eliminating most diseases, mortality rates from all causes of death would have to decline at all ages by 55% and at ages 50 and over by 60%. In fact, these increases have not occurred since 1990, and future gains in life expectancy are expected to be very small and at a much slower pace, because they will depend on dramatic biomedical and technological breakthroughs that provide cures for the diseases and disorders of aging itself (Olshansky et al., 2001).

Factors that influence life expectancy:

- Medical progress
- Reductions of environmental pollutants
- Decline in smoking, drinking, and drug abuse
- Increase in number of people willing to change their lifestyle

Gender Differences

One of the interesting questions of longevity is why women throughout the world outlive men by 4 to 10 years. Although more males are conceived than females, the female survival advantage begins at conception and increases throughout life. More spontaneous abortions, miscarriages, and stillbirths are male, and as shown in figure 1.7, the ratio of males to females decreases throughout life. James V. Neel of the University of Washington was quoted as saying, "We really are the weaker sex, biologically less fit than females at every step of the way" (Holden, 1987).

years if major known risk factors, such as smoking, high cholesterol, high blood pressure, and obesity, were eliminated. Dramatic changes in the life expectancy of women have accompanied the technological advances in the monitoring of childbearing. Figure 1.6 shows the distribution of deaths at all ages per 100,000 females for the cohort born in 1900 and the hypothetical distribution for the cohort born in 1985, represented by a dashed line (Olshansky et al., 1990). Note that the life expectancy of the 2000 cohort (77 years) is 30 years longer than that of the 1900 cohort (47 years). In the 1900 cohort, a sharp increase in deaths occurred in women at childbearing age, approximately ages 16 to 25, and the majority died between the ages of 50 and 70. A large percentage of the causes of death for these women was infectious disease. The 1985 cohort, conversely, is almost free of these causes of death and will die of chronic diseases between the ages of 70 and 100. The curve shown by dotted lines represents a hypothetical life span as the average approaches 100 years, perhaps because of medical breakthroughs and dramatic changes in lifestyle. In this figure, the theoretical estimates for average life span are 80 to 100 years.

Whether life expectancy at birth will continue to increase is a topic of hot debate in gerontology. The attention of researchers interested in extending life expectancy has turned to finding ways to eradicate

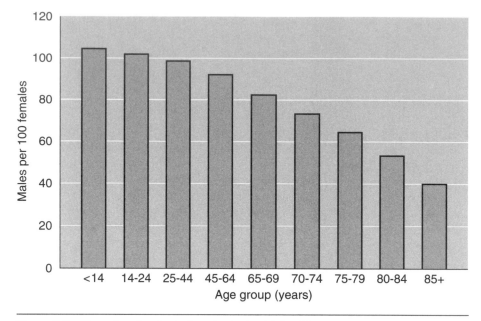

Figure 1.7 The ratio of males to females in the United States.
Data from Crandall 1991.

The gender gap was significant at the beginning of the 20th century and widened considerably until approximately 1970, at which time it leveled off. Average life expectancy of a boy born in 2001 is 74 years, whereas that of girl born in the same year is 80 years. The gap has not increased within recent years, at least partly because the life expectancy for females is leveling off. However, the Census Bureau projects that in 2050, 61% of those over 85 will be women.

In 1987, the gender gap was intriguing enough to be the subject of a conference sponsored by the National Institute on Aging. At this international conference, a great many scholars discussed biologically and behaviorally known facts that could explain the gender gap, but they could not draw any satisfactory conclusions. Many of the conferees expressed the belief that it would be a long time before the gender gap is fully understood. Why do women live longer than men? Several explanations, which may be categorized as genetic, hormonal, or social, have been proposed.

Genetics Theory

One argument for why women live longer is that because women have two sets of the female-determining X-linked genes, cells can operate on instructions from genes on either X chromosome. If a male has an X-linked gene for a recessive gene disease such as muscular dystrophy, he will develop the disease because the gene is on the only X chromosome he has. But if a woman has an X-linked recessive gene,

theoretically she could function on the other X chromosome, which may be free of the X-linked disease-producing gene. For this reason, males have more gender-linked recessive gene diseases. As long ago as 1953, Montague, in his popular book, *The Natural Superiority of Women*, made this argument. Some suggest that this same type of argument might be made if an X-linked gene or gene system related to longevity is someday identified, or if some aspect of the replication and repair mechanism of cells is X chromosome-linked. Although the X-linked gene argument continues to be intuitively compelling, it is probably too simplistic in its present form. As has been emphasized by many, one of the X chromosomes in most women is inactivated, so women really are operating on a single X chromosome, just as are men. However, another hypothesis has been that longevity is influenced by differences in the male Y chromosome.

Hormonal Differences

Another explanation for the greater longevity of women is based on the observation that women do not die in their 50s and 60s from heart disease at the percentages that men do. Until 2001, estrogen, the hormone responsible for female characteristics, was thought to protect against heart disease by lowering levels of low-density lipoproteins (LDLs) and increasing levels of high-density lipoproteins (HDLs), which protect against the development of atherosclerosis. This theory, which had reached the level of dogma, was dealt a severe blow, however, by papers published from the Women's Health Initiative study (Chlebowski et al., 2003). At present, many physicians are no longer automatically prescribing estrogen supplements to postmenopausal women. Androgens, the male hormones, lower the protective HDLs and raise the atherosclerotic-inducing LDLs. Androgens also increase aggressive and combative behavior, which are associated with automobile accidents and other types of violent death.

Hormonal differences also affect the immune system. Females have greater and faster immune responses to foreign objects in the blood, a beneficial effect in youth in terms of warding off antigen-produced diseases. For example, the results of research on mice have suggested that the greater immune activity may provide greater resistance to the development of tumors. In general, women are more frequently sick than men as they age, but their illnesses tend to be chronic and debilitating rather than fatal. The faster response of the female immune system is detrimental in terms of autoimmune diseases. Thus, diseases in which the immune system of an individual attacks him- or herself, such as arthritis, lupus, and myasthenia gravis, are much more prevalent in women. As the immune system ages, it becomes less and less accurate in identifying foreign versus self-produced antigens, and thus the autoimmune system is more likely to attack its own host.

Social Explanations

The different social roles and behaviors of males and females in society are also used to explain the gender gap. These explanations center on the disparate work roles and responsibilities of men and women and gender-related differential health habits such as smoking and the use of health resources.

During the first three quarters of the 20th century, females generally were in less dangerous and stressful environments. Boys were more likely to have serious or fatal accidents than girls, and, although the work-related responsibilities of women are increasing, men continue to hold a high percentage of working positions in which job-related stress is high. Historically, women in the first half of their lives have always been less subject to violent death attributable to war, homicide, suicide, or accident. Even in the 1991-92 Persian Gulf War, in which women made up a larger proportion of the U.S. military than ever before, they were for the most part limited to supportive stations in combat zones. Insurance rates attest to the fact that generally women do not drive automobiles as fast, nor are they as accident prone, as men. These social role disparities are slowly changing, but they exist at present.

Until relatively recently, women have always participated less than men in the high-risk habit of smoking. There is much controversy over whether the difference in smoking habits of men and women can account for a substantial portion or all of the gender gap. One argument used to support this hypothesis is that the gender gap is larger in the working class, and smoking is more prevalent among blue-collar males than any other group. Miller and Gerstein (1983) have gone so far as to say that the different smoking habits of the two genders may account for

all of the gender gap. Miller and Gerstein challenged many of the studies that found a large gender gap because these authors claimed that smoking was not a well-controlled factor; that is, former smokers were not identified and distinguished from nonsmokers. Miller and Gerstein (1983) suggested that if these analyses are done, when the number of women smokers catches up with that of men, the gender gap almost disappears. Miller (1986) insisted that if the male–female longevity difference is plotted over 6 decades, this difference follows smoking trends. Before World War I, few men smoked and the gender gap was small. During and after World War II, smoking became popular, many men smoked, and the gender gap began to climb. African-Americans also began to smoke in larger numbers and their gender gap increased. Women, as depicted in the advertisement, "You've come a long way, baby!" began to smoke in much greater numbers in the late 1970s and 1980s, after which time the gender gap began to attenuate. By 1980, African Americans were smoking as much as Caucasian Americans, which was reflected by the gender gap. The 1964 Surgeon General's Report on the dangers of smoking motivated more Caucasians than African Americans to stop smoking, and this too is reflected in a racial gap.

Another way that scientists have tried to explain the gender gap is by studying nonsmoking populations of men and women so that smoking is not a factor. Among the nonsmoking populations of the Irish in Slieve Loughner, Ireland, and the Amish in Lancaster County, Pennsylvania, men tend to live as long as or longer than women (Casey & Casey, 1971). However, in several studies in which smoking was well controlled and in studies of other nonsmoking populations, these claims were refuted (Friedman et al., 1979). Although many agree that "women who smoke like men will die like men" and the gender gap trend seems to be decreasing, others in the research community believe that smoking may account for only 50% to 75% of the gender gap (Enstrom, 1984), with genetics and hormonal differences also contributing.

Another social explanation of why women live longer than men is that women tend to have more contact with the health system. They are more consistent in having annual medical examinations and quicker to go to the doctor if a symptom appears. They also are more social and are more likely to have friends who can assist them in their health needs.

An irony of the gender gap is that although women live longer and use the health care system more, they have more acute illnesses and nonfatal chronic conditions (figure 1.8). Older females have a higher

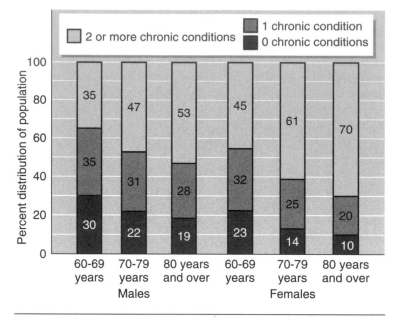

Figure 1.8 Percent distribution of population 60 years and older by number of chronic conditions, according to age group and gender, in the United States, 1984.

Adapted from Guralnik et al. (1989).

incidence of arthritis, sinusitis, colitis, soft tissue disorders, and chronic constipation. Conversely, older males experience more emphysema, heart disease, and cerebrovascular disease. Older women as a group presumably experience more emotional stress, exercise less than men (Holden, 1987), have high incidences of disability, and are more dependent.

It is clear that descriptive analyses have produced a wealth of information about aging. From studies of the human survival curve and comparisons of it with the survival curves of other species have come the concepts of primary and secondary aging, the rate of aging, maximum life span potential, average life span, and life expectancy. The curious gender difference in life expectancy also has been revealed. But these descriptions only inform researchers about what appears to exist; these descriptions do not explain why aging takes place.

What Causes Aging?

Throughout recorded history, humans have tried to understand why people age, partly out of curiosity, but more urgently because most humans would like to discover a way to stop, slow, postpone, or reverse aging. One of the motivations for searching for immortality is that many, if not most, humans suffer from thanatophobia—a fear of death—and

therefore one of the great quests of science has been to extend the maximum life span. Hippocrates (460-377 B.C.) is credited with being the first to propose a theory of aging—that aging is an irreversible and natural event caused by the gradual loss of body heat. Galen (A.D. 130-201) expanded this theory by suggesting that age-related changes in the body humors began early in life and that these changes gradually caused a slow increase in dryness and coldness of the body. Roger Bacon (1210-1292), in his monograph "Cure of Old Age and Preservation of Youth," subscribed to the Greek belief that aging was caused by a loss of body heat, but Bacon was the first to suggest that this process might be slowed by good hygiene. He also was the first to articulate the "wear and tear" theory of aging, that continual abuses and insults to body systems eventually age them.

Erasmus Darwin (1731-1802) thought that aging was attributable to a loss of irritability in nervous and muscular tissue. By this time, many scholars were attributing aging to a loss of some type of vital force or physical essence that was necessary for intrinsic energy. A popular theory in the late 19th century was that aging was caused by intestinal putrefaction, which led Charles Brown-Sequard (1817-1894) to inject animal testicular extracts into his own body when he was 72 years old in an effort to postpone aging. Because he died 5 years later, it is safe to say that his efforts were unsuccessful.

By the mid-19th century, the anatomic and physiological changes in the major organ systems were being systematically documented, and it was agreed that with time cells eventually die and are not replaced. But serious and prolific scientific interest in the causes of aging and the aging process is a relatively recent phenomenon. The term *geriatrics*, described for the first time by Ignatz Nascher as a medical specialization on aging processes, was not coined until 1914 in the title of his book *Geriatrics: The Diseases of Old Age and Their Treatment* (1914/1979). The first geriatric medical journal began publication in 1945, and the first gerontology conference on aging was held in 1950. In the United States, serious interest in a medical phenomenon is usually expressed by the creation within the National Institutes of Health of an institute dedicated to the topic, yet the National Institute on Aging was not created until 1974. The realization that the baby boomers of this country will begin to reach retirement age in 2010 has greatly stimulated the interest in the effects of aging on all aspects of life. Research on aging is increasing as each year passes. The questions researchers hope to answer are, What determines the average life span of a population? What determines the life span of an individual? To what maximum could the life span of humans be extended?

Because even the definition of aging is controversial, it may seem premature to develop theories of aging before a consensual definition is articulated. Nevertheless, theories abound. Modern theories of aging, a consequence of dramatic advancements in science and technology, are sophisticated and complex and beyond the scope of this book, but a brief summary is appropriate. One way to organize these theories is to divide them into three major categories: genetic theories, damage theories, and gradual imbalance theories.

Genetic Theories

The most extreme genetic theorists propose that the entire process of aging, from birth to death, is programmed by our genes. Age-related events such as puberty and menopause are markers of the biological clock programmed into each cell. In these theories, life span, as well other age-related events, may be controlled by one or more specific, positively acting genes (either major or minor) operating independently or with others for longevity. Some have even proposed a "death gene" that programs early death. However, as Miller (1999) so eloquently pointed out, a death gene is not logically possible because natural selection only retains genes that enhance the survival of the species. Carriers of a "death gene" would not have a selective advantage and would eventually be lost to the population. As yet, no longevity genes have been identified. A less extreme view is that one or more

genes dictate cellular aging within the nucleus of the cell or that certain genes are expressed or repressed during the normal developmental process of living.

Another theory that has been proposed is that DNA mutations of the mitochondria (the energy producers of the cells) build up during an individual's lifetime, thus causing aging (Miguel, 1991). Recently, using highly sophisticated DNA microchip technology, Ly and colleagues (2000) observed that the aging process was accompanied by an increasing number of errors that occurred during the cell division process. After comparing cell division characteristics in normal young, middle-aged, and old persons and persons with Hutchinson-Gilford progeria (a disease that appears to accelerate aging), they proposed that the errors that occur during cell division lead to chromosomal pathologies that in turn result in a dysregulation of the genes involved in the aging process.

One of the most well-known expressions of a genetically based theory was formulated by Leonard Hayflick in 1977. What is now called the **Hayflick limit** states that cells will divide and reproduce themselves only a limited number of times and that this number is genetically programmed. Thus, the physiological age of the cell (the number of divisions left before it stops reproducing) is determined by the genetic material in the nucleus of the cell, and just as the process of puberty is "turned on" during the growth period, the process of senescence is turned on at some point in middle age. Hayflick later suggested that evidence is overwhelming that aging and the determination of longevity, or a sort of "cell clock," occur within the cell (Hayflick, 1994). The **telomere** hypothesis suggests a mechanism by which this clock might work. At the end of each chromosome in dividing cells is a region called a telomere, which is a piece of DNA that contains no genetic information. With each replication of the chromosome, the telomere

Two Diseases That Mimic Aging

The mechanisms of two diseases are of great interest to scientists today. In both diseases, the ravages of age begin occurring at very early ages. In Werner's syndrome patients, their hair unexpectedly begins to gray, their muscles weaken, their skin loses its resilience, and they begin to contract one or more diseases generally associated with old age: cataracts, cancer, heart disease, diabetes, or others. Werner's syndrome has been attributed to the mutation of one gene, and because this gene is also associated with cancer, it may provide insights into the cellular mechanisms of aging (Pennisi, 1996). Progeria, also caused by gene mutation, has similar results except that the aging symptoms begin in early childhood, making very young children look like their grandparents. These children generally die before they are 15 years of age and before they can pass the gene on to their children. Thus, progeria is very rare; perhaps only 30 children in the world have it. Researchers (e.g., Ly et al., 2000) are intensely studying the cell replication behaviors as a possible window to understanding cellular aging.

shortens. Because this process happens at a fixed rate, it has been proposed as the clock that times the cell's death. This theory is far from proven, but many researchers believe it is promising.

Genetic theories are not accepted by many researchers, who argue that the heritability of longevity only accounts for 15% to 30% of the variance in humans (e.g., Ljungquist et al., 1998). Other geneticists point out that genetic markers cannot correlate very well with longevity in a population that is so narrowly defined and relatively homogeneous (i.e., only like-sexed fraternal human twin pairs). Of course, genetics must play a role in longevity, otherwise the great disparity between a housefly that lives only about 3.5 months and a Bristlecone pine tree that lives more than 5,000 years would not exist. The controversy regarding genetic theories rages on unabated.

Damage Theories

These theories are based on the concept that chemical reactions that occur naturally in the body begin to produce a number of irreversible defects in molecules. In addition, the body is under assault daily from chemical damage that may occur from polluted air, from the food or other substances eaten, from tobacco smoke, from products of the body's own metabolism, or just from the repetitive stress of muscle and cartilage moving against bone. The suggestion by proponents of these damage theories is that if chemical damage could be minimized, the aging process could be slowed and people would live longer. A prominent example of this type of theory is shown in figure 1.9. Johnson (1985) suggested that, beginning at birth, microinjuries are unavoidable, universal, and ubiquitous. In the first box of the figure are examples of small insults (viruses, trauma, free radicals) that are a result of metabolic products, background environmental radiation, and a high body temperature, which encourages molecular instability. Repeated small insults eventually lead to injury, which either is repaired or results in a loss of function. The body's natural repair processes can either be overwhelmed or become less effective with aging. If the repair processes cannot keep up with the injuries, a system failure occurs. Loss of function therefore occurs throughout life, but because of the great redundancy in physiological systems, a system failure does not occur until a considerable amount of function has been lost. Johnson also argued that if a disease is defined as "a gradual accumulation of incompletely repaired injuries attributable to countless microinsults," then aging per se may be viewed as a disease. A similar view to this is that every adapta-

tion that the body makes to insults or to deviations from homeostasis takes energy and that the accumulation over time of these efforts exacts a toll on the body that could be described as the **allostatic load**. The allostatic load is a cumulative, multisystem view of the physiological toll that may be exacted on the body through attempts at adaptation (Seeman et al., 1997). Another explanation is that "the strain on the body produced by repeated ups and downs of physiologic response, as well as by the elevated activity of physiologic systems under challenge, and changes in metabolism . . . can predispose the organism to disease" (McEwen, 1998).

A prominent example of damage theories is the cross-linkage theory. Some highly reactive cellular components made up of atoms or molecules have chemically active sites that can link to the DNA helix within the cell. When one of these cross-linking agents attaches to a strand of DNA, the body's defense mechanism cuts out the piece of corrupted DNA (where the agent is connected) and then repairs the strand using the other strand of the helix as a template. But if the repair process is too slow, or if the cross-linked agent also connects to the corresponding

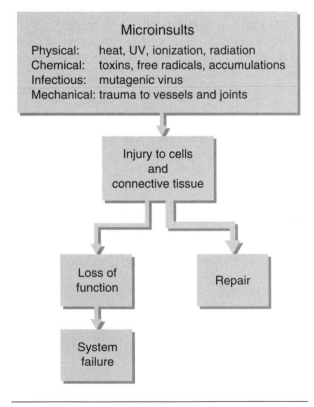

Figure 1.9 The damage-inflicted model of aging. UV = ultraviolet.

Reprinted, by permission, from H.A. Johnson, 1985, Is aging physiological or pathological? In *Relations between normal aging and disease*, edited by H.A. Johnson (Philadelphia, PA: Lippincott, Williams, and Wilkins).

site on the other DNA strand, then this site is cut out of both DNA strands. Thus, no template is available and the damage cannot be repaired. As cross-linking occurs between these molecules, large tangles form, thus obstructing metabolic processes and the intracellular transport of nutrients and information. Because cross-linking occurs on the strands of the DNA helix itself, a very small input can result in a very large change.

Detrimental cross-linking of proteins may also occur in the presence of excessive levels of the blood sugar, glucose. One of the most stressful internal changes that occurs with aging is an increase in blood glucose. The increase occurs because receptors in the pancreas, which supplies insulin to remove glucose, become less sensitive to circulating levels of glucose. Researchers have shown that glucose can randomly attach itself chemically to places on proteins and nucleic acid where it is not normally found. When this happens, it triggers a series of chemical reactions that cross-link proteins in undesirable ways. Supporters of the cross-linkage theory believe that regardless of how cross-links are made, the random attachment of proteins and the development of large tangles of malfunctioning molecules accumulate over time and lead to many of the problems and systems that are associated with aging: stiffening of tissue, rigidity of blood vessels, tight ligaments and muscle tendons, cataracts, atherosclerosis, and many more. Although this theory has many advocates, it is not universally accepted because it is based primarily on deduction, with no real experimental evidence showing that cross-linking actually obstructs metabolic processes or causes the formation of faulty molecules (Hayflick, 1994).

Many cross-linking agents are molecules called free radicals, which are products of oxygen metabolism. These chemical compounds contain an unpaired electron in an outer orbital and thus are able to link to tissue and cause damage. This damage theory is called the **free-radical theory**. Free radicals oxidize and attack other cellular components, causing alterations and malfunctions that accumulate throughout life. Eventually, so much cellular damage occurs that the cell dies, a scenario that occurs in more and more cells as ones ages.

A suggested strategy for reducing free radicals and thus slowing the rate of aging is the consumption of supplementary doses of vitamin E and perhaps C. Vitamin E and C are antioxidants and are proposed to attack and destroy the damaging free radicals continually created in the body. The enzymes glutathione, superoxide dismutase (SOD), and catalase also destroy free radicals. A number of scientists are studying this strategy, but no clear evidence exists in humans to support the use of these vitamin supplements as anti-aging agents. Another cross-linking agent is aluminum, a metal that is plentiful in the environment and used in many common products (e.g., cans, cookware). Several scientists have proposed that the intake of aluminum is highly damaging and contributes to aging (Bjorksten, 1989; Ganrot, 1986). Most scientists agree that free radicals exist, but not all agree that free radicals play a central role in aging. Although it has been shown many times that animals fed antioxidants live longer than those that eat usual diets, researchers have not met the major criterion for showing that antioxidants affect the aging process, that is, that antioxidants increase the life span. Researchers have only shown that antioxidants increase the life expectancies of animals. Nevertheless, this theory is currently one of the most heavily researched theories.

Gradual Imbalance Theories

Gradual imbalance theories state that the central nervous system, the endocrine system, and the immune system, which are highly integrative and work together, gradually begin to fail to function. Not only do they begin to fail, they may age at different rates, producing an imbalance among the systems as well as reduced effectiveness within each system. Both the central nervous system and the neuroendocrine system serve as regulators and integrators of cellular functions and organ systems. Failures of the immune system challenge these control mechanisms and leave older individuals vulnerable to diseases of many types. Because aging is more apparent when complex coordination and integration of systems are required for proper function, many researchers have proposed that a general aging theory can be developed through a better understanding of these control mechanisms. This is not a novel idea, because Frolkis proposed as early as 1968 that death occurs when one or more of these regulatory processes fail (Frolkis, 1968). Evidence continues to accumulate that regulatory processes seem particularly vulnerable to aging.

The neuroendocrine regulatory systems integrate cellular, tissue, and organ activities and enable the body to adapt to real or perceived environmental challenges, such as increases or decreases in temperature, increases in physical work, or psychological threats. The neuroendocrine system requires the proper functioning of both the central nervous system and the endocrine system. Hypothalamic releasing and inhibiting hormones secreted by the hypothalamus of the brain regulate the pituitary gland. The pituitary gland in turn regulates the thyroid, the adrenal gland, and the release of the sex hormones, estrogen and testosterone. Thus, the pituitary gland controls the release of human growth hormones, thyroid hormones, and glucocorticoids, which in turn control metabolic rate. The thyroid hormone is not really a regulatory hormone, but it interacts with other hormones to enhance their functions; for example, it enhances the actions of growth hormone, cortisone, and estrogen. When thyroid hormone is insufficient, as in hypothyroidism, aging symptoms are accelerated. Thyroid hormone replacement therapy, however, reduces or eliminates these symptoms of increased aging. The hypothalamus–pituitary axis has been a prime target of aging theories, and it has even been postulated that within the hypothalamus resides some type of "biological clock" that controls the rate of aging.

The observation that adequate levels of estrogen in females seem to protect against some symptoms of aging, for example, deterioration of muscular strength, also implicates the neuroendocrine system. After menopause, when estrogen levels decrease sharply, biological aging accelerates. If the control processes of these regulatory hormones break down, an imbalance occurs, further stressing the control mechanisms. A regulatory system out of balance causes malfunctions in each of its components, and each malfunction places an even greater stress on the other components of the system. Thus, age-related changes in certain aspects of the neuroendocrine control mechanisms result in initial endocrine imbalances, producing other physiological and metabolic imbalances that further alter control mechanisms. Eventually the balance of many hormonal and physiological systems is disrupted, a result that Finch (1976) called a cascade of metabolic disturbances described as aging symptoms.

Gradual imbalance theories also include immunological theories. The ability of the immune system to produce antibodies and certain types of T cells declines, the proportions of certain types of T cells change, and these declines are related to dysfunction in the thymus. The thymus, along with bone marrow, is a major component of the immune system. Because the shrinkage of the thymus is correlated with aging and also with declines in the immune system, Nabarra and Andrianarison (1996) suggested that the thymus is really an aging clock that quantifies age-related changes in the immune dysfunction. A special case of the immunological theory of aging is the **autoimmunity theory**. Proponents of this theory propose that during aging, the immune system, which normally attacks foreign substances such as viruses or cancerous cells in the body, loses the capacity to distinguish foreign antigens from normal body materials. Antibodies are formed that react with normal cells and destroy them or that fail to recognize and destroy the small detrimental mutations that occur in cells. This is called autoimmunity, doubly lethal because the immune system not only becomes less protective against foreign objects but actively begins to destroy its host. According to this theory, autoimmunity may be the underlying mechanism of aging. However, this theory suffers from several criticisms. First, animals differ greatly in the development of their immune systems, yet aging is universal, differing only in rate. Second, autoimmunity is tied to pathology of the immune system, and these models do not provide close fits for theoretical models of primary aging as a normal process. Third, manipulations of the immune system have not been shown to change the normal rate of aging. No one doubts that deleterious changes occur to the immune system during the passage of time; the criticism is targeted to the concept that immune dysfunction is the underlying, single cause of aging.

Although genetic, damage, gradual imbalance, neuroendocrine regulatory, and autoimmunity theories of aging have been discussed independently, almost everyone agrees that they are not independent of each other. Some aspects of these theories are complementary rather than exclusive: A gene, perhaps related to immune function, becomes defective, rendering it more vulnerable to free radical attack, which in turn disturbs the neuroendocrine immunity balance. Thus, aging occurs because of interactions among genetic, damage, and system theories. This is shown in figure 1.10, where genetic and environmental stresses are shown affecting the life maintenance reserve, which when compromised leads to death (Jazwinski, 1996). Complicated though the process of aging is, the search for and understanding of its basic mechanism have intensified over the past several years. The "Holy Grail" for researchers in gerontology is to find a way to retard or stop the aging process. The search continues unabated, and some success has already been achieved.

Can the Aging Process Be Slowed?

If the aging process could be stopped, people could live indefinitely, but present knowledge indicates that this is impossible. It does not even appear possible to extend the maximum life span potential by any significant amount in the near future. Remember the earlier discussion on aging processes versus the

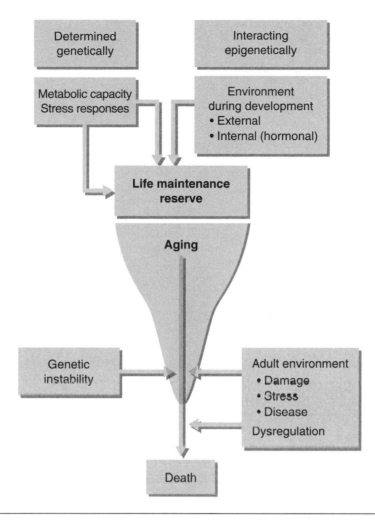

Figure 1.10 How genetic and environmental processes may affect the life maintenance reserve. The factors that affect aging are genetic, epigenetic, and environmental. Limiting factors for longevity are metabolic capacity, efficiency of stress responses, and dysregulation.

Reprinted, by permission, from S.M. Jazwinski, 1996, "Longevity, genes, and aging," *Science* 273: 57.

process of aging. To change aging processes would require changing the rate of aging, and that has only been shown to be possible in a few animal species. However, it is possible, by some behavioral interventions, to slow the process of aging (rate of secondary aging); that is, fewer people would die at ages younger than the average human life span. If almost everyone lived to the full human life span, an ideal situation from a survival perspective, the shape of the human survival curve would be more like a rectangle (figure 1.2, p. 7). If everyone adopted a healthy lifestyle, the change would consist of eliminating accelerated aging.

Having a rectangular human survival curve means maximizing the number of persons who approach the average life span of humans (85 years) by eliminating chronic diseases and accidents. This was expressed not as survival data but as mortality data

in figure 1.6 (p. 11). In this scenario, almost everyone would live until he or she was very close to the average human life span, somewhere between the ages of 75 and 90. Many would exceed the average life span age. Factors that influence the shape of the human survival curve are medical progress, reductions of levels of environmental pollutants, a decline in the rates of smoking, drinking, and drug abuse, decreases in the rate of violent crime, and increases in the number of people willing to make lifestyle changes that promote longevity. Mortality rate has also been associated with health, general activity level, quality of life, independence, cognitive function, demographic indicators, and happiness. Three factors—improving nutrition and decreasing the total amount of food consumed, maintaining adequate general activity, and performing moderate amounts of physical exercise—have been of particular interest

Beware of "Anti-Aging" Products and Lifestyle Changes!

As more and more people grow older, the market for anti-aging products is exponentially increasing. Consequently, 50 world-renowned scientists agreed that a position paper needed to be written to protect people against those who would try to benefit from people's desire to postpone old age.

> "There has been a resurgence and proliferation of health care providers and entrepreneurs who are promoting anti-aging products and lifestyle changes that they claim will slow, stop, or reverse the processes of aging. Even though in most cases there is little or no scientific basis, the public is spending vast sums of money on these products and lifestyle changes, some of which may be harmful."

From Olshansky and colleagues (2002).

to those who wish to decrease secondary aging and thus increase life expectancy.

Caloric Restriction (Undernutrition)

Caloric restriction is the only strategy that appears to alter the rate of aging. In this strategy, the major nutrients, minerals, and vitamins that are necessary for health are maintained in the diet, but the total amount of food is reduced to about two thirds of normal consumption. This strategy, tested largely in rats, has been successful. It has been shown with little doubt that rats fed only two thirds of the food that they would normally eat live longer than rats that eat as much as they want. Food restriction lengthens their life whether implemented early or late in the life span and positively affects 80% to 90% of processes that have been studied. Examples are behavior and learning, immune responses, gene expression, enzymatic activities, hormonal actions, glucose intolerance, DNA repair capacities, and rates of protein synthesis. In a primate colony that has been studied longitudinally for almost a decade, the results seem to be following those found in rodents (Kemnitz et al., 1993; Weindruch, 1995). The primates on food restriction have decreased blood glucose and insulin concentrations, improved insulin sensitivity, and lower body tem-

peratures. The proposed mechanisms by which this strategy works are that energy that would have been used for reproduction or for unstimulated levels of cellular proliferation and other processes is redirected into essential maintenance and repair processes of the organism. In addition, caloric restriction may cause global changes in gene expression that result in greater longevity (Walford & Crew, 1989).

The results of caloric restriction studies with rats have been so striking that a few scientists have advocated caloric restriction for humans. The strongest proponent of this life extension technique is Dr. Roy Walford, a biochemist at the University of California at Los Angeles, who at one time personally followed a food restriction diet by eating only every other day (Walford, 1983). However, the application of this strategy to humans has evoked some highly negative reactions among the scientific community, with criticisms centering on the great differences between rats and humans. The food that the rats in these studies had been eating, detractors say, was extremely high in protein and was developed to encourage rapid and artificial growth. It was, they claim, developed to produce large numbers of rats that grew fast but didn't necessarily live a long time. The calorie-restricted diet purported to extend their life span (the rats were fed only every other day) was beneficial only because it enabled the rats to live to their normal average life expectancy. It did not, detractors claim, increase the maximum life span of the species. Nevertheless, the effect on extending the life span is so well documented in rats and other animals that it is used as a biomarker of aging, and any theory of aging must pass the test of accounting for caloric restriction before it can be considered viable.

General Activity Level

The general activity hypothesis has been prevalent in the gerontological community for almost 30 years. The theory states that persons who are more generally active live longer than their sedentary counterparts. Unlike the food restriction hypothesis, which has been experimentally verified many times, the general activity hypothesis is based mainly on anecdotal and associative information. No one has ever shown that general activity actually alters the rate of aging, but it does seem to enable more people to achieve their maximum life span potential. This theory is understood by almost all lay people, and in fact individuals who are exceptionally old often attribute their longevity to staying active. Subjects over the age of 85 listed activity ("hard work," exercise, and keeping active, physically and mentally) as first on their list of secrets to long life (Hogstel & Kashka, 1989). Their other "secrets" were heredity, lifelong good health, strong religious beliefs, a positive attitude toward self and others, abstinence from alcohol, smoking, and drugs, good nutrition, a good support system (parents, spouse, or children), helping others, adequate rest and sleep, and use of health care resources.

Activity inventories have been developed to assess the activities of individuals in three categories: interpersonal activities (family and friend involvement, community or voluntary organization activity), physical or manipulative activities (household activities, exercise habits), and intellectual or solitary activities (Arbuckle et al., 1986/1987; Stones & Kozma, 1986). Many researchers have found that in both community and institutional settings, activity level is a potent predictor of survival. Indeed, in an institutional setting, a young age and a high level of activity were the strongest predictors of survival (Stones et al., 1989). General activity was an even higher predictor than health status in these institutionalized subjects, and the authors concluded that "mortality was found to relate more to lifestyle than to ill health" (p. P78). Conversely, other investigators have failed to find a relationship between general activity level and mortality rate (Lee & Markides, 1990). An obstacle that makes it difficult to clarify the relationship between general activity level and mortality rate is that investigators of the various studies use different activity inventories, so they may not be assessing similar activity constructs. The subjects in their samples are also different. For example, unlike most other samples, which are largely Caucasian, 70% of the sample in the Lee and Markides study (1990) were Mexican Americans. Thus, the consensus of researchers provides cautious support for the notion that general activity level is a factor in longevity.

Physical Activity

It is now generally accepted that chronic and systematic exercise throughout life, when accompanied by reasonable health habits, increases life expectancy. Increased longevity in exercised animals compared with sedentary animals has been shown many times (Drori & Folman, 1976; Edington et al., 1972; Goodrick, 1980; Retzlaff et al., 1966; Sperling et al., 1978), and Holloszy (1993) concluded from a minireview of the role of exercise in longevity of rats that exercise does indeed counteract the deleterious effects of a sedentary life combined with overeating. Exercise made it possible for more rats to live to an old age. One dissenting group of researchers found no significant effect in rats, but in this study the exercise activity was voluntary and started from mid- to late life (Goodrick et al., 1983).

The results of human studies also support the exercise–longevity relationship (Rakowski & Mor, 1992). The mean life expectancies of 2,613 men who had represented Finland in Olympic or international competition were categorized by type of sport activity and occupation. Life expectancies for the total group were higher than those of nonathletic referents (Sarna et al., 1993). Life expectancies were longest for the endurance athletes, followed by the team and then power athletes (figure 1.11). This order was observed for those athletes who were clerical workers and skilled and unskilled laborers but not for those who had been executives. The authors offered no explanation for this exception. Also, the results from a 32-year longitudinal study of highly fit male amateur ice-skaters in The Netherlands, who are capable of ice-skating for 8.5 hr or more, supported the conclusion that these men have a longer life expectancy than the average population, although curiously this did not extend to the professional ice-skating racers in the study (van Saase et al., 1990). However, it is not athletic status per se that confers additional years to life but rather the amount of habitual activity in which individual participate throughout their lives. Also, much more moderate levels of exercise have been shown to extend the life span of individuals.

One of the most definitive studies to support the idea that physically active individuals live longer was a study of 17,321 Harvard graduates aged 35 to 74 (Lee et al., 1995). In the mid-1960s, these investigators used a detailed questionnaire to determine the general health and living habits of these graduates and followed them through 1988. Physical exercise level was expressed in calories expended per week, and the participants were divided into quintiles on the basis of their energy expenditure and compared on all-cause mortality. Those men who exercised vigorously (activities requiring >6 metabolic equivalents [METs], i.e., running, swimming, tennis) lived longer than those who did not. The intensity of their energy expenditure was inversely related to their mortality rate, except in the two highest categories, which were both associated with expending at least 12,600 **kilojoules (kJ)** per week. All-cause mortality was not decreased in those who participated in nonvigorous activities (<6 METs, i.e., slow walking, light household activities). More recently, Vita and colleagues (1998) divided 1,741 older university alumni into low-, moderate-, and high-risk groups on the basis of smoking and exercise habits and an estimate of body fat. The first measures of these variables were made in 1962, and the researchers began measuring the variables again annually in 1986. The low-risk

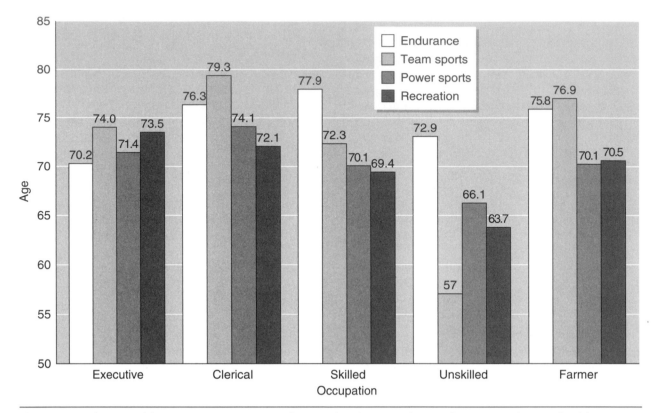

Figure 1.11 The mean life expectancy estimates at the age of 20 for 2,613 former champion male Finnish athletes, compared with 1,712 referents, categorized by the sports they participated in and the occupations that they held for the longest period in their lives. Sports groupings were arbitrarily formed by the researchers to represent the type of training needed for maximum performance in the sport (aerobic, anaerobic, or mixed). Lifelong physical activity was estimated by a self-report questionnaire. Occupation was coded for that in which the subject stayed the longest in his life.

Reprinted, by permission, from S. Sarna et al., 1993, "Increased life expectancy of world class male athletes," *Medicine and Science in Sports and Exercise* 25: 237-244.

group, which had the highest exercise activity and the lowest body fat, extended their longevity from 1 to 4 years. The results from these studies as well as others (e.g., Paffenbarger et al., 1984) indicate that habitual exercise is related to longevity, but athletic status per se is not. The mortality rates of former athletes were similar to those of nonathletes. If the athletes remained active after graduation, their mortality rate was decreased, and if they became sedentary, their mortality rate increased. The inescapable conclusion is that the benefits of exercise and physical activity cannot be stored for a later date. The number of additional years of life projected on the basis of physical activity is probable only so long as the individual remains active.

A surprising result of this study was that exercise also seemed to have the beneficial effect of countering some diseases. Hypertensive men who exercised had half the mortality rate of hypertensive men who did not exercise. The mortality rate of smokers who exercised was 30% less than that of smokers who did not exercise.

The definitive study of exercise and mortality comes from a group of researchers at the Institute for Aerobics Research in Dallas, Texas, who documented the relative risk for mortality of several factors in more than 30,000 men and women (Blair et al., 1996). The strength of this study is that "fitness" was quantified by $\dot{V}O_2$max (described in detail in chapter 4), along with many other demographic and health attributes, for all of the subjects. The subjects were grouped into five categories, ranging from those who were sedentary to those who ran 30 to 40 miles a week (figure 1.12; Blair et al., 1996). Men who were in the lowest fitness category died at 3.5 times the rate of the most fit men. For women, the difference was even greater; those in the least fit category died at a rate 4.5 times greater than women in the highest fit category. Both men and women in the least fit category had higher incidences of cancer as well as cardiovascular disease.

A new finding that emerged from this study that may have particular relevance to the elderly is that the most important predictor of longevity was *not being*

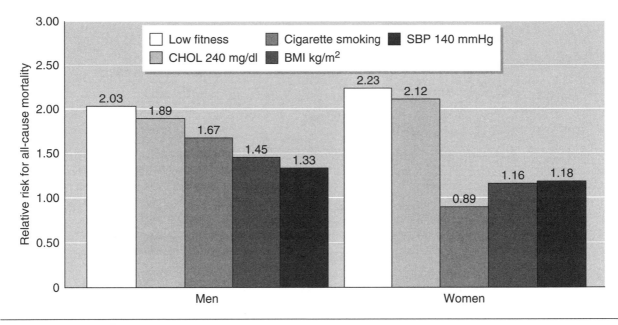

Figure 1.12 Relative risk of death from all causes for men and women, Cooper Institute for Aerobics Research. SBP = systolic blood pressure; CHOL = cholesterol; BMI = body mass index; SBP = systolic blood pressure.

Reprinted, by permission, from S. Blair et al., 1996, "Influences of cardiorespiratory fitness and other precursors on cardiovascular disease and all-cause mortality in men and women," *Journal of the American Medical Association* 276: 205-210.

in the lowest fit category. Higher levels of fitness were associated with increasing longevity for women but not for men. That is, the researchers concluded that in men, systematic exercise at relatively low levels will increase longevity almost as much as more intensive exercise. The data over the past 20 years have demonstrated clearly the importance of physical activity to decreasing all-cause mortality rate. These data led to the recognition of physical activity as the fourth independent risk factor for cardiovascular disease by the American Heart Association in 1992 and the consensus public health recommendations for physical activity in 1995, culminating in the Surgeon General's Report on Physical Activity and Health in 1996. The Surgeon General's report emphasized two important findings. First, demonstrated health benefits occur at a "moderate" level of activity, and therefore it is recommended that every adult accumulate at least 30 min of moderate activity each day (e.g., walking briskly for 30 min per day). Second, although physical activity does not need to be vigorous to provide health benefits, the amount of health benefit is directly related to the amount of regular physical activity (U.S. Department of Health and Human Services, 1996).

Adults should accumulate 30 min or more of moderate-intensity physical activity each day to optimize health.

From U.S. Department of Health and Human Services (1996).

To this point, discussions of aging have centered on the quantity, or length, of life. It is important to remember, however, that these results are specific to survival and do not necessarily speak to quality of life. Higher levels of systematic exercise provide many benefits other than just staying alive. Higher levels of cardiorespiratory and neuromuscular strength and flexibility enable any individual to be more generally active and expand the range of activities in which one can participate. These contributions of exercise-induced health and physical fitness and their role in psychological and social dimensions of life are discussed in more detail in chapters 9 and 10.

How Does Physical Aging Affect Quality of Life?

Modern medicine, science, and technology have been triumphant in the United States in bringing the majority of infectious and endemic diseases and nutritional deficiencies under control. The positive benefit of this major accomplishment is that a very high proportion of people born in this country can expect to live a very long time. The consequence of this increased longevity is that degenerative diseases have become our largest health care problem. The negative impact of a longer life span for mentally competent individuals is the potential for suffering

Table 1.3 **Accumulative Increases in Chronic Disease**

Age (years) Stage	20 Start	30 Noticeable	40 Subclinical	50 Problematic	60 Severe	70 Terminal
Emphysema	Smoking	Mild airway obstruction	X-ray hyper-inflation	Shortness of breath	Recurrent hospitaliza-tion	Chronic irreversible oxygen debt
Diabetes	Obesity	Glucose intolerance	Elevated blood glucose	Sugar in urine	Medication required	Blindness Neuropathy
Osteoarthritis	Abnormal cartilage staining	Joint space narrowing	Bone spurs	Mild joint pain	Moderate pain Stiffness	Disability
Atherosclerosis	Elevated cholesterol	Appearance of small plaques	Larger plaques	Leg pain with exer-cise	Angina pectoris	Heart attack

blindness, deafness, arthritis, osteoporosis, diabetes, hypertension, heart disease, incontinence, and physical frailty, and it many times becomes questionable whether life can be enjoyed fully under these morbid conditions that constrain activities so much.

Morbidity

Morbidity is the absence of health, and all too frequently it is a condition in which many frail elderly live for a long time before they die. Sometimes it is caused by terminal or chronic illness. The term *morbidity* is used to describe the condition in which an individual is so physically or mentally disabled by chronic disease that he or she becomes immobile and dependent on the care of others. The "five Ds" of morbidity are discomfort, disability, dependency, doctor problems, and drug interactions (among multiple medications). The major chronic diseases that eventually lead people into a condition of morbidity are atherosclerosis, cancer, osteoarthritis, diabetes, emphysema, and cirrhosis of the liver. These diseases generally start early in life and progress throughout the life span.

Even during youth, some degenerative changes begin to take place, but the body is able to compensate for the slight loss of function, particularly in the neuromuscular system. The great redundancy in this system suppresses overt symptoms for some time. Eventually, however, the pathologic changes become sufficiently extensive and the disease becomes symptomatic, leading inexorably to a morbid condition in which survival is dependent on extensive use

of medical support systems. Table 1.3 shows the average age at which symptoms of these chronic diseases begin to appear. Chronic diseases go through roughly six stages: the beginning, noticeable, subclinical, problematic, severe, and terminal stages. Many times individuals have one or more of these diseases, with each disease exacerbating the effects of the other. Living with multiple chronic diseases predisposes an individual to a very poor quality of life, which could contribute to the significantly higher suicide rate among these cohorts. The 65 and older age group accounts for only 13% of the U.S. population, but they account for 20% of all suicide deaths. Suicide in the aging population is discussed in chapter 10.

The social consequences of an unhealthy aged population are great. Not only does such a society have a large number of miserable and unproductive citizens and their extended families, but the financial burden on society as a whole is staggering. The financial burden is determined by the total number of elderly in the society and the percentage of these elderly who are incapacitated or ill. If the least conservative estimates are used, by the year 2040 the average life expectancy of older people could increase 20 years. Some projections are that by the middle of the 21st century, there will be 16 million Americans over 85 years of age. In addition, by 2040 there may be 94 million adults over the age of 65 who have chronic diseases or conditions (Gill, 2002). Prognosticators also say that the average 65-year-old will spend 7.5 years of his or her remaining 17 years living with some functional disability (Wilkins & Adams, 1983). If the present rate at which people

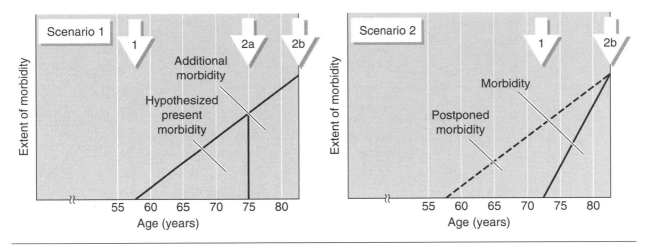

Figure 1.13 The compression of morbidity. The future of population health depends on relative movement of the two arrows: Arrow 1 represents the average age at initial onset of disease or infirmity, and Arrows 2a and 2b represent average age at death.

Adapted, by permission, from J.F. Fries, L.W. Green, and S. Levine, 1989, "Health promotion and the compression of morbidity," *The Lancet* 8636: 481.

are being added to the category of those experiencing morbidity is projected to the future, a 600% increase in health costs will occur. By 2040, Medicare costs, in constant 1987 dollars, will rise sixfold, dementia will ultimately afflict 28% or more of the elderly, and 800,000 hip fractures can be expected annually (Schneider & Guralnik, 1990). Social and medical programs are directly linked to the size and health status of the elderly population of a society. Thus, it is not only the number of years that seniors live but the way they live their remaining years that will determine the quality of life not only for them but for all Americans.

Compression of Morbidity

Given the projections for the number of individuals experiencing morbidity and the fact that raising the life expectancy ceiling is producing relatively fewer gains, the emphasis in gerontological research has shifted from lengthening life to increasing years of health. The goal is to compress the period of time in which individuals live in a state of morbidity. If the results of scientific advances and medical technology only increase the life span 15 or 20 years and in so doing merely increase the number of years of pain and suffering, then few individuals would accept that as a desirable goal. Figure 1.13 illustrates the concept of the **compression of morbidity**. First, the hypothesized present morbidity is shown for an average life span of 76 years (averaging male and female life expectancies), with an increasing number of the population experiencing morbidity, beginning at about age 55. Scenario 1 shows a hypothetical situation in

which life span is extended to age 85 through technological advances and medical breakthroughs, but the onset of morbidity begins at about the same average age. In this situation, which is clearly undesirable, more people experience morbidity for a longer time, because more people live longer, but the average age of onset and the morbidity slope remain the same. Extension of years of life without changes in health habits would only expand the period of morbidity. But extension of years of life accompanied by changes in health habits can compress the period of morbidity, as shown in Scenario 2. Because chronic diseases begin early in life and develop gradually, a healthy lifestyle can prevent or greatly postpone the start of some of these chronic diseases, such as adult-onset diabetes, emphysema, cirrhosis of the liver, and heart disease. Thus, the start or appearance of noticeable symptoms of those diseases would be postponed to a later age.

As shown in figure 1.14, the longer diseases are prevented, the less time an individual would experience morbidity in the terminal years. Individuals who practice sound health habits and prevent the onset of chronic disease for many years may never experience morbidity. For example, one of the positive outcomes for a group of healthy older adults who participated in a 2-year program of aerobic exercise was that as a group they evidenced a delay in the onset of cardiovascular disease symptoms (Topp et al., 1989). It is highly probable that a healthy lifestyle may also prevent or delay the threshold stage of other diseases such as osteoarthritis and some types of cancer.

Some gerontology scholars argue that a compression of morbidity cannot occur, and others argue

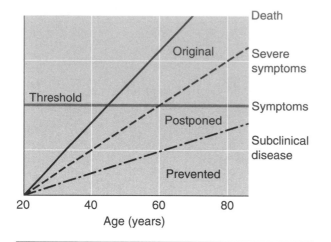

Figure 1.14 Schematic of the hypothetical development of chronic illness. The universal, chronic diseases begin early in life, progress through a clinical threshold, and eventuate in disability or death. Altering the rate (slope) at which symptoms develop postpones the clinical appearance of the illness, thus "preventing" it.

Adapted, by permission, from J.F. Fries and L.M. Crapo, 1981, *Vitality and aging* (New York: Freeman), 7.

vigorously that it can. The doubters see no evidence that individuals who change their lifestyle may experience a lower incidence of morbidity; they argue that even if there were evidence, the majority of individuals will not or cannot change their lifestyles. Fries (1980), however, summarized several large studies in which substantial reductions in morbidity were accomplished by education and the initiation of health promotion programs. The evidence from these studies showed that for each hour of exercise a week, there was a 10% improvement in reported health status. There were health risk reductions (19%) and a significant reduction in work time lost after 6 months of these health promotion programs. Doctor visits and hospitalization time also decreased. An important point that Fries made in his review of these studies was that the average rate of death did not decrease as a result of these health promotion studies, but the morbidity markers did significantly decrease, and thus the quality of life was increased for many of the program participants. In a study by Vita and colleagues (1998), a group of older adults who did not smoke, had good exercise habits, and had low body fat not only extended their longevity from 1 to 4 years but also decreased their morbidity in the last year of life by 50%. The most recent follow-up of these data continues to corroborate the value of self-care lifestyle health habits. Persons with better health habits survived longer, and disability was postponed and compressed into fewer years at the end of life (Fries, 2002). In addition, Rowe (1997)

summarized evidence that supports the compression of morbidity hypothesis. The incidence of arthritis, dementia, hypertension, stroke, and emphysema has decreased over recent years. In the most recent survey, 89% of 65- to 74-year-olds reported no disability, 40% of those over 85 years were fully functional, and the percent of those living in long-term care centers decreased from 6.3% (1982) to 5.2% (1997).

The results of several large population studies "make a compelling argument for the reduction and postponement of disability with healthier lifestyles as proposed by the compression of morbidity hypothesis" (Hubert et al., 2002, p. M347-M351).

The doubters are also concerned that fixing the responsibility of a contemporary illness on the behavior of individuals amounts to "blaming the victim," which is not consistent with the caring goals of service professions. However, the preventive contributions of good health habits and their effects on the quality of life outweigh their effects on the quantity of life, and individuals must take responsibility for the quality of their own lives. It is important for the health professions to develop and enhance life-extending strategies, but only if professionals also provide strategies that enable people to live as well as they can while continuing to be the best they can be. Of course, for individuals to optimize their abilities, they must actually use these strategies.

Quality of Life Components

In 1990, the Anna and Harry Borun Center for Gerontological Research of the University of California, Los Angeles, sponsored a symposium titled "Measuring the Quality of Life in the Frail Elderly." At that pioneering conference, it was generally agreed that 11 factors constitute quality of life for the frail elderly. The factors of cognitive and emotional function reflect everyone's desire to maintain productivity, independence, and an active interaction with the environment. Life satisfaction and a feeling of well-being represent emotional control and mental heath. Economic independence, although not essential, has the potential of enhancing quality of life. Social function, recreation, and sexual function enable people to enrich their lives. These factors, which are also highly relevant to healthy older persons, are shown in figure 1.15. But it is also clear that the physical dimension of life, which includes health, physical function, and energy and vitality, contributes in a very significant way to quality of life for the elderly. It is noteworthy

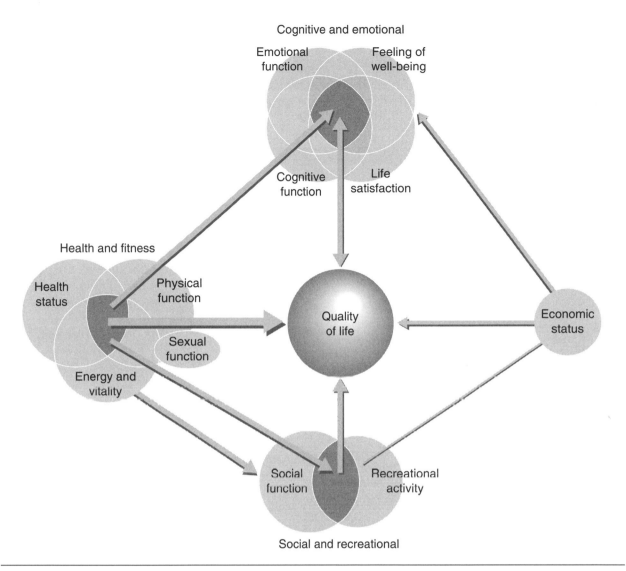

Figure 1.15 Factors affecting the quality of life. These factors are shown as three major constellations: cognitive and emotional, health and fitness, and social and recreational. Economic status also contributes in many direct and indirect ways but is deemed less important by older adults.

that of the 11 factors thought to be essential for a high quality of life in the last years, four of these relate to the physical dimension.

Health status, energy and vitality, and physical function, which support the execution of physical tasks, are generally taken for granted by the average young person, but age-related deficits in performance, which begin to concern middle-aged adults, become of greater concern to the young-old and grow to be a primary concern to some old and most of the oldest-old. Physical ability is the basis for performing the activities of daily living, such as walking, eating, bathing, and dressing; job-related tasks, such as typing, writing, lifting, and reaching; and participation in sport and recreational pursuits. This strong contribution of health, energy and vitality, and physical

function to the quality of life is shown in figure 1.15 by the broad line connecting the health and fitness cluster to the quality of life sphere. The integrity of these three factors has a profound influence on one's active life expectancy.

Mortality is associated with

- health and general function and
- quality of life (independence, cognitive function, and happiness).

Active life expectancy is a term coined by Katz and his colleagues (1983) that combines mortality and disability data. Active life expectancy refers to the number of remaining years of life that an individual may expect to be able to conduct the basic activities of daily living (ADLs). The ADLs are activities such as walking, dressing, bathing, eating, and getting up from a bed or chair. Individuals who cannot carry out these activities are in a state of morbidity, are dependent on others, and do not have a high quality of life by most people's standards.

Physiological changes accompany aging, and these changes eventually constrain motor performance. However, it is difficult to distinguish physiological changes attributable to aging per se from those attributable to declining physical activity, decreases in motivation, lower societal expectations, and the occurrence of disease. Many exercise physiologists suggest that most symptoms that people (especially those 50-75 years of age) attribute to aging are really the result of the "rotting, corrosion, and rust" that develop in a stagnant system. The dimensions of the physical components also extend directly to other facets of the quality of life. These are shown in figure 1.15 (p. 27) by thinner lines that depict the relationship to mental functions (cognitive and emotional function, life satisfaction, and feelings of well-being) and social function. The interrelationships of the physical dimension with mental and social dimensions are explored in chapters 9 and 10.

Quality of life is the difference between active living and just being alive.

Health and Fitness Contributions in Different Age Categories

Because the physical dimension is so inextricably interwoven with other human life dimensions, and because health and physical activities have a high probability of contributing to the compression of morbidity in the population, good health habits and consistent exercise are beneficial for everyone. Individuals of all ages gain better health, higher levels of physical function, and emotional and mental benefits from habitual physical activity and good health habits. But the primary contribution of consistent physical activity for quality of life varies with age. These differences are summarized in table 1.4. In children, adolescents, and young adults, physical activity contributes to growth, development, refinement, and self-knowledge of abilities and skills. In middle-aged adults and the young-old, good health habits and exercise can maintain near peak performance and postpone premature aging. For the old, consistent physical activity can substantially enhance the quality of life, enabling the elderly to continue to participate in many of the most enriching experiences of life. The effects of preventive health measures on quality of life may outweigh their effects on quantity of life.

Table 1.4　The Role of Physical Activity in Life Stages

Description	Age (years)	Role of physical activity
Infant	0-2	Mobility
Child	3-12	Mobility, developing identity, self-esteem, recreation, social interaction
Adolescent	13-17	Developing identity
Young adult	18-24	Self-esteem, recreation, social interaction
Adult	25-44	Recreation, self-esteem, social interaction
Middle-aged adult	45-64	Self-esteem, maintenance (function, job)
Young-old	65-74	Maintenance (mobility, job), recreation, social interaction
Old	75-84	Mobility, ADL, eating, bathing, dressing, walking, social interaction; IADL, e.g., cooking, washing clothes
Old-old	85-99	Mobility, ADL, independent living
Oldest-old	100+	Mobility, ADL, independent living

Note: ADL = activities of daily living; IADL = instrumental ADL.

Factors That Optimize Successful Aging

- Avoiding disease (health):
    Blood pressure (diastolic and systolic)
    Blood lipid profile
    Adiposity
    Pulmonary function
- Engagement with life:
    Social activities
    Club activities
    Volunteer work
- Maintaining high cognitive and physical function:
    Fitness (aerobic and muscular endurance, upper and lower body strength, flexibility, balance)
    Sleep
    Diet
    Absence of drug abuse
    Controlled alcohol use
    Controlled stress

From Rowe and Kahn (1998).

Health and fitness in 70-year-olds provide them with the vitality to hike, ski, swim, take walking tours, and deal with the physical demands of shopping, traveling, or socializing. Physical capacity in the oldest-old is the difference between mobility and helplessness, between maintaining independence and being dependent on others, and eventually between life and death.

It is customary to think of physical capacity and performance as improving through the early years, peaking in the third decade, and then declining linearly until death. However, each person is a unique individual, and the interaction of aging and life experiences decreases the consistency of performance within individuals and increases the differences among individuals on many variables across the life span. The differences in physical function of old adults are striking. Capacities range from the frail older adult living in a long-term care facility, who experiences severe difficulty walking, bathing, and dressing, to an 80-year-old living independently, who can run a 26.2-mile marathon race in a masters track meet. The concept of "average" ability for a specific age group becomes less and less appropriate for individual performance with increasing age.

SUMMARY

Life can be described in terms of quantity (how long it is) and quality (how satisfying it is). Quantity is described by several different terms: the maximum life span potential, operationally defined by the longest living survivor of the species; the average life span, which is the average age by which almost all of the members of a population are deceased; life expectancy, which is the average number of years of life remaining for an individual; and the rate of aging, which is the change in organ and system function over time. Another important definition is that of birth cohorts, which include all people born within a similar time frame. The most visible cohort is that of the baby boomers, who are an example of a birth cohort born between the years of 1946 and 1960.

The life expectancy of humans has almost doubled since the beginning of the 20th century, but the average life span has remained relatively stable. The number of individuals over the age of 80 will increase dramatically between now and the year 2025, but the fastest growing age group will be the centenarians, those more than 100 years old.

Several theories, which can be categorized as genetic, damage, or gradual imbalance theories, have been developed to describe and understand aging. These age theories have been developed in hopes of attaining the major goal of the life sciences and professions: to rectangularize the human survival curve. Three factors that contribute to increased life expectancy are food restriction (undernutrition), general activity level, and physical exercise. Activity level and exercise result in more adults living longer, not an increase in the maximum human life span. An interesting aspect of the human survival curve is the gender gap. Women throughout the world outlive men by 4 to 10 years. Theories proposed to account for the gender gap include genetics, hormonal differences, and social behavioral differences (primarily smoking habits).

Quantity of life is only of value, however, if the quality of life is endurable, and the goal of extending the life span is only viable if a reasonable quality of life can be maintained throughout the terminal years. Maintaining health and postponing the onset of debilitating disease as long as possible are called compression of morbidity.

The quality of life in the elderly, particularly the frail elderly, is affected by 11 major factors: health status, physical function, energy and vitality, cognitive function, emotional function, life satisfaction, a feeling of well-being, sexual function, social function, recreation, and economic status. Most of these factors highly interact with each other. Of particular interest in this book is the substantial contribution that health and fitness, physical function, and energy and vitality can make to the quality of life.

REVIEW QUESTIONS

1. How many differences exist among the demographic profiles (shown on page 9) of the United States, Japan, and Cambodia? What are the factors that contribute to these differences? What are the implications of the dramatically different distributions of age groups among the three countries?

2. In humans, which of the following is affected most by a lifetime of physical activity and why: life span, life expectancy, or maximum life span?

3. List four types of evidence that support the caloric restriction hypothesis as an extender of life span.

4. What are the social consequences of a society in which 20% of the population are more than 65 years of age and a large portion of them have multiple chronic diseases and conditions?

5. What are the three major categories of aging theories, and how are they conceptually different?

6. Can the aging process be slowed?

SUGGESTED READINGS

Olshansky, S.J., Hayflick, L., & Carnes, B.A. (2002). No truth to the fountain of youth. *Scientific American, 286*, 92-95.

Olshansky, S.J. (1998). Confronting the boundaries of human longevity. *American Scientist, 86*, 52-61.

Rusting, R.L. (2002, December). Why do we age? *Scientific American*, pp. 130-141.

Individual Differences

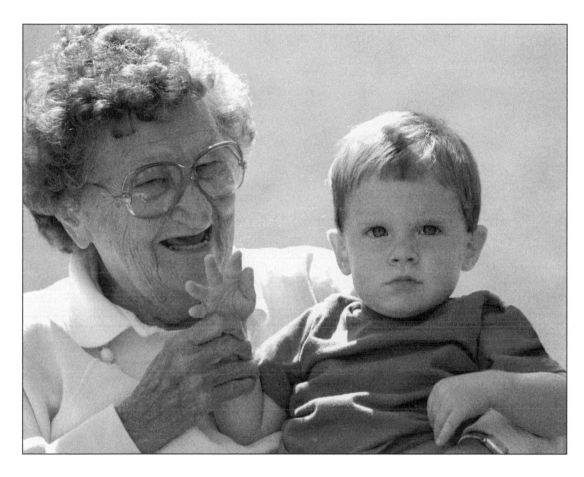

The objectives of this chapter are

- to explain between-group, within-group, and within-individual variability;

- to discuss several sources that contribute to the individuality of older adults;

- to provide examples of how gender, culture, education, and socioeconomic factors play a role in making all of us different;

- to clarify how research design, test selection, and test administration can affect the appearance and interpretation of individual differences; and

- to describe the concept of biological age and how it contributes to individual differences.

Aging is an individual experience, because people differ not only in their attributes and behaviors but in the way these change over time. Two older adults may be so different that one seems to be 40 and the other 80 years old. One is wheelchair bound, whereas the other runs marathons. One is an active heart surgeon, and the other cannot find his way home. One is an internationally famous comedian, and the other does not speak to anyone. The results of hundreds of experiments and research projects using both human and animal subjects have shown that chronological age is not a good predictor of function or performance for an individual on most variables. Aging is a highly personal process, with individuals not only being different from each other but also having physiological systems that age at different rates. The average blood pressure, for example, gradually increases in an age cohort as time passes. But when individuals are measured longitudinally, blood pressure does not increase at all in some people. In those whose blood pressure is unchanged, however, other systems may deteriorate more rapidly. Also, random variations in many physiological variables are frequently seen in individuals throughout their life span, so the differences observed among individuals over time do not remain entirely stable.

Several other factors contribute to individual differences. The assessment of aging rate may be influenced by the measurements taken or the tasks used for testing. Each individual begins life with different attributes and behaviors and with aging rates that differ for different systems, and these attributes and their aging rates also interact with the measurements made. The result is a unique aging pattern for each person. **Individual differences,** the term used to describe the great **variability** among people, describes a phenomenon that is just as much a hallmark of aging as the concept of age-related functional decline. Considering that individual differences exist among the elderly, it is no wonder that chronological age is such a poor predictor of function for an individual.

Assessment of Individual Differences

The differences that exist among people are measured by determining the spread of scores on a particular variable from the mean (average) score for that age group. Figure 2.1a shows the range of performance on a hypothetical strength test for individuals of different ages. The filled circles indicate the average score for each age group, but the unfilled circles show the strength score of each person in each age group. Notice that in this particular example, no single person has exactly the mean score. The mean adequately represents the amount of force that most of the members of each age group can produce, but it cannot accurately predict each individual's score. In some individuals, such as subjects 26 and 27, the mean is a very poor estimate of their strength. Subject 27 has strength-trained all his life and consequently has superior scores not only for his age group but for persons in the other age groups as well. Subject 26, an extremely sedentary individual, has a very low level of strength. This individual's strength is extraordinarily different from that of others in his age group.

The amount of individual difference (interindividual variability) among people in an experimental group is measured by the standard deviation *(SD)* of the scores about the mean *(M)*. The standard deviation roughly represents an average of the distances of the subjects' strength scores from the mean score of the age group. Standard deviation is calculated by

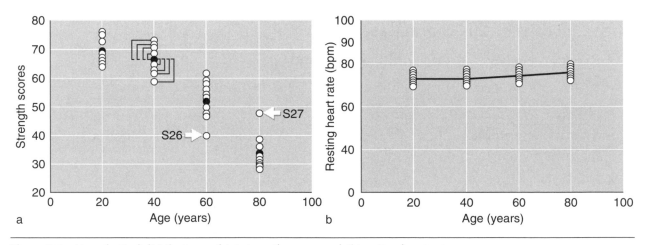

Figure 2.1 Hypothetical distributions of *(a)* strength scores and *(b)* resting heart rate.

taking the square root of the variance, which is the sum of the squared difference of each score from the group mean divided by the total number of subjects in the group.

$$\sqrt{(\sum x^2/N)}$$

A mean score is calculated statistically. It is possible that not a single person in the sample has a score that is also the mean score.

The distance of each score from the mean is shown by the brackets in the 40-year-old group (figure 2.1a). The greater the spread of scores from the mean, the more different the members of the group are and the less accurate the mean is in estimating individuals' strength. Figure 2.1b shows a hypothetical distribution of resting heart rates. Resting heart rates do not change significantly with age, and the standard deviations are small. In this figure, two points are important: First, the magnitude of individual differences varies with the attribute or function being measured. Physiological variables tend to have smaller individual differences than do performance variables. Second, particularly in variables with large individual differences, the means do not accurately predict the individual scores.

Because they arise from different sources, between-subject differences are larger in older ages in many variables. For example, human gestation requires 280 ± 5 days, onset of menarche occurs at 151.8 ± 14.1

Coefficient of Variation

The CV [(SD/M) · 100] is a way to assess the relative variability that exists within several distributions of scores, each of which have different units of measure. When we discuss the standard deviation of each distribution as a function of its mean, the magnitudes and discrepancies of means are neutralized.

months, and age at menopause is 50 ± 8 years (Baker & Sprott, 1988). Psychomotor test scores (figure 2.2) are examples of variables on which the individual differences increase with age. The average **coefficient of variation (CV)** [(SD/M) · 100] across six psychomotor tasks for 20-, 50-, 60-, and 70-year-olds is shown in figure 2.2a. The standard deviations are larger in the older age groups. Reaction time, measured in cross-sectional studies, also increases in individual differences as age increases (Botwinick, 1973; Fozard et al., 1976; Hertzog, 1985). In figure 2.2b, individual differences in choice reaction time (CRT) are shown across five age groups (Spirduso et al., 1990). The coefficient of variation reveals that large individual differences exist among a group of 8-year-olds, that the individuals in the 12- and 20-year-old groups are the most alike, but that individual

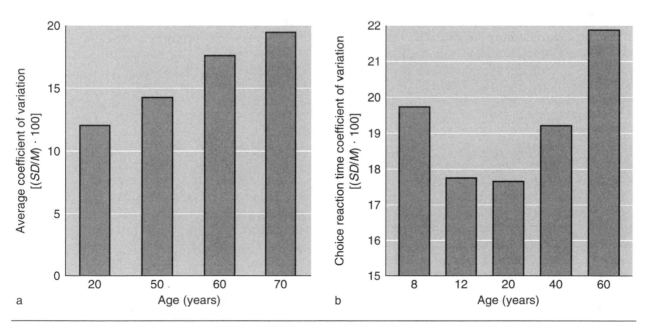

Figure 2.2 Average coefficients of variation (CV) for (a) six psychomotor tasks and (b) a choice reaction time test. In (a) the tasks were stationary tapping, between-target tapping, simple reaction time (foot), discrimination reaction time (foot), trail making, and digit-symbol substitution. In (b) the task was a two-choice reaction time paradigm.
Data from Light and colleagues (1996).

differences are also substantially larger in the oldest two age groups.

The larger between-subject variability in older people seen in reaction time data could be attributable either to a larger range of reaction times or to a more highly skewed distribution, that is, one in which just a few individuals are either much faster or much slower than the group as a whole. But the greater differences that exist among older adults are not a statistical artifact. When reaction times are measured longitudinally, individuals appear to become more different from each other. Individuals stay at about the same place in the distribution from one longitudinal measure to the next, but the distance among them increases. For example, individual differences in 8 of 15 variables measured six times over a 13-year period were maintained throughout the period studied (Maddox & Douglass, 1974). In 5 of the 15 variables analyzed in those longitudinal studies, the between-subject variance increased with increasing age. However, individual differences do not increase on all variables with aging. Body weight, perhaps because of selective mortality, is an example of a variable on which individual differences are stabilized throughout the life span.

Sources of Individual Differences

Individual differences arise from many sources. Individuals inherit different attributes, behaviors, and predispositions, and a lifetime of interacting with the environment and developing unique compensatory behaviors magnifies these differences. People differ in age, weight, height, gender, skin color, eye color, strength, intelligence, and a host of other variables, each of which alone and in combination contributes to individual differences. Additionally, physiological systems age at a different rate for each person. Also, as people grow older they perform less consistently on many types of tests. Gender, cultural differences, education, and socioeconomic status are additional sources of individual differences. Finally, the research designs used in gerontology research also contribute to the observations of individual differences.

Sources of observations of individual differences:

- Genetics
- Variations in lifestyle
- Disease
- Gender

- Differential rates of aging of different systems
- Culture, society, and education
- Within-individual biological variability
- Research design and process
- Compensatory behaviors

People are born with unique **genotypes** (genetic makeup), which vary on several dimensions and in hundreds of attributes. Not only are many individual differences in attributes and function genetically expressed, but behavioral genetics studies of children have shown that social and physical activity habits are also strongly determined by heredity (Buss & Plomin, 1984). Studies of adult twins have indicated that the genetic influence on physical activity persists into the second half of the life span (Plomin et al., 1988). In other words, some patterns of behavior with which individuals interact with their environment are relatively stable throughout the life span, and many lines of evidence suggest that these patterns may reflect individual differences in the propensity for certain behaviors that originate in genetic inheritance and early experiences (Stones et al., 1989).

Although people tend to stereotype the elderly, older adults exhibit more individual differences than young adults do. Every year that passes in a person's life provides more unique experiences, more opportunities for gene expression, more opportunities for environmental influences, and more exposure to possible accidents. In a sense, the older people become, the more unique they become.

Research on aging animals strongly supports the role of genetics in aging (Collier & Coleman, 1991). Same-aged mice and rats of different strains age differently in different tasks. Aging mice of some strains lose the capacity to balance on a moving rod but retain the ability to find an underwater target better than do mice of other strains. Individual differences in behavior are therefore partially a function of inherited traits but also partially shaped by a genotype that predisposes individuals to interact with their environment in certain ways. The abilities that they have and their predispositions to maximize their talents and compensate for their inadequacies allow wide disparities of function to occur among individuals. For example, the aging of a system, such as the cardiovascular system, is modified by the use of medications and alcohol, by smoking, by diet and exercise habits, by the incidence of disease, and by social factors. The different interactions, partly genetic, that people exhibit also increase individual differences. Genetic interactions with environmental experiences have also been demonstrated in animal research. Mice that were handled daily by technicians during the first 3 weeks of their lives managed stress better as they aged than did nonhandled mice (Levine, 1962).

Disease and Aging

People differ in the extent to which they experience disease, because each unique genotype supports different types and frequencies of inherited pathologies, different vulnerabilities to certain environmental challenges, and different levels of immune system effectiveness. Clearly, disease accelerates aging in some systems, and stress on these affected systems eventually stresses other systems. Events such as a heart attack, an environmental toxic stress, or the onset of depression following the death of a spouse can radically affect behavior and thus the aging process. In Johnson's (1985) model of aging (see figure 1.9, p. 16), diseases such as diabetes or cardiovascular disease would exacerbate injuries to cells and connective tissue and accelerate the loss of function of a system. Although it has not been possible to measure the different time courses of, reaction to, frequency of, and intensity of disease among people and predict life span, it is likely that these pathologies are related to biological aging and account for some of the individual differences that are seen in physical function of the elderly. As will be seen later, lifestyle and environmental effects interact with genotype to influence the presence and severity of disease and pathology.

Differential Aging of Body Systems

Another contributor to individual differences is the different rate at which physiological and behavioral systems age within the individual. The deterioration of systems is progressive but does not occur at the same rate across all sensory modalities and physiological systems.

Even in a single system, for example, the cardiovascular system, age differences in maximum heart rate are small but inevitable in the active older adult, but other cardiovascular components such as stroke volume and submaximal cardiac output are not noticeable. Fast-twitch muscle fibers become harder to recruit, but slow-twitch fibers age very slowly. Some aspects of psychomotor function, such as long-term memory, are maintained, whereas others, such as rapid decision making, deteriorate. In a longitudinal study, Schaie (1990) observed that no subjects universally declined on all abilities monitored (verbal meaning, spatial orientation, inductive reasoning, and number and word fluency). In addition, age-

Classic Individual Differences Research Study of Nathan Shock

One of the most famous early studies of aging was the classic graph published by Shock in 1967 (figure 2.3). He showed that nerve conduction velocity is about the same throughout the life span, but maximal breathing capacity is greatly different in people of increasingly older decades. Vital capacity also is very different in people of different ages, but the age differences in cardiac index are much less. In summary, age decade-related differences are system specific.

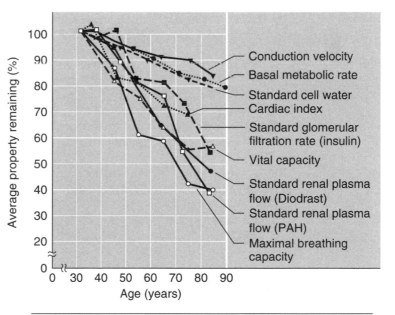

Conduction velocity
Basal metabolic rate
Standard cell water
Cardiac index
Standard glomerular filtration rate (insulin)
Vital capacity
Standard renal plasma flow (Diodrast)
Standard renal plasma flow (PAH)
Maximal breathing capacity

Figure 2.3 Age differences in physiologic functions from age 30. Data are derived from cross-sectional studies.

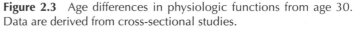

Reprinted from "Physical activity and the rate of aging" by N.W. Shock, 1967, *Canadian Medical Association Journal*, 96, p. 836. Copyright 1967 by the Canadian Medical Association. Reprinted by permission of the publisher.

Table 2.1 **Patterns of Change with Age**

Change pattern	Example
1. Stability, absence of change	Resting heart rate, some personality factors
2. Disease-related changes	Careful health screening showed that plasma testosterone does not decline in healthy men, contradicting earlier research. Thus, apparent age-related declines in testosterone are likely to be disease-related.
3. Steady decline in function in healthy persons	Creatinine clearance
4. Disease-accelerated aging of a system that declines in healthy persons[a]	The decline in forced expiratory ventilation, which is inevitable even in healthy individuals, is exacerbated by the development of ischemic heart disease.
5. Changes that occur precipitously in old age	Dementia (These changes are often expressions of disease.)
6. Compensatory changes	Frank-Starling mechanism to maintain cardiac output during exercise represents the body's attempts to maintain function with advancing age.
7. Cultural changes	Reduction of dietary cholesterol has nothing to do with aging but represents a change in behavior that influences other patterns.

Note: Data from Shock et al. (1984).

[a]From Fozard, Metter, and Brant (1990).

related change in different systems can follow different patterns of decline, shown in table 2.1.

Within-Individual Variability in Aging

Another source of individual differences is **within-individual variability,** or subject consistency. When researchers measure functions or behaviors of subjects, they hope that their measurement represents the true value of that function or behavior. But true scores of a function or behavior can only be estimated by obtaining two or more measurements from the same subject and calculating the average of these observations. The amount of variation that occurs in several measures of a variable from the same subject is called the within-subject variability. This variation is described by the standard deviation of all the subject's trials about the subject's mean. The principle is the same as that used to determine individual differences within a group: To determine individual differences, the average distance of each person's score from the mean of the group is calculated. To determine within-subject variability, the average distance of each score of a person from the person's own mean is calculated.

A comparison of between-individual variability (individual differences), within-individual variability (consistency), and between-group differences is shown in figure 2.4. In this figure, the data from performances on six different trials of a reaction time task are shown for each of 20 individuals in three different age groups. Each cluster of symbols represents the six trials of an individual shown on the x-axis. Because this is a time score, a high score represents slow performance and a low score represents fast performance. A horizontal line indicates the mean of the 20-year-old age group. Each individual trial is shown as a function of the 20-year-old mean (trial score minus the mean). The subjects are ranked from 1 to 20 on the basis of their within-individual variability. Thus, the trials of individuals to the extreme left of each figure are tightly clustered, and those at the extreme right are extremely varied. Several important points about aging and variance can be seen in this figure. First, individuals differ considerably in how spread their trial scores are. Those at the left of the figure react within almost the same time on every trial (within-individual variability). Second, individuals in each age group vary considerably in how close they are to the 20-year-old mean (**within-group variability**; individual differences measured by the standard deviation). Some individuals are very close to the 20-year-old mean, and others are very far away from it. Even in the 20-year-old group, a few of the individuals' times are substantially slower than

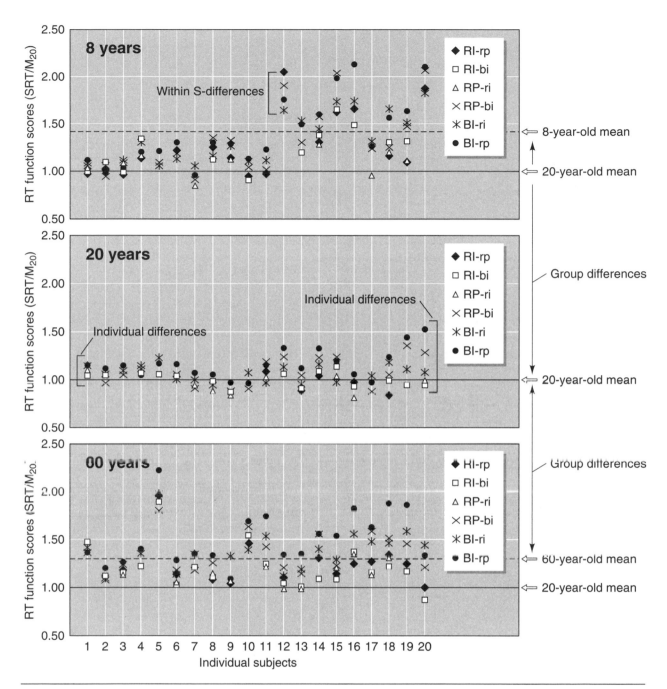

Figure 2.4 Reaction time (RT) data obtained from 8-, 20-, and 60-year-old females and calculated as a function of the 20-year-old mean (RT [8, 20, 60] / mean [20]). Subjects chose two of three combinations of fingers to make the reactions. RT reactions were made by RI = right index finger, RP = right pinch, and BI = bilateral index fingers, when paired with another finger combination. Uppercase (RI) indicates the finger combination used to make the reaction, and lowercase (ri) indicates that this was the finger combination paired with the primary task. In a block of 20 trials, stimuli indicated reaction with either RI or RP, whichever combination was indicated by the stimulus. The RI times were obtained when the stimulus light indicated to react with RI (RI-rp), and the RP times were those taken when the stimulus indicated an RP (RP-ri). The horizontal solid line across each graph is the 20-year-old mean, and the dashed line is the age group mean. Subjects are ordered across the x-axis according to their within-subject variability, so that those subjects who provide similar reaction times for all six tasks (or all six trials if these were trials) are more toward the left of the graph, and those who have great variation across the tasks (or trials) are more toward the right of the graph.

the group mean. Third, **between-group variability,** or age group differences, is very apparent in both group comparisons and within-group variances. At least half of both the 8- and the 60-year-old group individuals exhibit a very large spread in their six times, and in the 8-year-old group, half of the individuals are very far away from the 20-year-old mean. Almost all of the 60-year-old individuals exhibit more variability among their six trials and are also considerably slower than the 20-year-old mean.

In some variables, within-subject variation is very small. Multiple measures of nerve conduction velocity, for example, provide almost identical values unless the measurements are taken at different times of the day. If resting heart rate is measured 10 times for 1 min, the result will not be identical on all 10 trials, but the measures will be very close. Within-subject variability may occur because of the nature of biological oscillating systems, **stochastic** (random) **processes,** or it may be caused by errors of measurement. In other variables, such as reaction time, the responses of subjects are so variable that a large number of trials have to be taken so that the average or median of these trials can be used to estimate the subject's true response speed. Subject motivation, fatigue, and learning and the experimental use of different strategies on different trials explain some of the within-subject variability in these behaviors.

The extent to which within-subject variability is stable throughout the life span probably differs with the function measured. Conflicting results have been obtained for reaction time. Within-subject variabil-ity stayed the same over a 13-year period with six measures of reaction time according to Maddox and Douglass (1974) but increased with age according to Fozard and colleagues (1976).

Variations in Lifestyle

Variations in lifestyle also contribute to individual differences. In different combinations and at different levels, people adopt positive health behaviors that are known to optimize physical and mental function and to postpone or avoid disease, such as good diets and ample physical activity and sleep. Similarly, they participate in negative behaviors such as smoking, drinking alcohol in excess, taking excess medications, indulging in drugs, and putting themselves into situations that cause their stress levels to skyrocket. Adults also differ greatly in the extent to which they selectively maintain different functions through training or practice. For example, some play contract bridge weekly, which maintains memory and reasoning but not reaction time (Clarkson-Smith & Hartley, 1990). Others play racquetball, which may maintain reaction time but perhaps not the ability to reason. The social and personal lifestyles that people adopt also influence their health and performance as they age (Stones & Kozma, 1986).

These lifestyle differences may not actually alter the rate of aging, as defined in chapter 1, but the differences in lifestyles can make a big impact on function and ultimate disability. As shown in figure 2.5, lifestyle affects both reserve and disease. Positive

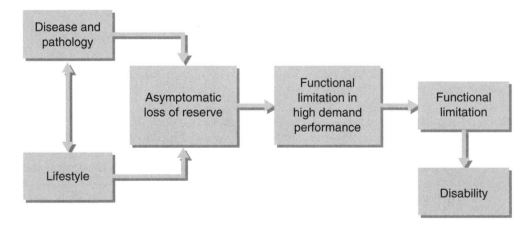

Figure 2.5 A model of disease and pathology, originally proposed by Nagi (1991) and later adapted by Rikli and Jones (1997), is shown slightly modified. In this model, as time passes in the human life span, disease and lifestyle affect the loss of reserve, even if symptoms of poor health or function are not apparent. Lifestyle also significantly interacts with disease. As time continues to pass, asymptomatic losses of reserve give way to functional limitations, but only in high-demand performances. Thus, an individual may appear to have no cardiorespiratory problems, until the individual runs for a bus or has to walk up a steep hill. Finally, these functional limitations give way to limitations in performing ordinary household tasks and activities of daily living, eventually leading to disability.

health behaviors postpone, lessen, or avoid disease and also help to maintain reserve, even before symptoms of disability can be observed. The maintenance of reserve also maintains performance at a higher level, so that reactions to emergencies or high-demand situations are adequate, postponing physical limitations and disability for as long as possible.

Compensatory Behaviors of Older Adults

One of the necessities of life is to learn to compensate for inadequacies and to develop strategies that maximize personal goal acquisition. Young people develop compensatory strategies to achieve their objectives if they are lacking in relevant talents or skills. Adults develop compensatory strategies when they begin to lose skills or talent. For example, older adults adjust to handling heavy objects by switching to larger muscle groups and by adopting a more biomechanically optimizing posture. As typists grow older, they learn to anticipate what is to be typed to compensate for their slower eye–hand coordination. They begin cognitively processing the typing of a letter or character earlier than young subjects so that their performance is not hampered by their slower central nervous system function (Salthouse, 1988). The magnificent human cognitive intellect provides behavioral flexibility, that is, the ability to choose different strategies, which adds to the plasticity of the system. But in so doing, it also adds to the individual differences that are observed in groups of people.

Gender, Cultural Differences, Education, and Socioeconomic Status

Gender differences in physiological function and psychosocial role expectations are great and contribute substantially to individual differences in aging on some physical dimensions. For example, women tend to live longer than men, but they have more debilitating diseases than men. Women have more osteoarthritis and osteoporosis than men, both of which impair physical function. Women lose muscle mass at approximately the same rate, but they start the decline at a much lower level, so that sarcopenia (muscle wasting) is much more severe in women. The combination of more debilitating disease and higher levels of sarcopenia results in a much greater difference in physical function of men and women over the age of 70. Only 33.2% of men over 70 have difficulty with one or more activities of daily living (walking, climbing stairs, stooping, crouching, kneeling, reaching

up), whereas 50.3% of older women have difficulty with these (Older Americans, 2000). Women use health care resources more than men (Pescosolido, 1992), whereas men have fewer debilitating diseases in the very old age categories; all are examples of gender as a source of individual differences.

Cultural and subcultural differences exist in all aspects of life. Cultural membership affects personality, patterns of familial and friendship interaction, the ways people cope with and adapt to perturbations of their environment, and also the way people age (Jackson et al., 1990). Cultural membership affects eating behaviors (diet and pattern of eating) and participation in negative health behaviors (smoking and alcohol and drug use). More specifically, cultures have specific views of the role of physical activity in the lives of members, and members of the culture have strong expectations concerning which physical activities are appropriate for different age groups. Cultural and subcultural expectations of the value of hard work, financial success, social success, and "appropriate" work activities can affect psychological stress levels. Individual differences in youth and middle age may also be accentuated with increasing age, because in many cultures social constraints on older people are relaxed. Older people in most cultures have more freedom to behave in the ways they want to behave.

Finally, the social theory of **cumulative disadvantage** suggests that the quality of life in older decades is influenced heavily by social factors relating to development in different cohorts (O'Rand, 1996). The social roles of millions of women as caregivers disadvantage them in the labor market and depress their financial incomes, which influences their health. Social, educational, economic, and political factors contribute to racial disparities in health care and development of self-care health behaviors.

Yet another source of individual differences is education. The vastly different educational backgrounds of 70- and 80-year-olds compared with 20-year-olds make it exceptionally difficult to understand age-related cognitive changes that are independent of educational background. If researchers simply compare 20- and 80-year-olds' cognitive performance, they also compare groups that have vastly different educational experiences. Conversely, if researchers match for educational level, so that they only study subjects who have the same amount of education, they are studying a group of 80-year-olds who represent a population more educationally elite than that of the 20-year-olds. This is particularly true when studying females. So few women went to college in the 1930s that any 80-year-old women who did represents a population with a very different intellectual and personality profile. The influence of educational level is not isolated to cognitive tests. It is also related to many types of physical performance as well.

Socioeconomic status (SES) provides an entirely different environment for individuals and is thus another source of individual differences. A good example of this is the interaction between SES and obesity. Obesity is more prevalent in people who have lower incomes, who tend to eat cheap, filling, fat, fast foods in large portions. Those at high SES levels are more likely to eat light, delicate, lean foods and to exercise.

Socioeconomic status can also bias a researcher's analysis of some variable if low-income older adults who are financially stressed volunteer for a study just because of the monetary incentive, whereas young adults volunteer to participate in the study for reasons other than financial incentive.

How Research Design Affects Our View of Individual Differences

The study of individual differences in aging, and particularly the rate of aging for individuals and groups, is not as straightforward as it might seem. The appropriate design for such study appears intuitively to be a longitudinal design, in which the same people are measured on a particular variable over a number of years. But people live too long for this to

Sources of Individual Differences Interact With Each Other

A good example of how sources of differences exert their influences together is the interaction of gender and cultural influences on exercise habits. In America today, exercise is viewed as a desirable health habit and both women and men are encouraged to exercise daily by health professionals and their peers. However, in many cultures, exercise is viewed as admirable and necessary for men but unsuitable for women. In these cultures, women who insisted on exercising would be ostracized. Unless their daily work involved long-lasting physical activity throughout the day or intensive physical work, it is unlikely that they would be as healthy and as physically fit as the men in that society.

be feasible in most instances. It would be extremely costly, and many of the subjects would outlive the researcher. The design used by most investigators is the cross-sectional research design shown in figure 2.6, in which people of different ages are compared. A longitudinal design (row 6, which is shaded) involves measurement of the same people, the 1920 cohort, in the years 1970, 1980, and 1990, and 2000. A cross-sectional study (column 5, far right) involves

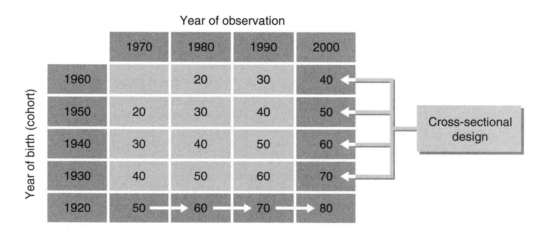

Figure 2.6 Comparison of cross-sectional and longitudinal research designs. In cross-sectional research designs, measurements are down a column (i.e., in 1970, 20-, 30-, 40-, and 50-year-olds would be measured). Those who are 30 are different people from those who are 40, and so on. A longitudinal analysis involves measuring the same people in one or more birth cohorts over several years (i.e., the 1930 cohort would be measured in 1970 at age 40, again in 1980 at age 50, again in 1990 at age 60, and yet again in 2000 at age 70).

Adapted from "Research Methods" by J. Botwinick. In *Aging and Behavior* (p. 389) by J. Botwinick (Ed.), 1984, New York: Springer.

measurement only in the year 2000, of people born in 1960 (40-year-olds), 1950 (50-year-olds), 1940 (60-year-olds), and 1930 (70-year-olds). Some combinations of cross-sectional and longitudinal designs over limited time periods have also been used, but these combinations comprise a very small percentage of research studies.

The cross-sectional design, however, is not a good design for determining individual differences on many variables for several reasons. First, cross-sectional analyses can only assess age differences, not age changes. Second, old and young people do not volunteer and remain in studies in the same percentages. Third, the pattern of mortality, disability, and health status in aging adults affects the results. Fourth, the number of subjects in the various age groups is usually unequal, with far more younger than older subjects. Fifth, the sampling techniques to acquire older subjects for study may be different than those techniques used to obtain young subjects.

> Cross-sectional analyses only assess age differences, not age-related changes.

Age Differences Versus Age Changes

Individuals age at different rates, but it is not possible to measure the rate of aging of selected functions unless the same individuals are measured over an extended period of time. Most of the information about capacities and abilities at various ages comes from cross-sectional studies in which variables are measured in individuals of different ages. Thus, oxygen consumption is said to "decline" with increased age, because the average oxygen consumption values are lower in the older groups. However, these are age differences not age changes. The results of longitudinal studies, such as the Baltimore Longitudinal Study of Aging and the Duke Longitudinal Studies I and II (Palmore, 1970, 1981), produced similar descriptions of age changes that occur in healthy adults. When individuals are measured longitudinally for a period of time, relatively few of them actually follow the means that are plotted for a variable from cross-sectional studies (i.e., studies of different people at different ages). Even fewer would follow the average sample means derived cross-sectionally for several different parameters. Graphs of average aging patterns provide only a rough approximation of the actual pattern of aging followed by an individual. Thus, the researchers involved in the Baltimore and the Duke studies concluded from their analyses that cross-sectional studies are not very accurate in predicting individual aging patterns. It is all too easy to fall into the trap of interpreting differences between age groups as age-related changes, but as noted in the discussion of selective mortality, such interpretations can lead to completely inaccurate conclusions.

> When individuals are measured longitudinally for a period of time, relatively few of them actually follow the means that are plotted for a variable from cross-sectional studies.

Differential Attrition of Subjects

Subjects drop out of studies for a variety of reasons; they may become sick, disabled, or disinterested. Whatever their reasons, they represent a very different sample of their age group than those who continue in a study. Those who remain in studies typically have higher self-reported measures of physical health, psychological well-being, life satisfaction, self-esteem, and social support—all factors that describe successful aging. The dropouts generally participate less in personal, recreational, and social–interpersonal activities (Powell et al., 1990) and exhibit more incidence of depression than the remaining research participants. Clearly, studying individual differences among age groups can be affected if the older groups include people who are successfully aging, whereas the younger groups contain a mixture of those who will successfully age and those who will not. Many older people who are unhealthy or who feel that they cannot perform as well as their peers may refuse to participate in a study or may refuse to return as a subject for the second or third testing in a longitudinal study. If these older people are accurate in their self-evaluation, then the scores from those who return for testing will overestimate the abilities or functions of people of that age group and may artificially reduce the individual differences observed.

Selective Mortality

Another problem that occurs when averages are taken cross-sectionally from different age groups is that the results can be distorted by **selective mortality.** Selective mortality describes the phenomenon that only a "select few" live to be 80 or 90 years old. More than half of a birth cohort die before their 70th birthday. Some of those who are measured in their 30s and 40s in present experiments will not live to be 70, whereas the 70- or 80-year-olds in the study obviously already have lived that long. Consequently, the comparisons that are drawn between 20-year-olds and 70-year-olds are on a mixture of select and nonselect 20-year-olds with only select 70-year-olds. The 70-year-old sample may have smaller individual differences because of

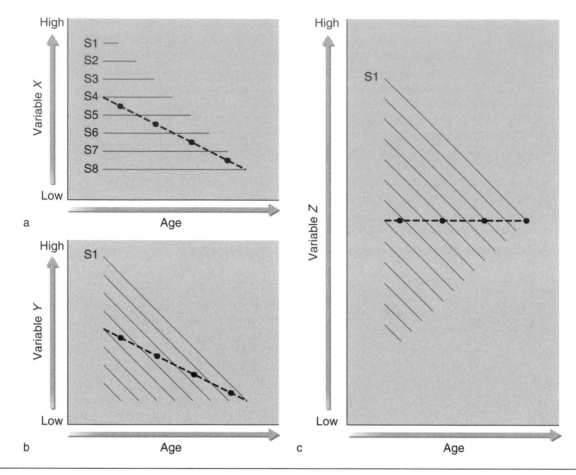

Figure 2.7 *(a)* Confounding effect of selective mortality on inferences about age changes. Each solid line segment represents the pattern of change in an individual (in this case there is no change with aging, and death occurs at the end of the line). High values for X are assumed to be deleterious. The closed circles represent mean values obtained in a cross-sectional study; the dashed line connecting these dots then correctly represents age differences among age groups, but the inference that age changes were occurring in individuals would be erroneous. *(b)* Confounding effect of selective mortality on the magnitude of age changes. A floor effect or lethal limit is assumed for the variable. In this case, the dashed line representing age differences underestimates true aging. *(c)* Confounding effect of selective mortality as a result of which age changes are not revealed in cross-sectional studies. A lethal limit that varies with age is assumed. In this case, the dashed line shows no age differences, although there were large age changes in individuals.

Adapted from Shock et al. 1984.

the selective process. Figure 2.7 shows how selective mortality in cross-sectional studies can mislead researchers in hypothetical situations in which (a) no change occurs with aging, (b) a "floor effect" exists, and (c) a lethal limit varies with age. Each filled circle is a hypothetical mean that represents a different group of adults who happen to share the same chronological age. Connecting them implies a continuity from one decade to the next, which does not exist.

Unequal Numbers of Subjects in Age Groups

It is difficult to find older adults who are willing to be tested. The more difficult the test and the more

energy it requires, the less easy it is to convince older adults to participate. Also, as discussed previously, more older adults than younger adults may drop out of an experiment. Consequently, in most research projects, the number of subjects dwindles for each increasingly older age group. For example, a study of young, middle-aged, and old adults may have 50 young adults, 32 middle-aged adults, and 18 old adults. But compounding this inequality of sampling is the fact that the age ranges are also usually unequal. The young group may have an age range of 9 years (20-29), the middle-aged group an age range of 13 years (40-53), and the old group, often referred to as the 60+ group, a range of 23 years (60-83). Thus, the individual differences within each age group increase with increasing age, contaminating the results of the age group comparisons.

The smaller number of subjects in the oldest age group not only contaminates the age group comparisons by compromising the statistical analyses but also represents a situation in which the population of one age group—the oldest age—is less represented than the other two age populations. Consider the measurement of muscular strength: A researcher wishing to know how aging affects the maximum amount of weight a man can lift analyzes the records of weightlifting contests. But the number of 20-year-old men who weight train and compete in weightlifting is many times larger than the number of 70-year-old men who compete. The 20-year-olds' weightlifting records, because they are obtained from a much larger number of contestants, probably estimate the population mean for that age group more reliably than the 70-year-olds' records do for their age group. So few old individuals participate in strength and power athletic events that the records surely must underestimate the upper limits of human strength and power in the 7th, 8th, and 9th decades. This problem is discussed in more detail in chapter 12, which compares the numbers of competitors in each age group with their average times (figure 12.13, p. 299) for a rowing ergometer competition.

Researchers generally are reluctant to force elderly adults to do anything that is against their desires, so most investigators are left to recruit only those old adults who volunteer to serve as subjects. Volunteers of any age, by their nature, are different from randomly selected subjects on a wide variety of variables. Young volunteers have been shown from various studies to be more sociable, to have a greater need for social approval, to be more easily influenced by the presence and opinions of others, and to be more intelligent. Females tend to volunteer in greater numbers for research projects that are relatively standard or unthreatening, whereas males volunteer more frequently for experiments that are more unpredictable.

Studies of aging tend to be studies of volunteers, and this is another source of individual differences that is independent of aging effects. Furthermore, when recruiting old adults as subjects for research, many investigators are tempted, for ease of testing, to use intact groups of people such as college faculty members, residents of nursing homes, retirement communities, or long-term care facilities, Veterans Administration hospital outpatients, members of garden clubs, or participants of social service groups, such as Meals on Wheels. Although such groups are more convenient to measure, the very factors that

caused them to be in those groups also contribute another source of individual differences that can contaminate the comparisons made with younger groups.

Can the Process of Studying People Influence Individual Differences?

If we are to understand the effects of aging on various behaviors by comparing older adults' performances to those of younger adults, the comparison must distinguish between the performer's competence and his or her assessed performance. This distinction is not a serious problem in the measurement of many physiological variables, such as blood proteins, muscle tissue composition, or bone calcium analysis, although some variables, such as oxygen consumption and blood pressure, thought by some researchers to be totally free of psychosocial influences, are not. In most behavioral assessments, however, the participants must voluntarily produce a good effort. The difference between their true abilities and their test performance is most apparent in behavioral variables when the subject must produce his or her best effort. Examples of this type of variable are tests of memory, reaction time, balance, and strength. Larger individual differences in older groups compared with younger groups on these types of measurements arise from several sources, thus making the comparison of age differences more difficult to understand.

Two prime behavioral characteristics long thought to inflate individual differences in performance are intrinsic motivation (need achievement and anxiety) and self-efficacy. Several researchers have reported in the psychological literature that older adults are not as motivated as young adults to do their best in performance tests; adults' need for achievement declines with age (e.g., Verhoff et al., 1984), whereas the anxiety related to testing increases. How need achievement and anxiety interact depends on the type of test. For example, women in their 70s may have little interest in producing the highest strength score within their capability, but they may be very interested in providing a good short-term memory performance. The women want to prove to themselves and to others that their memory is still excellent. A 20-year-old man, on the other hand, may be relatively disinterested in a short-term memory test, which he may consider irrelevant to anything he cares about, but may be very anxious to produce the highest muscular strength performance he can. In this example, age and gender account for large individual differences, but the different motivations these subjects have with regard to the test variables also contribute to the individual differences seen in their performances. Kausler (1990), however, pointed out that although differential age-related motivation effects on performance are almost dogma in the gerontological field, few investigators have addressed the issue. Results from these studies were contradictory and inconsistent, and he concluded that the results were so ambiguous that neither need achievement nor anxiety appeared to account for the age differences in performance. Nevertheless, because it has been well established that motivation influences performance at any age, and because inadequately or unequally motivated subjects contribute artificially to the individual differences seen, the conscientious reader of research must consider whether the research and measurement procedures were designed so that any differences seen are related to age and gender, not to motivation.

Self-efficacy is an individual's perception of his or her capability to execute a certain behavior successfully. It may be considered a "situation-specific" measure of self-confidence. Self-efficacy is not related to the skills an individual possesses but rather to that individual's perceived confidence about his or her skills. It is affected by performance accomplishments, vicarious experiences, verbal persuasion (social

expectations), and physiological arousal (Bandura, 1977). The strongest source of efficacy information is performance accomplishments. In the previous example, a 75-year-old woman who is to be tested on strength and short-term memory has probably not been tested in more than 50 years on any type of test. When she was young, it was not "proper" for young ladies to exhibit strength; thus, she may never have been tested on strength and she probably has no feeling for a maximum strength effort. Conversely, the 20-year-old man's memory has been tested in every school class he has taken for the past 12 or more years. He has found many ways to test his strength against his peers and may even have taken weight training classes in school. Thus, the confidence that he brings to the testing situation is likely to be very different from the confidence that an older woman feels when entering the laboratory.

If tests are short and completed in 1 day for a shotgun type of experiment, it is unlikely that the older subjects will be able to approach the tests with the same confidence in their ability that younger adults have. Older people are also more likely than younger people to attribute poor performance to their own ability, which further detrimentally affects self-efficacy and interacts with task performance (Lachman & McArthur, 1986). Yet individual differences in the variable of interest may be more related to the scores of the older subjects being con-

A Portrait of "Successful Aging"

At 101, Constance Douglas Reeves mounted her horse and rode to the side of the line of young girls saddled up for their 2-hr horseback riding class at Camp Waldemar in Kerrville, Texas. "Let's move 'em out," she called, leading what must have been well over the thousandth class she's taught over 70 years. While Connie was studying at the University of Texas Law School, a young and handsome Jack Reeves, a professional rodeo cowboy, swept her off her feet. They married and together ran a 10,000-acre ranch in the winter, raising sheep, goats, and cattle. During the hot summer months, they taught riding classes 6 hr a day, 6 days a week. That included herding the horses from ranch to camp, caring for them, and managing all the equipment. Constance taught four generations of young girls how to ride, which earned her a place in the National Cowgirl Hall of Fame and the Cowboy Hall of Fame. She was the oldest living cowgirl in either Hall.

At 93, Connie was on a trail ride showing the new instructors the idiosyncrasies of the riding trails when her horse brushed into a hornets' nest, setting the hornets into a full-stage attack on Connie and her horse. The horse bolted, throwing her to the ground, leaving her with multiple stings, a broken wrist, five broken ribs, and a partially collapsed lung. Two months later, she was back in the saddle teaching.

At 101 this tough and energetic centenarian wore cowboy shirts, pants, and her special Cowboy Hall of Fame blue boots right up until the last time that she tumbled from her horse and wound up in the hospital. There, she contracted pneumonia and died. She was blessed with good genes, but the more than half a century of riding, working the ranch, staying active, and being around young people played a large role in maintaining her mobility and sharp thinking. Connie's photo is featured on the cover of this book.

taminated by intimidation rather than to true age differences.

Biological Age

Individual differences are nowhere better represented than in the concepts of biological or functional age. Casual observations of people provide ample evidence that individuals differ dramatically in the way they age. Some individuals seem very young for their chronological age, whereas others appear to be much older than their age-group peers. This is implied when a woman is described as "aging gracefully" or a man is told that he doesn't look his age. The observation seems straightforward enough, but how can it be defined and measured?

Determining biological age would require measurement of the gradual breakdown and decline of physiological and cognitive systems irrespective of chronological age, so that an assessment could be made of how far an individual is along the life course. Obviously, individuals differ greatly in their chronological age at death, but they may not differ substantially if age were represented by the biological status of physical systems. The issue is a very complex one, however, further complicated by the fact that the gerontological scientific community has been unable to develop a consensual definition of aging. The time-related decline of physical systems clearly interacts with environmentally induced, as well as hereditary, disease processes (Ludwig & Smoke, 1980). Yet theorists continue to disagree as to whether the results of disease processes should be included in a definition of aging.

The concept of biological age is not new. Historically, scientists have assessed biological age in children by measuring skeletal and dental characteristics. The chronological ages at which different children develop the same bone maturation markers are quite different. Sexual maturation has been measured by anthropometrics, and physiological and physical changes have been associated with puberty and menopause. The accuracy of these measures is clearer in children, however, and the measurements themselves tend to be more useful for determining landmark stages of development than for quantifying the slow, progressive changes in the physical dimension associated with adult aging.

Definition of Biological Age

Biological aging is the process or group of processes that causes the eventual breakdown of mammalian homeostasis with the passage of time. It is expressed as a progressive decrease in viability and an increase in vulnerability of the body with the passage of time, both of which lead eventually to death. In this sense, biological aging refers to the organism as a whole. Biological aging can only be inferred from measurements of variables that represent physical and mental functions, and because it is correlated with chronological aging in the general population, people tend to think of biological age and chronological age as being synonymous. Everyday observations, however, which quickly reveal that some individuals do not appear to be as "old" in some behaviors as others of the same age, have led researchers to seek a measure of biological age that is independent of chronological age. Such a measure could be used as a **biomarker of aging.** The essential criteria for biomarkers are that they be able to determine the rate of change in a function or performance that is related only to the passage of time and not to disease processes and that they be measured without altering the basic biological processes and behavior of the individual. Biomarkers also should reveal directional change—decreased viability and increased vulnerability to death with increasing chronological age.

Desirable Features of Useful Biomarkers

1. Biomarkers should be able to be assessed in a nonlethal manner in animal models and should not cause trauma in humans.
2. Biomarkers should be highly reproducible and reflect physiological age.
3. The function examined should display significant alterations during relatively short time periods.

The clinical functions being measured should be important to the effective maintenance of health and function (Sprott, 1999, p. B464).

Several biomarkers, none of which meet all of these criteria, have been proposed on the basis of research on lower life forms. In a hypothetical example, if a nematode (a type of worm) has a life span of 60 days and is observed to wiggle 60 times a minute when touched with a pencil on its first day of life, 59 times a minute on its second day and so on, with the wiggles decreasing by 1 wiggle a minute each day of its life, one would only have to touch any nematode and count the wiggles per minute to know how many days of life remained. It would not be necessary to know the date of birth. In this case, the wiggles-per-minute behavior would be a perfect biomarker, for it would predict the age and the time of death for members of that species. This type of biomarker seems unattainable in humans at the present time.

Researchers had hoped for a biomarker or combination of biomarkers that represents a point on the life course of an individual that would be relatively independent of chronological age. Unfortunately, the aging process in humans is more complicated and complex, and a biomarker of aging that can meet all the criteria mentioned here has been elusive.

Measurement of Biological Age

Without the ability to measure humans on one or more variables throughout the life span, most researchers resort to chronological age as the criterion. The method used to derive most biological age scores is to calculate how far an individual deviates from the average score for his or her age group. Those individuals whose score is higher than the average for their age group are said to be "older" than those whose scores fall below the average. Figure 2.8 shows average choice reaction times (CRTs), which become slower with age, for individuals aged 20 through 80 on a hypothetical test. The average CRT (shown by open circles on the graph) is 310 ms for 20-year-olds, 340 ms for 50-year-olds, and 368 ms for 80-year-olds. The CRT of a 50-year-old female is represented by a filled circle and that of a 60-year-old male by a filled square. The 50-year-old's CRT is faster (lower time) than the average for her age group; indeed, her CRT is identical to the average CRT of women who are 30 years old. Thus, according to her CRT, she is biologically younger than her age cohort. Conversely, the 60-year-old male's CRT is slower (higher time) than the average for his cohort. His CRT is equivalent to the average for 80-year-olds; thus, on this CRT variable, he is biologically older than his age group.

Biological age scores can be calculated for any variable by correlating the scores of the subjects with their ages. This procedure produces an equation that describes the linear relationship between age and the variable for all subjects in the group as a whole:

$$Y = a + bX$$

where Y = the predicted scores, a = a constant representing the magnitude of the scores, b = the change in variable scores with the change in age, and X = the age of an individual subject.

Using the correlation be-tween performance and age, we can determine an individual's biological age on a particular variable by substituting the individual's age for X in the equation and predicting Y. Then the individual's actual score on the variable is subtracted from the predicted score, yielding the biological age score. Thus, biological age can be determined for many variables.

Scores on tests are converted to standard scores for comparative purposes so that distributions of scores from several tests will have the same standardized means and standard deviations. (Statistically, this also eliminates the need for the constant in the equation.) The scores are transformed further so that for all variables, scores above the mean represent being biologically older (i.e., exhibiting poorer function) and scores below the mean represent better or younger function or performance. If an individual's score on a variable is exactly the same as the average for his or her age group, the predicted score also would be the same and that individual's biological age would be 0, or the same as his or her age group. Individuals of

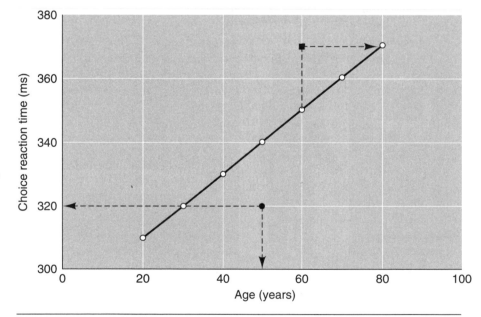

Figure 2.8 The calculation of biological age scores from the correlation between age and choice reaction time. The diagonal line represents the correlation between age and choice reaction time. Individuals whose scores are above the line, that is, higher than the average for their age group, have a higher (older) biological age. Individuals whose scores are lower than the average for their age group have lower (younger) biological ages.

vastly different ages—even 20-year-olds and 60-year-olds—can have the same biological age on a variable, because the biological score is a measure only of their performance relative to the mean of their own age groups. That is, biological age calculated in this way is a measure of an individual's aging status relative to his or her cohort age group. It is not a measure of the rate of aging of a person on that variable.

Animal research, however, has also provided persuasive evidence that chronological and biological aging can be very different. In addition to showing that same-aged animals lose abilities differentially, many investigators have shown that biological age can be manipulated by caloric restriction, by regulating glucocorticoid function, and by administering certain molecular compounds (Collier & Coleman, 1991). These three types of manipulation have resulted in rats achieving substantially longer life spans. The entire volume (54A) of the *Journal of Gerontology: Biological Sciences* (1999) consists of research articles that chronicle the progress of science in identifying biomarkers.

Limitations of the Biological Age Concept

The biomarker concept is now accepted by a large majority of the scientific and policy-making communities, but not by all (Sprott, 1999). When individuals appear as healthy as people half their age, or when their performance scores on physical fitness, strength, or reaction time tests are better than those of much younger people, it is tempting to say, "He has the body of a man half his age," or "That 60-year-old woman can run as fast as most women half her age. She has the legs of a 30-year-old!" But several objections have been raised against both this type of metaphoric explanation and the underlying assumptions of the concept of measuring biological age.

First, theories of biological age, especially those that suggest the existence of a single biological age score, assume the existence of a general aging factor, that is, a uniform rate of aging across different systems. Almost all gerontology researchers have abandoned hope of finding a single biomarker. Thus, extending the metaphor used previously, the tacit assumption would be that a woman who has the legs of a person half her age would also have the kidneys and brain of a person half her age. Yet, the research evidence discussed at the beginning of this chapter does not support the existence of a single aging process. Shock's (1967) classic work (figure 2.3, p. 35) exemplified this, and the fact that aging occurs at different rates in different systems has been

confirmed many times. Costa and McCrae (1980) analyzed changes in several anthropometric and laboratory variables over 5- and 10-year periods and found no evidence for a single aging factor. Also, if there were a unitary biological rate of aging, the correlations among physiological function and test performances should be higher with each other than they are with chronological age. Yet, this pattern of correlation among functions does not occur. In most test batteries for humans, age correlates more highly with each item than the items do with each other.

Second, the metaphor of a 60-year-old man with the heart of a 30-year-old implies that such a man could live as many more years as a 30-year-old. That is, with the average biological limit for life span (discussed in chapter 1) at 85 years, this 60-year-old could expect to live 55 more years. This would make him (and all others at his biological age) 115 years old at his death, almost surpassing the world record of human longevity. This prospect is highly unlikely.

Third, most critics of multiple regression research on biological age find it ironic that researchers use test batteries composed of attributes and performances because they are dissatisfied with chronological age as a marker of biological age. Yet, these researchers base the validity of their biomarkers on the correlation of these markers to chronological age!

Finally, people who are biologically younger than their peers should age at a slower rate on tests of functional capacities measured over time, but Costa and McCrae (1985) suggested that the individual differences seen in an age group are more likely attributable to differences in initial levels, the presence or absence of illness, or measurement error than to a hypothetical rate-of-aging factor. Costa and McCrae suggested that, rather than postulating a single, unicausal process of aging, researchers should emphasize the interacting influences of biological processes, social forces, and health behaviors of individuals.

One way that researchers have addressed these criticisms is by foregoing attempts to determine a unitary measure of biological age and, instead, designing biological age test batteries to determine the biological age of a system by testing several organs and systems. Multimeasure scores are thought to be more predictive because they are more likely to represent higher order function. An example of a test battery to assess the rate of aging of brain function might include tests of memory, processing speed, attention, executive function, and sensorimotor processing. The biological age scores of individuals at different ages are compared and analyzed collectively, because the scores are all calculated as scores relative to the mean of their age groups. Similarly, the biological age scores of all variables can be analyzed simultaneously, because the biological age scores are derived from standard scores.

Those who design biological age test batteries establish criteria for selection to determine which variables should be included in the test batteries. For example, the following criteria were used by Borkan and Norris (1980):

1. The variables should show a clear directional trend (either positive or negative in slope) during adulthood that is evident in both cross-sectional and longitudinal data.

2. A cross-sectional score on a particular parameter should primarily be the result of change over time rather than genetic endowment, measurement error, or daily or short-term fluctuation.

3. The variables selected should cover a wide range of physical functions and not be restricted only to known deleterious aspects of aging (Borkan & Norris, 1980, p. 178).

In some of the biological age profile approaches, statistical techniques have been used to determine how highly each variable in the test battery is correlated with age. Stones and Kozma (1988) proposed a tech-

nique for computing biological age in which the relative contribution of each variable to biological age is estimated statistically. Similarly, Chodzko-Zajko and Ringle (1989) used a statistical technique to weight the variables in their Index of Physiological Status.

Borkan and Norris (1980) extended the notion of a biological age by developing a biological age profile for individuals. A biological age score for each variable in their battery was determined for each subject, and a biological age profile was established. An example of the biological age profile for one of their male subjects is shown in figure 2.9. The standard biological age score of 0.0 represents a score for this individual that is exactly the same as his age group. (Recall that biological age is derived by subtracting an individual's measured score from the score predicted for him from the group equation.) His biological age on six variables (maximum breathing capacity (MBC), systolic and diastolic blood pressure, hemoglobin count, globulin, auditory threshold, and visual acuity) is almost exactly 0.0 on the y-axis, meaning that his function on these variables is at the average for his age group. All variables for which his biological age is older than that of his age cohort appear as points above the line, and variables on which he has a younger biological age score appear below the line. In this example, his status relative to his

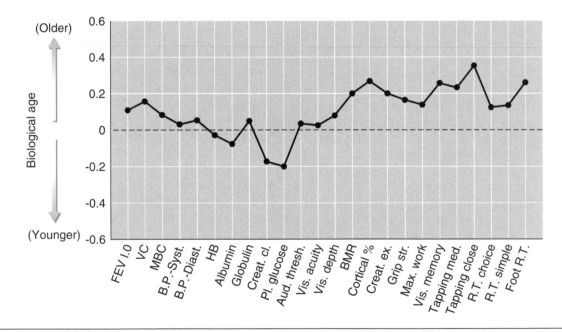

Figure 2.9 Biological age profile of a single individual. This profile demonstrates that an individual may be biologically older on some parameters than others. FEV 1.0 = forced expiratory volume in 1 s, VC = vital capacity, B.P. Syst = systolic blood pressure, B.P. Diast = diastolic blood pressure, HB = hemoglobin, Creat. cl. = creatine clearance, Pl. glucose = plasma glucose, Aud. thresh. = auditory threshold, Vis. = visual, BMR = basal metabolic rate, Creat. ex. = creatine excretion, str. = strength, max. = maximum, R.T. = reaction time.

Reprinted, by permission, from G.A. Borkan and A.H. Norris, 1980, "Assessment of biological age using a profile of physical parameters," *Journal of Gerontology* 35: 180.

peers is considerably younger for two variables, creatinine clearance and plasma glucose, but he seems to be considerably older on 11 other variables, particularly those that represent neuromuscular and central nervous system function. Borkan and Norris (1980) hoped to account for the discrepancy in system aging rates by using this profile strategy.

One way to validate the use of biological age scores as biomarkers would be to obtain scores on the variables of the biological age test battery, wait several years, and then compare the biological age scores of those subjects who were deceased with those who survived. If the concept of biological age is valid and if the biological age test battery scores reliably measure biological age, then those who had younger biological age profiles could be expected to live longer than subjects whose biological age profiles were older than those of their age group. This was the strategy used by Botwinick and colleagues (1978). They began their study by developing a potential biological age battery composed of psychological variables, such as demographic factors; cognitive, perceptual, and psychomotor abilities; personality and morale factors; and health and social activities. One of their analyses revealed that, taken together, eight of the performance measures correctly

classified 71% of the living subjects and 64% of the deceased. None of the variables had any predictive value when used as a single predictor.

The Borkan and Norris (1980) biological age test battery included only tests of physiological and neuromotor function and excluded assessments of personality factors. They also used deceased-survivor status as a criterion, and their efforts to predict whether subjects were in the deceased or survivor group appear in figure 2.10. The deceased group's biological age scores were significantly greater on nine of the test battery variables (shown by an asterisk on the graph). Their biological age scores were especially higher on systolic blood pressure and ventilation, measures of blood proteins (serum albumin and globulin), and four behavioral measures of central nervous system function (two speed-tapping and two reaction time tasks). The five variables on which the group was biologically younger did not statistically differ from the average. Thus, the ability of 9 of the 24 variables to differentiate significantly survivors from decedents supports the concept of biological age and suggests that these nine variables operating together may have some clinical usefulness for determining aging. These nine variables also seem intuitively useful as biological

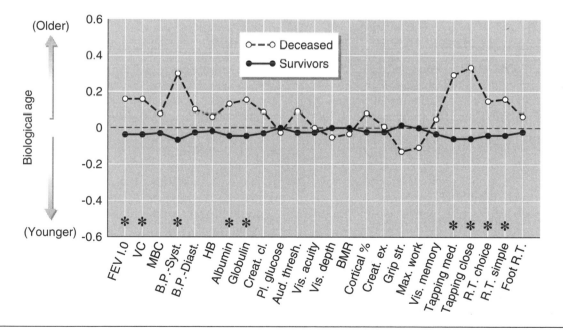

Figure 2.10 Biological age profile comparison of deceased and surviving study participants. Dashed line represents mean biological age scores of 166 men who died since being measured in the Baltimore Longitudinal Study on Aging. Solid line represents mean scores for all other participants (n = 922) who were alive in 1977. Parameters marked with an asterisk represent significantly different mean scores. FEV 1.0 = forced expiratory volume in 1 s, VC = vital capacity, B.P. Syst = systolic blood pressure, B.P. Diast = diastolic blood pressure, HB = hemoglobin, Creat. cl. = creatine clearance, Pl. = plasma, Aud. thresh. = auditory threshold, Vis. = visual, BMR = basal metabolic rate, Creat. ex. = creatine excretion, str. = strength, max. = maximum, R.T. = reaction time.

From "Assessment of biological age using a profile of physical parameters," by G.A. Borkan and A.H. Norris, 1980, *Journal of Gerontology*, 35, p. 181. Copyright 1980 by The Gerontological Society of America. Reprinted by permission.

age scores, because other researchers have found them to be interdependent (see chapter 9).

Webster and Logie (1976) took the opposite approach and found that a group of exceptionally healthy women had lower predicted biological ages than a group of women rated merely average in health. Webster and Logie's biological age test battery included chronological age and several physiological variables.

The biological age batteries developed for humans to date have not improved much on chronological age as a descriptor of the aging process, nor can they successfully predict aging rate. No unitary biomarker has been identified that can predict aging of individuals across several physiological and psychological systems. Nevertheless, biological age test scores have been successful in distinguishing groups that seem to age at different rates. Genetic research also is following lines of inquiry that may lead to the discovery of some causal factors for aging. Because there has been some limited success, and progeria (a disease characterized by acutely accelerated aging) and genetic research seem promising, it is likely that researchers will continue to search for multimeasure human biomarkers that will describe aging and predict the rate of aging.

Importance of Individual Differences in Understanding Aging Research

Aging is a very personal, individualized process, and averages of function and behavior for different chronological age groups are just that—averages. As pointed out in figure 2.1 (p. 32), averages do not accurately estimate the capacities of many individuals. Nevertheless, comparisons of the function and performance of individuals serve many important purposes in biological, psychological, and social sciences. Professionals such as nurses, psychologists, physical therapists, social workers, and health promotion specialists need estimates of abilities of various age groups in order to maximize their services. Consequently, a great many average values of function and performance for different chronological ages are available in the literature, and these will be discussed throughout this book. Average values provide an idea of the capacities of a large number of people at a given age, but the student of aging and the professional should interpret all of these from within the framework of individual differences.

SUMMARY

Aging is a highly individual process, with individuals aging at rates that may be very different than the rates of others at the same chronological age. Indeed, individual differences are just as much a hallmark of aging as age-related decline in function. Individual differences are measured by calculating the standard deviation of the individuals within the group of people measured. Individual differences also can be displayed graphically and analyzed as a cumulative frequency distribution.

The many sources of individual differences include genetic differences, disease, and different rates of aging of physiological and biological systems within individuals. Variations in lifestyle and compensatory behaviors of older adults also create differences. Other sources are gender, culture, education, and socioeconomic status.

Time-related changes in function and performance follow different patterns: no change (stability), disease-related change, steady decline in function, precipitous expression of disease, compensatory change, and cultural changes. This diversity of ways that change can occur (or not occur) within and among individuals increases individual differences.

The research designs used to study aging and the research process itself sometimes magnify individual differences. Then, too, older people are less consistent in their performance than younger people, which means more differences in older groups than in younger groups.

Biological age has been used as a descriptor to explain the individual differences seen on variables within chronological age groups. Biological age is defined statistically as the distance of an individual from the mean of the chronological age cohort. It has been calculated as a value derived from the linear relationship between the scores on a variable and the age of the subjects. Individuals whose scores on a variable are higher than the average of their age group are described as older for their age than those whose scores fall below the average. Biological age test batteries have been used to develop profiles of aging on variables known to be related to chronological age. These test batteries and profiles have been used successfully in a few studies to predict longevity and the presence of health risk factors.

Although the evidence from animal research supporting the concept of biological age is compelling, it is not without its critics when used in the context of human age. The notion of biological age assumes an underlying general age factor, which has not been supported by research on humans. The fact that different systems age at different rates in different people leads many scientists to believe that the notion of a unicausal mechanism controlling the rate of aging is too simplistic and that it will be many years before the mechanisms of aging are discovered.

REVIEW QUESTIONS

1. How does genotype influence individual differences? What environmental factors interact with genotypes to influence behavior?

2. Volunteers 70 to 85 years old were recruited in a middle- to high-income neighborhood by an advertisement in a senior activity center newsletter to be subjects in a study of the effects of health promotion classes on self-reported health indicators and psychological well-being. Young adults 20 to 30 were recruited from a church congregation in the same neighborhood. Considering the research process by which these subjects were obtained and the type of questionnaire that they were likely to have completed, how representative of 70- to 85- and 20- to 30-year-olds would you consider this sample to be? What factors other than chronological age might influence the findings of this study?

3. The differences in physical function among adults in their 70s and 80s are in general greater than those in their 40s and 50s. Some in the older decades are totally physically dependent, and a few can play tennis, hang glide, or complete a marathon. Other than chronological aging, what factors contribute to these differences in physical function?

4. If a biological age marker could be identified, of what value would it be? Why are so many scientists pursuing the concept of biomarkers?

SUGGESTED READINGS

Cromie, W.J. (1998). Why women live longer than men. *Harvard University Gazette*. October. Available: http://www.news.harvard.edu/gazette/1998/10.01/WhyWomenLiveLon.html [05.29.04]

Sprott, R.L. (1999). Biomarkers of aging. *Journal of Gerontology: Biological Sciences, 54A*, B464-B465.

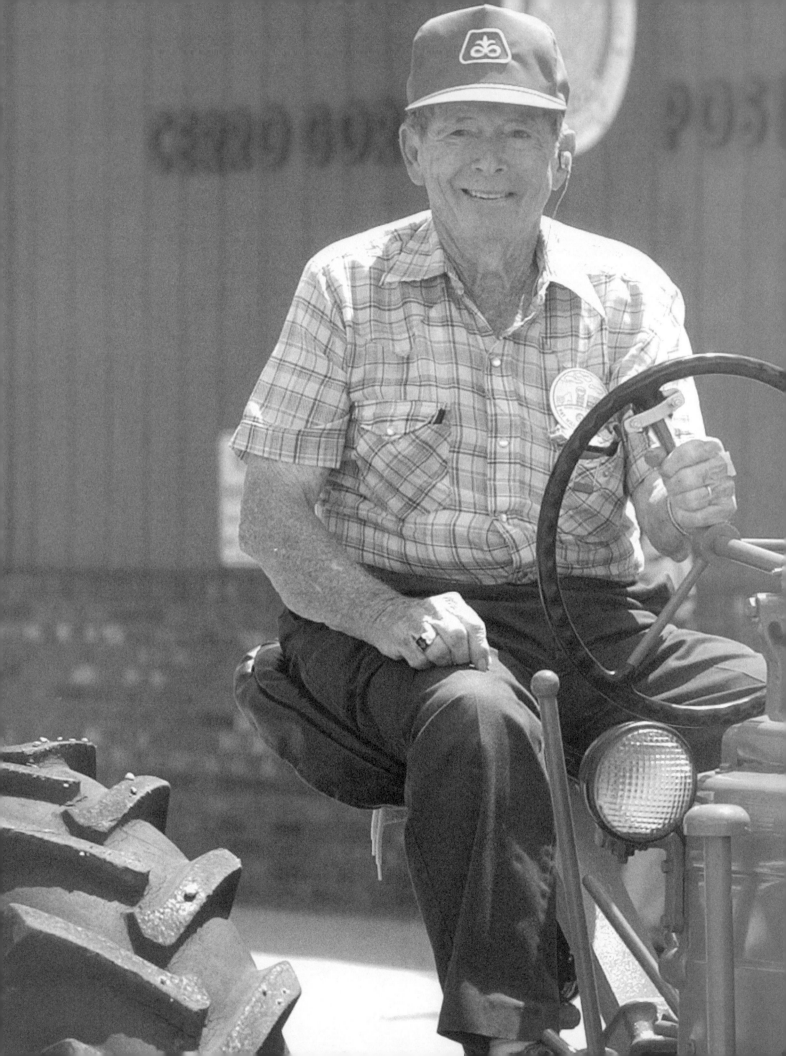

PART II

Physical Changes in Structure, Capacity, and Endurance

Physical Development and Decline

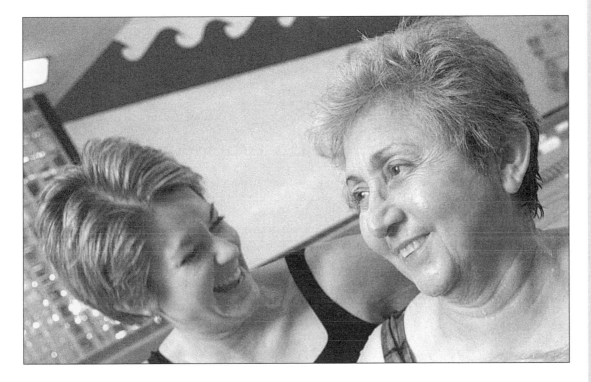

The objectives of this chapter are

- to summarize changes in height, weight, and body mass index across the life span and discuss factors that affect these changes;

- to identify the major changes in body composition in older adults and discuss factors that might modify these changes;

- to describe bone changes with aging and discuss factors that affect bone health;

- to summarize joint changes with normal aging and osteoarthritis and the effects of exercise on joint structure and function; and

- to describe changes in skin with aging and what can be done to slow the aging effects.

When a baby is born, one of the first things that people ask is, "How much does he weigh?" or "How long is she?" As the child grows, family and friends mark the progression with measurements of height and weight. One of Norman Rockwell's wonderful covers for the *Saturday Evening Post* showed a father's annual ritual of recording his son's growth by adding a pencil mark on the wall. Throughout the growth and development phase of life, the various changes of size are important and are often recorded. At maturity, except for some concerns about increases in body weight, social interest in changes in physical dimensions decreases. But although physical dimensions may not be measured and publicly recorded or announced, the age-related changes in body dimensions and composition do not stop. For most people, height and weight continue to change with increasing age. Body composition, primarily the composition of bone, fat, and muscle, also changes both absolutely and relatively. The range of motion of the joints is also affected by time and disuse. The skin undergoes profound age-related changes. This chapter describes the age-related changes that occur in these basic physical components of the body, discusses some of the pathologies that interact with aging, and illustrates the role that physical activity plays in these age-related changes.

Changes in Body Shape

The dimensions of the body are obtained by **anthropometry,** the branch of science dealing with the measurement of the human body. Height and weight are two of the most easily obtained anthropo-

metric measures, and therefore they have been used extensively in screening and monitoring programs. They are usually made in centimeters (2.54 cm = 1 in.) and in kilograms (1 kg = 2.2 lb). In addition to measures of height and weight, anthropometric dimensions include many breadths (e.g., the breadth of the hips), segment lengths (e.g., leg length), and circumferences (e.g., the circumference of the waist). These are often used to estimate the general shape and composition of the body.

Height

Height, also known as stature, is usually measured in centimeters (cm) or inches (in.) and refers to the distance from the floor to the top of the head without shoes. Height is distributed approximately normally (on a bell-shaped curve) at each age, except that the population has a few more tall than short people. Average heights and weights by age for American males and females are shown in figure 3.1. In males, height increases until about age 20 and declines slowly, with a loss of about 4% seen by the age of 70. Females reach their peak height somewhat sooner, between ages 16 to 18 years, and then their height gradually declines with a loss of about 3% by 70 years of age (Chandler & Bock, 1991; Frisancho, 1990).

In each of the eight cross-national comparison studies of community-dwelling older adults, 60 to 89 years of age, a decline in height was found in all three decades (60s, 70s, and 80s; Launer & Harris, 1996). Loss in mean height ranged from 1.9 to 6.7 cm across the 3 decades. Height measured longitudinally from 17 different Caucasian populations was remarkably consistent by gender in the age-specific rates of height

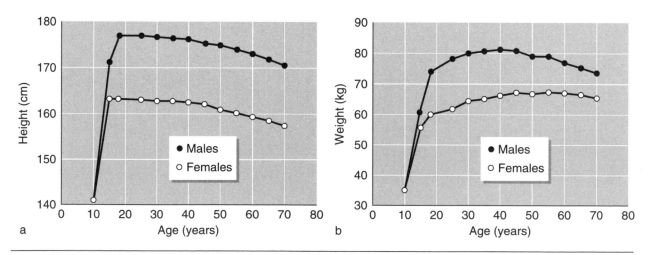

Figure 3.1 (a) Body height and (b) weight of males and females. Standard errors are so small that they are not visible in this figure.

Adapted from Frisancho (1990).

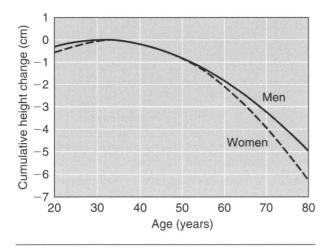

Figure 3.2 Cumulative height change in men and women from young adulthood to old age. The solid line represents a combination of the age-specific rates of height loss from 13 studies of men; the dashed line represents a combination of the age-specific rates obtained from 11 studies of women.

Reprinted, by permission from J.D. Sorkin, D.C. Miller, and R. Andres, 1999, "Longitudinal changes in the heights of men and women: Consequential effects on body mass index," *Epidemiologic Reviews* 21: 256.

loss (Sorkin et al., 1999). Height changed little in these populations until age 40, when both men and women exhibited a 1-cm loss per decade in height for the next 2 decades (figure 3.2). The change in height for women in their 60s and 70s was greater than for the men, averaging about 1.5 cm in the 60s and 2 cm during the 70s. The loss in height with age for both men and women is probably attributable to vertebral compression, changes in height and shape of the cartilaginous discs between the vertebrae, loss of muscle tone, and postural slump (World Health Organization, 1998b). The accelerated rate of loss in stature for older women, compared with men, could be attributable to hormonal, diet, weight, and physical activity differences as well as the fact that more women than men develop **osteoporosis,** a degenerative bone disease. Osteoporosis is discussed in more detail later in this chapter.

Height loss of about 1 cm per decade occurs during the 40s and 50s with accelerated height loss after age 60 in both genders but to a greater extent in women.

Weight

The topic of weight is always of interest to people, and the "ideal" weight for an individual is much debated. The U.S. Department of Agriculture (1995) suggested that the phrase "healthy weight" should replace the phrase "ideal weight," because what is "ideal" is more difficult to define and measure, whereas a "healthy weight," the weight that is associated with the lowest mortality and morbidity rates, is more clearly articulated. Ranges of healthy weights, based on an individual's height, are shown in table 3.1 (U.S. Department of Agriculture, 1995). Individuals with low muscle and bone mass should use the low end of the range, and individuals with high muscle and bone mass should use the high end. Deciding on a healthy weight for an individual is important, but the fact remains that the prevalence of obesity is on the rise around the world (Popkin & Dorak, 1998) and in the United States has increased dramatically in recent years.

Data from the National Health Examination Survey (NHES I) in the 1960s and the National Health and Nutrition Examination Surveys (NHANES) in the 1970s, 1980s, and 1990s included information on weight by age and gender. As seen in table 3.2, the prevalence of obesity, based on age- and gender-related prevalence, has increased for all ages from 1960 to 1994 and is higher in women than men. The increase in obesity in men, over this 34-year period, ranges from a 25% increase in 20- to 29-year-olds to a 115% increase in 50- to 59-year-olds. For women, the largest increase in obesity, 139%, occurred in 20- to 29-year-olds, with less increase in obesity seen in the older age groups.

The average body weight of American females continues to increase until 45 or 50 years of age, at which point it stabilizes until about age 70. Males follow a similar increasing weight pattern up to age 40, followed by a plateau until age 55 and then a slow, gradual decline in weight (figure 3.1; Frisancho, 1990). This pattern of weight loss at 65 or 70 years of age can be explained in three ways. One explanation is called "selective survival" and refers to the possibility that the obese young and middle-aged persons die prematurely and therefore what remains is a selection of individuals who have maintained their weight with age. A second possible explanation is called the "cohort effect," which means that the older people come from cohorts in which obesity was less common. Finally, there is the possibility that the loss of weight after age 65 is truly attributable to the aging process. Support for this final explanation is found in the fact that in indigenous, non-European populations, the increase in weight during middle age is not seen, but a decline at older ages still occurs (Launer & Harris, 1996).

Data for those more than 80 years of age were obtained only in NHANES III. In this old-old age group, there was a relatively low prevalence of obesity compared with younger ages. Two possible explanations

Table 3.1   1995 USDA Healthy Weight Ranges

Height (no shoes)	Frame (mm) (medium) Male	Female	Weight (lb) (without clothes) Range	Midpoint
4'10"		57-64	91-119	105
4'11"		57-64	94-124	109
5'00"		57-64	97-128	112.5
5'01"	64-73	57-64	101-132	116.5
5'02"	64-73	57-64	104-137	120.5
5'03"	67-73	60-67	107-141	124
5'04"	67-73	60-67	111-146	128.5
5'05"	67-73	60-67	114-150	132
5'06"	67-73	60-67	118-155	136.5
5'07"	70-76	60-67	121-160	140.5
5'08"	70-76	60-67	125-164	144.5
5'09"	70-76	60-67	129-169	149
5'10"	70-76	60-67	132-174	153
5'11"	70-79	64-70	136-179	157.5
6'00"	70-79	64-70	140-184	162
6'01"	70-79	64-70	144-189	166.5
6'02"	70-79	64-70	148-195	171.5
6'03"	73-83	64-70	152-200	176
6'04"	73-83		156-205	180.5
6'05"	73-83		160-211	185.5
6'06"	73-83		164-216	190

Note: Weight ranges are for men and women. People with low muscles and bone mass should use low end of weight range, and vice versa. For same size, values below the range are rated "small" and above "large."

Adapted from U.S. Department of Agriculture (1995).

adults (World Health Organization, 1998b). Morley (1996) reported that involuntary weight loss occurs in approximately 13% of those more than 65 years of age. When a precipitous loss in weight occurs, the loss is unexplainable in about 24% of cases, but other sudden losses have heralded the onset of cancer (16%), depression (18%), gastrointestinal ailments such as ulcers (11%), an overactive thyroid gland (9%), neurological problems (7%), and the effects of or responses to medications (9%) (Thompson & Morris, 1991). Therefore, the involuntary loss of weight in older adults should be closely monitored.

Although there is growing concern in the United States about obesity, particularly the increase in children and young adults in the last 20 years, the unusual or sudden loss of body weight in the elderly also is a cause for concern.

Body Mass Index

Measures of height and weight are frequently combined to yield a measure known as the body mass index (BMI). To calculate BMI, simply divide body weight in kilograms by height, in meters squared, to obtain BMI (kg/m^2). The higher the BMI, the more likely an adult is to have a high proportion of fat. However, in

are immediately apparent. One is the selective survival effect, and the other is that the loss of weight in the old-old age group may be attributable to the higher frequency of diseases in this group (Kotz et al., 1999).

Although there is growing concern in the United States about obesity, particularly the increase in children and young adults in the last 20 years, the unusual or sudden loss of body weight in the elderly also is a cause for concern. Involuntary loss of weight is the single best predictor for risk of death in older

young weight-trained individuals, greater muscle mass also could be associated with a high BMI. Higher BMIs are positively associated with increased incidence of cardiovascular disease, diabetes, hypercholesterolemia, hypertension, and certain cancers (American College of Sports Medicine, 1998).

Although BMI is not a direct measure of fatness, and it is not very sensitive to redistributions of fat, it can be used as a proxy for relative fatness and is a more accurate measure of total body fat than weight alone.

Table 3.2 Prevalence of Obesity Stratified by Age and Gender in the United States From 1960 Through 1994

Age (years)	NHES I, 1960-1962 (%)	NHANES I, 1971-1974 (%)	NHANES II, 1976-1980 (%)	NHANES III, 1988-1994 (%)
Men				
20-29	9.0	8.0	8.1	12.5
30-39	10.4	13.3	12.1	17.2
40-49	11.9	14.2	16.4	23.1
50-59	13.4	15.3	14.3	28.9
60-69	7.7	10.3	13.5	24.8
70-79	8.6	11.1	13.6	20.0
80+	NA	NA	NA	8.0
Women				
20-29	6.1	8.2	9.0	14.6
30-39	12.1	15.1	16.8	25.8
40-49	17.1	17.6	18.1	26.9
50-59	20.4	22.0	22.6	35.6
60-69	27.2	24.0	22.0	29.8
70-79	21.9	21.0	19.4	25.0
80+	NA	NA	NA	15.1

NA = not available; NHES = National Health Examination Survey; NHANES = National Health and Nutrition Examination Survey. Obesity defined as body mass index >30. Prevalence for ages 70-74 years.

Modified from K.M. Flegal, M.D. Carrol, R.J. Kuccnavski, et al.: Overweight and obesity in the United States: Prevalence and trends, 1960-1994. *Int. J. Obes. Relat. Metab. Disord.* 22: 39, 1998.

With worldwide rates of obesity increasing steadily, the National Institutes of Health (NIH) and the World Health Organization (WHO) recently adopted similar body weight guidelines for overweight and obesity that are based on BMI (table 3.3). Overweight is defined as a BMI of 25 to 29.9 kg/m², with those having a BMI of 30 or greater being classified as obese. Further subclassifications of obesity based on BMI include mild (30-34.9), moderate (35-39.9), and severe obesity (>40). Recent researchers have documented the presence of abdominal obesity as an additional indicator of morbidity and mortality, so further stratification based on waist circumference is seen in table 3.3. A large waist circumference was found to be a better predictor of all-cause mortality, at least in nonsmokers, than high BMI or a large waist–hip ratio (Seidell & Visscher, 2000). It is not only the additional fat that increases risk for disease but also the location of that additional fat on the body.

Table 3.3 Disease Risk Associated With Body Mass Index and Waist Circumference

Classification	BMI (kg/m²)	Disease risk relative to normal weight and waist circumference[a] Men ≤40 in. (101.6 cm) Women ≤35 in. (88.9 cm)	>40 in. >35 In.
Underweight	<18.5		
Normal (desirable)	18.5-24.9		
Overweight	25.0-29.9	Increased	High
Obesity			
I Mild	30.0-34.9	High	Very high
II Moderate	35.0-39.9	Very high	Very high
III Severe	≥40	Extremely high	Extremely high

[a]Disease risk for type 2 diabetes, hypertension, and cardiovascular disease.

Modified from U.S. Department of Health and Human Services (1998).

www.nhlbi.nih.gov

Cross-sectional normative data on measures of body composition by decade, including total body weight, muscle mass and fat mass, for males and females in the Baltimore Longitudinal Study of Aging are shown in figure 3.3 (Muller et al., 1996). Muscle mass was computed as a function of urinary creatinine excretion to height ratio and fat mass was estimated from skinfold measurements. A sedentary lifestyle and easy access to high calorie foods explain much of the increase in body weight and adiposity, as shown by BMI or % body fat, in both men and women up through middle age. This increase in body fatness puts individuals at risk for diseases such as hypertension, cardiovascular disease, diabetes, some forms of cancer, and osteoarthritis (American College of Sports Medicine, 1998). In men, there is a decrease in body weight after the fifth decade and this is primarily due to a decrease in muscle mass. However, in very old men, those in their eighties and nineties, both muscle and fat mass decrease thus resulting in a large decrease in body weight. Women increased

body weight through the sixth decade, primarily to a continuous increase in fat mass, and the fluctuations in fat mass are the major influence on body weight, though muscle mass does continue to decline.

> Both men and women lose muscle mass after 25 years of age but also put on fat during the next 3 decades, so there is little change in BMI.

The relationship between BMI and mortality was examined in an extremely large prospective study of more than 1 million adults in the United States who were followed for 14 years (Calle et al., 1999). Men and women who never smoked and were disease free at the study's start experienced the greatest health risk from excess weight (figure 3.4). In healthy people, the lowest point of the curve for BMI and mortality occurred between a BMI of 23.5 and 24.9 for men and 23.0 and 23.4 for women, with a gradient of increasing risk associated with moderate overweight. White men and women in the highest BMI (>40) had

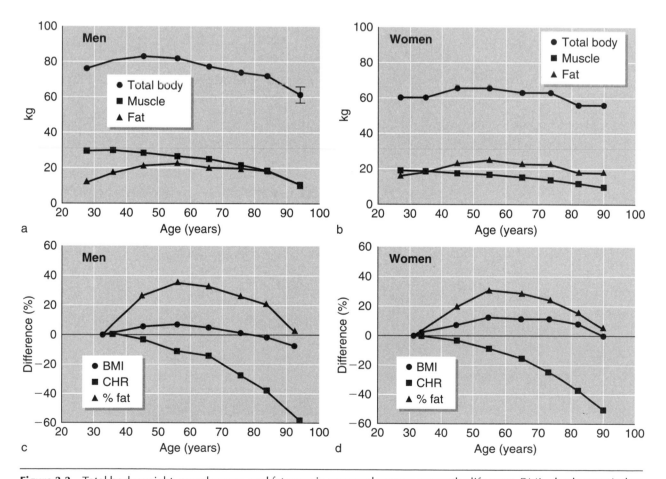

Figure 3.3 Total body weight, muscle mass, and fat mass in men and women across the life span. BMI = body mass index; CHR = ratio of creatine excretion to height, which is a measure of muscle mass.

Reprinted from *Seminars in Nephrology*, Vol. 16, D.C. Muller et al., The effect of age on insulin resistance and secretion: A review, pgs. 289-298, Copyright 1996, with permission from Elsevier.

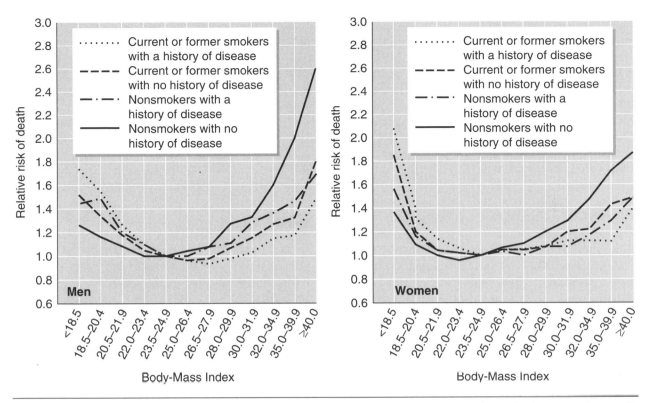

Figure 3.4 Multivariate relative risk of death from all causes among men and women according to body mass index, smoking status, and disease status. The four subgroups are mutually exclusive. Nonsmokers had never smoked. The reference category was made up of subjects with a body mass index of 23.5 to 24.9.

Reprinted, by permission, from E.E. Calle et al., 1999, "Body-mass index and mortality in a perspective cohort of U.S. adults," *The New England Journal of Medicine* 341: 1097-1105. Copyright © 1999, Massachusetts Medical Society. All rights reserved.

a relative death risk equal to 2.58 (men) and 2.00 (women), compared with counterparts with a BMI of 23.5 to 24.9 (relative risk of 1.0). Although the shape of the curves was similar for all groups, with the lowest relative risk of death seen for those with BMI between 22 and 26, the risk of death increases for underweight and overweight individuals, particularly current smokers. This is probably because the risk of illness and death cannot be separated from the effect of smoking and disease on BMI.

BMIs are often measured in large population studies because of the simplicity of measurement and calculation and the low cost. BMI also has an advantage over relative weight, such as that used for the Metropolitan Life Insurance tables, because those tables were developed primarily from white, higher socioeconomic status populations and have not been altered to reflect body fat content accurately in the public at large. However, the BMI has some limitations in classifying individuals into categories of normal, overweight, or obese, particularly in older adults. For example, BMI overestimates body fat in persons who are very muscular, can underestimate body fat in persons who have lost muscle mass

(older adults) or in persons with edema, and can be inaccurate in very short persons (<5 ft [152 cm]). Gallagher and colleagues (2000) developed provisional equations and tables for linking current BMI guidelines with predicted percentage body fat. They reported greater fatness in older adults, even after controlling for BMI. An important and unanswered question is whether greater fatness in older adults poses additional health risks.

Changes in Body Composition

Determining age-related developmental changes in body size (i.e., height and weight) or weight relative to height (BMI) is inadequate for understanding the actual changes that occur, because the body is composed of many different tissues. Adults may have the same weight and height but have very different body compositions. One person may be very muscular and lean with a substantial percentage of the weight coming from metabolically active muscle tissue, whereas another may be very sedentary and pudgy with a large percentage of the weight accounted for by inert fat tissue. Even within individuals, changes in body composition occur over time with changes in nutrition, physical activity, and aging. A 40-year-old former athlete may actually weigh less than she did when she competed as a youth but, because of inactivity and 20 years of aging, may wear a skirt size larger than the one she wore in earlier years. She has traded muscle, which weighs more but is more compact, for fat, which weighs less but takes up more space.

Body weight is a general descriptor of an individual's total body mass, whereas body composition includes information on various components. The body, most often, is partitioned into two distinct compartments: **fat mass** and **fat-free mass** (McArdle et al., 2001). Fat mass (FM) plus fat-free mass (FFM), which is made up of water, protein, and bone mineral, equals total body mass. Many techniques are available to estimate FM and FFM, but all involve indirectly measuring either FM or FFM and deriving the other by subtraction. More specific descriptions of body fat, such as isolating internal abdominal or visceral fat from subcutaneous, appendicular, or truncal fat, can be made by more sophisticated and expensive laboratory instrumentation. Women and men differ significantly in relative quantities of specific body composition components in that the reference man is taller and heavier, his skeleton weight is greater, and he possesses a larger muscle mass and lower body fat content than the reference woman (table 3.4; McArdle et al., 2001).

Changes in body composition with aging have been increasingly recognized as a potentially modifiable factor in the quest for optimal health, function, and longevity. Although body composition, as well as the age-related changes in it, has a strong genetic component, it is also influenced by environmental factors. The primary influences are diet, disease, and physical activity. For example, failure to consume sufficient calories and protein in the diet can limit the development of muscle tissue or negatively influence the maintenance of muscle tissue, and failure to have adequate calcium in the diet has a major negative impact on bone formation and remodeling. Diseases such as osteoporosis drastically affect bone, and it has been well established that consistent, daily physical activity of a moderate intensity plays an important role in promoting bone health, maintaining muscle mass, and reducing the accumulation of body fat.

Age-related changes in body composition have important implications for successful aging. Such changes alter the pharmacokinetic and pharmaco-

dynamic properties of drugs, so that dosages and schedules that are appropriate for young individuals are not appropriate for older adults. Because changes in body composition are related to disease and function, it is useful to monitor changes. For a variety of reasons, older adults eat less as they age, and it is easy for them to become undernourished. Careful monitoring of BMI and body composition can prevent malnutrition and simultaneously provide information about the effectiveness of maintenance, reduction, and weight gain programs.

Body Fat

Body fat generally has negative implications in the United States because so many people have more of it than they wish, and they are constantly bombarded by media messages that emphasize these negative aspects. Diets and other schemes to lose fat are a way of life for millions of people. But a certain level of fat is necessary for normal function. Fat is a source of energy, a storage site for some vitamins, and a necessary component of cell membrane integrity. Fat provides padding, cushions shocks, serves as packing or filler around structures, and acts as an insulator to slow heat loss. Of course, the insulating property of fat is a negative factor when the environment is hot and the dissipation of body heat is desirable.

Body fat is of two types: essential fat, which is necessary for normal function of the central nervous system and other organs of the body, and storage fat, which is fat stored in adipose tissue. The reference woman has considerably more total fat than

Table 3.4 **Body Composition for a Young Reference Man and Woman**

	Man	Woman
Age (years)	20-24	20-24
Stature (cm)	174	164
Mass (kg)	70	57
Fat-free mass (%)	85	73
Muscle (%)	45	36
Bone (%)	15	12
Remainder (%)	20	25
Total body fat (%)	15	27
% storage fat	12	15
% essential fat	3	12

Reprinted, by permission, from W.D. McArdle, R.I. Katch, and V.L. Katch, 2001, *Exercise physiology: Energy, nutrition, and human performance* (Philadelphia, PA: Lippincott, Williams, and Wilkins).

the reference man because more fat is needed for specific functions that are related to reproduction. Consequently, percent body fat norms are different for men and women (table 3.4).

Body Fat Measurements

Estimates of body fat can be grouped into field (clinical) and laboratory measurements. In clinical situations, skinfold measurements, made with calipers, are most often used to predict body fatness and are reasonably accurate if the clinician is well trained. The skinfold measurement is made of the thickness of a double fold of skin, along with the adipose tissue that lies immediately beneath it, at critical sites such as above the front of the hip, the abdomen, the upper thigh, below the shoulder blade, and the back of the upper arm. When performed correctly, skinfold measures provide an estimate of percent body fat that has a high correlation with other more expensive measures of body fat such as underwater weighing and dual-energy X-ray absorptiometry (DEXA; Nieman, 2003). However, the regression equations for predicting percent body fat from skinfold measures are population specific, and few of the studies that developed the equations included adults over the age of 65 years. Therefore, using skinfolds to measure body fat in older adults, even with skilled clinicians, may not be as accurate as in younger adults.

Several laboratory procedures are available for determining body fat. They include hydrodensitometry, air plethysmography, bioimpedance, DEXA, computed tomography, and magnetic resonance imaging. The most widely used laboratory procedure for measuring body density is hydrodensitometry (underwater weighing). Densitometry is considered the "gold standard" for estimating body composition and is used to determine the validity of clinical measures such as skinfolds. A relatively new laboratory technique used to measure body volume through air displacement, rather than water displacement, is the air plethysmograph, referred to as the BOD POD Body Composition System (Life Measurement, Inc., Concord, CA). The BOD POD uses the same two-component model as underwater weighing but is based on air displacement rather than water displacement. The majority of studies have shown that air displacement plethysmography is an accurate and suitable alternative to underwater weighing (Fields et al., 2002). This method has several advantages over hydrostatic weighing in that it is quick (about 5 min), is relatively simple to operate, and can accommodate special populations such as

children, older adults, obese persons, and disabled persons, because the physical demands and the instructions are minimal.

Another recent technique, bioelectrical impedance analysis (BIA), passes a harmless 50-kHz current (800 µA maximum) through a person and measures the resistance to electrical current; different tissues, such as fat, have a greater electrical impedance than fat-free mass. Several sources of measurement error are possible with the BIA method including differences in BIA analyzers from different companies and the client's state of hydration, which is of particular importance in older adults. When these sources of error are controlled, the BIA method has similar accuracy to the skinfold method but may be preferred with older adults because it does not require a high degree of technician skill and it is more comfortable and less intrusive.

The advent of DEXA in the late 1980s created much excitement among body composition researchers because this method allows simultaneous measurement of three components of the body (fat, bone mineral, and nonbone lean tissue). DEXA is safe (involves a low dose of radiation), is quick (10-20 min), and requires little cooperation from the subject, making studies of children, older adults, and individuals with disease much easier than other methods. Most researchers have concluded that DEXA is a precise method and correlates highly with results from underwater weighing. The major limitations of DEXA include the high cost of the equipment and the fact that the models on which the equations are based assume constant hydration in fat free soft tissues.

Although available for more than 25 years, computed tomography (CT) was only minimally applied in body composition research because of expense and radiation exposure. The introduction of magnetic resonance imaging (MRI), and the technical refinements to CT that followed, however, led to the widespread use of these methods in assessing body composition. Both CT and MRI produce cross-sectional images of different tissue components at predetermined anatomic locations. MRI uses extremely high magnetic fields and radio waves to translate the differential energy released from tissues into colorful images. It is particularly useful for differentiating between soft tissues of the body, such as muscle and fat. Both the CT and MRI imaging methods are based on mechanistic models that have no known age dependence and are the most fully accepted methods of estimating the important visceral adipose tissue compartment (Heymsfield et al., 2000). This means that CT and MRI techniques are used for determining intra-abdominal fat, which is now thought to be more related to health than total amount of body fat.

> The measurement of skinfolds is the most often used clinical measure for determining body fat, whereas DEXA is a widely accepted laboratory measure that determines amount of bone, nonbone lean tissue, and body fat.

Body Fat Distribution

Recent research indicates that where excess fat is deposited may be even more important for predicting morbidity and mortality than increased body fatness per se. People who have more of their fat deposited in abdominal areas rather than the hip and thigh areas (centralized adiposity) are at increased risk for cardiovascular disease, diabetes, high blood pressure, stroke, arthritis, sleep apnea, and mobility impairments (Fiatarone Singh, 1998). On average, males and females differ in the way they store fat, and these differences begin early in life (Baumgartner et al., 1986). At about 9 years of age, boys begin to deposit more fat in the abdomen (centripetal fat pattern), whereas girls begin to deposit more fat in the hips and legs (Durnin & Womersley, 1974; Malina & Bouchard, 1991). These two gender-differentiated patterns, which become more pronounced with puberty and maturation, are called the android (male) and the gynoid (female) fat patterns. Men depicting the typical android pattern are sometimes described as apple-shaped, because their fat is primarily stored on the trunk, chest, back, and abdomen, whereas women depicting the gynoid pattern are described as pear-shaped and are characterized by greater fat deposition on the hips and legs (Bray, 1985; Kissebah et al., 1989; Gillum, 1987). These different fat patterns can be differentiated by measuring the ratio of waist-to-hip circumference or by the waist circumference by itself (Kotz et al., 1999). Waist-to-hip ratios that exceed 0.8 for women and 0.95 for men are related to increased risk of death, even after one adjusts for BMI (Despres, 1997). As shown earlier (table 3.3, p. 59), overweight individuals who also have a waist circumference of 40 in. (102 cm) for men or 35 in. (89 cm) for women have increased risk for all-cause mortality (U.S. Department of Health and Human Services, 1998). It appears that fat cells in the abdominal area tend to be more active (releasing and taking up fat molecules) than those in the gluteal and femoral areas. Therefore, when the supply of abdominal fat is too great, the cells release their fat into the vessels that supply blood to the liver. Fat that travels to the liver is linked to negative health consequences (Rebuffé-Scrive et al., 1990). Abdominal

fat deposition, as measured by CT or MRI, is a better predictor of health risk than is the waist-to-hip ratio (Kotz et al., 1999).

> Increased deposition of fat in the abdomen is associated with increased mortality and morbidity.

Fat Mass Changes With Age

Increasing body fat and decreasing muscle mass (sarcopenia) are both hallmarks of the aging process (Evans & Campbell, 1993). However, most of our knowledge regarding age-related patterns of changes in body composition is derived from cross-sectional studies, and few of these include adults over 60 years of age. Most researchers have documented increases in body weight and fat mass (FM) throughout middle age, with body fatness stabilizing or declining after 60 years of age. Obesity is a major public health problem in the general population, particularly because it has doubled in the past 30 years, but weight loss in older adults appears to have more detrimental effects on health and physical function than does an equivalent amount of weight gain (Hughes et al., 2002). Longitudinal studies of body composition in men over age 60 have consistently found a greater loss of FM than FFM, but there are few data on women and so a consistent pattern cannot be described. In a recent longitudinal study, 73 women and 53 men (average age 60 years) increased their fat mass 7.5% over 10 years (Hughes et al., 2002). However, women who were premenopausal at baseline gained significantly more weight and fat mass over the 10 years compared with the women who were postmenopausal at baseline. No age-related effect was observed in men.

Not only does percent body fat increase with age, it is slowly and progressively redistributed. In older adults, intra-abdominal fat tends to increase and subcutaneous fat on the limbs tends to decrease (World Health Organization, 1998). Younger women have lower intra-abdominal fat than younger men, but with age the intra-abdominal fat increases until absolute amounts of intra-abdominal fat are similar between men and women in their 7th decade (Hunter et al., 1996; Hunter et al., 1997). The accumulation of intra-abdominal fat begins in the late 20s and continues through the 60s, but about 40% of the increase in intra-abdominal fat occurs by the 5th decade (Schwartz et al., 1990). Abdominal obesity increases cardiovascular disease risk and is thought to be the first step in a series of events that leads to insulin resistance, glucose intolerance, abnormal lipoprotein–lipid profiles, and hypertension. This constellation of risk factors is sometimes called the metabolic syndrome (Muller et al., 1996).

Fat-Free Mass Changes With Age

Fat-free mass (FFM) includes nonfat components of the body: muscle, skin, bone, and organs. FFM is most often estimated by subtracting FM from the total body mass, but FFM of specific components of the body also can be estimated. The FFM of organs can be measured by imaging techniques, such as MRI and DEXA (discussed earlier). DEXA is a particularly good measurement tool for body composition because it simultaneously measures body fat, bone mineral, and nonbone lean tissues (Nieman, 2003). Another term often used interchangeably with FFM is lean body mass (LBM), which includes essential fat in addition to FFM, but FFM is the term used in this book. *Sarcopenia*, a word coined from the Greek meaning "flesh loss," refers to the age-related decline in muscle mass. Sarcopenia poses significant health risks for older adults, including impairment in maximal aerobic capacity, glucose intolerance, lower resting metabolic rate, immune dysfunction, slower gait speed, and functional dependency (Fiatarone Singh, 1998).

FFM peaks in the 20s or 30s, followed by a steady decline with age in both men and women (Muller et al., 1996). The loss of FFM is primarily attributable to the wasting of muscle tissue, muscle atrophy (figure 3.3, p. 60). Because most of our knowledge about aging effects on FFM is derived from cross-sectional studies, and few of these have included individuals over the age of 70, the rate of loss of FFM with age is not well documented. Losses of 5% per decade in men and 2.5% per decade in women have been reported, although a longitudinal study showed a 2% loss in men over a 10-year period with no decline in women, of the same age, over that same period of time (Hughes et al., 2002; Rudman et al., 1991). What is clear is that skeletal muscle atrophy, or sarcopenia, is highly prevalent in older adults, as high as 40% in those more than 80 years of age, and is strongly associated with weakness, disability, and morbidity (figure 3.5). Older adults at greatest risk for disability are those who are simultaneously sarcopenic and obese, and the prevalence of this combination of low muscle mass and excess fat increases with age from about 2% in those 60 to 69 years of age to about 10% in those more than 80 years old (Baumgartner, 2000).

Factors Influencing Fat Mass and Fat-Free Mass Change With Aging

Although genetic factors certainly are involved in the FM and FFM changes with aging, research suggests that regular exercise is important in the achievement and maintenance of optimal body composition with aging. The primary goals of any intervention would be to prevent or treat sarcopenia, reduce or redistribute FM, and prevent or treat osteopenia (bone loss, to be discussed later in this chapter).

Recent reviews comparing aerobic exercise with resistance exercise training to determine the effects on body composition of older adults supported the following conclusions: (a) aerobic training was effective in reducing weight and FM in 20 of 22 studies, and greater amounts of weight and FM were lost as the total number of exercise sessions increased; (b) fat loss for men and women occurred preferentially in the central regions of the body, but the effects of exercise on body fat distribution may be different in men and

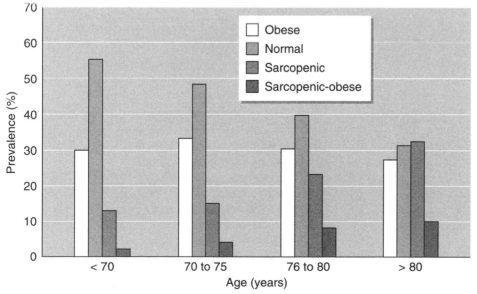

Figure 3.5 Prevalences of obesity, sarcopenia, and sarcopenic obesity by age in the combined New Mexico Elder Health Survey and New Mexico Aging Process Study.

Adapted from Baumgartner (2000).

women because the waist-to-hip ratios decreased in the men but stayed the same in the women; and (c) aerobic exercise was not an effective intervention for increasing muscle mass in older adults because this mode of exercise does not provide a strong enough stimulus to promote muscle growth (Fiatarone Singh, 1998; Hurley & Hagberg, 1998; Toth et al., 1999).

Resistance exercise also was effective in decreasing FM in older adults, with the loss of 1 to 2 kg of body fat for individuals completing resistance or aerobic training programs lasting 12 to 52 weeks. Unlike aerobic exercise, resistance exercise increased FFM in most studies conducted in older adults, and this increase ranged from 1.1 to 2.1 kg. Protein supplementation, however, did not augment these body composition changes beyond those attained with a normal diet. Energy needs during resistance training increase by about 15% in healthy elderly people, and therefore an increase in food intake may be necessary to stabilize weight.

More information is needed to refine the exercise prescription, including mode, intensity, duration, and frequency, for older adults who want to lose body fat. Does greater loss occur with a single 30-min bout of aerobic exercise, or is it better to do three bouts of 10 min? Is it better to do high-resistance strength training or lower resistance strength or power training for optimizing body composition? The role of exercise intensity, particularly in older adults, is unclear.

> Research suggests that regular aerobic and resistance exercise is important to achieve and maintain optimal body composition with aging.

Another way to determine the relationship between exercise and body composition is to study the percentage of body fat of masters athletes who train and compete in different sports. The body composition of 756 masters competitors is shown in table 3.5. These older individuals, who participate in extremely vigorous activities (distance running, cycling, canoeing) occurring over a relatively long time period, tend to have lower relative fat mass than people who participate in sports requiring relatively less energy expenditure over a shorter time period (racket sports, team sports). All competitors are on the lower end of body fat percentages compared with

Table 3.5 Body Build of 756 Masters Competitors

Event	Men			Women		
	Height (cm)	Lean body mass (kg)	Body fat (%)	Height (cm)	Lean body mass (kg)	Body fat (%)
Short-distance track	173.4[a]	58.6	19.7	165.7	43.1	28.8
Long-distance track	175.7	60.5	18.3	163.2	41.7	23.5
Short-distance swim	176.4	62.6	20.4	164.6	45.0	27.2
Long-distance swim	177.9	63.9	19.2	166.7	45.1	28.6
Cycling	175.0	61.4	17.2	166.9	48.2	25.9
Racket sports	174.8	61.0	21.6	161.0	43.6	29.5
Rowing	179.9	64.8	20.4	—	—	—
Canoeing	177.2	64.8	17.9	165.5	44.6	26.9
Sailing	174.8	59.3	19.3	168.1	47.0	32.9
Synchronized swimming	—	—	—	161.9	41.7	30.4
Team sports	176.3	64.0	22.2	—	—	—
Fencing	—	—	—	157.7	42.6	30.5

[a]The highest and lowest values in each column are underlined.

Reproduced, with permission, from T. Kavanaugh and R.J. Shephard: Can regular sports participation slow the aging process? *Phys Sportsmed* 1990; 18(6): 94-104 © 2004 The McGraw-Hill Companies. All rights reserved.

physically inactive adults of the same age, but they have higher body fat percentages than young athletes. In a review of six studies, Pollock and colleagues (1987) found that the body fat of masters runners was 5% to 10% higher than that of elite young runners. Two longitudinal studies that examined body composition changes in senior track athletes and elite runners reported increases of only 2% to 3% per decade in the body fat of athletes who remained highly and moderately active, whereas those who had lower activity levels or were inactive exhibited an increase of 4% to 6% per decade in body fat (Pollock et al., 1997; Trappe et al., 1996). Although FFM decreased across the 20-year study in all the athletes, those who began weight-training exercise were able to better maintain both FFM and strength and to show a greater arm bone mineral density.

In addition to exercise, changes in body fat and muscle mass during aging may be produced by changes in sex hormones or changes in growth hormone (GH) levels. Rudman and his colleagues (1991) discovered that men who took GH supplements for 18 months increased their FFM by 6% and the sum of 10 muscle areas by 11%, while decreasing their fat mass by 15%. These changes, however, were accompanied in some subjects by unpleasant side effects such as carpal tunnel syndrome and painful enlargement of the breasts. Both the positive changes and negative side effects disappeared 3 months after participants discontinued the GH supplement. A recent double-blind, placebo-controlled, parallel-group trial of GH and sex hormone administration in healthy older adults, 65-88 years of age (estrogen for women and testosterone for men) was conducted to determine the effects of these hormones on body composition and strength (Blackman et al., 2002). The researchers found that GH, with or without sex hormones, in both women and men increased FFM and decreased FM. The magnitudes of the changes in FFM and FM were similar to those reported after 6 months of exercise training three times per week. Testosterone plus the GH increased muscle strength and cardiovascular endurance in men but not in women. However, the adverse effects were frequent and included glucose intolerance and diabetes. Because of these serious adverse effects, GH interventions in older adults should be confined to controlled research studies, and the long-term efficacy of such treatment is questionable.

Changes in Bone

The skeleton not only provides structural support for the entire body but also serves as a reservoir for minerals and fat, a site for red blood cell production, a support for delicate tissues and organs, and a lever for muscles that allows for movement and speed. Nature selects materials and structures with properties that meet the contradictory needs of strength and lightness. Major quantitative and qualitative changes occur in bone tissue during growth and maturation, but bones eventually become fragile. Maintenance of bone health throughout the life cycle is essential, because a decline in skeletal integrity increases the risk of osteoporosis and bone fracture. The combination of good nutrition and exercise produces healthy bones in youth, and higher peak bone density is associated with a reduced risk of bone fracture in later life. This section examines how age-related bone changes are measured, how bone changes with age, factors that influence bone health, the relationship between muscle strength and bone health, and the prevention of and treatment of osteoporosis.

Measurement of Bone

Bone is a living tissue that undergoes a continuous cycle of bone building by osteoblasts and bone resorption by osteoclasts. Measures of bone integrity include bone mass (the amount of bone), bone

---

Assessing Aging Effects on Bone

We can assess changes in bone by looking at rate of bone gain or loss and changes in bone geometry, as described in this table.

Bone gain, bone loss	Net increase or decrease in bone mass from Time 1 to Time 2
Bone maintenance	No change in bone mass from Time 1 to Time 2, or if less bone loss is observed than might be expected according to the age of the subject
Rate of bone gain or loss	Change in mass over change in time
Changes in bone geometry	Thickness and number of trabeculae Thickness of cortical bone

---

mineral content (BMC; the amount of calcium, phosphorous, magnesium, boron, and manganese), bone mineral density (BMD; the amount of calcium or minerals per unit volume of bone), bone geometry (internal structure of bone), and rate of bone loss.

Assessments are made more frequently in forearm (radius), femur, and spinal (lumbar) bones. Measurements of bone parameters in one bone do not always correlate well with measurements in other bones. Although there is no precise measure of bone strength, BMD is the measure of bone mass most often reported in study of bone changes with aging, and it is believed to account for approximately 70% of bone strength (National Institutes of Health, 2001a).

Bone measurements are specific to the bones that are being measured because different bones are exposed to different weight-bearing stresses, and age-related changes in bone are not equally distributed across bones.

Methods used to measure bone integrity include dual energy X-ray absorptiometry (DEXA), mentioned earlier as a method for measuring FFM and FM, quantitative computer tomography and qualitative ultrasonometry. DEXA is the most widely used and best validated tool available. Hip BMD is the best predictor of hip fracture, and spine BMD is the best predictor of spinal fractures (National Institutes of Health, 2001b). Quantitative computer tomography is used to measure the actual volumetric density of bone, irrespective of bone size, and can distinguish between cortical and trabecular bone tissue. However, quantitative computer tomography costs more and involves higher radiation exposure than DEXA. Qualitative ultrasonometry has been recently introduced and is popular because of its ease of use, low cost, lack of radiation, and portability. Unlike the other two measures, it provides measures of bone quality.

Bone Changes Throughout the Life Cycle

There are two types of bone tissue: cortical (compact) bone and trabecular (cancellous) bone. Cortical bone is relatively dense and solid and forms the shaft of long bones such as the humerus and femur. Trabecular bone, or spongy bone, is much less dense because it is formed from struts called trabeculae and is found in the ends of the long bones, where bones are not stressed as heavily or where stresses on the bone arrive from difference directions. Some bones, such as those in the spine and hips, have a higher proportion of trabecular than cortical bone.

Throughout life, bone, which is a living tissue, continually undergoes a process of remodeling, in which old bone is replaced by new bone. Every 10 years, this remodeling replaces the entire skeleton. The changes in bone that occur over the life span are diagrammed in figure 3.6. Two mechanisms that principally determine adult bone health are peak bone mass (PBM), which is achieved during growth and early adulthood, and the rate of bone loss with advancing age, with the menopausal years being a time of considerable concern for women. In children, old bone is resorbed, but because new bone is formed at a faster rate, total bone increases linearly with a 40% to 70% increase in bone mass during puberty. However, this increase in bone mass during puberty varies according to skeletal site. Bone mass continues to increase until peak bone mass is achieved around age 30 for both males and females. During childhood and young adulthood, bones are reshaped through specific, local stresses, such as the widening and increase in robustness of the bones of a tennis player's playing arm (Huddleston et al., 1980; Jones et al., 1977), a baseball player's throwing arm (Watson, 1973), and a soccer player's legs (Karlsson, 2000). Such differences are related to the level of resistance encountered by the bone daily during weight bearing, chronic use, or training. Thus, the bones of weightlifters are stronger and thicker than the bones of joggers, whose bones are stronger than those of swimmers (Nillsson & Westlin, 1971). Some investigators believe that the modeling process provides a larger bone "bank" or reserve above the needs of normal daily activity (Frost, 1989). This reserve might postpone the inevitable onset of microfractures at an older age (Schultheis, 1991).

Two mechanisms that principally determine adult bone health are peak bone mass and the rate of bone loss with advancing age.

What happens to bone formation with aging, and how are males and females different? The average woman attains a peak bone mass that is generally about 10% below that of a man's. Toward the end of the third decade, the rate of formation fails to keep pace with resorption, and bone loss of approximately 0.7% to 1% a year occurs up until age 50 for both women and men. Bone loss in women increases to about 2% to 3% per year beginning at menopause and continues for 5 to 10 years. On average, women may lose between one third to one half of the BMD during menopause. Data show that the rate of bone loss increases in the 8th and 9th decades in women and men. The change in the ratio of formation to resorption is said to become uncoupled. Although this uncoupling process is not well understood, some possible expla-

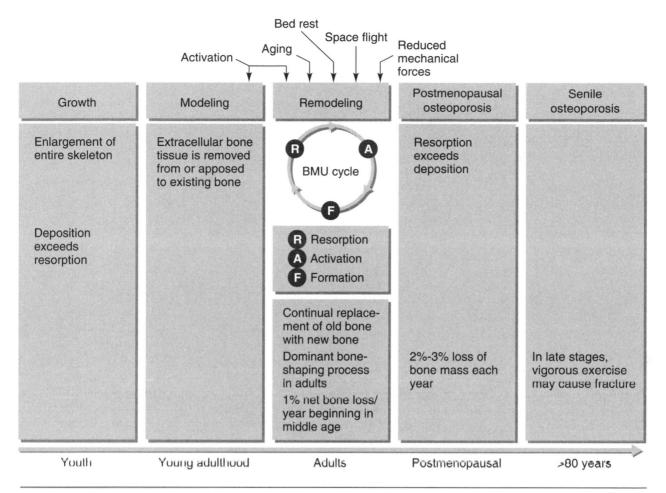

Figure 3.6 Changes in bone over the life span. BMU = basic multicellular units, which are groups of cells that work together. Within a BMU, osteoclasts (cells that resorb bone) and osteoblasts (cells that form bone) interact in a cycle of activation, resorption, and formation.

nations, all age related, include changes in calcium-regulating hormones, decreased perfusion of bone tissue as a result of changes in bone blood flow, changes in the properties of bone mineral material, and a decrease in the number and metabolic activity of the cells that produce bone (Kiebzak, 1991).

The balance between resorption and formation of bone differs substantially not only in different bones (e.g., weight-bearing vs. non-weight-bearing) but also in different bone tissue. For example, cortical bone in the vertebral body of the spine declines in men slightly (10%) from 30 to 80 years, but the decline of this same cortical bone in women is 30% over the same 50 years (Seeman, 2002). However, trabecular bone density of the vertebral body declines much more than cortical bone in men (55%) and in women (65%) over this same 50-year period.

Major architectural and other compensatory changes occur within the bone during aging when resorption occurs at a faster rate than formation.

A remodeling cycle occurs over 3 to 6 months, but because remodeling is slower with increased age, microfractures accumulate. Eventually, the accumulation of microfractures compromises the integrity of the bone, and a major bone fracture occurs. Aged bone actually becomes more highly mineralized, causing it to be more brittle and vulnerable to fatigue and microfractures. However, because bone also becomes more porous and there is actually less bone in older people, measurements of bone mineral content are always lower in aged samples than in younger ones. BMD is related to bone strength, but the architecture of the bone or bone quality, such as the trabecular thickness and the perforations in the trabecular network, is also important (Mosekilde, 2000).

Factors Influencing Bone Health

Two types of factors affect bone health with age: non-modifiable factors such as gender and ethnicity, and modifiable factors such as hormones, diet, exercise, and body weight.

Gender and Ethnicity

Men have larger and denser bones than women at every age (figure 3.7; Looker et al., 1997). At the age of 30, men have a 10% higher peak bone mass than women and this gender difference increases with age, so that men have a 20% higher peak bone mass than women after menopause. Men produce an age-related compensatory increase in bone size (increase in cross-sectional area of the vertebral bodies) that is not observed in women. After 50 years of age (menopause), the bone architecture of women has a higher tendency than that of men to change. For example, more disconnections of the horizontal trabecular struts are seen. This leads to more pronounced deterioration of the network in women and thereby a greater loss of bone strength (Mosekilde, 2000). Individuals with BMD below 0.65 g/cm² are classified as having poor bone quality that can lead to osteoporosis. On the average, men do not reach this threshold until age 80 although women may reach it as early as 50 years of age.

Ethnicity is associated with differences in BMD, with most investigators reporting higher BMD in African Americans and Mexican Americans, lower BMD in Asian Americans, and intermediate BMD in Caucasian Americans. The Study of Women's Health Across the Nation (SWAN), a recent large,

multiethnic, community-based study investigating a wide range of characteristics as women age through menopause, found that unadjusted lumbar spine and femoral neck BMD were the highest in African American women, next highest in Caucasian Americans, and lowest in Asian American women (Finkelstein et al., 2002). However, the ethnic patterns of BMD changed when the effects of selected anthropometric and lifestyle variables (notably body weight) on BMD were analyzed. After these adjustments, BMD remained highest in African American women, but there was no significant difference in BMD among the remaining ethnic groups. The researchers also examined BMD in a subset of women weighing less than 70 kg and found that the only ethnic difference that remained, after the adjustments, was that Caucasian Americans had lower BMD than the other three groups. Other studies report that Mexican American women have BMDs between those of Caucasian American and African American women. Limited available information for Native American women suggests that they have lower BMDs than white non-Hispanic women (National Institutes of Health, 2001a). Variations in bones assessed during the study and the difficulties of categorizing individuals' ethnicity make determining ethnic differences in bone integrity difficult.

Lifestyle Choices

Three major factors that influence bone health in older adults and can be modified by lifestyle choices

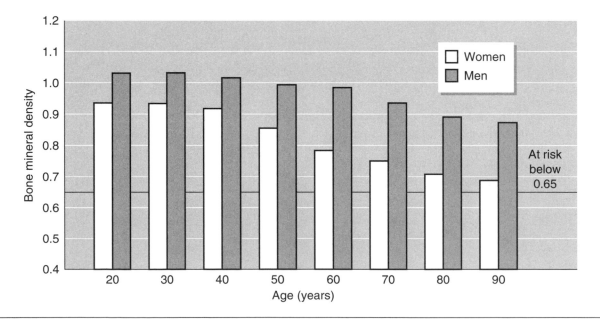

Figure 3.7 Changes in the average bone mineral density of the hip with age in white women and men in the United States.

Reprinted, by permission, from A.C. Looker et al., 1992, "Prevalence of low femoral bone density in older US adults from NHANES III," *Journal of Bone Mineral Research* 12: 1761-1768.

What Research Indicates About Ethnicity and Bone Mineral Density

This table summarizes data from a variety of studies on bone density among African American, Caucasian, Asian, Mexican American, White non-Hispanic, and Native American groups.

Source	Highest BMD	Intermediate BMD	Lower BMD
Majority of studies	African American	Caucasian	Asian
SWAN (Finkelstein et al., 2002)	African American	Caucasian	Asian
SWAN, adjusted for body weight (Finkelstein et al., 2002)	African American	No difference between Caucasians and Asians	
Other studies	African American	Mexican American women	Caucasians
NIH (2001)		White non-Hispanic higher than Native American women	

Note: BMD = bone mineral density, SWAN = Study of Women's Health Across the Nation, NIH = National Institutes of Health.

include hormones, diet, and exercise. Aging is associated with declines in the sex steroids estrogen and testosterone and the adrenal androgen dehydroepiandrosterone (DHEA). These hormonal changes, particularly the decline in estrogen in women, are associated with accelerated bone loss over the 8 to 10 years following menopause. Dietary deficiencies, primarily related to low intake of calcium- or vitamin-D-rich foods, and decreased physical activity also have been shown to affect the development and maintenance of bone.

Hormonal Changes

In normal healthy women, menopause is probably the best predictor of bone mineral loss (Hagino et al., 1992). Menopausal-related hormonal changes, especially the decrease in estrogen, result in a rapid increase in the processes that deteriorate bone, and, simultaneously, the cells that manufacture bone are impaired. These changes also may contribute indirectly to bone loss, because estrogen depletion reduces absorption of calcium in the intestine (Schultheis, 1991). Also, calcitonin and some vitamin D metabolites, hormones that regulate calcium homeostasis in bone, decrease with age. A decrease in these hormones, and the age-related increase in parathyroid hormone, favor bone resorption over bone formation (Kiebzak, 1991). Even in men, estrogen is the sex steroid most strongly associated with bone density of the spine, hip, and forearm, although testosterone level is related to higher BMD (Greendale et al., 1997). Thus, for both women and men, estrogen appears

to have important skeletal effects on bone health with aging.

So the question on the mind of women entering menopause, or the change in life, is whether taking hormones, such as estrogen, will decrease menopausal symptoms and maintain bone density or increase adverse events that outweigh the therapy's benefit. These adverse effects of hormone replacement therapy (HRT) have received much recent attention because of the results of several large randomized control trials in women, such as the Women's Health Initiative (WHI; Writing Group for the WHI Investigators, 2002) and the Heart and Estrogen/progestin Replacement Study (HERS; Hulley et al., 1998). HRT, a combination of estrogen and progestin, has been recommended for women with a uterus to relieve menopausal symptoms and to prevent many chronic conditions such as osteoporosis and heart disease. Because approximately 38% of women in the United States use HRT, the latest findings that 5 or more years of HRT use increases the risk of heart disease, stroke, blood clots, breast cancer, and cholecystitis (inflammation of the gall bladder) is of considerable concern. However, prevention of osteoporosis and fractures with HRT use is supported by results from the WHI and several consistent, good-quality observational studies of HRT and bone health. Prevention of colon cancer is also well supported by WHI and other studies, whereas the effects of HRT on dementia need further research (Nelson et al., 2002). Overall, mortality rate is not higher in HRT users. The *Journal of the American Medical Association* published a "Patient Page" suggesting that all women, before deciding whether to take HRT, should discuss their personal health history, symptoms of menopause, and risk for osteoporosis, heart disease, and breast cancer with their personal physicians (Torpy et al., 2002).

Diet

Good nutrition is essential for normal growth and development, and a balanced diet, adequate calories, and appropriate nutrients are the foundation for development and maintenance of all tissues including bone. Calcium is the nutrient most important for attaining peak bone mass and for preventing and treating osteoporosis. Many adults, particularly women, tend to have inadequate calcium, vitamins, and minerals in their diets. Part of the explanation is that many older adults simply lose interest in food and consume so little that they cannot get as much of these essential nutrients as they need. Another reason is that the dietary patterns of the elderly often do not include milk and other calcium-rich foods. Also, older adults lose some ability to produce, through sun exposure to their skin, the vitamin D metabolites so important to calcium utilization in bone.

Sufficient data exist to recommend specific dietary calcium intakes at various stages of life, as shown in the sidebar. Vitamin D is required for optimal calcium absorption and is also important for bone

---

Recommended Dietary Calcium Intakes for Various Ages

This table summarizes recommended dietary calcium intake and percentage of the populations meeting these recommendations. There is no data available for the 70+ age group.

Age	Amount	Percent of U.S. populations meeting requirement
Children 4-8 years	800 mg/day	
Adolescents 9-17	1300 mg/day	25% boys; 15% girls
Adults	1000-1500 mg/day	50%
Adults, 70+	??	

From National Academy of Sciences (1997).

---

health. An intake of 400 to 600 IU/day of vitamin D has been established for adults (National Institutes of Health, 2001b). Findings from the National Diet and Nutrition Survey of older adults found that 97% of free-living older adults and 99% of institutionalized older adults had vitamin D intakes that were below the reference nutrient intake with one-third of the institutionalized older adults being vitamin D deficient (Finch et al., 1998). Other nutrients such as caffeine, phosphorous, and sodium can adversely affect calcium balance, but their effects disappear in individuals with adequate calcium intakes. One area of increasing interest is the positive association reported between high intakes of fruits and vegetables and bone health. The evidence that high intakes of fruits and vegetables reduce obesity and heart disease and improve bone health encourages this lifestyle choice for individuals of all ages.

Exercise

Exercise is expected to have a beneficial influence on the maintenance of bone, because bed rest, immobilization, and disuse of muscles are disastrous for bone mineralization (Schneider & McDonald, 1984; Weinreb et al., 1989). Subjects of one study lost 1% of bone a week and only regained it at a rate of 1% a month (Krolner & Toft, 1983). The evidence from spaceflights, for both experimental animals and human astronauts, was that an unabated loss of bone, attributable to a lack of mechanical stress (i.e., gravity) on the bone, occurred during all flights. NASA-sponsored studies of bed rest have shown that calcium and bone mineral are lost steadily throughout the period of immobility. Yet when mobility is reinitiated, the recovery of bone components is much slower than was the rate of bone loss (LeBlanc & Schneider, 1991). Indeed, exercise may be critically important in increasing bone formation, because the effect of weight-bearing loading is essential for bone formation, whereas calcium supplements and estrogen treatment only slow down bone resorption (Franck et al., 1991; Heaney, 1986). Both muscular contraction and gravity apply force to bones that influences the structure and integrity of the bone.

The prevention of osteoporosis, like many chronic diseases, is more effective when started early. The results of many cross-sectional investigations have found that individuals, who engage in regular weight-bearing exercise, particularly those participating during childhood, have greater bone mass than sedentary people. However, exercise is not a natural panacea, and inherent subject selection bias of cross-sectional studies supports the need for controlled, randomized exercise intervention trials that use subjects of all ages and both genders. Both resistance and endurance exercise programs have been shown to enhance bone density of young women in a site-specific manner. For example, high-impact endurance training increased femoral neck but not radius BMD in 35- to 45-year-old women (Heinonen et al., 1996). Few intervention trials have been reported with young men, but one investigator who followed the marathon training of young men for 9 months reported a larger change in calcaneal BMD of consistent runners compared with nonexercising controls (Williams et al., 1984). Only a few researchers have examined effects of endurance training in perimenopausal women on BMD, and the results have been mixed. Clearly, more research is needed to determine the type, frequency, and duration of exercise in perimenopausal women that will produce the greatest positive effect on bone health.

Several studies have examined resistance exercise effects on bone health in postmenopausal women. One of the first studies examined the effects of one year of high-intensity strength training on the bone health, muscle strength, and dynamic balance in postmenopausal women. The study found that resistance exercise preserved bone density and improved muscle mass, strength, and balance (Nelson et al., 1994). There was also an increase in spontaneous physical activity in the strength trained women, despite instructions not to alter their habitual activity levels. The results of studies in which postmenopausal women wore a weighted vest and performed jumping exercise have been mixed, but when these interventions were done 3 times per week for 32 weeks a year for 5 years, BMD was maintained in the exercise group while the control group lost 3-5% over the 5 years (Snow et al., 2000). A recent study examining the effects of a 2-year intense exercise program in postmenopausal osteopenic women, the Erlangen Fitness Osteoporosis Prevention Study (EFOPS), reported that the general purpose exercise program, with special emphasis on bone density, significantly reduced bone loss, back pain, and lipid levels and increased strength and endurance (Kemmler et al., 2004).

The time required for bone to undergo a full modeling or remodeling cycle in response to altered patterns of loading, as might be experienced in an exercise training program, is approximately 4 and 6 months. Therefore, exercise interventions less than 6 months in duration may not accurately reflect either the effectiveness of the exercise stimulus or the relative responsiveness of bone to loading. Also, the magnitude of bone response to exercise likely depends on an individual's initial bone mass, with

the greatest gains seen in individuals with very low initial bone mass. Other key exercise-related factors that affect bone health with exercise include the intensity, duration, and mechanical stress that are put on the bone during the exercise. Long-term resistance training programs in postmenopausal women have been shown to increase or maintain BMD of the whole body, lumbar spine, proximal femur, and radius (Beck & Marcus, 1999). Long-term endurance training programs (7-18 months) with postmenopausal women generally have resulted in increases or maintenance of BMD, compared with bone losses in control subjects. These changes were seen in whole body, lumbar spine, proximal femur, radius, and calcaneus. No randomized, controlled interventions trials of this nature have been conducted in men.

Even after considerable research, no consensus has developed with regard to the precise intensity, frequency, duration, and type of exercise that most benefits bone. Although resistance training and high-impact endurance exercises, such as running, stair climbing, and jumping, have the most positive impact on bone health, these activities also increase the risk of cardiovascular stress and falls. These types of exercises also have a greater attrition rate than lower-intensity exercise programs. It is clear that individuals with advanced osteoporosis should not engage in high-impact activities or deep forward flexion exercises such as rowing. Finally, the debate over which exercise is best for bone health misses the more important point that the adult populations of most Western industrialized societies are relatively sedentary. The effects of aging on physical activity patterns are dramatic, with more than 50% of those 65 to 74 years old and almost 66% of those over the age of 75 years reporting no leisure-time physical activity (U.S. Department of Health and Human Services, 2000). Therefore, the most effective recommendation is one that will increase the overall level of activity of an inactive person to any degree and that also will be associated with the greatest long-term compliance. Walking, perhaps with a weighted vest, remains a very attractive option for older adults because it has cardiovascular and neuromuscular benefits and may also have a positive effect on bone.

Interactions Among Exercise, Hormones, and Diet

Although the relationship between exercise and bone loss seems compelling, it is far from straightforward and probably depends greatly on hormonal status and calcium. For example, Drinkwater (1986) found that although women athletes who had menstrual cycles monthly had vertebral densities well above those of inactive women, the bone densities of amenorrheic athletes, those who had a cessation of monthly menstrual cycles for at least 3 consecutive months, were actually lower than those of the controls. Presumably these amenorrheic athletes trained as intensely and as often as the eumenorrheic athletes, but the exercise did not protect them from bone loss. Similarly, fitness and vertebral bone mineral density were moderately and positively correlated in young eumenorrheic women but not in amenorrheic women (average age 59 years) who completed an exercise program (Kirk et al., 1989). Some studies of HRT in menopausal women have found that exercise enhances the bone-conserving effects of HRT (Kohrt, Ehsani, & Birge, 1998), whereas other studies have found otherwise (Heikkinen et al., 1991). Hormone and exercise interactions have not been studied effectively in men, and there is a great need for more research in women.

What about the interaction between calcium and exercise? Specker (1996) reviewed 17 studies on this topic and found that exercise affects BMD only when mean calcium intake surpasses 1,000 mg/day and that the effect is more pronounced in the lumbar spine than at the radius. However, others have not found a significant interaction effect of exercise and calcium supplementation. Perhaps age, hormonal status, calcium intake before supplementation, and type, intensity, and frequency of exercise affect this interaction. Clearly more research is needed on this topic.

Relationship Between Bone and Muscular Strength

Bone mass and muscle mass develop together during youth and decline together during aging. Frost (2000) argued that mechanical factors, such as muscle strength and physical activity, not nonmechanical factors, such as age, gender, hormone levels, and diet, have the greatest influence on bone health. For example, years after a paraplegic has experienced complete paralysis, the bones in the paralyzed lower extremities, but not in the normal upper extremities, have lost 40% of the bone mass. Loss of muscle strength precedes the loss of bone, and the recovery of muscle strength precedes the recovery of bone mass. The delay between loss of bone and muscle is substantial, reflecting the different rates of adaptation of these two tissues. In men and women aged 61 to 84 years, several measures of strength are correlated with spinal bone density (Bevier et al., 1989; Halle et al., 1990). Grip strength is correlated with forearm and spine density, but back strength is

the best predictor of bone density in elderly men. Body mass also significantly predicts bone density in elderly women, perhaps because the greater the body mass, the greater the gravitational and stress forces on the bones. Although muscular strength correlates positively with bone density, increases in bone density cannot necessarily be inferred from increases in muscular strength (Pocock et al., 1988). It seems most likely that bone loss is truly a multifactorial phenomenon, and the loss of mechanical stimulation as a consequence of declining muscle strength will prove to be one of several important contributors.

Loss of muscle strength precedes the loss of bone, and the recovery of muscle strength precedes the recovery of bone mass.

Bone Fractures

Many factors contribute to bone fracture (figure 3.8). One of the most important of these factors is the age-related decrease in bone mass that makes adults vulnerable to bone fractures, particularly those of the hip, wrist, and vertebrae (Nevitt, 1999). As individuals age, some bone loss is inevitable. Bone mass, the rate of bone loss, body mass index, and chronological age all significantly predict fractures. Chronological age is a somewhat better predictor of bone fracture than direct measures of forearm bone mass (Hui et al., 1988), and bone mass predicts fractures better than the rate of bone loss (Gardsell et al., 1991). BMI is inversely related to risk of bone fracture so that women with very low BMIs have almost twice the risk of fracturing a hip than do women with higher BMIs. The excess weight of women with high BMI places a greater than average mechanical stress on some bones, perhaps slowing the rate of bone loss (Harris et al., 1992). Then, too, women with fatter hips have more protection against damage when they fall. Bone fractures are a serious threat because the lifetime risk of having any type of fracture for a 50-year-old white woman is 70% and fractures are a major contributor to morbidity and to the high cost of medical care (Nevitt, 1999). The incidence of hip fractures in women is twice that of men. Furthermore, a substantial percentage of women who experience a hip fracture will never regain their mobility, and as many as two out of five may die from complications of the fracture. There is strong evidence that that a physically active lifestyle reduces the risk of hip fractures by 20% to 40% (Gregg et al., 2000). A recent publication from the Nurses' Health Study found that for every 1 hr per week increase in walking, at an average pace, there was a 6% reduction in risk for hip fracture (Feskanich et al., 2002).

Definition and Prevalence of Osteoporosis

Osteoporosis is a crippling disease characterized by low bone mass and microarchitectural deterioration of bone tissue that increases bone fragility and the risk of bone fractures. This disease involves decreased bone mass and poor structural quality of the bone. The incidence and prevalence of osteoporosis increase with age, and it affects women much more than men. Because there is no accurate measure of overall bone strength, BMD is used as a proxy measure. In 1994, the World Health Organization established BMD measurement criteria, using the BMD of young adult women at the age of peak bone mass as the standard, that allowed diagnosis of osteoporosis before a bone fracture occurs (National Institutes of Health, 2001b). Osteoporosis was defined as a BMD that is 2.5 standard deviations below the mean for young women, whereas osteopenia was defined as BMD values between 1.0 and 2.5 standard deviations below the mean for young women. For each standard deviation below peak bone mass, a woman's risk of fracture approximately doubles. In the United States, osteoporosis is associated with 1.5 million fractures of the spinal bones, hips, forearms, and other bones in those 45 years of age and older. Primary osteoporosis, bone loss attributable to aging, may occur in two types: type I osteoporosis (postmenopausal), which is the accelerated decrease in bone mass (3-7% per year for the 5 years after menopause) that occurs when estrogen levels decrease after menopause; and type II osteoporosis (age-related), which is the inevitable loss of bone mass with age and occurs in both men and women. Secondary osteoporosis may develop at any age as a consequence of hormonal, digestive, and metabolic disorders, as well as prolonged bed rest and weightlessness (spaceflight).

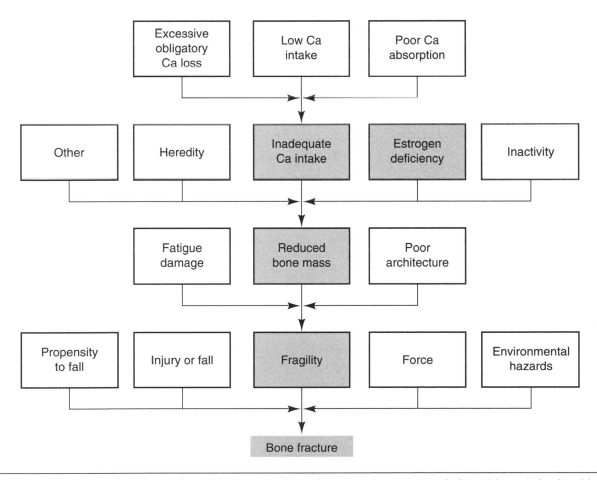

Figure 3.8 Factors that contribute to bone fracture. The shaded boxes are factors particularly problematic for the elderly. Ca = calcium.

Adapted, by permission, from R.P. Heaney, 1992, "Calcium in the prevention and treatment of osteoporosis," *Journal of Internal Medicine* 231: 169-180.

For each standard deviation below peak bone mass, a woman's risk of fracture approximately doubles.

Factors That Increase Risk of Developing Osteoporosis

Certain people are more likely to develop osteoporosis than others. Factors that increase the likelihood of developing osteoporosis are called "risk factors." Nonmodifiable risk factors for osteoporosis include age, gender, body size, ethnicity, and family history. The older you are, the greater your risk of osteoporosis, and women have a greater risk than men. Women are more at risk for osteoporosis than men for several reasons. Women generally consume less calcium in their diets because they are more likely to avoid milk products, which they perceive as fattening. Many women are chronic dieters; thus, they do not consume enough food to ensure an adequate calcium intake. Women never attain the peak bone mass of men, and because women live longer than men they have more bone loss attributable to aging. They may also deplete some body calcium during pregnancy and lactation. Finally, women experience a sharp decline in estrogen during menopause, which increases the risk for osteoporosis. Thus, many factors converge to predispose women to lose more bone tissue than men do. Small, thin-boned women are at the highest risk, and African American women, although they have the lowest risk of any ethnic group, are still at significant risk. Finally, susceptibility to fracture may be hereditary.

Osteoporosis—Facts and Figures

- Osteoporosis affects 44 million Americans, 68% of whom are women.
- One out of every two women and one in eight men over the age of 50 will have an osteoporosis-related fracture in their lifetime.
- Osteoporosis is responsible for more than 1.5 million fractures annually.
- Estimated national direct expenditures (hospitals and nursing homes) for osteoporosis and related fractures are 14 billion each year.

From National Institutes of Health Osteoporosis and Related Bone Disease—National Research Center. www.osteo.org.

Modifiable Risk Factors for Osteoporosis

- Hormonal levels, particularly low estrogen
- A diet low in calcium and vitamin D
- Lack of weight-bearing physical activity
- Having an eating disorder such as anorexia
- Certain medications, such as glucocorticoids or anticonvulsants
- Cigarette smoking
- Excessive use of alcohol

People whose parents have a history of fractures also have reduced bone mass and may be at risk for fractures.

Modifiable risk factors for osteoporosis are listed in the sidebar, with the three most important being hormonal levels, diets low in calcium and vitamin D, and lack of weight-bearing physical activity. As mentioned earlier, low estrogen levels as are found in young women who are amenorrheic or in older women at menopause, and low estrogen and testosterone levels in men are associated with increased risk of osteoporosis. These hormones are needed by the body to maintain bone absorption and formation so that bone loss does not occur. However, there must be sufficient calcium and vitamin D in the diet along with stress on the bone, produced by weight-bearing exercise such as walking and weightlifting, to maintain optimal bone health.

Medications for Prevention and Treatment of Osteoporosis

Currently, alendronate, raloxifene, risedronate, and estrogen are approved by the U.S. Food and Drug Administration (FDA) for the prevention of osteoporosis and for the treatment of postmenopausal osteoporosis. Calcitonin also has been approved for the treatment of postmenopausal osteoporosis. Only alendronate is approved for the treatment of osteoporosis in men. Both alendronate (brand name Fosamax) and risedronate (brand name Actonel) are medications from the class of drugs called bisphosphonates. The bisphosphonates are currently considered the best estrogen alternatives to maintain or build healthy bone (Rosen, 2003). The side effects from these medications are uncommon but may include abdominal or musculoskeletal pain, nausea, heartburn, or irritation of the esophagus. Raloxifene (brand name Evista) is from a new class of drugs called selective estrogen receptor modulators (SERMs), which have been shown to have beneficial effects on bone mass and bone turnover and can reduce the incidence of vertebral fractures. Side effects are uncommon with Raloxifene but include hot flashes and deep vein thrombosis. Another medication approved for treatment of osteoporosis is calcitonin, a naturally occurring nonsex hormone involved in calcium regulation and bone metabolism. It can be taken as an injection or nasal spray, but an injection of calcitonin may cause an allergic reaction and unpleasant side effects including flushing of the face and hands, urinary frequency, nausea, and skin rash. Although HRT has been shown to protect against osteoporosis, the recent studies showing a small but significant increase in breast cancer, heart attack, stroke, and blood clot risk for women taking HRT support the use of other medications discussed previously instead of HRT for the prevention of osteoporosis (Rosen, 2003).

Aging Joints: Coping With the Interface of Aging Bones, Muscles, and Tendons

One of the most important functions of bone is to provide structural support for the entire body. However, support without mobility would leave us little better than statues. Body movements must conform to the limits of the skeletal system, and these movements are restricted to joints or articulations—where two bones meet. Some joints are interlocking or immoveable, such as the sutures in the skull, whereas other joints, like synovial joints of the shoulder or hip, permit a wide range of movements. Synovial joints typically are found at the end of long bones, such as those of the upper and lower limbs. Under normal conditions, the bony surfaces do not contact one another because special articular cartilages cover the ends of the bones. These cartilages act as shock absorbers and help reduce friction during movement. A joint capsule composed of a thick layer of dense connective tissue surrounds the synovial joint. A synovial membrane lines the joint cavity but stops at the edges of the articular cartilages. Synovial fluid, produced by the synovial membrane, fills the joint cavity and serves several functions. The synovial fluid provides lubrication, nourishes the articular

cartilage, and serves as a shock absorber when the joint is compressed, as would occur at the hip joint during walking or running. The synovial membrane also contains the nerve endings that signal pain when insults to the joint occur. In addition to the synovial joint structure, stability at the joint is provided by cartilage pads within the joint cavity, such as the menisci in the knee, ligaments that connect bone to bone, tendons that attach muscle to bone, and bursae. Bursae are fluid-filled pockets in connective tissue that are found around most synovial joints and help reduce friction during movement and absorb shock.

Joints are subjected to heavy wear and tear throughout life, and problems with joint function are relatively common in older adults. **Rheumatism** is a general term that indicates pain and stiffness affecting the skeletal or muscular systems. Arthritis encompasses all the rheumatic diseases that affect synovial joints. **Arthritis** often involves damage to the articular cartilages, but the specific cause can vary. For example, arthritis can result from bacterial or viral infection, injury to the joint, metabolic problems, or severe physical stress. Osteoarthritis, also known as degenerative arthritis, is the most common arthritis in the United States for those age 65 and older. Osteoarthritis is discussed in more detail later in this chapter. Rheumatoid arthritis is an inflammatory condition that affects roughly 2.5% of the adult population. In some cases, this condition occurs when the immune response mistakenly attacks the joint tissues.

Description and Measurement of Flexibility

Flexibility refers to the range of motion around a single joint or multiple joints. Flexibility depends on the state and condition of the soft tissues of the joint, tendons, ligaments, and muscles. When these tissues are soft and pliant, the joint is allowed its full range of motion. Muscle is thought to be the most important and modifiable structure for improving flexibility (Nieman, 2003). Flexibility is maintained in a joint by using the joint and by participating in physical activities that move the joint through its complete range of motion. When a joint is relatively unused, the muscles that cross it shorten, thus reducing its range of motion. Joint flexibility is crucial for effective movement. It would serve little purpose to have strong bones and muscles if the bones cannot be moved through their range of motion enough to manipulate objects or to locomote. Therefore, flexibility, along with cardiovascular endurance, body composition, and muscular strength, is considered an essential component of health-related physical fitness.

Flexibility is specific to each joint of the body, and flexibility at one joint does not necessarily indicate flexibility in other joints. There is also no general flexibility test for the whole body. Flexibility is most often measured as a health-related fitness component by using the sit-and-reach test. The sit-and-reach test is singled out because it has been noted in some clinical settings that people with low back problems lack flexibility in the low back and hamstrings. The test is performed by having the person being tested perform a warm-up that involves brisk walking or stationary cycling before performing the test. The person then removes his or her shoes and sits facing the flexibility box, with knees fully extended and feet flat against the box. The person reaches directly forward, as far as possible along the measuring scale, extends forward maximally four times, and then holds the position of maximum reach for 1 to 2 s. The score is the most distant point reached on the fourth trial, measured to the nearest centimeter (Nieman, 2003). Rikli and Jones (2001) modified the sit-and-reach test to the "chair sit-and-reach test" as part of their Senior Fitness Test. Their modification allows the person being tested to remain seated in a chair and uses an 18-in. ruler to measure how far beyond their toes the person can reach.

Upper body flexibility is important to activities of daily living such as reaching and grasping. The most frequent measure of upper body flexibility involves measuring range of motion at the shoulder joint. The Senior Fitness Test uses the "back scratch test," a modified version of a clinical test that has been used for years by clinicians, for evaluation of general shoulder range of motion. This assessment is performed in a standing position. The preferred arm is raised, elbow bent (pointing upward), and the hand reaches down across the middle of the back as far as possible. At the same time, the other arm is extended up behind the back, palm facing outward, in an attempt to touch the fingers of the other hand. A ruler is used to measure the distance between fingers of the two hands. Performance charts that include values (including normal range, above average, below average, and at risk for loss of functional mobility) for older adults by 5-year increments beginning with 60- to 64-year-olds are given for all the assessments included as part of the Senior Fitness Test (Rikli & Jones, 2001). The scores from the Senior Fitness Test provide good gender and age comparisons because the norms are based on scores from thousands of independently living older adults across the United States.

In a clinical setting, flexibility is generally measured with a goniometer, which is essentially a movable protractor with two long arms. If the two arms are stretched out to make a straight line, they measure 180°. If they are positioned to make a right angle, they measure 90°. Using the goniometer, we can determine flexibility at the fingers, elbow, shoulder, ankle, knee, and hip. The measures of flexibility in the fingers, elbow, and knee are primarily in one anatomical plane. Shoulder and hip joint movements, however, are three-dimensional. Shoulders and hips are attached to limbs that can flex and extend, but they can also abduct (move away from the body) and adduct (move toward the body) in another plane.

Loss of flexibility not only reduces the amount and nature of movement that can be made at a joint but also increases the possibility of injury to the joint or to the muscles crossing the joint. Inflexibility can lead to muscle strains or to muscle, tendon, or ligament damage or detachments. In older adults, lower body flexibility is particularly important for good mobility, including bending, lifting, reaching, stooping, walking, and stair climbing (Badley et al., 1984; Konczak et al., 1992). Sufficient upper body range of motion is needed for functional tasks such as zipping a back zipper, putting on or removing garments over one's head, reaching for a seat belt, placing something high on an overhead shelf, or removing a wallet from a back pocket.

Maximum range of motion is achieved in the mid- to late 20s for both men and women and gradually deceases with age (20-30% between 30 and 70 years of age), but the loss with age is more rapid in some joints than others (Bell & Hoshizaki, 1981). Similar declines are seen in men and women, though women are more flexible than men throughout life (Holland et al., 2002; Rikli & Jones, 1999). Spinal flexibility, particularly trunk extension, shows the greatest declines with age. Hamstring and lower back flexibility, as measured by the YMCA sit-and-reach test in 33,000 participants from YMCA centers across the United States, declined about 1 in. (2.54 cm) per decade (15% loss per decade) in both men and women (Golding & Lindsay, 1989)

> Flexibility, as measured by the sit-and reach test, decreases approximately 15% per decade in both men and women, but greater losses in trunk extension are reported in older adults.

What changes occur in spinal flexibility with age? Figure 3.9 includes data on spinal flexibilities of women ages 20 through 84 (Einkauf et al., 1987). The greatest aging effects were seen in extension of the spine, with the 70- to 84-year-old age group exhibit-

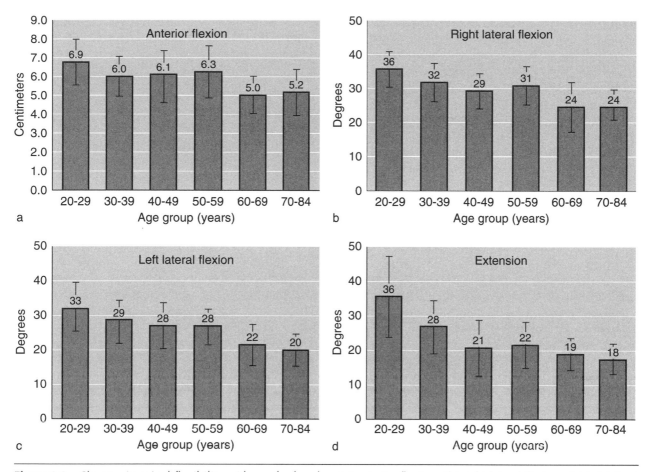

Figure 3.9 Changes in spinal flexibility with age for females: *(a)* anterior flexion, *(b)* right lateral flexion, *(c)* left lateral flexion, *(d)* extension. Bar graphs represent means and standard deviations by age group.

Reprinted from *Physical Therapy* with the permission of the American Physical Therapy Association.

ing a 50% loss in extensor flexibility compared with the 20- to 29-year-olds. The losses with age were least severe in anterior flexion (bending forward). The authors interpreted these results as consequences of the types of daily activities in which most people participate. Few occasions arise in the course of daily life to lean backward, whereas many activities of daily living involve leaning forward. In addition, most daily activities such as eating, reading, knitting, and cooking predispose people to use neck, shoulder, and arm flexion rather than extension. Finally, as people age their balance is compromised, and they are much less likely to lean backward—and probably less likely to "stretch themselves" to lean backward in a laboratory test of flexibility.

The ankle joint also loses flexibility with aging. From the age of 55 to 85, female subjects lost about 50% of their range of motion in their ankle joints whereas male subjects lost about 35% (Vandervoort et al., 1992). Age-related weakness in the muscles that flex the ankle upward (dorsiflexors), and an increase in muscle resistance of the calf muscles attributable

to loss of compliance of the connective tissue of old muscles, mean that the ankle is not flexed as much during walking. Decreased use eventually leads to a loss of range of motion at or about the ankle joint, which when added to the age-related strength losses increases the risk for falling.

Exercise Effects on Flexibility

Much of the loss in flexibility with age may be attributable to inactivity; thus, daily activity involving moving joints throughout the range of motion should maintain or improve flexibility with age. Some researchers have examined general exercise interventions, including various combinations of aerobic training, strength training, dance, calisthenics, and t'ai chi, and their effects on range of motion. However, the ability to determine the effects of these general exercise programs on flexibility is complicated by the fact that many of these studies included stretching as part of the training regime, making it difficult to determine which of the exercises performed contributed to the changes in flexibility (Hurley & Hagberg, 1998). One innovative group examined the effects of 12 weeks of t'ai chi training on several fitness parameters including trunk flexibility in men and women 58 to 70 years of age (Lan et al., 1998). Trunk flexion increased 11° (21%), an amount that was significantly different from controls, who did not change over the 12-week study. However, because kyphosis (forward flexion of the upper spine) increases with age, improvements in trunk extension would be of greater benefit to older adults and this was not assessed in this study.

Few researchers have examined specialized stretch interventions to increase flexibility in older adults despite the decrements in joint range of motion seen with age (American College of Sports Medicine, 1998). Most of the studies involved small groups of older adults with short (6- to 10-week) interventions. One well-controlled study examined the effects of a specialized stretching training in a group of 20 older adults (mean age 71.8 years) randomly assigned a control or an experimental group (stretch training) for 10 weeks (Rider & Daly, 1991). The supervised stretching program took place 3 days per week, 30 to 40 min per session, and consisted of sit-and-reach maneuvers, knee tucks to the chest and pelvic lifts from the supine position, and back extension movements from the prone position. All stretches were held for 10 s with three repetitions. The experimental group improved in low back and hamstring flexibility (sit-and-reach) by 4.2 cm (25%) and spinal extension (prone hyperextension) by 7.2 cm (40%), but the control group did not change. This along with the other limited data would indicate that flexibility can be increased by range-of-motion exercises in healthy older adults and that such exercises should be included in any exercise program for older adults who want to improve mobility. However, specific "dose-response" guidelines (i.e., how many repetitions of the stretch, how long to hold the stretch, what specific stretches to do) are not yet available.

Osteoarthritis: Description, Risk Factors, and Causes

Arthritis encompasses all the rheumatic diseases that affect synovial joints and always involves damage to the articular cartilages. When the articular cartilage is damaged, it begins to break down and the cartilage changes from a slick, smooth gliding surface to a rough network of bristly collagen fibers. This bristly network of fibers increases friction, damaging the cartilage further so that eventually the articular surface may completely disappear, so that the two bones are articulating directly with each other. Immobilizing a joint is one of the causes of these degenerative changes. When motion ceases, so does circulation of synovial fluid, and the cartilages begin to suffer.

Osteoarthritis (OA), or degenerative joint disease, is one of the most prevalent chronic diseases, and the most common form of arthritis. OA is a leading cause of disability in the United States, affecting more than 21 million persons, most of whom (74%) are women (Arthritis Fact Sheet, n.d.). OA affects approximately one out of every two adults over age 65 and 85% of those 75 years of age and older (American Geriatrics Society Panel on Exercise and Osteoarthritis, 2001). OA accounts for more trouble with climbing stairs and walking than any other disease and is the most common reason for total hip and total knee replacements (Felson et al., 2000). OA can range from mild to very severe and affects hand as well as weight-bearing joints such as the hips, knees, feet, and back. It most often develops in joints that are injured by repeated overuse in the performance of a particular task or a favorite sport or from carrying around excess body weight. OA can be defined by symptoms and pathology. Injury or repeated impact wears away the hyaline articular cartilage with concomitant changes in the bone underneath the cartilage, including development of bone spurs, and in the soft-tissue structures in and around the joint. These structures may include inflammation of the synovial membrane, laxity in the ligaments, and weak muscles around the joint. Usually the first symptom a person has with OA is pain that worsens following exercise or immobility.

> Osteoarthritis affects approximately one out of every two adults over age 65 and 85% of those 75 years of age and older.

The causes of OA are not completely understood, but it seems clear that heredity, environmental, and lifestyle factors are involved. As with atherosclerotic heart disease, the risk of developing symptomatic OA is influenced by the presence of multiple risk factors. Some risk factors such as age, gender, and family history cannot be modified, whereas others such as obesity, muscular weakness, heavy physical activity, and inactivity are modifiable. Reducing or eliminating these risk factors may reduce the symptoms and disability associated with OA. Nevitt and his colleagues (2002) compared the prevalence of hip OA among 1506 adults over 60 years of age in Beijing, China, with two samples from the United States, those over the age of 65 from the Study of Osteoporotic Fracture (SOF) and those 60 to 74 years of age from the first National Health and Nutrition Examination Survey

(NHANES) population. The authors reported prevalences of 0.9% in Chinese women versus 3.8% to 5.5% in the samples of American women and 1.1% in Chinese men versus 4.5% reported for the sample of American men. Also, prevalence of OA with age did not increase in the Chinese population. These results indicate that hip OA was 80% to 90% less frequent in the Chinese than in white persons in the United States. The authors proposed that these cultural differences in hip OA prevalence could be attributable to differences in physical activities, a lower prevalence of obesity in the Chinese, and genetic factors. Perhaps the amount of squatting, a traditional resting and working posture in China, along with the additional walking involved in daily life helps to maintain the strength, endurance, and flexibility of the muscle, tendons, and joints at the hip and thereby helps prevent OA.

> Hip osteoarthritis was 80% to 90% less frequent in the Chinese sample of older adults than reported for older adults in the United States.

Age is the most consistent risk factor for OA, with the prevalence for OA greater after the age of 40 in women and 50 in men. Women more often have OA of the hand and knee, whereas the prevalence of hip OA is higher in men. Prospective, longitudinal studies, such as the 30-year Framingham Knee Osteoarthritis Study, which examined the relationship between body weight and OA, indicate that overweight men and women are at higher risk for OA than normal-weight individuals (Felson, 1997). However, randomized clinical trials have provided evidence that a reduction in OA symptoms is correlated more strongly with reduced body fat mass than with reduced total body weight (Toda et al., 1998). Moderate amounts of physical activity do not increase the risk for OA, but participation in occupations requiring strenuous physical activity or intense competitive sports activity throughout life may contribute to the development of OA (Felson, 1997). Other risk factors for developing OA include muscular weakness and reduced joint proprioception. Quadriceps weakness is common in individuals with knee OA, and this weakness is associated with joint instability and a reduced shock-absorbing capacity (Hurley & Hagberg, 1998). These people's muscles are probably weak because they avoid loading painful joints. However, quadriceps weakness is strongly associated with knee OA even in older adults without a history of knee pain. Therefore, quadriceps weakness not only is a consequence of knee OA but

is also a risk factor for knee OA (Ettinger et al., 1997; Slemenda et al., 1997).

Although no definitive treatment or cure for OA has been identified, the management of OA includes patient education, therapeutic modalities, exercise, and medications in parallel. The goals of treatment include reducing pain, maximizing functional independence, and improving quality of life within the constraints imposed by both OA and other comorbidities. The management of OA should be adjusted to the needs of the individual and should follow an algorithmic approach developed by the American Geriatrics Society Panel on Exercise and Osteoarthritis (2001). Flexibility, strength, and endurance exercises along with thermal modalities, such as ice or heat, are important nonpharmacological interventions.

Exercise Effects on Osteoarthritis

Little evidence suggests that exercise training can affect the pathological process of OA, but the evidence is clear that exercise training does not exacerbate pain or disease progression and can decrease pain and improve function (American Geriatrics Society Panel on Exercise and Osteoarthritis, 2001). In fact, regular physical activity can lead to the same physical, psychological, and functional benefits observed in the general population. One of the most important benefits of exercise training is improved strength, balance, and postural stability, which may reduce falls in this at-risk population (Ettinger et al., 1997; Messier et al., 2000). Both aerobic and strength training programs effectively improve physiological parameters related to functional capacity in older adults with OA. The increased strength and flexibility derived from exercise training programs can reduce pain. If the exercise is aerobic and is continued long enough, weight loss can occur, which will reduce the forces produced at the joints and thereby reduce pain.

Exercise also can increase a sense of well-being (chapter 11). Joisten and Albrecht (1992) suggested that appropriate sports activities could provide this very important benefit for arthritic patients. These authors pointed out that arthritis often diminishes the self-assurance and self-image of those with the condition, but the improvements in physical appearance, mood, or feeling that accrue from participation in physical activity counteract those diminished feelings. Sports activities are also excellent activities to involve individuals with arthritis disabilities in social interactions, situations that these people tend to avoid.

Many people have questioned whether a lifetime of heavy running aggravates and stresses joints to such an extent that runners develop OA. Information regarding the relationship between running and OA is scant, but the data does not support a negative effect on joints from regular running (Lane et al., 1986; Panush et al., 1986; Puhl et al., 1992). Running did not accelerate the development of OA in runners between the ages of 50 and 72 years (Lane et al., 1993). Lane and colleagues compared the incidence of bone spurs, sclerosis, and joint space narrowing in the same subjects between 1984 and 1989. Although the incidence of OA increased in both groups, the runners had not developed more arthritis than the nonrunners.

Skin: Taking the Brunt of the Environment for Years

The skin, or cutaneous membrane, is probably the most closely watched yet underappreciated organ of the body. It is the only organ we see every day, almost in its entirety. However, the skin has more than a cosmetic role, because it protects the body from environmental hazards, helps regulate body temperature, and contains sensory receptors that provide considerable information about the outside world. It is the interface between the internal body and the external world. The sense of touch, which comes from receptors in the skin, contributes important information that enables people to manipulate objects and maintain their balance. Touch also provides important, unique information about the environment. Babies want to touch and hold every object they see because they learn more about it through touch than by just seeing it, and this need to touch does not change over the life span. The skin is also important in communication. Touching, whether it is soft and gentle, direct, or harsh, conveys emotional expressions, and because emotional changes cause rapid circulatory adaptations, observing people's skin conveys information about their emotional state. Persons who are highly agitated or stressed may exhibit large red blotches across their necks and faces. Everyday speech conveys these observations: "He was so mad he was red-faced." "She was as white as a sheet." "You can talk until you are blue in the face and you won't convince him!"

Skin Composition

The skin is composed of two parts, the **epidermis,** the superficial epithelium, and the **dermis,** the underlying connective tissues. Although it is not usually considered to be a part of the skin, the **subcutaneous layer** separates the skin from the deep fascia around other organs, such as muscles and bones, and contains a large number of adipose (fat) cells. The fat cells provide padding, cushion shocks, act as an insulator to slow heat loss through the skin, and serve as packing or filler around structures.

The epidermis is composed of four to five layers with the top layer (skin surface) containing 15 to 30 rows of flattened, dead, and interlocking cells that form an extremely important barrier to the external environment. The innermost layers of the epidermis are living cells, which proliferate and reproduce. The cells in each successive layer of the epidermis are less and less able to reproduce themselves, so that those in the outer layer of the epidermis are dead cells, sloughed off daily.

The dermis, which is much thicker than the epidermis, lies immediately underneath the epidermis and contains collagen and elastic fibers that surround blood vessels, hair follicles, and nerves as well as sweat and oil glands. The interwoven collagen fibers provide considerable strength to the skin, and the extensive array of elastic fibers enables the skin to stretch and recoil repeatedly during normal movements. Oil (sebaceous) glands lubricate the skin and help keep it pliable. Nutrients are provided to the skin by the arteries located in the dermis and subcutaneous layers. Circulation to the skin is tightly regulated for two reasons. First, skin circulation plays a key role in thermoregulation, the control of body temperature, which helps individuals acclimate to hot or cold environments. When core body temperature increases, increased circulation to the skin permits the loss of excess heat via sweat produced by the sweat glands. Approximately 2 to 4 million sweat glands are distributed throughout the surface of the body. When body temperature decreases, reduced circulation to the skin promotes retention of body heat. The second reason skin circulation is strictly controlled is because total blood volume is relatively constant so that an increase in blood flow to the skin means a decreased blood flow to some other organs. Therefore, the circulatory, nervous, and endocrine systems work together to regulate blood flow to the skin while maintaining adequate blood flow to other organs and systems.

Skin Changes With Age

Skin is the tattletale of aging, and the media depicts the "beautiful" people as having flawless skin. Of course, photos of magazine models, with their airbrushed, poreless faces, are very different from the real-life versions. Aging, particularly of the skin, is fought aggressively every step of the way. Many people use the general appearance of the skin to estimate the overall health and age of a person, and clinicians can use the appearance of the skin to detect signs of underlying disease. For example, skin color changes from the presence of liver disease.

Some of the changes in the skin that occur with age include thinning of the epidermis and dermis, change in the collagen and elastic fibers in the dermis, reduced blood supply to the skin, and decreased activity of the oil and sweat glands.

Because the skin is constantly exposed to environmental stresses, such as ultraviolet radiation, heat, wind, chemicals, toxins, and mechanical pressure, it reveals its age. Of these environmental factors, the most consequential is sun exposure (Fusco, 2001). Some of the changes in the skin that occur with age include thinning of the epidermis and dermis, change in the collagen and elastic fibers in the dermis, reduced blood supply to the skin, and decreased activity of the oil and sweat glands. This decrease in sebum (oil) production with increasing age causes the skin to become dry and scaly. The decrease in activity of the sweat glands with aging makes it more difficult for older adults to dissipate heat and regulate core temperature. Living in hot, humid climates without the assistance of air conditioning can be life-threatening to older adults because of their decreased ability to regulate body temperature.

The decrease in activity of the sweat glands with aging makes it more difficult for older adults to dissipate heat and regulate core temperature.

The epidermis and dermis components of the skin thin with age. The aging epidermal cells do not reproduce as rapidly because blood profusion of these tissues decreases with age. The organization of the epidermal cells throughout cell turnover is not maintained well; consequently, skin cells become haphazardly grouped together and become dryer and rougher. Because of a preponderance of dead, scaly cells on the surface of the skin, the skin may become chalky in appearance.

Aging is also accompanied by a breakdown of collagen and elastin fibers, so that the dermis becomes weaker, thinner, and less pliable. The collagen fibers coarsen and collect in bundles. The elastin fibers become more cross-linked and more calcified (Par-

tridge, 1970). These changes in the resiliency and compliance of the skin can be observed by pinching a fold of skin on the back of the hand. Hold the skin in the pinch for a few seconds and then let go. The skin will return to its original shape, and the location of the pinch can no longer be seen. If 20 people representing ages 20 to 80 were to do this "pinch test" simultaneously, the 20-year-old's skin would return to normal almost instantaneously after releasing the skin, but the location of the pinched skin of the 80-year-old might be visible 10 or 15 s after release.

Contributing to these age-related changes in the quality of skin is that the circulation to the dermis decreases and becomes less efficient. The result of these inevitable age-related changes in the characteristics of skin is that it becomes paler, wounds do not heal as quickly, and the skin becomes more vulnerable to sun damage, less able to produce sweat, less efficient at thermoregulation, more permeable, and less able to produce an inflammatory response.

As skin becomes less and less resilient and compliant, losing tone and elasticity, the constant displacement of skin that occurs at joints and other places where the skin is pushed together or folded (e.g., when people smile, laugh, frown, and express other emotions) results in wrinkles. Each time a young person quits laughing, the skin that has been displaced returns to its original position. After thousands of laughs and many years, however, a stiffer, dryer, less elastic skin does not return as easily and begins to form folds. Consequently, wrinkles of skin, which begin forming early in life, become more and more visible. Wrinkles reflect the predominant positions of skin. Thus, people who frown most of the time have frown wrinkles on their foreheads, and people who smile most of the time have smile wrinkles around their mouths. Exposure to the sun accelerates the development of wrinkles, because the sun damages skin and makes it dryer. The constant squinting of the eyes and furrowing of the brow by people who are in the sun for long periods of time create large, multiple wrinkles in their skin.

Substantial evidence is available that smoking will age facial skin. In fact, the "smoker's face," with its yellowish skin and spiraling orbital lines, can be a deterrent to the aging person who does not want wrinkles. Early studies showed that while one is smoking there is a 30% decrease in oxygen to the skin (Fields, 2000). Nicotine and other by-products of smoke also affect the skin through the microvasculature. Individuals who have smoked for many years have skin that appears much older than their chronological age.

Above all, the sun has the greatest impact on aging skin. The sun has been linked to damage and proliferation of blood vessels, production of brown spots, thinning of the skin, fine and coarse wrinkles, texture changes, fragility of the skin, precancers, and ultimately cancers (Fields, 2000). Warren and colleagues (1991) used high-resolution facial photography, image analysis instrumentation to measure elasticity and histologic examinations to compare the faces of young (aged 25-31 years) and older (aged 45-51 years) women who had been exposed to either less than 2 hr of sun a week or greater than 12 hr of sun a week for the previous year. The researchers did not find a significant effect of chronic sun exposure on the elasticity, skin color, or wrinkles of the young women, but the results for the older women were very different. In the older high-sun-exposed group, significantly more wrinkles and less elasticity were present. Also, the older high-sun-exposure group was perceived by a panel of 24 untrained women judges, 20 to 60 years old, to be significantly older than the older women who were exposed to the sun very little. Perceived age and facial wrinkles were strongly correlated ($r = .85$), supporting the well-known observation that those with a high prevalence of facial wrinkles are perceived to be older than their chronological age. Comparing one's facial or hand skin to skin in areas never exposed to the sun further supports the fact that sun exposure is detrimental to skin.

Fortunately, sun damage can be prevented by the proper use of sunscreen, by wearing hats and protective clothing, by avoiding or limiting outdoor activities, and by some medications. For most effective protection, at least 1 oz (30 ml) of sunscreen (SPF 15 or higher) is needed to cover a person before sun exposure. Most people use only about one fourth that amount, and reapplication is needed every 2 hr. Wearing a hat will protect the face and should be a habit of individuals of all ages. People should avoid being outside during the times of the strongest sun exposure, 10 A.M. to 2 P.M., to help reduce sun damage to the skin. The only FDA-regulated drug therapy for the reversal of skin aging is tretinoin 0.05%, marketed as Renova (Fields, 2000). This can be applied as a cream and has been proven to change the function and structure of the skin so that there is an improvement in fine lines, brown spots, and texture of the skin. However, some undesirable side effects include scaling and redness. It has been suggested that postmenopausal estrogen use may prevent some of the negative changes associated with aging skin. The first large population-based study of the relationship between estrogen use and skin aging reported that postmenopausal estrogen use was associated with a 25% to 30% reduction in dry skin and skin wrinkling (Dunn et al., 1997). However, more longitudinal research is needed to further document this finding.

SUMMARY

Aging is associated with visible and sometimes dramatic changes in the body. Indeed, the relentless decline of the physical body is perhaps the most routinely used marker of chronological age. Both men and women lose height, but women lose more, faster. Losses of bone and the compression of cartilage between the vertebrae cause women especially to lose height and to develop the dowager's hump characteristic of osteoporosis. Both men and women gain weight until late middle age, at which time women's weights stabilize, then decline after 70 years of age, whereas men's weights decline after age 55. Although body weight stabilizes or declines in the later years, body composition continues to change. Younger men and women have about 15% to 25% body fat and about 36% to 45% muscle. Beginning in the late 20s and 30s, the ratio of body fat to muscle steadily increases. Muscle mass is lost and body fat increases, until average men and women in their 70s have between 30% and 40% body fat. The redistribution of body fat and muscle and the loss of height

result in a body mass index that continues to climb with age until about 70 years of age. The percent body fat and amount of fat free mass can be profoundly affected by the amount and type of physical exercise that a person experiences.

Bone loss begins to occur in the mid- to late 20s in everyone, regardless of gender, race, or geographic location. Losses occur in bone mass, bone density, and bone geometry, largely attributable to hormonal changes, dietary deficiencies, and physical inactivity. Women lose more bone faster than men, because they begin with less bone mass and they experience a more drastic hormonal change with age. Bone losses can be attenuated by hormonal therapy, diet, and exercise. Hormone replacement therapy has been the most effective way to prevent excessive bone loss in postmenopausal women, but increasing evidence has been found that exercise in postmenopausal women, particularly resistance training and weight-bearing aerobic exercise such as walking, can retard bone loss. Certain medications (in women) combined with an exercise program and a diet that includes all of the required nutrients, especially calcium, appears to be the best preventive measure against bone loss, osteoporosis, and bone fractures. Osteoporosis is a crippling disease characterized by low bone mass and microarchitectural deterioration of bone tissue that increases bone fragility and the risk of bone fractures. The factors that prevent bone loss—hormone replacement, diet, and exercise—are the same ones that reduce one's risk for osteoporosis. Bone loss is a major concern, because 50% of women and 13% of men in the United States will experience an osteoporosis-related fracture sometime in their life.

Another physical loss with age is that of flexibility. The range of motion at most joints is severely curtailed if stretching exercises are not performed regularly. Another factor that reduces flexibility is the development of OA, a degenerative disease of the joints in which the cartilaginous and ligamentous components of the joint become damaged, causing substantial pain and impaired mobility. Exercise is one part of a comprehensive arthritis treatment plan that includes rest and relaxation, proper diet, medication, instruction about proper use of joints and ways to conserve energy, and the use of pain relief methods. The best exercise program for those with OA is one that includes range of motion, strengthening, and endurance exercises. These exercises maintain or increase muscle mass as well as optimize body weight and range of joint motion, thus reducing workload at the joint.

In addition to the visible changes in physical appearance that occur, age-related changes in body composition also have implications for physical function and health. The redistribution of and increase in fat and the loss of muscle mass result in a substantial decrease in aerobic capacity. These changes in body composition in combination with the loss of bone mass and the development of osteoporosis and OA can result in decreased function of muscles (e.g., decreased strength) and organs (e.g., kidney and liver malfunction). Finally, increased body fat, particularly upper body or abdominal fat (expressed by higher BMIs), is associated with increased risk for cardiovascular disease and diabetes and earlier mortality.

The last physical changes discussed in this chapter were those that occur to the skin. Skin is the tattletale of aging—of all the physical changes that occur, those to the skin are the most obvious. Much of the damage that occurs to the skin over a lifetime is attributable to sun exposure; consequently a substantial amount of age-related skin degradation can be prevented by protecting the skin from the sun.

REVIEW QUESTIONS

1. Graphically depict changes in height, weight, and body mass index across the life span and describe several factors that might affect these changes in older adults.

2. What changes in fat mass and fat-free mass occur after age 25? Older adults who have excessive intra-abdominal fat are at increased risk for what? Why is there a concern if older adults experience a sudden weight loss?

3. Those at greatest risk for increased disability and mortality are those with sarcopenia and obesity. Explain what is meant by this statement and what can be done to prevent sarcopenia and obesity.

4. Why is the use of growth hormone for increasing fat-free mass and decreasing fat mass not recommended at this time?

5. What factors affect bone health and risk for osteoporosis?

6. Describe the change in flexibility with aging. Why should strengthening of the trunk extensors and stretching of the trunk flexors be important components of an exercise program for older adults?

7. What can be done to decrease the aging of skin?

SUGGESTED READINGS

Beck, B.R., & Snow, C.M. (2003). Bone health across the lifespan—Exercising our options. *Exercise and Sport Sciences Reviews, 31*, 117-122.

Karlsson, M. (2004). Has exercise an antifracture efficacy in women? *Scandinavian Journal of Medicine and Science in Sport, 14*, 2-15.

National Institutes of Health. (2001). NIH Consensus Development Panel on Osteoporosis Prevention, Diagnosis, and Therapy. *Journal of the American Medical Association, 285,* 785-795.

Nelson, H.D. (2002). Assessing benefits and harms of hormone replacement therapy: Clinical applications. *Journal of the American Medical Association, 288,* 882-884.

Rosen, C.J. (2003). Restoring aging bones. *Scientific American, 288,* 70-77.

World Health Organization. (1998). *Obesity: Preventing and managing the global epidemic. Report of a WHO consultation on obesity.* Geneva, Switzerland: World Health Organization.

Cardiovascular and Pulmonary Function

Holden MacRae
Pepperdine University

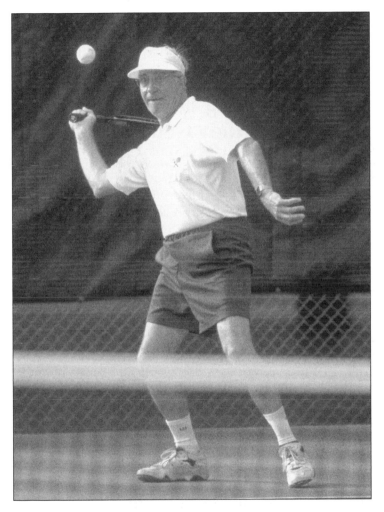

The objectives of this chapter are

- to describe the changes in the structure and function of the cardiovascular system with age;

- to detail how aging affects the structure and function of the respiratory system; and,

- to clarify the extent to which regular physical activity may postpone age-related declines in the cardiovascular and respiratory systems.

Heart disease has been the leading cause of death for persons 65 years of age and older for the past 2 decades, accounting for nearly a million deaths in 1997. Approximately 35% of all deaths are attributable to heart disease, including heart attacks and chronic ischemic heart disease. Other important chronic diseases among persons 65 years of age and older include stroke, chronic obstructive pulmonary diseases, diabetes, and pneumonia or influenza. As seen in table 4.1, four of the top five causes of death are attributable to deterioration in the cardiovascular and respiratory systems, and this is seen across ethnic groups. How aging affects the cardiovascular and respiratory systems, and how regular exercise helps maintain the function of these systems, will be the focus of this chapter.

The capacity to perform physical work draws on the function of several interrelated and interdependent systems. The structure and function of the heart, lungs, arteries, and veins and the ability of these systems to use oxygen to produce energy over an extended period are crucial to independent physical functioning. In youth, routine activities of daily living place minimal physical demands on these systems, and therefore physical capacity differences between physically fit and nonphysically fit young persons are not obvious. These differences only become observable when dynamic physical exertion is demanded, such as dashing up a long flight of stairs, loading heavy boxes onto a vehicle, or running a mile. With increasing age, however, less physically demanding tasks require increasingly more of the physical work capacity reserves, particularly for those who are sedentary. Early in life, increased age provides developmental processes necessary to reach the peak potential of physical performance. After the second decade of life, however, aging begins to erode many functions, whereas exercise training enhances the function of physiological systems. Aging and chronic exercise, therefore, drive several key body functions in opposite directions. Aging degrades the systems that support physical work capacity, whereas systematic exercise generally enhances these systems. Therefore, the amount of physical activity in one's lifestyle is a highly significant determinant of individual differences in the physical work capacity of older adults.

> Four of the top five causes of death in adults are attributable to deterioration of the cardiovascular and respiratory system. Aging and disuse degrade these systems, whereas systematic exercise generally enhances them.

Aging Effects on the Cardiovascular System

The cardiovascular system is responsible for transporting all the substances essential for cellular metabolism and for protecting the body against blood loss (clotting) and foreign microbes or toxins introduced into the body. To maintain homeostasis, the cardiovascular system must deliver oxygen and nutrients and remove waste products from all living body cells. The cardiovascular system can be compared to a cooling system in a car, with the basic components including the circulating fluid (blood), a pump (heart), and an assortment of conducting pipes (arteries and veins). The optimal functioning of each of these components is necessary for maximal health, physical function, and quality of life. In resting conditions, such as being seated in a chair, cardiovascular parameters in a healthy adult change so little with aging, except for systolic **blood pressure**, that they are adequate to meet the body's need for blood pressure and blood flow (Gerstenblith et al.,

Table 4.1 Leading Causes of Death for Persons 65 Years of Age and Older in the United States

White	African American	American Indian	Asian/Pacific Islander	Hispanic
1. Heart disease	Heart disease	Heart disease	Heart disease	Heart disease
2. Cancer	Cancer	Cancer	Cancer	Cancer
3. Stroke	Stroke	Diabetes	Stroke	Stroke
4. COPD	Diabetes	Stroke	Pneu/influenza	COPD
5. Pneu/influenza	Pneu/influenza	COPD	COPD	Pneu/influenza

Note: COPD = chronic obstructive pulmonary disease; Pneu = pneumonia.

Data from Sahyoun et al. (2001).

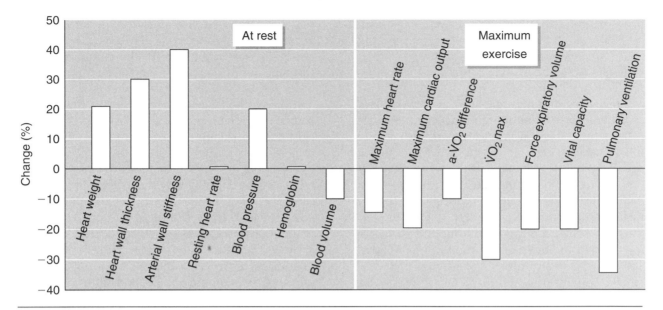

Figure 4.1 Changes in selected measures of cardiovascular and respiratory function in sedentary, untrained older adults.

1987; Lakatta, 2002). The cardiovascular response to exercise, however, is greatly reduced in the average older adult. The contrast in aging effects on resting and exercise cardiovascular performance can be seen in figure 4.1, where resting parameters change only moderately but some of the exercise responses decline substantially.

Differences in cardiovascular function between older and younger individuals have been extensively described in the literature. However, confusion often arises in interpreting these differences because of a failure to acknowledge, or to control for, interactions among age, disease, and inactivity. Genetic components of age, disease, and inactivity, which remain largely unknown, complicate the picture even more.

Heart Structure and Control

The primary structural changes of the aging cardiovascular system include an increased thickening of the walls of the blood vessels and left ventricle, an increased stiffness in the aorta and arterial tree, and an increase in size of the left atrial chamber of the heart (Lakatta, 2002). There is some evidence of a decrease in heart cell number and enlargement in heart cell size, which might modify contractility of the heart, but these changes are not thought to lead to functional abnormalities in most older adults.

With advancing age, the internal layer of the large arteries (tunica intima) thickens and fragments, a process similar to what occurs in early stages of atherosclerosis. Recent epidemiological evidence

suggests that the thickening of the vessel walls is a strong predictor of stroke and cardiovascular disease (O'Leary et al., 1999). The left ventricle of the heart, which pumps blood to all portions of the body except the lungs, increases in wall thickness approximately 30% between the ages of 25 and 80. This change may occur as a compensation for the age-related increases in systolic blood pressure (Fleg, 1986; Lakatta, 1990). As blood pressure increases, the heart muscle has to work harder. The heart muscle, like an arm or leg muscle, hypertrophies with additional work, and thus the ventricle walls grow thicker. However, the ventricular cavity dimensions and systolic ventricular function during rest, as a result of either aging or regular physical activity, are unaffected by the ventricular wall thickening.

The aorta and the arterial tree become thicker and less compliant (increase stiffness) with aging, a factor that contributes to increased systolic blood pressure and imposes a greater load on the heart (Fleg, 1986). In healthy sedentary men and women, there was a 40% to 50% mean decrease in carotid artery compliance between those 25 and 75 years of age (Tanaka et al., 2000). Very small arteries, the arterioles, also become less responsive during physical activity to neurohumoral cues for dilation, thus remaining inappropriately constricted. These changes, plus increased peripheral resistance, are the major contributors to the development of high blood pressure, also known as **hypertension** (Safar, 1990). Despite these age-related changes, heart function in the nondiseased aged individual is adequate for resting and light physical work. The development of **atherosclerosis**, however, significantly alters cardiovascular structure and function in most aged people and, in combination with hypertension, forces the cardiovascular system to work under a substantial stress even during relatively light physical work.

Efficient communication between the nervous and cardiovascular systems is required for optimal physical function. This communication occurs largely via the autonomic nervous system, which acts through parasympathetic and sympathetic nerves. Parasympathetic nerve fibers innervate the pacemaker of the heart, releasing acetylcholine, which slows the heart rate. Sympathetic nerve fibers innervate the heart muscle itself and release norepinephrine, increasing the rate and force of contractions. Sympathetic activation also stimulates the adrenal medulla to release epinephrine and norepinephrine (catecholamines). Resting levels of norepinephrine are not higher in older persons, but when measured during submaximal and maximal exercise, norepinephrine levels are elevated compared with those of younger people. Conversely, epinephrine levels are higher in older persons under all conditions: resting, submaximal exercise, and maximal exercise (Fleg et al., 1985).

With aging, the heart and vasculature become less sensitive to stimulation via the catecholaminergic hormones; thus, the aging heart cannot achieve the maximum heart rate levels that were possible during youth. Cardiovascular adaptation to the onset and offset of exercise also slows. The age-related impairment of hormonal response is an important limiting factor of cardiovascular performance during physical stress. In fact, this loss is thought to be one of the primary changes in cardiovascular function that occurs with aging in normal individuals who are free of cardiovascular disease (Lakatta, 1986).

Total peripheral resistance represents the ease with which blood can flow from the smallest arteries (arterioles) into the capillaries. Enlarging the radius of the arterioles decreases total peripheral resistance. Total peripheral resistance increases about 1% a year with aging, even in the absence of coronary artery disease, attributable partly to increased rigidity of arterial vessels and partly to decreased biochemical mechanisms of vasodilation. Regulation of vasodilation is via α- and ß-receptors. α-receptors are found on all smooth muscle cells in the walls of the arterial tree, whereas there are very few in the heart itself. Thus, α-receptor-mediated activity primarily assists the blood vessels in constricting through smooth muscle contraction, whereas ß-receptor-mediated stimulation causes smooth muscles to relax and blood vessels to dilate. With aging, the arterial wall smooth muscle becomes less sensitive, largely attributable to a decreased number of ß-receptors, and hence less responsive to the dilator effects of catecholamines. α-receptor-mediated responsiveness of the vasculature appears to remain intact (Lakatta, 1986), but the decrease in ß-receptors changes the balance between α- and ß-receptor function, so that peripheral vasculature tends toward vasoconstriction, thus increasing total peripheral resistance. One of the consequences of this increase in total peripheral resistance is a chronic increase in mean arterial pressure.

Age-related changes in neural control mechanisms of the arterial tree are also seen in **postural hypotension,** which is the result of a loss in responsiveness of homeostatic reflexes. When young individuals rise quickly from a supine or seated position, their heart rate and blood pressure also increase to ensure an adequate blood supply to the brain. Baroreceptors in the aortic arch and the carotid sinus are sensitive to changes in blood pressure and initiate reflex cardiovascular responses such as an increased heart rate to maintain systemic blood pressure. These baroreflexes assist in maintaining blood flow to vital organs when systemic blood pressure suddenly decreases. When many older adults move suddenly from a lying to a standing position, however, the baroreflexor response is inadequate, and systemic blood pressure decreases substantially. This condition, postural hypotension, causes dizziness, confusion, weakness, or fainting. Age-related declines in baroreceptor reflex function occur even if the lack of response is not severe enough to be expressed as postural hypotension. Postural hypotension is fairly common in older adults, ranging from 22% to 30% in the young-old and 30% to 50% in those more than 75 years of age (Docherty, 1990).

Increased arterial wall stiffness and thickness, a decline in hormonal sensitivity, an increase in total peripheral resistance, and decreased responsiveness to homeostatic reflexes occur in the aging cardiovascular system.

Heart Function

The function of the heart is a major player in the quality of life that adults can enjoy in their older decades. In fact, for many of the oldest-old, the function of their heart is a central focus. Descriptions of function include heart rate, stroke volume, cardiac output, the arteriovenous oxygen difference, and the maintenance of proper systolic and diastolic blood pressure.

Heart Rate

The average resting heart rates of older adults are not significantly different from those of young adults, although the younger heart rates are more variable (Lipsitz, 1989). The maximum rate at which the heart can beat during heavy exercise, however, decreases about 5 to 10 beats a decade (Shepherd, 1987), and no amount of training seems to be able to halt this inevitable decline. This aging effect reflects reduced medullary outflow of sympathetic activity (depressed ß-receptor-mediated stimulation) and occurs similarly in men and women (Seals et al., 1994).

The average maximum heart rates of young (aged 24-28) and older (aged 50-68) trained and untrained men, taken from 15 research studies, are shown in figure 4.2. In all of these studies, the maximum heart rate was higher for the young men than for the older men, and exercise training did not affect maximum heart rate in the young or older men. Estimation of maximum heart rate is one of the most commonly used values in clinical medicine and physiology, because maximum exercise testing of older individuals is not feasible in many settings. Maximal heart rate is often estimated using the age-predicted equation of 220 – age. However, a combined meta-analytic and laboratory-based study revealed that this equation underestimates maximal heart rate for those individuals over 40 years of age. As such, the regression recommended for maximal heart rate is 208 – 0.7 × age in healthy adults over 40, and this estimation is independent of gender and habitual physical activity status (Tanaka et al., 2001).

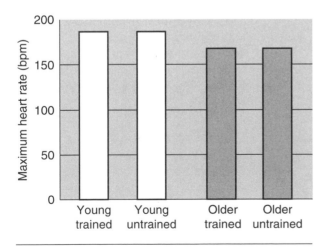

Figure 4.2 Maximum heart rate for young and older, trained and untrained men. Age means and standard deviations were young trained = 27.1 ± 2.4; young untrained = 26.4 ± 2.0; older trained = 61.6 ±4.9; older untrained = 59.1 ± 8.9.

Stroke Volume

Stroke volume (SV) is the amount of blood (in milliliters) that is pumped from the heart with each beat. The heart has the ability to regulate the strength of its own contractions. If a greater amount of blood is returned to the heart from the peripheral circulation, it increases the amount of blood in the heart's ventricles and stretches the heart wall. The heart responds by contracting more vigorously. In this way, the heart can respond to increased work demands by increasing the SV. Stroke volume in the aging heart has been reported to decrease moderately, but this observation is questionable because the subjects studied were not screened for coronary artery disease. In studies where subjects were screened to exclude coronary artery disease, resting supine SV showed little change with aging in men or women (Lakatta, 2002).

Cardiac Output

Cardiac output (Q) is the total amount of blood ejected from each ventricle of the heart in 1 min expressed in liters per minute ($L \cdot min^{-1}$). In exercise, cardiac output represents the ability of the cardiovascular system to deliver oxygen and nutrients to the exercising muscles. Cardiac output also can be expressed relative to body size (divided by an estimate of body surface area). This ratio is called the cardiac index. Maximum cardiac output is calculated by multiplying the total amount of blood that can be ejected in one heart contraction (the maximum SV) by the total number of times the heart can beat in one time period (the maximum heart rate). The higher the volume of blood pumped to the periphery, the greater the potential for oxygen transport and uptake. At rest, the cardiac index of healthy 80-year-olds is not different from that of 20-year-olds, but during exhaustive upright exercise there is a 25% decrease in cardiac index in the older adults compared with young adults (Lakata & Sollott, 2002).

> Resting heart rate, stroke volume, and cardiac index show little change with age in healthy older adults. However, maximal heart rate declines about one beat per year after age 20, and the cardiac index, during maximal exercise, is reduced by approximately 25% in healthy men and women in their 80s compared with healthy 20-year-olds.

Using the Oxygen That Is Circulated: The Arteriovenous Oxygen Difference

At the tissue level, some of the oxygen carried by arterial blood diffuses from the capillary, where it is highly concentrated, across the capillary membrane to the active tissue. There, oxygen is consumed and carbon dioxide is generated when food (glucose and fats) is metabolized to provide usable energy. Therefore, blood that has traversed the tissue capillary bed and entered the veins has less oxygen. The **arteriovenous oxygen difference,** or (a-$\bar{v}$)O$_2$ difference, is the difference between the amount of oxygen transported in the arterial blood and the amount transported in the mixed venous blood. At rest, the oxygen content of arterial blood is around 20 ml · 100^{-1} ml of blood, whereas the mixed venous blood has an oxygen content of around 15 ml · 100^{-1} ml of blood. Thus, the resting (a-$\bar{v}$)O$_2$ difference is 5 ml · 100^{-1} ml of blood. This value reflects the amount of oxygen extracted by the tissues of the body. Little information is available on the effects of aging on (a-$\bar{v}$)O$_2$ difference at rest or during exercise. It appears that resting (a-$\bar{v}$)O$_2$ difference decreases with increasing age, so that the resting values for a 65-year-old male are approximately 20% to 30% lower than those of a 25-year-old male. Maximal (a-$\bar{v}$)O$_2$ difference values for older men and women performing heavy exercise are also lower than (a-$\bar{v}$)O$_2$ difference values for young adults by approximately 10% to 12% (Spina, 1999).

Blood Pressure

Arterial blood pressure reflects the combined effects of arterial blood flow per minute (cardiac output) and the resistance to that flow offered by the peripheral blood vessels. At rest, the highest pressure generated by the heart during ventricular contraction is referred to as **systolic blood pressure,** which provides an estimate of the work of the heart and the force that blood exerts against the arterial walls. During the heart's relaxation phase, when the aortic valves close, the natural elastic recoil of the arterial system provides a continuous head pressure. This maintains a steady flow of blood into the peripheral blood vessels until the next surge of blood. This relaxation phase is referred to as the **diastolic blood pressure** and is indicative of peripheral resistance encountered, or the ease with which blood is circulated to organs or muscles from the arterioles into the capillaries.

With aging, systolic and diastolic blood pressures are increased because of (a) arteries that have become hardened with fatty material deposited within their walls or thickened connective tissue layer or (b) arteries that offer excessive resistance to peripheral blood flow because of neural hyperactivity or because of kidney malfunction (McArdle et al., 2001). A systolic pressure greater than 140 mmHg or a diastolic pressure greater than 90 mmHg is viewed as borderline high blood pressure (hypertensive). At least 60% of men and close to 70% of women over age 65 have hypertension (National Center for Health Statistics, 2001). This percentage is alarming, because 65% to 70% of fatal and nonfatal cardiovascular events occur in hypertensive individuals (Klag et al., 1990). A high resting systolic pressure is also related to postural hypotension, which is one of the causes of falls in older adults (Harris et al., 1991). Postural hypotension, discussed earlier in this chapter, occurs when an individual suddenly changes position (e.g., stands up from being seated for a while) and the blood pressure to the brain cannot be adequately maintained, so the person may become dizzy or faint, leading to a fall. Controlling hypertension in older adults is important for optimizing health and preventing heart attacks and falls.

Exercise Effects on the Cardiovascular Function of Older Adults

An important ingredient for healthy aging is to maintain a physically active lifestyle (Shiraki et al., 2001). Regular physical activity or exercise reduces the risk for morbidity and mortality from cardiovascular disease, cancer, high blood pressure, osteoporosis, bone fractures, diabetes, and depression (American College of Sports Medicine, 1998b; Paffenbarger & Lee, 1996). Consistent exercise also

National Heart, Lung, and Blood Institute 2004 Blood Pressure Guidelines

This table presents ranges for normal through Stage II hypertensive blood pressure.

Blood pressure status	Systolic blood pressure (mmHg)	Diastolic blood pressure (mmHg)
Normal	<120	<80
Prehypertensive	120-139	80-89
Stage I	140-159	90-99
Stage II	>160	>100

From Joint National Committee on Prevention, Detection, Evaluation and Treatment of High Blood Pressure (2004).

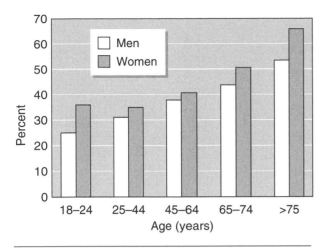

Figure 4.3 Percent of adults who are inactive (i.e., never engage in any physical activity for as long as 10 min at a time) by age and gender: United States, 1997–1998.

is associated with improvements in body composition, fitness, longevity, ability to perform activities of daily activities, and management of arthritis or other conditions that might limit physical activity (DiPetro, 1996; Shepherd et al., 1995). Unfortunately, adults become less physically active with age so that by 75 years of age, 54% of men and 66% of women report no physical activity (figure 4.3). This means that these older adults never engage in any leisure-time physical activity for as long as 10 min at a time. Women are less physically active than men across the life span.

The recruitment of skeletal muscle during exercise results in an increase in oxygen consumption (VO_2) so that energy in the form of adenosine triphosphate can be generated from the catabolism of carbohydrate and fat. The more intense the level of exercise, the greater the oxygen requirement. VO_2 increases as a linear function with increasing exercise intensity and will reach a maximal value ($\dot{V}O_2$max) at exhaustion. The $\dot{V}O_2$max, used interchangeably with **maximal aerobic capacity** or aerobic power, reflects the maximal rate at which oxygen can be taken up, distributed, and used by the body during exercise that engages a large muscle mass. Every individual has a functional limit of the cardiovascular system; that is, during progressively increasing exercise stress, the cardiovascular system will no longer be able to increase delivery, distribution, exchange, and return of blood. This functional limit occurs at the $\dot{V}O_2$max and is a reproducible characteristic of an individual (as are height and weight) that varies little on a day-to-day basis. $\dot{V}O_2$max is viewed as the single best variable to define the overall physiological changes that occur with aging (Mazzeo et al., 1998). However, determining the effects of age on

$\dot{V}O_2$max is confounded by a number of factors, such as the physical activity of the individual, underlying coronary artery disease, and gains in body weight, particularly body fat (Spina, 1999).

$\dot{V}O_2$max, in cross-sectionally derived averages from sedentary adults, declines approximately 1% per year for each year after age 25. Figure 4.4 shows $\dot{V}O_2$max values, gleaned from many studies in the literature, for four categories of physical activity: athletes, physically active adults, short-term trained adults, and sedentary adults. It is very clear from this graph that $\dot{V}O_2$max declines with aging, irrespective of the amount of training that an individual undergoes. All of the regression lines in figure 4.4 have a downward slope. This decline in $\dot{V}O_2$max with age is even greater when measured in longitudinal research designs than when measured in cross-sectional designs, probably because subjects at older ages who volunteer to be measured in cross-sectional fitness studies tend to be more physically fit than those who do not volunteer. This is an example of the discussion in chapter 2 about how system decline appears to be different depending on the research study design (figure 2.7b, p. 42). Extrapolating this average rate of decline shown in figure 4.4 reduces aerobic capacity by age 100 to a level in which the maximal oxygen consumption would be equivalent to resting oxygen consumption in a 20-year-old adult. As such, the ability of very old individuals to perform even the most basic activities of daily living can be severely compromised.

A minimum $\dot{V}O_2$max of 13 ml $\cdot$ kg^{-1} $\cdot$ min^{-1} is considered necessary for independent living. The decreased $\dot{V}O_2$max that accompanies aging may accelerate from age 65 to 75 and again from 75 to 85. Thus, if the downward slope of $\dot{V}O_2$max in figure 4.4 is followed to these older ages, it is apparent that the

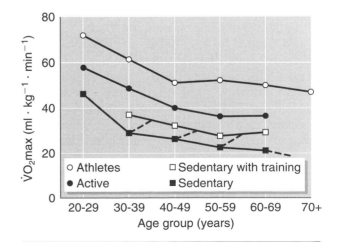

Figure 4.4 Average maximal oxygen consumption by age and physical activity level.

oxygen delivery and utilization system of many of the least fit older individuals falls below the minimum necessary to maintain an independent lifestyle (Shepherd, 1987), and many 65-year-old sedentary people are poised perilously near the edge of disability.

A number of early studies suggested that endurance training in older men and women did not improve their $\dot{V}O_2$max. However, these studies generally were very short or included low-intensity exercise. Later studies showed that longer endurance training programs of moderate to high intensity elicited increases in $\dot{V}O_2$max in older adults similar in relative magnitude to those seen in young adults. The effects of endurance training on $\dot{V}O_2$max in sedentary, active, and masters athletes of different ages are presented in figure 4.4. Training in older persons raises the overall level of maximal oxygen consumption, in some cases higher than the values seen in much younger individuals. Thus, trained adults at any age are on a higher parallel-aging curve than untrained individuals. The highest levels of $\dot{V}O_2$max, at any age, are those exhibited by competitive runners who maintain an intense, daily training schedule and who compete regularly. The studies on "masters athletes" are discussed in more detail later in this chapter. The "sedentary with training" line in figure 4.4 shows that when middle-aged or older individuals begin a training program, they can achieve improvements similar to young adults, ranging from 10% to 30%, depending on intensity and duration of training (American College of Sports Medicine, 1998b; Hagberg et al., 1989; Spina, 1999). The "sedentary with training" group line represents the average of the improvements made by sedentary older groups in several different studies. The small dotted lines that go from the "sedentary" to the "sedentary with training" lines represent the improvements that might be predicted for sedentary groups at each age who undergo exercise-training programs.

Older individuals do not achieve the same absolute gains in maximal oxygen consumption (milliliters per kilograms per minute) that younger people achieve, but their relative gains (percent increase) are very similar. Even the oldest age groups respond favorably to physical conditioning if the exercise programs are individually prescribed, cautiously increased, and carefully supervised by professionals. In nursing home residents and frail but independent elderly, who have been sedentary all their lives, even low-intensity programs provide an adequate training stimulus for increasing $\dot{V}O_2$max (Binder et al., 2002).

It is clear that older adults can derive great benefits from a consistent exercise program. The American College of Sports Medicine in their position stand on physical activity and older adults stated that contraindications to exercise in frail and extremely old adults are not different from those applicable in younger, healthier adults and "in general, frailty or extreme age is not a contraindication to exercise" (1998b, p. 1001). But to maintain aerobic capacity, exercise must be performed throughout life. Marti and Howald (1990) showed that even former highly trained runners decreased in aerobic capacity and increased body fat if they did not continue training.

Shepherd (1987) suggested that an increase in $\dot{V}O_2$max of 20% is not trivial. He maintained that a gain of this size "offers the equivalent of 20 years of rejuvenation—a benefit that can be matched by no other treatment or lifestyle change" (1987, p. 5).

Changes in Cardiac Output and (a-$\bar{v}$)O$_2$ Difference in Response to Exercise Training

In healthy older adults, cardiac output (heart rate and SV) and (a-$\bar{v}$)O$_2$ difference respond to exercise in a manner similar to that of young adults. Heart rate is generally elevated in anticipation of an exercise bout. That is, the heart rate may be elevated by as much as 20 to 30 beats · min^{-1} before the onset of exercise attributable to an increase in the activation of the sympathetic nervous system. Release of both norepinephrine from sympathetic nerve endings and epinephrine from the adrenal medulla contributes to the elevated heart rate in anticipation of the onset of exercise. Once exercise begins, heart rate increases in proportion to the intensity of exercise will stabilize if the exercise intensity is low but will take longer to plateau if the exercise intensity is high. The increase in heart rate will plateau, as the individual approaches exhaustion, indicating that the maximal heart rate has been reached. Longitudinal assessment of changes in maximum heart rate with age demonstrate that maximum heart rate declines with advancing age and this decline is not attenuated by exercise training (Hawkins et al., 2001; Kasch et al., 1999; Katzel et al., 2001; Pollock et al., 1997). Unlike the heart rate response to exercise, SV increases linearly with increasing exercise intensity but only up to heart rates of around 110 to 120 beats · min^{-1}. Increasing exercise intensity beyond this heart rate leads to only small increases in SV.

One of the consequences of exercise training, particularly endurance training, is that the sinus node of the heart is hyperpolarized by the increased release of acetylcholine attributable to a higher tone (increased firing rate) of the parasympathetic vagus nerve. Additionally, this type of exercise training also decreases resting sympathetic nerve activity. The observed effect of these nervous system adaptations is a reduction in the resting heart rate. Resting heart rates in healthy endurance-trained individuals are typically around 50 beats $\cdot$ min^{-1}. However, values below 30 beats $\cdot$ min^{-1} have also been reported. The consequence of this lower resting HR is that resting SV increases to around 100 ml $\cdot$ beat^{-1} in men and 80 ml $\cdot$ beat^{-1} in women after a period of endurance exercise training. An unresolved issue related to this observed increase in SV is whether the bradycardia (slow HR, i.e., HR below 60 beats $\cdot$ min^{-1}) resulting from endurance training "causes" a larger SV, or whether the heart improves its contractility, thereby increasing SV and thus requiring a lower rate of contraction to achieve the resting cardiac output.

The major component mediating the decline with age in $\dot{V}O_2$max is a decline in cardiac output, a function of the decrease in maximum heart rate and SV. Additionally, there is a decline in $(a-\bar{v})O_2$ difference. Although endurance training has been shown to improve aerobic capacity, regardless of age, the mechanisms involved in the training-induced increases in $\dot{V}O_2$max appear to be different for older men and women, even when the increases in $\dot{V}O_2$max with training are similar. In older men, approximately two thirds of the increase in $\dot{V}O_2$max is attributable to an increase in cardiac output with the other one third attributable to greater $(a-\bar{v})O_2$ difference. However, in women, the increase in $\dot{V}O_2$max is solely attributable to peripheral adaptations, that is, an increase in $(a-\bar{v})O_2$ difference (Spina, 1999). This gender difference reported in older adults is not seen in younger men and women, who respond to training with similar adaptations. The differences in the response of maximal cardiac output of older postmenopausal women, compared with older men and young men and women, suggest that sex hormones may play a role in normal cardiovascular adaptations to training. For example, in one study older women did not develop the same left ventricular hypertrophy in response to exercise training that has been reported in young men and women and older men (Spina, 1999). However, further research is needed to adequately determine why there is the gender difference in older adults who undergo endurance training.

Improvement in $\dot{V}O_2$max with endurance exercise training in older men is attributable to augmented cardiac output and $(a-\bar{v})O_2$ difference. In contrast, the increase in $\dot{V}O_2$max in older women is solely caused by peripheral adaptations, that is, $(a-\bar{v})O_2$ difference.

Few researchers have longitudinally examined the effects of age on aerobic capacity and the mechanisms responsible for these changes. One longitudinal study stands out, however, because the effects of two endurance training programs separated by a period of 30 years were analyzed (McGuire et al., 2001). In 1966, five healthy 20-year-old men underwent 3 weeks of bed rest followed by 2 months of intensive exercise training, resulting in an 18% increase in $\dot{V}O_2$max. Thirty years later, when these men were in their 50s, they were reassessed and trained for 6 months using a similar exercise-training program. After the 6 months of endurance training, $\dot{V}O_2$max increased by 14%, and thus aerobic capacity was returned to the pretraining levels exhibited 30 years earlier. However, despite the improvement in aerobic capacity with training, no individual attained the $\dot{V}O_2$max that was achieved after training 30 years earlier. The mechanism responsible for the recovery of $\dot{V}O_2$max in these 50-year-old men was predominantly a peripheral adaptation to training, that is, an increase in the maximal $(a-\bar{v})O_2$ difference. In contrast, maximal cardiac output was unchanged over the 30 years even though maximal heart rate declined by 12 beats $\cdot$ min^{-1}. Maintenance of maximal cardiac output was

Sexual Function and Physical Activity

A recent study examined the association between age and erectile dysfunction in 31,742 men, aged 53 to 90, a cohort in the Health Professionals Follow-up Study. When men with prostate cancer were excluded, the prevalence of erectile dysfunction in the previous 3 months was 33%. There was a 10-fold increase in relative risk for erectile dysfunction in the 80-year-old men compared with those in their early 50s, regardless of health states or previous erectile function. The modifiable health behaviors most strongly associated with maintenance of good erectile function were physical activity and leanness. Men who had no chronic medical conditions and engaged in these healthy behaviors had the lowest prevalence of erectile dysfunction (Bacon et al., 2003).

therefore accomplished by an increase in maximal SV. The authors concluded that 3 weeks of bed rest when the subjects were 20 years old had a more profound impact on the men's cardiovascular power than 30 years of aging.

Exercise Training Effects on Blood Constituents, Flow, and Pressure

The ability to transport and deliver oxygen to organs and tissues is also dependent on the number of red blood cells and hence hemoglobin content of the blood. **Anemia** is prevalent among older individuals, especially those over age 70, but it is difficult to tell whether the decline in hematocrit and hemoglobin values is a function of aging or of other more indirect factors. In a review of 1,024 medical history charts, 17.7% of males and 8.4% of females were classified as anemic (Timiras & Brownstein, 1987). A major cause of anemia in older individuals is change in diet, which may entail not only a decrease in total calories per day but also changes in types of food consumed. Many older people, especially those living alone, are challenged by loss of appetite, impaired mobility to obtain groceries, reduced income to purchase food, and lowered capacity to cook, just to name a few. Other age-related contributors to anemia may be unrecognized internal bleeding or deterioration of gastrointestinal absorption of iron or vitamin B_{12}. Some evidence suggests, however, that mean hemoglobin levels are not different in older adults, except in males over 85, and should not be expected to change with advancing age.

Frequency of exercise, rather than intensity, is more important for optimizing blood pressure. Daily exercise is the most beneficial activity.

Endurance training greatly improves peripheral blood flow, regardless of age or gender. Hagberg and colleagues (1985) reported that the peripheral resistance of older male masters athletes who had engaged in strenuous physical training for many years was nearly 30% lower during exercise than that of their sedentary age-matched peers. This response of the peripheral vasculature to training also occurs rather quickly in both young and old adults. After only a few months of training, sedentary older subjects can achieve the same peripheral blood flow responses to exercise that are exhibited by highly trained older road racers (Martin et al., 1990). The physical conditioning of the peripheral vasculature is related more to the occurrence of physical activity per se than to a high exercise capacity (Martin et al., 1991). Of course,

in older individuals who have pathological peripheral circulation conditions such as phlebitis or intermittent claudication, peripheral blood flow is impaired and exercise capacity is limited.

Regular aerobic exercise has been shown to be effective in reducing high blood pressure in older adults. Immediately following an exercise bout, the systolic blood pressure of hypertensive men falls below pre-exercise values by 20 to 30 mmHg and that of normotensive men by 8 to 12 mmHg. This effect lasts approximately 2 hr in healthy individuals and as much as 12 hr in hypertensive individuals (Nieman, 2003). One potential mechanism for this postexercise hypotensive effect includes relaxation and vasodilation of the blood vessels in the legs and visceral organs. Body warming effects, local production of certain chemicals, decreases in nerve activity, and changes in certain hormones and their receptors also may cause blood vessels to relax after an exercise session. The American College of Sports Medicine and others conclude that people with mild hypertension can expect systolic and diastolic blood pressure to decrease by 8 to 12 mmHg and 6 to 10 mmHg, respectively, in response to exercise. This effect is independent of changes in body weight or diet. Most studies show that exercise training improves blood pressure among hypertensives and that this improvement occurs within the first few weeks. The important exercise criterion is frequency rather than intensity, with daily exercise being most beneficial (American College of Sports Medicine, 1998a).

Mechanisms by Which Exercise May Reduce Resting Blood Pressure

1. Decreases resting heart rate
2. Decreases resting cardiac output
3. Decreases total peripheral resistance
4. Decreases plasma norepinephrine levels
5. Decreases peripheral sympathetic nervous system stimulation
6. Alters renal function, which lowers blood pressure
7. Decreases body weight and body fat

From American College of Sports Medicine (1993).

Heart Disease

Heart disease, or cardiovascular disease (CVD), comprises more than 20 diseases of the heart and its blood vessels and includes diseases such as hypertension, coronary heart disease (CHD), and stroke. In this text, CVD and CHD will be used interchangeably. Although tremendous progress has been made in fighting CVD, it has been the leading cause of death among Americans in every year but one (1918) since 1900 (American Heart Association, 2001). From 1920 to 1950, deaths from heart disease rose sharply, primarily attributable to acute **myocardial infarction** (heart attacks) among men. The causes for this increase are unknown, but several factors may have contributed including the fact that Americans moved from farms into cities, began driving cars, and increased their consumption of saturated fats and cigarettes during this time. Since the 1950s the trend has reversed. The sharp increase of the earlier period has been followed by an equally sharp decrease in deaths from heart disease (National Center for Health Statistics, 2001). Since 1950, CVD death rates have decreased by 60%, illustrating one of the greatest public health successes of the 20th century. Men and women of all races shared in that encouraging downward mortality trend. Although estimates vary, about half of the decline in CVD mortality rates has been related to risk factor improvements and the other half to improvements in the treatment of CVD. However, even given these positive trends in CVD, the lifetime risk for developing CHD, for those 40 years of age and younger, is still very high, with one of every two males and one of every three females at risk for developing CVD (United States Department of Health and Human Services, 2000).

Risk factors are defined as personal habits or characteristics that medical research has shown to be associated with an increased risk of heart disease. The risk factors for heart disease and the percent of the U.S. population with each of the risk factors are shown in table 4.2. The danger of heart attack increases with the number of risk factors. Often people who have CVD have several risk factors, each of which is only marginally abnormal. Until 1992, the American Heart Association did not include physical activity in its list of major risk factors that could be changed. Most of the earlier studies showed that physically active, compared with inactive, people had a lower risk for CVD, but critics contended that other important factors, such as diet and family history, were not controlled. In 1987, a landmark review article was published by the Centers for Disease Control, in which 43 studies were reviewed, and not one reported a greater risk for CVD

among physically active individuals (Powell et al., 1987). Sixty-six percent of the studies supported the findings that physically active individuals, compared with inactive, have less CVD. The average relative risk of death attributable to CVD is approximately 45% less in those individuals considered physically active compared with their inactive counterparts (Manson et al., 1992).

One of the most important reasons why active people have less CVD is that other risk factors are typically under control as well. For example, relatively few active people smoke cigarettes, are obese or diabetic, have high blood **cholesterol,** or experience high blood pressure. Active people have lower blood triglycerides and more high-density lipoprotein cholesterol, and they generally report less anxiety and depression (Williams, 2001). There are other important reasons why regular exercise is identified with lower CVD risk. **Coronary arteries** of endurance-trained individuals can expand more, are less stiff in older age, and are wider than those of unfit subjects (Haskell et al., 1993; Seals, 2003; Tanaka et al., 2000). Also, there is some evidence that exercise may decrease the potential for clot formation; thus, with larger, more compliant coronary arteries and a diminished likelihood of forming clots, the active individual of any age is at a lower risk for a heart attack. Additionally, the heart muscle itself becomes bigger and stronger with regular exercise.

Table 4.2 **Risk Factors for Heart Disease**

Major Risk Factors	% U.S Adults With Risk Factor
Can be changed	
1. Cigarette/tobacco smoke	24
2. High blood pressure (>140/90 mmHg)	28
3. High blood cholesterol (>240 mg · dl⁻¹)	21
4. Physical inactivity	40
5. Obesity (BMI >30 kg · m⁻²)	23
6. Diabetes	6
Cannot be changed	
1. Heredity	
2. Being male	
3. Increasing age (>65 years)	13

BMI = body mass index.
Data from American Heart Association (2001).

Achievable Reductions in Heart Disease Risk

As shown in this table, lifestyle changes can effect reductions in heart disease risk.

Risk factor modified	Independent contribution of each risk factor to decrease risk
Quitting cigarette smoking	50-70% decrease within 5 years
Decreasing high blood pressure	2-3% decrease for each 1 mmHg decrease in diastolic BP
Decreasing blood cholesterol	2-3% decrease for each 1% decrease in cholesterol (in people with elevated cholesterol levels)
Becoming physically active	45% decrease for those who maintain active lifestyle
Maintenance of ideal body weight	33-55% decrease for maintaining ideal weight vs. obesity

Note: BP = blood pressure.

From Manson et al. (1992)

What is clear from epidemiological studies is that an inverse, dose–response relationship exists between the volume of physical activity and all-cause mortality rates. These relationships have been demonstrated in men and women and hold for older (those over 60 years of age) as well as younger cohorts. Expending approximately 1,000 kcal · week^{-1} in exercise reduces mortality rate by about 30%, and a reduction of as much as 50% is seen in those who expend approximately 2,000 kcal · week^{-1}. This would be equivalent to walking 20 miles per week, or approximately 1 hr a day of walking. In one longitudinal study involving more than 25,000 men and more than 7,000 women, it was reported that low fitness level was a strong, graded, and independent risk factor for all-cause mortality in men and women (Blair et al., 1996; figure 4.5). Men in the lowest fitness category had an increase of 2.03 in relative risk of death, whereas the women in the low fitness category had a 2.23 increase in relative risk of death. Other risk factors, such as cigarette smoking, high systolic blood pressure, high cholesterol, and higher body mass index, were also associated with increased mortality risk in men, but only low fitness and cigarette smoking increased the risk of death in women.

Although CHD is still the number one cause of death in the United States, accumulating 30 min of moderate activity can greatly reduce one's risk for many diseases including CHD.

What exercise program will reduce the risk of CVD the most? An expert panel convened by the National

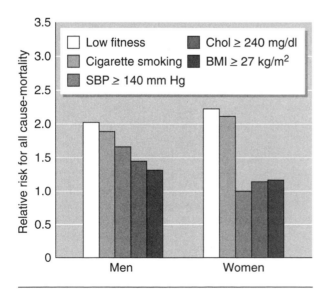

Figure 4.5 Relative risk of death from all causes for 25,341 men and 7,080 women. SBP = systolic blood pressure; CHOL = cholesterol; BMI = body mass index.

Data from Blair and colleagues (1996).

Surgeon General's Report on Physical Activity and Health: Key Messages for Older Adults

- Older adults, both male and female, can benefit from regular physical activity.
- Physical activity need not be strenuous to achieve health benefits.
- A moderate amount of activity can be obtained in longer sessions of moderately intense activities (such as walking) or in shorter sessions of more vigorous activities (such as fast walking or stair walking).
- Previously sedentary older adults who begin physical activity programs should start with short intervals of moderate physical activities (5-10 min) and gradually build up to the desired amount.
- In addition to cardiorespiratory endurance (aerobic) activity, older adults can benefit from muscle-strengthening activities, thereby reducing risk for falling and improving the ability to perform routine tasks of daily life.

From U.S. Department of Health and Human Services (1996).

Institutes of Health concluded that to reduce the risk of premature death, including death from CVD, exercise does not have to be structured or vigorous. The majority of the benefits of physical activity for children and adults can be gained by performing moderate-intensity activities for at least 30 min on most, preferably all, days of the week (NIH Consensus Development Panel on Physical Activity and Cardiovascular Health, 1996). This modest exercise prescription for preventing all-cause mortality is particularly encouraging for older adults. Older adults are encouraged to be physically active by routinely carrying out their daily activities with a minimum of assistance. These activities could include cleaning house, gardening, walking to the store, and taking the stairs whenever possible. However, there is also evidence that increasing physical activity up to 2,000 kcal · week^{-1} (approximately 20 miles of walking) is associated with lower mortality rate.

Aging Effects on the Respiratory System

Cells obtain energy primarily through aerobic metabolism, a process that requires oxygen and produces carbon dioxide as a by-product. The respiratory system, in conjunction with the cardiovascular system, provides a means by which oxygen is delivered to cells and carbon dioxide is removed. Age-related changes in the respiratory system include (a) changes in the structure of the lungs and airways, (b) changes in lung volumes, (c) impaired efficiency of gas exchange, and (d) alterations in the ventila-

tory pump. These changes in pulmonary function are determined by an interaction between internal (aging and genetics) and external factors (smoking, diet, exercise, and exposure to environmental pollutants). Some researchers contend that lung function declines the fastest of any organ with aging because of its continuous exposure to environmental pollutants, whereas others argue that lung function is the best maintained because of constant use.

Lungs and Airways

Morphological changes in the lungs have been widely observed in older adults. A decrease in alveolar surface area of about 15%, from age 20 to 70, reflects a reduction in the number of alveoli per unit of lung volume (Rossi et al., 1996). This causes an enlargement in terminal airspace, less surface area for gas exchange, and an increase in physiological dead space. After the age of 40, there is a slight increase in diameter of the large, central airways, with a decrease in diameter of the small airways (those <2 mm). These changes in airway capacity cause total flow resistance to either increase slightly or remain essentially unchanged with age. The major age-related physiological change in the lungs is the loss of elastic recoil. This loss of elastic recoil of the lungs, along with the increase in chest wall stiffness that occurs with age, increases the work involved in breathing, particularly at high rates of breathing.

Changes in Lung Volumes

The volume of air that is cycled through the lungs is customarily categorized into four major volumes:

tidal volume, inspiratory reserve volume, expiratory reserve volume, and residual volume. Tidal volume is the amount of air inspired and expired during normal, quiet breathing, whereas residual volume is the amount of air remaining in the lungs at the end of a maximal expiration. Inspiratory reserve volume is the extra volume of air that can be inspired with maximal effort after reaching the end of a normal quiet inspiration, and expiratory reserve volume is the extra volume of air that can be expired with maximal effort beyond the level reached at the end of a normal quiet expiration. Four capacities can be calculated from the sum of volumes:

Inspiratory capacity = tidal + inspiratory reserve

Functional residual capacity = expiratory reserve + residual

Vital capacity = tidal + inspiratory reserve + expiratory reserve volume

Total lung capacity = all four volumes

Lung volumes and capacities vary with age, body size, and gender and also may vary by ethnicity. The subdivision of lung volumes changes with age, mainly as a consequence of the loss of elastic recoil and increased chest wall stiffness. As seen in figure 4.6, residual volume and functional residual capacity increase about 25% with age, whereas vital capacity, the most widely measured lung capacity, declines 25% from age 40 to 80. Total lung capacity remains

constant throughout adult age, although a small reduction (5-10%) may be observed that is attributable to a decreased inspiratory muscle strength and decrease in statue. Two common measures of pulmonary function include the forced expiratory vital capacity (FVC) and the forced expiratory volume in the first second of expiration (FEV$_1$). A ratio of FEV$_1$/ FVC is used to diagnose obstructive disorders of the respiratory system, with a ratio of 7:10 (70%) representing the lower limit of the normal range. With aging, maximum pressures generated by full inhalation and expiration are significantly decreased, and even in apparently healthy older adults, the ratio of FEV$_1$/FVC may be as low as 55% to 65%, indicating that older adults do have limitations in respiratory function (Zaugg & Lucchinetti, 2000). Although age itself does not increase airway resistance at rest, the work of breathing may be elevated by 30% during exercise in older adults.

Gas Exchange in the Lung

Oxygen and carbon dioxide, driven by differential pressures, pass back and forth between the alveoli of the lungs and the blood, through the alveolar membrane. It is through this alveolar–arterial gas exchange that the body is able to move oxygen from the air into the lungs and then into the bloodstream, where oxygen is transported to all body tissues. Arterial oxygenation is progressively impeded with

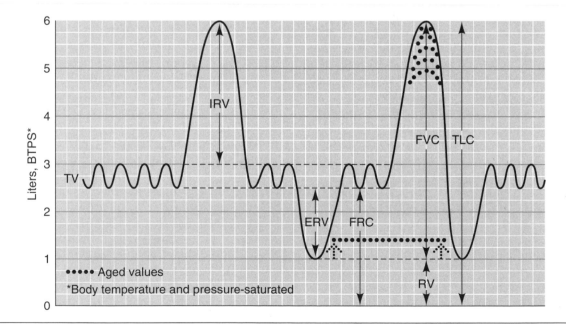

Figure 4.6 Changes in pulmonary volume with aging. BTPS = body temperature and pressure saturated; TV = total volume; IRV = inspiratory reserve volume; ERV = expiratory reserve volume; FRC = functional reserve capacity; RV = reserve volume; FVC = forced expiratory vital capacity; TLC = total lung capacity.

Adapted, by permission, from W.D. McArdle, R.I. Katch, and V.L. Katch, 1991, *Exercise physiology* (Philadelphia, PA: Lippincott, Williams, and Wilkins), 240.

increasing age, whereas carbon dioxide elimination is unaffected by aging. The greatest decrease in arterial oxygen tension is seen from 40 to 75 years of age with little change thereafter. This impaired oxygenation is primarily attributable to increased ventilation–perfusion mismatch rather than a decrease in diffusing capacity (Zaugg & Luccinetti, 2000).

Ventilatory Pump

Advancing age appears to affect all components of the ventilatory pump, including the chest wall, respiratory muscles, and respiratory centers. The stiffness of the rib cage increases with age perhaps because of other age-related changes including rib decalcification, rib cartilage calcification, changes in rib vertebral articulations, changes in the shape of the chest, and narrowing of the intervertebral disc spaces (Davidson & Fee, 1990). The respiratory muscles are the only skeletal muscle that must contract with a regular rhythm throughout life, yet they, like other skeletal muscle, are not spared the effects of advancing age. Inspiratory muscle strength decreases with age, but this loss does not appear to affect breathing at rest, exercise performance, or the ability to maintain or initiate a physically active lifestyle during old age (Brooks & Faulkner, 1995). However, because the oxygen consumption of the respiratory muscle decreases linearly with age, this may render these muscles more susceptible to fatigue when stressed

---

Age-Related Changes in the Respiratory System

The aging lung

- Reduction in alveolar surface area, which creates increased physiological dead space
- Reduction of lung elastic recoil

Lung volumes and maximal flows

- Decreasing vital capacity
- Increase in residual volume and functional residual capacity
- Decreasing FEV_1 and FEV_1/FVC ratio

The aging pump

- Increased chest wall stiffness
- Decreased respiratory muscle strength
- Decreased respiratory center sensitivity

---

by pulmonary disease. Control of ventilation is dependent on peripheral mechanoreceptors in the chest wall, lungs, and joints and on peripheral and central chemoreceptors. The respiratory response to hypoxia (low blood oxygen) is decreased by approximately 50% in the 70-year-old healthy individual and is primarily attributable to reduced central nervous activity and reduced neuronal output to respiratory muscles (Zaugg & Lucchinetti, 2000).

Respiratory Function During Exercise

Generally, in healthy individuals, the aged respiratory system functions very well under resting and moderate exercise conditions. Because maximal oxygen consumption is related to the amount of ventilation in the lungs, it might seem intuitive that respiratory function is an important limiting factor in maximal physical work capacity. However, the respiratory system is usually not the limiting factor in exercise performance. Healthy individuals terminate maximal physical work bouts because of the limitations of Q and $(a-\bar{v})O_2$ difference, not because of an inability of the respiratory system to provide oxygen to the blood. The lungs offer no major barrier to gas exchange, at least in individuals younger than age 70 who are free of respiratory disease. Furthermore, as in younger adults, older adults demonstrate a progressive increase in pulmonary ventilation during incremental exercise. Therefore, it appears that for older adults without respiratory disease, the respiratory system is not a limitation to exercise training and training may actually help maintain respiratory function with age, although more research is needed in this area.

> The respiratory system in older adults without respiratory disease is not a limitation to exercise training and may enhance respiratory function.

Preventing or Postponing Aging Effects on the Cardiovascular and Respiratory Systems

The evidence is quite clear that although aging inevitably impairs the cardiovascular and respiratory systems, a sedentary lifestyle accelerates that decline and appropriate physical activity postpones

How Exercise Can Change Your Life: A Personal Testimony!

Testimonials of dramatic improvements in the function and quality of life of diseased patients who begin a cautious yet habitual exercise program abound. A particularly striking example was described by Biegel (1984):

> Only five feet three inches [160 cm] tall and weighing 100 pounds [45 kg] for the past 40 years, Eula Weaver had developed cardiovascular disease and was treated for angina at age 67. At age 75 she was hospitalized with a severe heart attack; by age 81, she had developed an arthritic limp and had congestive heart failure, hypertension, and angina. When she began a regimen of dieting and walking at age 81, her limp limited her walking to 100 feet; the circulation in her hands was so impaired that she wore gloves in the summer to keep her hands warm. Gradually increasing her walking, she was able, by age 82, to be free of medications and her previous symptoms. After four years of increased activity, she participated in the Senior Olympics in Irvine, California, where she won gold medals in the half mile and mile running events. The following year, at age 86, she repeated those runs for another two gold medals. Each morning she runs a mile and rides her stationary bicycle 10-15 miles; three times weekly she works out in a gymnasium; and she follows a strict diet. (p. 31)

the impairment. The evidence for this comes from studies of exercise training and comparisons of adults who are physically active with those who are not. Also, the health and fitness of masters athletes give testimony to the beneficial effects of physical activity on these physiological systems.

Exercise and Physical Activity

Endurance training, such as walking, jogging, cycling, and swimming, is most beneficial for optimizing cardiovascular function and for decreasing risk for diseases such as cardiovascular disease, hypertension, dyslipidemia, and diabetes. A 50% to 80% reduction in lower body disability was found in older African Americans and Anglos who walked on a daily basis compared with their sedentary counterparts (Clark, 1996). Postponement in disability also was reported in runners over the age of 50 compared with age-matched community adults (Wang et al., 2002). Benefits in aerobic capacity and blood pressure with exercise training have even been found in older adults who begin their exercise after 80 years of age (Vaitkevicius et al., 2002). It is clear that endurance training improves cardiovascular and respiratory function, decreases risk for many diseases, and, perhaps most importantly, decreases disability in later life.

In addition to performing endurance training, older adults should include strength, balance, and flexibility exercises in their exercise programs. Strength training helps offset the loss of strength and muscle mass that typically is associated with aging and also improves bone health. Experts also recom-

mend balance training to improve postural stability and flexibility exercises to improve range of motion. It appears that the best exercise program includes all types of exercise such as endurance, strength, balance, and flexibility, but the exact frequency, intensity, and duration for older adults depend on the physical, cognitive, and emotional status of the older adults and their specific goals for exercise training. It is clear that daily physical activity is important for optimal physical and psychological function even for the extremely old and frail, although the goals of the exercise program as well as the exercises will be altered to accommodate individual disabilities (Mazzeo & Tanaka, 2001).

The best exercise program for decreasing morbidity and mortality rates and maintaining function in older adults is one that includes endurance, strength, balance, and flexibility exercises.

Masters Athletes

A masters athlete is an individual who competes in athletic events that are categorized by age. In most sports, the age categories for masters athletes begin at 50 years. Most masters athletes have been competing in sport all their lives, with a few initiating competition later in life. Although these athletes constitute a tiny percentage of the older adult population, it is not unusual to find 70- and 80-year-old men and women who have maintained a daily physical training schedule for many years. Consequently, these athletes who train, particularly in aerobic sports, such as running, cycling, and swimming, provide a "gold standard" against which age-related physical decline, not accelerated by physical disuse and disease, can be compared. Generally, athletes who aerobically train also adhere to other beneficial health habits, such as good nutrition, good sleep habits, and freedom from drug abuse. Thus, these masters athletes not only provide information about the heights of performance and physiological adaptation that are possible at advanced ages but also provide a source of inspiration to all aging individuals who realize that their physical abilities are weakening.

Although declines in maximum heart rate, maximal pulmonary ventilation, and maximal oxygen consumption are inevitable, and although these older athletes rarely continue to train as hard in their senior years as they did when they were competing 20- or 30-year-olds, they nevertheless come closer than any other group to being the models of how the human body can withstand the passage of time if it is well cared for and if exercise consistency and intensity are maintained. Discussions of training effects in this highly fit group, therefore, focus not on how much improvement can be made with exercise but rather on how intensive, systematic exercise can maintain cardiovascular function and aerobic capacity within the framework of an aging system.

There is one caveat: It cannot be assumed that the physical work capacity of all individuals, if they followed a similar lifestyle, would be similar to that of masters athletes, because about 40% of an individual's physiological athletic capacity is attributed to genetic factors. In addition, the extent to which individuals respond to physical training also has a genetic component (Bouchard & Malina, 1983). In other words, if some miracle occurred and every baby born today trained aerobically every day, the average VO$_2$ of 70-year-olds (assuming each baby lived to this age) in the year 2060 would probably be significantly lower than that of the average 70-year-old masters runner today, simply because today's masters runners probably are an elite and genetically talented group. Nevertheless, these people do provide evidence of the long-term benefits of aerobic training and good health habits.

Results from cross-sectional studies show that masters athletes who were still competing achieved dramatically higher $\dot{V}O_2$max than former athletes and sedentary individuals (see figure 4.4, p. 93). Cross-sectional data indicate that the decline in $\dot{V}O_2$max for men is about 1% per year after 25 years of age. Some researchers suggest that highly trained endurance athletes and moderately trained fitness

participants who maintain high-intensity training may experience less decline in aerobic capacity than sedentary individuals (Wilson et al., 2000). Recent longitudinal studies of changes in the cardiovascular system from 8 to 33 years in masters athletes have shown changes in $\dot{V}O_2$max ranging from 0.28% to 2.6% per year (Hawkins et al., 2001; Kasch et al., 1999; Katzel et al., 2001; Pollock et al., 1997). The major determinants of changes in $\dot{V}O_2$max with age were the initial level of aerobic power and the subjects' reduction in activity level. There are several possible reasons for the wide discrepancy in the findings of these longitudinal training studies of $\dot{V}O_2$max in masters athletes: (a) The training intensity, duration, and frequency were based on self-report; (b) the ages of the individuals when they were first tested were different; (c) the number of years and amount of training over those years were different; and (d) the body composition changes (i.e., increase in body fat and decrease in muscle mass) in the subjects were different. One thing is clear. Even if the rate of loss in $\dot{V}O_2$max is not attenuated in masters athletes who continue their exercise training, these athletes still exhibit a higher $\dot{V}O_2$max than older adults who never trained or individuals who trained earlier in life but quit training as they aged.

The encouraging aspect of these studies of highly trained aged competitors is that a decade of aging (50-60) may have little effect on a highly exercised cardiovascular system. The $\dot{V}O_2$max values of current masters athletes reveal strikingly youthful cardiovascular function. But for individuals who would like a quick and easy solution to aging, the results are discouraging in that they emphasize that the cardiovascular maintenance benefits of exercise are only effective as long as the exercise intensity is maintained. In fact, some measures of fitness decline by 50% within 3 weeks, and light or moderate exercisers who quit exercising may lose all exercise benefits within a few months.

To provide long-term benefits, exercise must become an integral, daily part of an individual's life.

Disuse, Bed Rest, and Deconditioning

Throughout this chapter, the positive effects of physical activity on the declines in cardiovascular and respiratory functions have been noted. However, the long-term negative effects of physical inactivity are so debilitating, not only for the cardiovascular system but also for the whole body, that further discussion is merited. Experiments on bed rest have shown that even a short period of physical inactivity, even in relatively young subjects, can have negative effects on cardiovascular function, blood pressure, and hormonal responses to exercise. Twenty days of bed rest in young adults led to a 25% decline in $\dot{V}O_2$max, whereas 4 months of detraining in older adults led to a complete loss of endurance training adaptations of the cardiovascular system (Saltin et al., 1968; Pickering et al., 1997). In the detraining study of 60-year-olds, there was an increase in $\dot{V}O_2$max of 16% after 16 weeks of supervised training on a cycle ergometer (Pickering et al., 1997). However, all of this gain in aerobic power was lost when the subjects were discharged from the study, even though they were strongly encouraged to keep training as regularly as possible. It appears that when the constraints and the social stimulation of the supervised exercise were withdrawn, the subjects did not maintain their exercise training and thereby lost all the benefit in $\dot{V}O_2$max they had gained through training. A lifetime of physical disuse can have catastrophic effects, eroding strength and mobility, and may eventually lead to frailty, immobility, and total dependency. To compound the problems of disuse, the low levels of daily caloric expenditure that accompany physical inactivity contribute to an increase in body fat, especially abdominal fat, and an increased ratio of body fat to muscle mass. An increase in body fat, particularly in the abdominal body, increases the prevalence of risk factors for atherosclerosis and type 2 diabetes.

Human frailty has three dimensions (Bortz, 1983), shown in figure 4.7. The first dimension, time, relentlessly drains energy and vitality. No one has yet found a way to halt the passage of time. Inevitably—for everyone—when enough time passes, death occurs. The second dimension, disease, is attributable to internal errors or external agents that damage body systems and lead to weakness, system fatigue, frailty, and eventually death. Through science and technology, miraculous preventives and cures for many diseases have been found. The third dimension, disuse, although far less publicized, is also significant in the transformation from robustness to frailty. In contrast to the previous two dimensions, disuse is controllable; the majority of individuals have, within some constraints, almost total control over the extent to which they use their mental, physical, and social capacities.

Information on the debilitating effects of disuse, which has largely surfaced from research on bed rest, water immersion, and weightlessness in space, is compelling. All of these conditions drastically alter three classes of stimuli that humans experience: hydrostatic pressure, compression force on long bones, and level of physical exercise (Greenleaf, 1984). Prolonged periods of sitting in recliners or on couches simulate bed rest, and transient bed-rest effects are easily seen. For example, when many older

Effects of Disuse: A Personal Testimony

Bortz (1983) articulated the deleterious effects that disuse has on the body from his personal experience with a leg broken during a skiing accident.

When the cast was removed, I found my leg giving all the appearance of the limb of a person forty or fifty years older. It was withered, discolored, stiff, painful. I could not believe this leg belonged to me. The similarity of changes due to enforced inactivity to those commonly attributed to aging was striking. And, in fact, if one were to go to all the standard textbooks of geriatrics and write down all the changes which seem to accompany aging, set the list aside, and then go to the textbooks of work physiology and write down all the changes subsequent to inactivity—and then compare the two lists, one would see that they are virtually identical. The coincidence is not random. It is intense. It forces the conclusion that at least part of what passes as change due to age is not caused by age at all but by disuse. (p. 2)

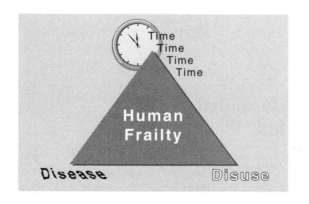

Figure 4.7 The three dimensions of human frailty: time, disease, and disuse.

people stand up from prolonged sitting or lying, the relatively sudden change in fluid compartment volumes lowers blood pressure so that they experience a light-headed sensation (postural hypertension). If the decrease in blood pressure is significant, they will faint (Convertino et al., 1984). Exercising the lower limbs assists in the venous return process, improving the blood flow and pressure needed to maintain adequate perfusion of the brain. Exercise also maintains important reflexes that compensate for changes in posture.

Especially in the elderly, three major problems develop from bed rest in healthy people as well as those confined for medical reasons: lung edema, venous and arterial thrombi, and hydrostatic

pneumonia (Booth, 1982; Greenleaf, 1984). Other symptoms associated with bed rest include bed sores, foot drop, general muscular weakness and atrophy, muscle shortening, knee joint stiffness, restriction of joint motion, loss of appetite, minor dyspepsia and heartburn, constipation and occasional intestinal obstruction, increased tendency for urinary calculi, and accentuation of symptoms during the course of multiple sclerosis and tabes dorsalis (Greenleaf, 1984).

The extent of the effects of disuse depends on the degree of disuse, but the results are clear. Disuse is devastating to the physical system, and even mild physical activity goes a long way in preventing some of the more serious disuse-precipitated diseases.

SUMMARY

The cardiovascular and respiratory systems are often front-page news because four of the five leading causes of death in the United States are attributable to deterioration in these two systems. In addition, the capacity to perform physical work is dependent to a large extent on the proper functioning of these two systems. Despite a large amount of research on the effects of aging on the cardiovascular system, it is still unclear to what extent the changes in this system are attributable to "normal" aging, physical inactivity, or heart disease. Some structural changes in the cardiovascular system with age include increased thickening of the walls of the blood vessels and left ventricular wall and increased stiffness in the arteries. Systolic and diastolic blood pressures increase with age, attributable primarily to a thickening and hardening of the aorta and arterial tree but also to an increase in total peripheral resistance. The heart and vasculature also become less sensitive to ß-mediated stimulation, and thus the aging heart cannot achieve maximum heart rate levels that were possible during youth. The heart rates of older people also remain higher and recover more slowly after maximal exercise. Postural hypotension, which predisposes an individual to dizziness, confusion, weakness, or fainting, increases with age but appears to be related more to high levels of systolic blood pressure than to aging per se. However, heart function in most older adults is adequate at rest. More structural and functional deterioration is attributable to pathological processes, such as heart disease, rather than the actual aging process.

A key ingredient of cardiovascular health is maintaining a physically active lifestyle. Regular physical activity reduces the risk for heart disease, hypertension, and diabetes and increases longevity

and decreases disability. The best measure of physical work capacity, $\dot{V}O_2$max, declines about 1% to 2.5% per year after age 25, with the decline being much less in chronic exercisers who maintain their exercise training across the decades. Many older chronic exercisers, even those over age 60, have a higher $\dot{V}O_2$max and can outperform many sedentary 20-year-olds in physical work capacity. The benefits that these exercisers receive include the following:

- Decreased resting heart rate but no change in maximal exercise heart rate
- Enhanced stroke volume, which assists in maintaining cardiac output
- Increased total blood volume and tone of peripheral veins, which reduce vascular resistance
- Decreased systolic and diastolic blood pressures
- Increased high-density lipoprotein cholesterol

However, the cardiovascular maintenance effects of habitual exercise are only effective as long as exercise frequency, duration, and intensity are maintained.

Cardiovascular disease includes more than 20 different diseases of the heart and blood vessels. Although cardiovascular disease death rates have decreased almost 50% in men over the last 50 years, cardiovascular disease is still the major killer of Americans, regardless of their ethnicity. The risk factors for heart disease include modifiable ones like cigarette smoking and physical inactivity as well as nonmodifiable ones like heredity and age.

Changes in the respiratory system with age include a reduction in elastic recoil of the lungs, a decrease in some volumes and capacities, particularly FEV_1, increased chest wall stiffness, decreased strength of the respiratory muscles, and decreased sensitivity of the respiratory centers in the nervous system. Despite these changes, in healthy individuals, the aged pulmonary system functions very well under resting and moderate exercise conditions. Even under heavy exercise conditions, pulmonary function is not usually a limiting factor in maximal physical work capacity. The limiting factor is more attributable to the limit that a decreased maximum heart rate places on cardiac output.

Habitual exercise both prevents and remediates cardiovascular disease, hypertension, and diabetes. In this sense it postpones many symptoms of aging in the cardiovascular and respiratory systems. Conversely, disuse, such as occurs during long periods of sitting in recliners or chairs or during bed rest, dramatically accelerates aging of most physiological processes. Masters athletes provide a gold standard of exercise habits and performance against which age-related decline that is not accelerated by physical disuse and disease can be compared.

REVIEW QUESTIONS

1. What structural and functional changes in the cardiovascular system are associated with "normal" aging?

2. Describe exercise affects on $\dot{V}O_2$max, maximal heart rate, cardiac output, $(a-\bar{v})O_2$ difference, and blood pressure in older adults.

3. What is heart disease, how common is it, and what are the major risk factors associated with this disease?

4. Describe the changes in the respiratory system with aging.

5. What has been learned from studies on masters athletes when compared with physically inactive older adults regarding effects on the cardiovascular and respiratory systems?

SUGGESTED READINGS

American College of Sports Medicine. (1998). Position stand: Exercise and physical activity for older adults. *Medicine and Science in Sports and Exercise, 30,* 992-1008.

Lakatta, E.G. (2002). Age-associated cardiovascular changes in health: Impact on cardiovascular disease in older persons. *Heart Failure Reviews, 7,* 29-49.

Mazzeo, R.S., & Tanaka, H. (2001). Exercise prescription for the elderly. *Sports Medicine, 31,* 809-818.

Rossi, A., Ganassini, A., Tantucci, C., & Grassi, V. 1996. Aging and the respiratory system. *Aging (Milano), 8,* 143-161.

Seals, D.R. (2003). Habitual exercise and age-associated decline in large artery compliance. *Exercise and Sport Sciences Reviews, 31,* 68-72.

Spina, R.J. (1999). Cardiovascular adaptations to endurance exercise training in older men and women. *Exercise and Sport Sciences Reviews, 27,* 317-332.

Muscular Strength and Power

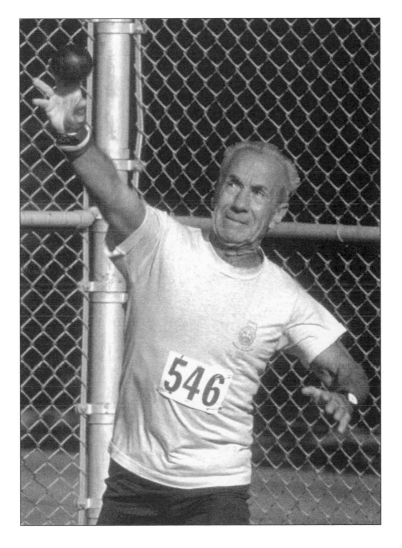

The objectives of this chapter are

- to describe the effects of aging on muscular strength and power,

- to detail the effects of resistance training on strength and power, and

- to explain the relationships among strength, power, and physical function.

The 700 skeletal muscles of the human body enable you to move, maintain posture, control reflexes such as swallowing and urination, and maintain body temperature. If muscles contract slowly they produce force (strength), and if they contract rapidly they produce power. The strength and power produced by these muscles are essential for many activities of daily living and are necessary for many job-related tasks and social activities. Moderate levels of strength and power are necessary for a surprising number of activities of daily living: carrying groceries and packages, lifting grandchildren, climbing stairs, and getting up from chairs or out of automobiles. Low to moderate levels of strength are necessary to retain certain types of jobs for those who wish to extend their work life beyond traditional retirement ages. Also, in older adults, strength plays a significant role in preserving the ability to participate in social activities, such as dancing and traveling, and to continue some lifelong hobbies, such as woodworking, painting, or gardening.

Muscular strength and power are important resources for all individuals, but these resources become even more important as individuals age. A substantial loss of lower body strength in the elderly not only impairs locomotion but also is associated with an increased risk of falling (Lord et al., 2003; Tinetti & Speechley, 1989). Adequate leg power may prevent a fall by enabling an individual to correct momentary losses of balance in time to prevent catastrophic falling events, and strength of the upper body musculature may reduce the amount of injury that results from a fall by breaking the force of the fall or by stabilizing the joints during the fall.

The first part of this chapter discusses the age-related changes that occur in muscular strength, the potential causes of these changes, and the role that resistance exercise plays in the acquisition and maintenance of strength. The second part of the chapter discusses the changes in muscle power with aging and the role of high-velocity resistance training on maintaining and improving muscle power in older adults.

Strength and Power

Skeletal muscle is the most abundant tissue in the human body, accounting for approximately 23% of a female's body weight and more than 40% of a male's (Nieman, 2003). Muscle size and function change dramatically across the human life span, with initial rapid increases attributable to growth and later more gradual decreases attributable to aging. Skeletal mus-

cles are affected by use, so that those muscles that are forcefully contracted become larger, which is called **muscle hypertrophy,** and those that are not used decrease in size and strength, called **muscle atrophy.** Muscular strength and power relate to the ability of muscles to exert maximal force. **Muscle strength** is defined as the amount of force that a muscle or group of muscles can produce with a single maximum contraction, but **torque** is the term used to describe the resulting amount of rotation of a limb, and the amount of torque depends on the angle of muscle tendon attachment, the length of the muscle, and its shortening velocity. **Muscle power** is the ability to generate force rapidly and is calculated as work divided by time (Brooks et al., 2000). Muscle strength is used when a person applies maximum force to try to lift a heavy box, whereas muscle power would be used if an individual runs up a flight of stairs as quickly as possible.

Types of muscle actions used in strength production include isometric and dynamic, with dynamic muscle action involving both concentric and eccentric actions. The term **isometric strength,** also called **static strength,** describes muscle activation in which no observable change occurs in muscle length. Isometric strength of the elbow flexors would be used to hold a tray of food as one carries it from the kitchen to the table. Isometric muscle strength is most often measured by a dynamometer, such as a handgrip dynamometer. **Isotonic,** or **dynamic, strength** involves a shortening and lengthening of muscles fibers so that movement of the skeleton occurs. **Concentric muscle contraction** occurs when the muscle shortens, creating tension in the muscle and causing joint movement. For example, a concentric contraction of the elbow flexors would be needed to lift a bag of groceries out of the cart at the grocery store. **Eccentric muscle contraction** occurs when external resistance exceeds muscle force and the muscle lengthens while developing tension. Lowering a bag of groceries to the ground or lowering a fork to the plate would involve eccentric contractions of the elbow flexors.

Measures of dynamic strength most commonly used today include 1-repetition maximum (1RM) and the use of an electromechanical accommodating resistance instrument called an isokinetic dynamometer. The 1RM refers to the maximum amount of weight an individual can lift at one time using proper form during a standard weightlifting exercise. This dynamic strength assessment technique can be safely used with all ages if proper protocol is followed. The isokinetic dynamometer allows for the generation of maximum force throughout the full range of joint motion at a pre-established velocity of limb movement. Therefore, strength assessment and training can be performed under either high-velocity (low-force) or low-velocity (high-force) conditions. The microprocessor that controls the isokinetic dynamometer gives details on the peak and average force generated throughout the range of motion. The isokinetic dynamometer is considered a safer way to assess strength than the 1RM, but it is a large, expensive piece of equipment and requires special training for the experimenter.

Muscle strength is the amount of force produced in a single maximum contraction of a muscle or muscle group, whereas muscle power is the ability to generate force rapidly.

Changes in Muscular Strength With Age

Maximal muscle strength is achieved in the 20s or 30s and then declines with age. The effects of aging on strength are affected by the type of strength measured (isometric vs. concentric vs. eccentric), the location of the muscles that are measured (upper vs. lower body), and the physical activity level and disease status of the individuals who are assessed. Cross-sectional data showing grip strength for males from 20 to 100 years of age are shown in figure 5.1. Isometric strength changes little until the 6th decade but then decreases

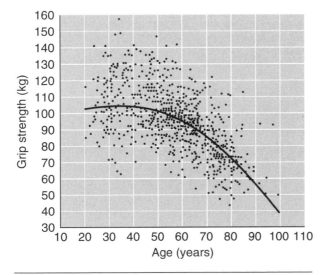

Figure 5.1 Grip strength of 847 males from 20 to 100 years of age.

Reprinted, by permission, from D.A. Kallman, C.C. Plato, and J.D. Tobin, 1990, "The role of muscle loss in the age-related decline of grip strength: Cross sectional and longitudinal perspectives," *Journal of Gerontology* 45: M83.

1.0% to 1.5% per year from 50 to 70 years of age and 3% per year thereafter (American College of Sports Medicine, 1998; Kallman et al., 1990; Vandervoort, 2002). Muscles of the upper extremities, such as handgrip muscles or elbow flexors and extensors, tend to change less with age than muscles of the lower extremities (Lynch et al., 1999).

When actual changes in handgrip strength of the general population are measured (longitudinal data), it is clear that people differ greatly in the amount of strength lost across the years (Kallman et al., 1990). Many of the older subjects in this sample lost less strength over a 10-year period than did middle-aged and young subjects, and about 29% of the middle-aged subjects and 15% of older subjects lost no strength at all over the 10 years. These findings are an excellent example of individual differences, which were discussed in chapter 2, and may be attributable to differences in the use of the handgrip muscles across the 10 years as well as differences in diseases, such as arthritis, that might affect the ability to produce maximal handgrip strength.

In a nationally represented sample of more than 6,000 community-dwelling adults over 70 years of age,

- 26% could not climb even one set of stairs without stopping,
- 31% had difficulty lifting 10 lb (a bag of groceries), and
- 36% reported having trouble walking several blocks.

From Stump and colleagues (1997).

Strength, as measured by a concentric (shortening) action, decreases with age in a manner similar to isometric strength, with the strength losses most dramatic after the age of 70 years. Many of the very old have lost so much lower body strength that they fall below minimum strength thresholds for some activities of daily living such as rising from a chair. At higher velocities of movement (power), the age-related deficit is even more marked and has a greater effect on activities of daily living including walking and stair climbing.

Strength decreases with aging have been found to be consistently less for the eccentric (lengthening) type of muscle action (Porter et al., 1997). The changes in muscle mass, contraction speed, and connective tissue, which reduce strength in the concentric action, seem to enhance muscle performance during eccentric contractions. Why aged muscle has this relative advantage to lengthen against resistance is unclear, but it is a phenomenon that might be considered when one is designing resistance training programs to improve strength in older adults. Perhaps eccentric exercises, which require less muscular effort and related cardiovascular response in older adults than concentric exercises, may lead to greater adherence to the exercise protocol.

> Most sedentary older adults exhibit a decline in strength of about 1% per year beginning in the 50s, with much steeper declines, approximately 3% per year, after 70 years of age.

A few researchers have examined longitudinal changes in dynamic muscular strength (Aniansson et al., 1992; Frontera et al., 2000; Hughes et al., 2001). In one study, both men and women (mean age 60 years at baseline) lost knee flexor and extensor strength similarly over 10 years, but the women lost almost no strength in their elbow flexors and extensors whereas the men lost 10% to 12% (figure 5.2). The reason for this variability in the response to aging of the different muscle groups in males and females is unclear, and more longitudinal data are needed. Perhaps the women used their upper body muscles more than the men so they maintained their upper body strength better. However, it is also possible that women are less able to produce maximal forces because of a lack of practice with such tasks and therefore the results of 1RM with women are not truly

maximal efforts. Another important gender difference in this longitudinal study of dynamic muscle strength was that the men exhibited a greater rate of decline (~60%) when their longitudinal data were compared with cross-sectional data. No such differences were seen in women. These longitudinal results support the idea that a decline in strength is not inevitable. Strength gains were observed for some individuals in all muscle groups tested. Depending on muscle group, 7% to 32% of the subjects showed positive changes over the 10-year follow-up period. This supports the longitudinal, isometric strength data mentioned earlier. The effects of age on strength, including differences in gender and study design, are summarized in table 5.1.

Why Strength Decreases With Aging

The decline in strength with aging is strongly affected by loss of muscle mass, called **sarcopenia,** a phenomenon that occurs even in masters athletes who train intensely. This process is not to be confused with the muscle atrophy that accompanies physical inactivity, because this type of atrophy can be reversed with resistance training. Sarcopenia reduces the size of the muscle mass that is contracting and therefore its strength. To a lesser extent, changes in muscle fiber characteristics, the nervous system, and muscle blood flow also decrease strength (figure 5.3). Increases in diseases, in addition to poor nutrition and decreases in physical activity levels, contribute directly to the declines in muscle strength as well as indirectly by increasing muscle atrophy and thereby decreasing muscle strength.

Muscle Atrophy

The strength an individual can produce depends substantially on the amount of working muscle that is brought to the task. Human skeletal muscle, regardless of gender, generates a maximum of 16 to 30 **newtons (N)** of force per square centimeter of muscle cross section (McArdle et al., 2001). In the human body, however, force-output capacity varies, depending on the arrangement of the bony levers and muscle architecture.

In general, differences in strength occur when individuals have a much larger muscle mass than other individuals. Males, for example, who on average are 50% stronger than females in upper body strength and about 30% stronger in lower body strength, also have greater muscle mass. Therefore,

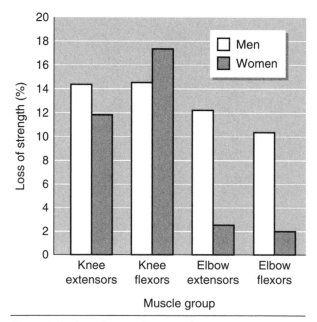

Figure 5.2 Loss in muscle strength (%) across 10 years for men and women.

Data from Hughes and colleagues (2001).

Table 5.1 Effects of Age, Gender, and Study Design on Strength

	Age effects	Gender differences	Cross-sectional vs. longitudinal
Overall body strength	> absolute loss in M than W > % loss in M than W in arm flexors and extensors = % loss in M and W in knee flexors and extensors	M > W	>loss in longitudinal for M
Upper vs. lower body strength	> loss in lower than upper for W = loss in M in upper and lower	> loss in W in knee flexion and extension than in elbow flexion and extension	M losses in knee flexion and extension 60% greater in longitudinal vs. cross-sectional W = loss in cross-sectional vs. longitudinal
Isometric, concentric, eccentric	Maintained better > rate of loss Maintained better	M > absolute strength than W	
Contraction velocity (power)	Power declines more than strength Loss of power in top 5% rowers < rest of field Power is more related to physical function than strength	M = W power losses in absolute loss (~4 W per year) W lose relative power > M 1.2% vs. 0.9%/year	
Muscle mass	Decline in both M and W over time 16% decline in mass with 25% decline in strength[b] 90% loss in strength accounted for by CSA of muscle	W have smaller % distribution of muscle in their arms W have < to lose and > to gain > % decline in M	
Physical activity	33% < 500 kcal per week in previous 12 months; 8% resistance training activities	M > PA M > decline in PA over time	
Resistance training	Related to muscle strength Neural > important than muscle CSA 20-30% increase in strength with only 2-6% increase in CSA[c]		
Muscle quality (specific force)	Reduction in in vivo strength to whole muscle size ratio[b]	M > W in single fiber max force[b], independent of fiber type or size	
Mechanisms	1. < gene transcription 2. slow protein turnover rate 3. post-translational modification		
Training-related muscle damage	= amount of focal muscle damage with heavy resistance training in O and Y men[b]	> damage in old W than in young W[b]	

Note: M = men; W = women; PA = physical activity; CSA = cross-sectional area; O = old; Y = young.
[a]Hughes et al. (2001); [b]Frontera et al. (2002); [c]Hakkinen et al. (1998).

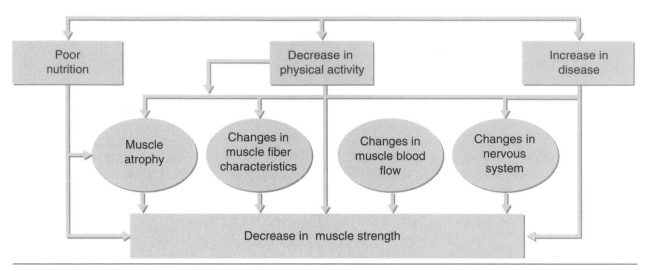

Figure 5.3 Factors that may cause loss of muscle strength with aging.

expressing strength in absolute values and comparing different ages, genders, or even changes over time is problematic because of the wide variety of size and structural differences. Ideally, measures of strength should be expressed per unit of muscle mass, but because this is a difficult measure to obtain in humans, researchers most often express strength relative to body weight or fat-free mass (FFM). We have already seen in chapter 3 that fat mass increases and FFM decreases with aging. Sedentary individuals lose large amounts of muscle mass over the course of adult life (20-40%), and this loss plays a major role in the similarly large losses in muscle strength observed in both cross-sectional and longitudinal studies (Kirkendall & Garrett, 1998). In addition to a decline in muscle mass, there is an increase in fat and connective tissue within the muscle belly in older people (Kent-Braun et al., 2000). In younger individuals, 70% of muscle is composed of muscle fibers, whereas in older adults only 50% of the muscle is made up of muscle fibers (Lexell et al., 1988).

The fact that muscle mass is a major determinant of the force-generating capacity of the muscle is demonstrated by high correlations between muscle mass and strength in both cross-sectional and longitudinal studies of adults (Frontera et al., 2000; Hughes et al., 2001; Lynch et al., 1999). However, loss of muscle mass with age does not explain all of the strength loss with age. Age-related changes in a longitudinal study were also influenced by the magnitude and direction of the body weight and muscle mass changes (Hughes et al., 2001). Changes in strength of upper and lower body muscle groups over a 10-year period were significantly and highly correlated (.40 to .95) with body weight changes in both men and women.

Changes in muscle mass were positively related to changes in muscle strength only in the lower body, and these relationships were much weaker (.10 to .30) explaining only a small part (5%) of the variance in knee strength observed. Therefore, change in muscle mass does not explain the majority of the change in strength seen with aging.

> Although sarcopenia accounts for a large amount of strength loss in aging adults, it does not fully explain the decline in strength with age.

Changes in Skeletal Muscle Characteristics

A muscle is organized into several subunits, shown in figure 5.4. The first subunit is the fasciculus, which is a packet of muscle fibers. Each muscle fiber (i.e., muscle cell) is a subunit composed of myofibrils, which are made up of myofilaments. Each myofilament is primarily made up of the proteins actin and myosin. An increase in muscle tension or force, as occurs in resistance training, provides the primary stimulus for skeletal muscle to increase in size (hypertrophy) as well as change neurologic factors. The mechanical stress on the muscle triggers signaling proteins in the muscle to activate the genes that stimulate protein synthesis. This accelerated protein synthesis increases the size of the muscle fibers and therefore increases muscle mass. Connective tissue proliferates and thickens to strengthen the muscle's connective tissue harness, improving the structural and functional integrity of tendons and ligaments. These adaptations are thought to protect joints and muscles from injury.

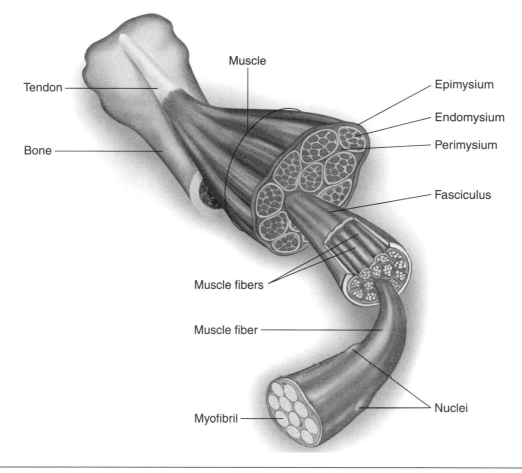

Figure 5.4 Schematic drawing of a muscle illustrating three types of connective tissue: epimysium (the outer layer), perimysium (surrounding each fasciculus, or group of fibers), and endomysium (surrounding individual fibers).

Reprinted, by permission, from National Strength and Conditioning Association, 2001, *NSCA's essentials of strength training and conditioning, 2nd ed.* (Champaign, IL: Human Kinetics), 4.

Muscle fibers are characterized by physiologists as slow- or fast-twitch fibers, with fast-twitch fibers being further subdivided into two groups. Slow-twitch fibers contract very slowly, using the aerobic energy system to drive the contractions. These fibers metabolize glycogen for energy, and, as long as the workload is at a relatively low to moderate intensity, energy can be supplied at the same rate at which it is being consumed by the fibers. Because slow-twitch fibers can maintain a balance between energy production and consumption at moderate workloads for a relatively long time, they are fatigue resistant and are called slow oxidative (SO) fibers. Morphologists (those who study cell structure, not function) call such fibers type I fibers. The body depends primarily on SO, or type I, muscle fibers when muscular contractions must be maintained for long periods, such as in long-distance running, cycling, or swimming as well as the ability to maintain upright posture.

Although muscles generally have a mix of both major types of muscle fibers, some muscles like the soleus, which is used almost exclusively in slow postural movements, are composed primarily of slow-twitch fibers.

Fast-twitch muscle fibers contract very rapidly, using energy derived from immediate stores of adenosine triphosphate (ATP) and from anaerobic energy processes to develop tension quickly. These anaerobic energy processes convert, via a short-term anaerobic process called glycogenolysis, some of the glycogen stored in the muscle to energy. Because of this capability, fast-twitch fibers are also called fast-glycolytic (FG) fibers, or type IIb fibers. FG, or type IIb, fibers contract two to three times faster than SO, or type I, fibers. Type IIb muscle fibers produce the rapid, powerful contractions needed for running sprint races and throwing a discus or shot put. The muscles that are used in these types of activities, especially the muscles of athletes who train in power events, have a high percentage of fast-twitch fibers. Some type II fast-twitch fibers contract at an intermediate speed and combine both aerobic and anaerobic properties. They are called fast oxidative-glycolytic, or type IIa, fibers.

Determining aging effects on the microstructure of the human muscle (fiber size, number, and arrangement) is difficult because the available techniques must be done on cadavers or are invasive and not completely free of discomfort. To obtain skeletal muscle tissue, a biopsy needle is used to remove a small amount of muscle. However, because this process is invasive, the needle must be small and the number of samples from each muscle must be kept to a minimum. Consequently, studies of human muscle characteristics are plagued with sampling problems. The amount of tissue available is usually only a few milligrams and contains only a few hundred muscle fibers. Recently several investigators, using either the in vivo biopsy techniques or analysis of cadaver specimens, have examined age-related changes in human quadriceps muscle, and a summary of their findings is presented in table 5.2. The findings from these studies are consistent in showing that sarcopenia is attributable to an overall loss in the total number of muscle fibers, both type I and type II, along with a significant reduction in the average size of type II fibers.

Another fundamental question is whether human skeletal muscle fiber-type composition changes with age. Some researchers maintain that with aging the number of type I fibers increases, but most favor the idea of no substantial change in fiber-type composi-

tion. A more recent suggestion is that what occurs is not so much an age-related change in the number of type I and type II fibers in the classic sense but more an obfuscation of the border between type I and type II fibers (Andersen et al., 1999). This means that in young adults, 10% to 20% of the fibers in the fiber pool have characteristics that would be considered type I or II (coexpression of two or more myosin heavy chain isoforms), whereas in the very old as many as 50% of the fibers in the fiber pool would be considered type I or II, neither strictly type I nor strictly type II. Muscle disuse, which often occurs with aging, has been suggested as an explanation for this increase in coexpression of fiber type, but findings that sedentary young people with knee arthritis and those who are paralyzed after spinal cord injury do not exhibit such coexpression do not support this hypothesis. A more likely explanation is that motor units are lost with age (discussed subsequently) which leads to denervation followed by reinnervation. This reinnervation would then cause a multiple number of fibers in the fiber pool to receive a different neural input, in contradiction to their myogenic lineage, thus providing the fiber with conflicting signals and eventually giving rise to a mixed expression of myosin isoforms.

Aging is associated with a decrease in the number of type I and II fibers, a decrease in size only in type II fibers, and a greater percent of fibers that appear as a cross between type I and II fibers (increased coexpression of fiber types).

Table 5.2 Age-Related Reductions in Human Quadriceps Muscle Fiber Number

Study	Gender	Age (years)	%↓ Type I	%↓ Type II
Larsson et al. (1978)	M	22-65	1	25
Essen-Gustavsson & Borges (1986)	M	20-70	15	19
	F	20-70	25	45
Lexell et al. (1988)	M	15-83	5	29
Hakkinen, Kallinen, et al. (1998) & H. Newton et al. (1998)	M	29-61	+8	10
Fiatarone Singh et al. (1999)	M and F	72-98	+7	60
Frontera et al. (2000)	M	65-77	22	2.5
Hikida et al. (2000)	M	58-78	24	40

Note: M = male; F = female.

Another possible reason for age-related muscle weakness is a change in **specific force,** that is, a reduction in the amount of force that each muscle fiber can produce (newtons of force per fiber cross-sectional area). The concept of specific force is very difficult to quantify in humans, but it has been attempted in intact humans by calculating "specific torque" (isokinetic torque in Newton-meters/lean mass), and it has been used as an indicator of **muscle quality** (Newman et al., 2003). Specific force was reduced 20% in older adults, and this reduction was proposed to be attributable to changes in muscle architecture (Young et al., 1985). Although specific force (tension) can be quantified more reliably in animal studies, answers from these studies are still unclear: some researchers have found age-related declines in specific force, whereas others have not (Brooks & Faulkner, 1988, 1994; McCarter & McGee, 1987). The mechanism of reduced specific tensions in rodent muscle is unclear, although it has been suggested that the contractile proteins, actin and myosin, change so that the development of cross-bridges is inhibited or the cross-bridges of the muscle fibers are not fully activated by calcium. There is, therefore, some support from animal studies for inherent changes in muscle fiber characteristics, which might explain some of the muscle strength loss with age, but these findings need to be replicated.

Another characteristic of neuromuscular function in aged animals is a change in contractile quality of the muscle, usually recorded as a slowed muscle contractile time and lengthened muscle relaxation time. In voluntary contractions, age-related reductions in the rate of force development as well as ability to accelerate the limb have been reported (Hicks et al., 1991; Larsson et al., 1979; Stanley & Taylor, 1993). Electrically evoked isometric contractile properties from various whole limb muscles from older humans usually exhibit reductions in maximal twitch tensions, and longer twitch contractions times are seen in most whole muscles and individual motor units (Doherty & Brown, 1997). It is also clear in humans that not all muscles are similarly affected by age, with greater age changes seen in lower body musculature.

Factors proposed to decrease muscle quality with aging include

- decreased proportion of type II muscle fibers,
- increased connective tissue,
- fatty infiltration, and
- altered muscle metabolism.

Changes in the Nervous System

Muscle fibers are innervated by a motor neuron, and the motor neuron, its axon, and all of the muscle fibers that it innervates are called a **motor unit.** The muscle fiber types are the same in specific motor units, so that motor units also can be categorized as slow oxidative, fast glycolytic, and fast oxidative-glycolytic.

Approximately 1% of the total number of motor units is lost per year, beginning in the third decade of life and increasing in rate after 60 years of age (Rice, 2000). This loss is thought to be attributable to the death of the motor neurons in the spinal cord. Surviving motor units, usually type I, increase fiber number by reinnervating some of the fibers that were innervated by a motor neuron that has died. Thus, the number of muscle fibers per motor neuron (the motor neuron innervation ratio) may increase in the aged adult. If the innervation ratio is substantially changed, fine control of muscle contraction (muscular coordination) may be impaired. The cause of this motor unit remodeling is unclear but it partially explains the functional and morphological changes in aging muscle.

Changes in Muscle Blood Flow— Capillarization

Another factor that could affect muscle strength is the number of capillaries per muscle fiber. The smallest arteries (arterioles) branch into even smaller, almost microscopic blood vessels called capillaries. Some capillaries are so small that they are microscopic, having a capillary wall only one cell thick and allowing only one blood cell to squeeze through them at a time. The larger the number of capillaries per muscle fiber, or the number of capillaries surrounding muscle fibers, the larger the **capillarity** and the better the oxygen exchange capacity. Capillarity declines with aging in very sedentary people (Cartee, 1994), and, hence, oxidative capacity declines. However, submaximal endurance-type training greatly increases the capillarity in muscle (as much as 34% in coronary patients), which in turn increases the tissue and blood oxygen exchange capacity (Ades et al., 1996). **Angiogenesis,** or the exercise-induced development of new capillaries, occurs in the elderly as well as in young individuals. In fact, the major exercise-induced improvements in aerobic capacity are attributed more to increases in mitochondria concentration and capillarity than to changes in blood flow capacity (Terjung et al., 2002). This is why walking is so valuable in the management of older adults who have intermittent claudication (poor peripheral circulation; Prior et al., 2003).

> Aerobic dysfunction of muscle in old adults seems to be much more related to sedentary behavior than to aging. "Some may consider the aged myocyte as a small, inactive, normal myocyte in need of activity!" (Terjung et al., 2002, p. 368)

Poor Nutrition and Physical Inactivity

Although muscle mass declines with aging, it declines significantly less in individuals who maintain a life-long practice of good nutrition accompanied by resistance training. Many elderly adults lose their interest in food, and as a result their nutritional status deteriorates. The combination of poor nutrition and physical inactivity can initiate a downward cycle of sarcopenia. As mentioned in chapter 4, the loss of muscle mass not only decreases the amount of strength and functional capacity of the individual but also accounts for some of the decreased aerobic fitness capability that occurs with aging. The primary measure of fitness, $\dot{V}O_2$max, is highly dependent on the amount of muscle working during the measurement. Thus, significant losses in muscle mass can result in a loss of physical function, fitness reserves, and, in time, the mobility that is essential for independent living.

Resistance Training for Strength

The effects of regular, systematic physical activity on the neuromuscular system of the aging adult are impressive, and the result of a well-planned, scientifically based, resistance training program can be spectacular. Of all the bodily systems, the neuromuscular system can demonstrate the most visibly dramatic difference between a completely sedentary, inactive person and a person who conscientiously trains. In figure 5.5, a series of photographs taken of Clarence Bass over a 45-year period clearly demonstrate the capacity of an individual to maintain muscle mass with training for many years. Over this period of time, he has maintained a lifestyle that includes resistance training, aerobic training, and an excellent diet ("Clarence Bass's Testing," 1993).

Differences in neuromuscular function can range from the 80-year-old who cannot lift a 10-lb (4.5-kg) weight to a person of the same age who can lift 200

What Type of Strength Exercises Should Older Adults Do?

Before the 1990s, exercise recommendations by professional organizations, such as the American College of Sports Medicine and the American Heart Association, emphasized aerobic or endurance exercise, such as walking, swimming, or cycling, as the main component of a fitness program with scarcely a word about muscular strength and power. However, the latest exercise recommendations for all ages, including older adults, include resistance training for muscle strength and power on equal footing with endurance exercises (American College of Sports Medicine, 1998).

lb (91 kg), and from an 80-year-old who cannot get up out of a chair to one who can run a 26.2-mile (42-km) marathon in the Senior Olympics. The muscular system is maintained to a great extent by the amount of daily physical activity an individual experiences, either in work or in leisure pursuits such as sports. The types of movements people make during their daily activities throughout their lives will determine the amount of functional capacity that they can maintain in their musculoskeletal system. Muscles that are never used will deteriorate with the passage of time. Individuals who are physically active and who make it a point to resistance train all of their muscle groups throughout the muscles' full range of motion will maintain an adequate amount of strength well into their senior years. Recent evidence also has shown that those adults who are the strongest in midlife have a two- to threefold reduction in risk of developing disabilities 25 years later compared with their weaker counterparts (Rantanen, 2003). Rantanen also reported that midlife grip strength predicted mortality rate in a group of initially healthy men, such that those with poorer strength at baseline were more likely to die over the 30-year follow-up period.

The muscular system is very responsive to strength training. The training effects are highly specific not only to the type of training, whether aerobic or resistance, but to the muscle that is being used and the way it is being used. Improvements in the amount of force that can be produced are relatively rapid, occurring within 2 months. Also, during this short period, visible changes occur in the shape and tone of body muscles. For these reasons, strength-training

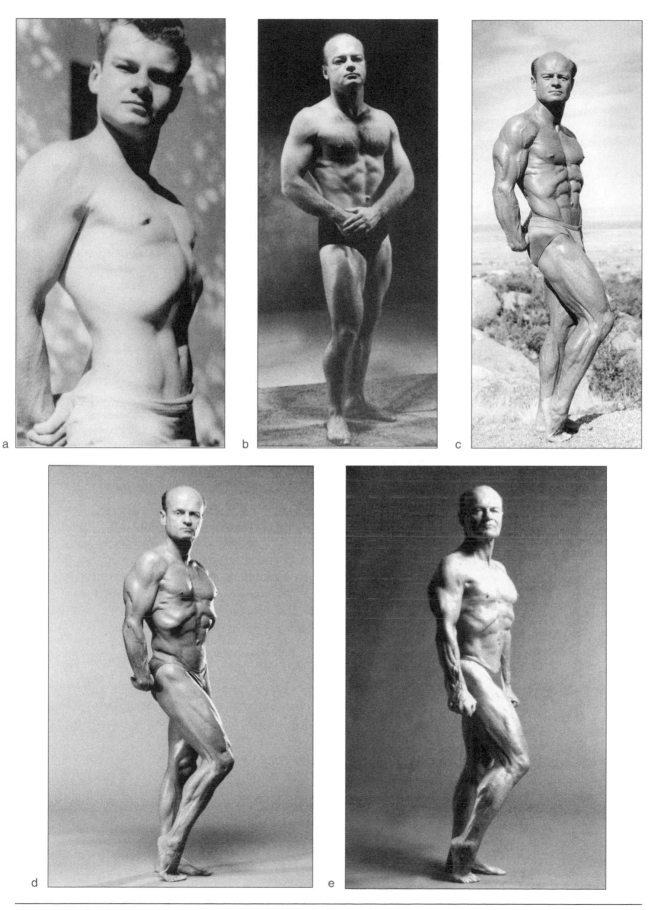

Figure 5.5 Clarence Bass at age (*a*) 15, (*b*) 31, (*c*) 43, and (*d*) 55, and (*e*) 60.

Courtesy of Clarence Bass, Lean for Life, Ripped Enterprises, 528 Clama NE, Albuquerque, NM 87108.

programs also may provide a psychological feeling of accomplishment for many elderly participants.

Individuals who remain physically active by participating in sports, or who work in a strength-demanding job, are stronger in measures of both isometric and dynamic strength than inactive adults, suggesting that the age-related decrements in muscle strength are a function of the type and amount of activity in which adults participate (Aniansson et al., 1983; Frontera et al., 1988). For example, amateur tennis players of both genders in their mid-60s had stronger knee extensors and flexors, when measured by an isokinetic dynamometer, than their sedentary counterparts (Laforest et al., 1990). Women who maintained a physically active lifestyle had higher levels of grip strength than sedentary women (Rikli & Busch, 1986). Adults who continue working at jobs that require strength above the levels required for a sedentary lifestyle generally maintain much higher levels of strength. For example, the grip strength of machine shop workers of various ages did not change at all over a period of 40 years (Petrofsky & Lind, 1975).

Research on the adaptive capacity of the aged human neuromuscular system to resistance training was first published in the 1980s. Frontera and colleagues (1988) shocked many people by reporting striking improvements in leg muscle strength (227%) and significant increases in muscle fiber sizes after only 12 weeks of high-resistance training in older men (average age 65 years). Following this study, Fiatarone and colleagues (1994) reported that nonagenarians (mean age 87) could improve muscle strength and mass after only 10 weeks of training. Since then, increasing numbers of researchers have documented the benefits of resistance training for older men and women, even in those older than 90 years of age. A selected sample of investigations that involved resistance training programs for older adults is summarized in table 5.3. All of these studies used high-intensity resistance training and examined strength changes of the quadriceps muscles—the most frequently studied muscle.

As shown, the typical duration of these resistance training programs was 10 to 12 weeks, with a few studies continuing longer. Strength changes were quite variable across studies, ranging from 28% to 152%, attributable to key design factors such as intensity of training, amount of direct supervision, baseline strength levels, age, and comorbidity conditions of the sample. One study that examined the

Table 5.3 Strength Gains of the Quadriceps Muscle Following High-Intensity Resistance Training in Older Adults

Study	N	Gender	Age (years)	Exercise movement	Duration (weeks)	Strength gains
Frontera et al. (1988)	12	M	60-72	Knee extension	12	1RM; 107%
Charette et al. (1991)	13	F	64-86	Leg press	12	1RM; 28%
Fiatarone et al. (1994)	100	M/F	72-98	Hip and knee extension	10	1RM; 113%
Lexell et al. (1995)	23	M/F	70-77	Knee extension	11	1RM; 152%
McCartney et al. (1996)	113	M/F	60-80	Leg press	84	1RM; 32%
Hakkinen, Kallinen, et al. (1998)	20	M/F	Mean = 70	Knee extension	26	1RM; 26%
Hunter et al. (1999)	11	M/F	64-79	Knee extension	12	1RM; 39%
Tracy et al. (1999)	23	M/F	65-75	Knee extension	9	1RM; 28%
Yarasheski et al. (1999)	12	M/F	76-92	Knee extension	12	1RM; 41%
Hagerman et al. (2000)	9	M	Mean = 64	Knee extension	16	1RM; 50%
Hortobagyi et al. (2001)	27	M/F	66-83	Leg press	10	1RM; 35%
Brose et al. (2003)	28	M/F	Mean = 68	Knee extension Leg press	14	1RM; 48% 1RM; 38%

Note: M = male; F = female; 1RM = 1 repetition maximum.

effects of a 2-year resistance training program in men and women, 60 to 80 years of age, found that strength continued to increase over the 2 years (increases ranging from 32% in leg press to 90% in military press) with no evidence of a plateau in the improvements (McCartney et al., 1996). These researchers also found that taking a 10-week break from resistance training between years 1 and 2 resulted in a loss of muscle strength of only 8%. Although researchers agree that to increase strength, overloading of muscle must occur, they disagree about the amount of overload that is needed for older adults to improve strength, muscle mass, and physical function. Some argue that only high-resistance training (i.e., 60-80% of 1RM for 6-10 repetitions) will increase strength and muscle mass and therefore will be of greatest benefit to independence and physical function (Fiatarone-Singh, 2002). However, there is evidence that even a modest 10% increase in strength, achieved by older adults who completed several months of low-resistance training (i.e., 30-50% of 1RM for 8-15 repetitions), was associated with improved physical function (Brown, 2000). More research is needed to clarify what type of training leads to the greatest benefits for the many different subpopulations of older adults with their many differences in physical function and diseases. Long-term adherence to resistance training also is an important consideration. The best resistance training program must be one that is efficacious but also one that will be followed by the population for which it is prescribed.

The two main factors that explain training-induced strength gains in young and older adults are increases in muscle mass (muscle fiber hypertrophy) and adaptations in the nervous system. Although adaptation in neural control is important for the improvements in strength during the first 4 to 8 weeks, significant muscle fiber hypertrophy occurs later on (Lexell, 2000). Typical training-induced increases in muscle cross-sectional area have been relatively moderate, ranging from 5% to 20%, even with the high-resistance training. Clearly, these muscle mass gains do not match the increases in observed strength, so other factors must be contributing to the increase in strength. Some of these other factors may be improved neural adaptations, improved "learning how to produce strength," increased expectations based on the increased strength experienced, and, finally, a higher motivation inspired by increases in strength with training (Fiatarone Singh et al., 1999; Hikida et al., 2000; Trappe et al., 2000).

A few studies have examined the effects of creatine supplementation in older adults who undergo strength training. The results have been mixed, with one study showing no additional benefits of creatine supplementation on strength gains or body composition and two studies finding that the supplementation was associated with significantly greater increases in fat-free mass and total body mass (Brose et al., 2003). The creatine appeared to be well tolerated by the older adults. Additional studies, with larger subject numbers, conducted over longer training and follow-up periods are needed to determine the safety and efficacy of creatine supplementation for older adults.

Muscle Hypertrophy

Most researchers, using muscle biopsy samples, have found that both muscle fiber types respond to high-resistance strength training with similar amounts of hypertrophy (Charette et al., 1991; Frontera et al., 1988; Hakkinen, Newton, et al., 1998; Hikida et al., 2000; Hunter et al. 1999). It also is important to remember that after 70 years of age, it is normal for muscle mass to deteriorate, so that simply maintaining tissue at that age is considered a benefit. Tracy and colleagues (1999) used magnetic resonance imaging techniques to evaluate in greater detail the effects of 9 weeks of resistance training on total quadriceps muscle volume, which amounted to 12% for both men and women 65 to 75 years of age. This is a much larger gain in muscle mass than the 2.7% increase found after 10 weeks of high-resistance training in a sample of much older (mean age of 87) and more frail residents of a long-term care facility (Fiatarone et al., 1994). However, the nonexercisers in that study lost 1.8% in muscle mass over the 10-week period. Maintenance of benefits from resistance training, as in any other exercise training regime, requires that the program be continued, but these initial gains can be sustained with a reduced exercise frequency of even once per week (Lexell et al., 1995; Taaffe et al., 1999).

High-intensity eccentric training may be an optimal way to provide a strong stimulus for muscle tissue adaptation in older adults, because it appears that the age-related changes in muscle mass, contraction speed, and connective tissue enhance a muscle's ability to achieve relatively high forces under lengthening conditions (Vandervoort, 2002). This high-force condition, in turn, has been reported to provide a powerful signal to the muscle's DNA molecular control mechanisms for cellular adaptations (Hortobagyi et al., 2001). One study in frail older adults, using high-intensity resistance that included an eccentric component, concluded that long-term adaptation to this type of training was characterized by muscle damage and repair cycles associated with large gains in strength (Fiatarone Singh et al., 1999). Muscle biopsy results indicate that the early adaptation to the progressive resistance training includes such muscle damage as a step in a remodeling process that ultimately leads to regeneration of skeletal muscle. The researchers also reported that the insulin-like growth factor 1 in their subjects' muscles following the training indicated that a mechanism of increased protein synthesis might be required for new or hypertrophied myofibril formation.

Logically, it seems that hypertrophy of muscle fibers must result from alterations in muscle protein synthesis, but our knowledge of the effects of training on protein turnover in older adults is limited. A recent study reported that the timing of protein intake after resistance training in older men was important for the development of hypertrophy in skeletal muscle (Esmarck et al., 2001). The authors found that the group of 70-year-old men who took an oral protein supplement immediately after resistance training experienced greater improvements in dynamic strength, muscle cross-sectional area, and lean body mass compared with a group that delayed the protein intake until 2 hr after their resistance training session. It appears that resistance training along with immediate protein supplementation is important for increasing lean body mass in older men.

Strength training by older adults substantially improves strength, and a lifestyle that incorporates strength training will surely maintain muscle mass to some degree. No lifetime longitudinal studies of the effects of resistance training on the maintenance of muscle mass have been conducted, however, so the extent to which strength training is effective is not known. Observations of aged weightlifters provide some evidence, but only force output, not muscle mass, is quantified in these competitive events. What has become clear is that endurance training alone cannot prevent the deterioration in muscle mass with age.

Physicians in the United States have been reluctant to recommend weightlifting and resistance exercise for older adults who have hypertension or a history of cardiovascular problems, and these physicians' concerns have extended also to their prescriptions for normal, healthy older adults. The concern has been that the high pressures that can develop within the chest cavity during contractions against heavy resistance could result in a great resistance to blood flow through the vessels in the thoracic cavity and precipitate cardiovascular or cerebrovascular accidents. However, Lewis and colleagues (1983) showed that not much difference exists in the blood pressure responses between isometric and dynamic exercises if similar activities are compared. Under the careful supervision of a physician, exercise physiologist, or rehabilitation

Precaution Before Prescribing Endurance Exercise for Frail Older Adults

Fiatarone Singh (2002) suggested that before using endurance training with a frail older adult, health care professionals should follow a simple rule. The frail older adult should be asked to rise from a chair, stand with eyes closed, open eyes, and then walk across the room. If the person has difficulty standing from the chair or has to use the chair arms to help push up, then strengthening exercise should be prescribed first. If there is impairment in standing balance, then balance exercises should be prescribed. Only if these first two tests are performed easily should endurance training be the first mode of exercise prescribed.

specialist, older adults who have a relatively low risk for cardiac problems and who have normal ventricular function could safely participate in strength and resistance training (Fiatarone Singh, 2002). Sufficient data from both epidemiological studies and experimental trials exist to warrant the training of all physicians, including geriatricians, in the basics of exercise prescription for health-related and quality-of-life benefits. Exercise advice should be specific in terms of modality, frequency, duration, and intensity and should be accompanied by practical implementation solutions and behavior support systems for monitoring progress and providing feedback.

Importance of Learning in Strength Training

Along with muscle hypertrophy and neural adaptations that occur with resistance training, there appears to be a large learning component that older adults undergo to produce maximal contractions. For example, it appears that older adults experience a large learning curve in their ability to switch movement patterns from concentric to eccentric. Some researchers were able to effectively increase ankle dorsiflexion in older adults by using an isokinetic, motor-driven dynamometer to rotate the subjects' ankle joints into plantar flexion while the subjects resisted with their dorsiflexor muscles as much as possible (Connelly & Vandervoort, 2000). However, the older adults underwent considerable learning with this task, progressing from an initial pattern of eccentric movements that were quite uncoordinated to a smoother and more effective torque generation pattern. This learning was most pronounced at high velocities. Maximal voluntary torque levels also improved, along with electromyographic evidence that the nervous system of the older adults adapted by learning to activate the dorsiflexor muscles at a higher intensity. This study, along with others, supports the idea that older adults improve intensity, steadiness of force development, and coordination of muscle activation levels after high-intensity resistance training. It also supports the translation of improved strength levels to functional mobility, as evidenced by tasks such as increased walking speed as well as improved ability to climb stairs and rise from a chair (Bassey et al., 1992; Fiatarone et al., 1994).

Muscular Power

The basic difference between strength and power is the speed at which a weight is lifted or force is exerted (force × velocity). **Power** is the work rate or the product of force produced and movement velocity. Generating peak power requires timing and coordination and a general assumption that participants are moving at their maximum velocity. Assessment of muscular power usually involves any all-out exercise of 6 to 8 s including stair sprinting and vertical jumps,

as well as sprint running (40-yd [36.5-m] dash), arm crank ergometry, and cycling tests. Isokinetic dynamometers are used to measure both strength and power as well. Several factors that are discussed throughout this book such as strength, speed, and coordination are primary contributors to peak power generation.

Changes in Muscle Power With Age

Age-related changes in power are about 6% to 11% per decade for absolute power and, if scaled to body size or mass (relative power), about 6% to 8% per decade. If individuals continue to train for power, such as competitive cyclists, the magnitude of decline is slightly less than that reported for the general population for absolute power (7.5% per decade), power scaled to body mass (7.6% per decade), and power scaled to lean thigh volume estimated and optimal pedaling velocity (3.5% per decade; Martin et al., 2000). The reduction in power for the general population versus elite cyclists emphasizes the importance of maintaining high levels of physical activity, particularly at high levels of intensity.

The decline in power with age is greater than the decline in strength. Despite a similar age of onset of decline, power declines at a 10% greater rate per decade than does strength (figure 5.6; Metter et al., 1997). Others have suggested that between the ages of

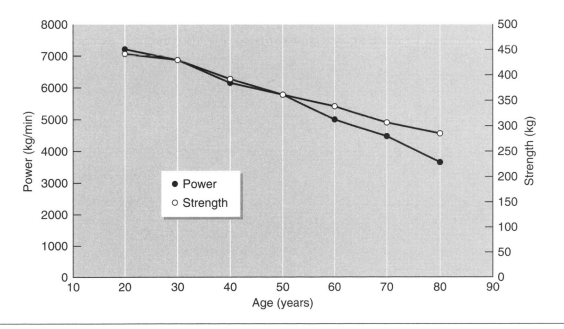

Figure 5.6 Longitudinal data for measures of strength and power for men followed for an average time period of 9.6 years. Both strength and power declined with age ($p < .001$), and power declined at a greater rate than strength ($p < .05$).

Journals of Gerontology. Series A, Biological Sciences and Medical Sciences by E.J. Metter. Copyright 1997 by Gerontological Society of America. Reproduced with Permission of Gerontological Society of America in the format textbook via Copyright Clearance Center.

60 and 89, the loss of power is accelerated, perhaps as high as 3.5% per year for leg extensor power (Skelton et al., 1995; Young & Skelton, 1994).

| Both strength and power decline with age, but power declines to a greater extent.

The percentage of decline reported also varies according to whether the study was cross-sectional or longitudinal. The difference in strength and power reported in longitudinal studies is frequently larger than that reported in cross-sectional studies (Metter et al., 1997; figure 5.7). The magnitude of decline may be related to the different types of subjects found in the two different study designs. For example, adults who choose to participate in a cross-sectional study may be more representative of "optimal agers," whereas individuals who participate in longitudinal studies may remain in the study through sickness, disease, depression, and minor injuries. These factors may be the explanation for older adults not participating in a cross-sectional study when given the opportunity.

Potential Causes for Age-Related Reductions in Power

The main determinants of maximal power, at least as reflected by an anaerobic cycling test, are the amount of muscle available (muscle volume) and the avail-

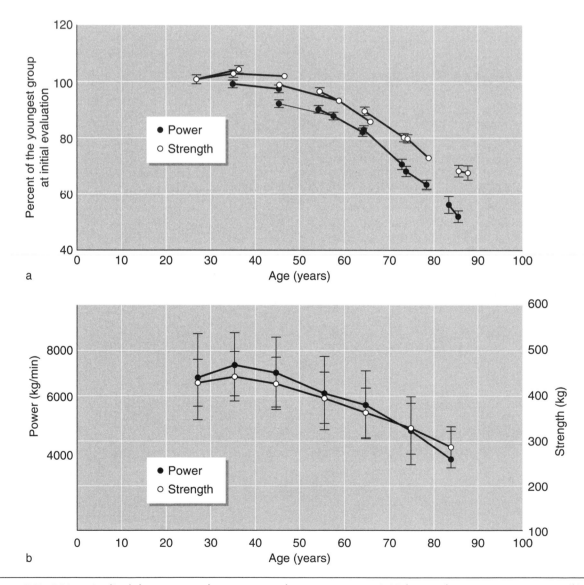

Figure 5.7 (a) Longitudinal data expressed as a percent of a young group at initial strength or power assessment; (b) cross-sectional data of men at seven different age decades.

Journals of Gerontology. Series A, Biological Sciences and Medical Sciences by E.J. Metter. Copyright 1997 by Gerontological Society of America. Reproduced with Permission of Gerontological Society of America in the format textbook via Copyright Clearance Center.

able fast twitch fibers in the muscle (Martin et al., 2000). If a muscle is highly trained throughout life so that the volume is maintained as high as possible and the muscle excitation is practiced frequently, age plays a very small role in the loss of power. As seen in figure 5.8, the effect of age on pedaling power of competitive cyclists looks huge if absolute power is predicted by age alone (82%). The effect is less if power is shown relative to body mass (~68%), it is dramatically less if the power is scaled to thigh volume (<20%), and it almost disappears (2%) if power is predicted by both thigh volume and maximal pedaling rate (an indicator of fiber type composition and function). Thus, the loss of power with age is primarily attributable to some of the mechanisms proposed to explain the loss of muscle strength: for example, sarcopenia, perhaps occurring more in fast-twitch fibers than in slow-twitch fibers, so that the rate at which muscle can be contracted is slower. In the highly trained competitive cyclists represented in figure 5.8, the loss of muscular power, when both muscle volume and contractile speed are considered, is only approximately 3% per decade, at least to the age of 70.

Power declines in aging average adults that are scaled only to body mass are about 6% to 11% per decade and presumably would be less if their contractile speed data were available. Nevertheless, aging inevitably reduces muscle volume, even in the trained athlete, and most researchers believe that although type I fibers decline, type II, fast-twitch fibers are selectively lost (Newton et al., 2002). This loss dramatically affects power, because type II fibers have been reported to have a peak power output that is four times that of type I fibers (Faulkner et al., 1986). The percentage of type IIa and IIb fibers in older adults was negatively correlated with age, even after a 72-hr mixed-method resistance training program (Newton et al., 2002).

However, these mechanisms cannot explain why absolute power losses observed in untrained adults are greater than strength losses after the 6th decade (refer to figure 5.6, p. 121). One explanation may be that although the same number of type IIb motor neurons is activated in a slow recruitment of maximum muscle force, the firing frequency of these type IIb fibers declines with aging, and they are unable to fire at the same high rates that they could at younger ages. The decline of neurological contractile mechanisms may accelerate in older decades (7th and older). Or, both the loss of type II fibers and slowing of firing frequency may accelerate in the older decades. This would explain the accelerated decline beginning around age 70 that is seen in performance records of elite athletes whose sports rely heavily on strength and power (see chapter 12 on weightlifting, power lifting, and sprinting performances).

Relationship Between Power and Physical Function

The maintenance of muscle power throughout life is important not just to older adults who wish to keep active in sports but to all older adults, even the oldest. The speed with which an individual responds to an unexpected event such as stopping abruptly to avoid an oncoming car, grabbing a handrail, recovering from a stumble, or pressing the brake pedal to avoid an accident is important, and the inability to perform these actions may have significant consequences. Power plays a significant role in the ability to correct for sudden losses of balance. Gradual age-related losses of power lead to an inability to correct for these temporary losses of balance, which in turn may result in a catastrophic fall. The strength and power of knee extensors and flexors and ankle plantar flexors and dorsiflexors are lower in fallers compared with nonfallers (Whipple et al., 1987). Thus, power is related to the ability to restore balance, and power training plays an important role in fall prevention programs. Recent studies comparing strength and power training programs have found power training to be more effective than strength training for improving physical function in community-dwelling older adults with muscle weakness (Miszko et al., 2003). Another study of 1,453 older adults in Italy found that leg power consistently explained more of the variance than strength did in several measures of physical performance (Bean et al., 2003). In fact, poor muscle power was associated with

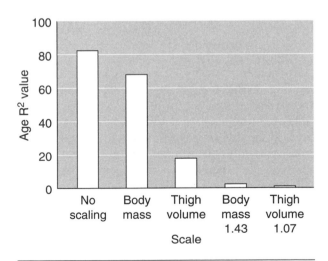

Figure 5.8 The effect of scaling lower limb power to body and specific muscle mass volumes.

Journals of Gerontology. Series A, Biological Sciences and Medical Sciences by J. Martin. Copyright 2000 by Gerontological Society of America in the format textbook via Copyright Clearance Center.

a two- to threefold greater risk for mobility impairments than poor muscle strength.

In perturbation paradigm studies, in which a jerk or a push is applied to make an individual lose balance and attempt to regain it, older adults have greater difficulty recovering from a perturbation, especially a backward perturbation. In particular, older adults responded to a backward perturbation with a compensatory step as opposed to the feet-in-place strategy used by young adults (Hall & Jensen, 2002). Older adults chose the compensatory step because it was less energy demanding than a feet-in-place response.

The maintenance of power also contributes to the maintenance of physical function in frail elderly adults. Bassey and her colleagues (1992) were among the first to demonstrate a relationship between functional status and power. In their study, the leg extensor power of frail nursing home residents was significantly correlated with functional measures such as chair-rising speed, stair-climbing speed, and walking speed (figure 5.9). In addition to the contribution that leg extension power makes to rising from a chair, leg extension power also enables old adults to step up on a high step such as might be encountered climbing into a bus (Skelton et al., 1994). When functional status (as measured by activities of daily living and mobility scores) was predicted from dynamic concentric strength, muscular power, muscular endurance, $\dot{V}O_2$peak, and habitual physical activity, only two of these, power and habitual physical activity, contributed independently to functional status (40% of the variance; Foldvari et al., 2000). Finally, the observation that older men and women who used assistive aids had less than half of the leg extensor power of those who did not need assistive devices strongly supports the proposal that in very old age, the maintenance of power, more than strength, is crucial to maintaining function in the lower extremities.

Resistance Training for Power

It is well known that resistance programs for strength are effective and safe for most elderly, from healthy community-dwelling individuals to frail populations. The amount of research on power training programs is not nearly as extensive as the research on strength training programs. The primary difference between strength training and power training is that in power training, the individual is asked to perform the concentric part of the weight lift as rapidly as possible, whereas little or no instruction related to the velocity of lift is given in strength training. The fact that power declines to a greater extent than strength has been known for quite some time; however, it was not until Bassey and colleagues (1992) established that a reduction in power has functional consequences that power training began to receive more attention. Since that study was published, the priority of establishing the efficacy and tolerance of power training programs for healthy, active, and frail populations increased among strength researchers.

The amount of strength and power that older adults have varies considerably and depends on individuals' characteristics and the type of strength or power that is tested. Initial baseline differences, subject characteristics, and the type of test used make a large difference in the degree of improvement that each person can expect following an intervention program (Newton et al., 2002). However, even though individual differences in power are great, most older adults can exhibit training adaptations toward faster, more powerful performance. Healthy older men have exhibited training effects as high as young men using 30% and 60% 1RM following a 10-week periodized resistance training program emphasizing muscle power, strength, and hypertrophy (figure 5.10; Newton et al., 2002). Not only are training adaptations possible and attainable, but increases as high as 141% (leg power following power training) at resistances set at 70% of body weight have been reported.

Is power training a necessary intervention, or can power be increased in an equally efficient manner through other types of intervention programs? According to the training specificity principle, physiological and functional adaptations are specific to the type of training used. Therefore, programs that do not emphasize high-velocity training may not lead to increases in power, at least not to the same extent.

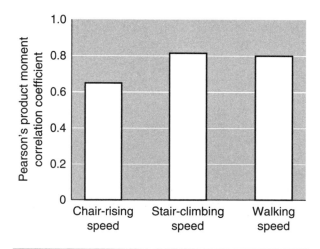

Figure 5.9 Relationship between leg extensor power and functional performance as indicated by chair-rising speed ($p < .001$), stair-climbing speed ($p < .001$), and walking speed ($p < .001$).

Adapted, with permission, from E.J. Bassey et al., 1992, *Clinical Science* 82: 321-327. © the Biomechanical Society and the Medical Research Society.

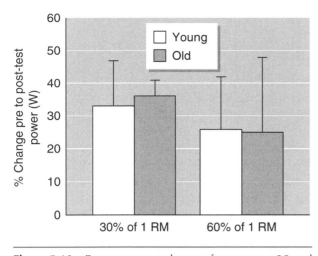

Figure 5.10 Pre- to posttest changes for power at 30 and 60% 1RM for young and old men.

Adapted, by permission, from R.U Newton et al., 2002, "Mixed-methods resistance training increases power and strength of young and older men," *Medicine and Science in Sports and Exercise* 34: 1372.

High-velocity training is an essential component for increasing power performance (Earles et al., 2001). In Earles and colleagues' study, two groups, a power and a walking training group, were exposed to a 12-week training program. Peak leg power increased significantly (22%) for the power training group but did not increase significantly for the walking training group (figure 5.11*a*). In addition, the power training group increased strength by 22% whereas the walking training group only increased strength by 12% (figure 5.11*b*). Thus, effective training interventions for power should incorporate exercises that have a high-velocity component.

Are strength training programs as effective as power training programs for increasing muscle power? The effectiveness of strength training programs to increase strength is well established, and the training procedures used to optimize strength gains have also been developed. Therefore, if existing strength training programs could be as effective at increasing power, then it would be practical to implement these programs to increase power performance. However, even though the results of strength training programs have been remarkable in developing strength (150% gains in frail older adults; Fiatorone et al., 1990), power increases following the same strength training protocol were much more modest (Fiatarone et al., 1994). Following a progressive resistance training program, strength was increased 100%, but stair-climbing power gains were much less robust (28%). These results have been corroborated by other researchers who have also found minimal to no gain in power following strength training programs (i.e., Joszi et al., 1999; Skelton et al., 1995). Conversely, high-velocity training has been shown in at

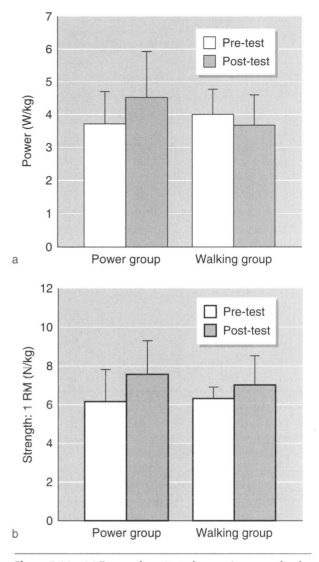

a

b

Figure 5.11 (*a*) Pre- and posttest changes in power for the power training group (*p* = .004) and the walking group (*p* > .05). (*b*) Pre- and posttest changes in strength for the power training group and the walking group (*p* > .0001)

Adapted from *Archives of Physical Medical Rehabilitation*, 82, D.R. Earles, J.O. Judge, and O.T. Gunnarsson. Velocity training induces power-specific adaptations in highly functioning older adults, pp. 872-878. Copyright 2001, with permission from American Congress of Rehabilitation Medicine and the American Academy of Physical Medicine and Rehabilitation.

least one study to be much more effective in increasing power and at least as effective as strength training in building strength (Fielding et al., 2002)

Even though research has shown compellingly that older adults can improve their power output with high-velocity training programs, many professionals are reluctant to implement these programs because older adults may not be able to tolerate high-velocity power training for an extended period of time, and the safety of such programs has not been determined for various age groups. Especially there is concern about implementing these types

Power Training Increases Strength

Fielding and colleagues (2002) found that high-velocity resistance training was more effective for increasing power and equally effective for increasing strength compared with low-velocity training. In this study, 30 women (aged 70 ± 1) with self-reported disability (preexisting functional limitations) were randomly assigned to a high- or low-velocity training group. This particular subject population was targeted because of their lower peak power compared with healthy, high-functioning adults. Subjects participated in a 16-week high- or low-velocity resistance training program at 70% 1RM (adjusted biweekly), during which they executed three sets of eight repetitions of bilateral leg press and left and right knee extension. The percent increase for peak power for the high-velocity group was twofold that for the low-velocity group for leg press and significantly more for knee extension (figure 5.12a). In addition, the gains in leg press and extensor strength were similar between groups (figure 5.12b). Also, strength gains were essentially the same, if not slightly greater, in the high-velocity group, suggesting that high-velocity training is effective for increasing both power and strength.

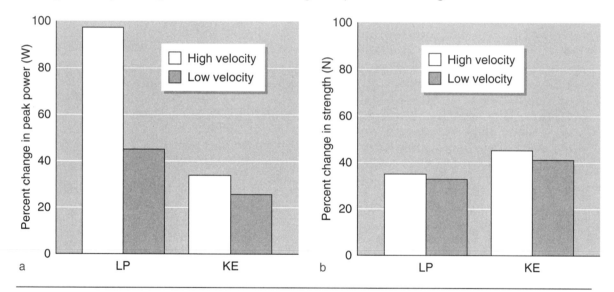

Figure 5.12 (a) Pre- to posttest change in power for leg press (LP; $p < .0001$) and knee extension (KE; $p < .001$) for high- and low-velocity training groups. (b) Pre- to posttest change in strength for LP and KE for high- and low-velocity training groups. Both groups increased muscle strength ($p < .001$). LP power increased significantly more in high- than low-velocity training.

Adapted, by permission, from R.A. Fielding et al., 2002, "High-velocity resistance training increases skeletal muscle peak in older women," *Journal of the American Geriatrics Society* 50: 655-662.

of programs for populations that are sedentary and have a low level of functioning. One study has addressed this issue. Fielding and colleagues (2002) specifically recruited old adults with functional limitations, physical disability, or a history of falls and found that these subjects could successfully complete and tolerate a high-velocity training program at 70% 1RM. The dropout rate of subjects from the high- and low-velocity groups was the same. Of the five subjects who dropped out, four did so because of pain associated with arthritis. However, several other participants who also had preexisting arthritic conditions remained in the study. An important key

to the success and safety of this intervention program for this low-functioning population is that the study was carefully designed by expert researchers in kinesiology and gerontology, and the participants were carefully supervised by knowledgeable professionals who had extensive training in this area.

Both strength- and power-training programs improve muscle strength, but only power training increases power output. However, knowledge about the safety of these programs and long-term adherence to the power training programs by older adults is limited.

SUMMARY

Both strength and power are essential to individuals across the life span because these factors are needed for many activities of daily living and are necessary for many job-related tasks and social activities. Declines of approximately 1% per year in strength begin in the mid-40s with greater yearly declines found in those over 70 years of age. Longitudinal studies show that men and women experience similar losses in lower body strength, but women show fewer declines in upper body strength with age than men. Isometric and eccentric muscle strength appears to decline less with age than does concentric strength. Much of the strength loss with age is attributed to a loss of muscle mass caused by an equal decline in number of type I and II fibers. There also is a decline in muscle fiber size, primarily in type II fibers. Although most investigators agree that an overall loss of muscle mass accounts for the largest portion of strength loss, it does not account for all of the loss. There are also changes in the nervous system with age including a loss of motor units, particularly fast-twitch units, and a larger innervation ratio in the motor units that remain. Declines in muscle blood flow with age may also explain some of the strength declines.

Chronic resistance training for strength enables individuals to maintain high levels of strength for many years and also provides individuals who have not been involved in strength training an opportunity to reverse many of the age-related deterioration processes that are observed in the muscles of sedentary people. Adults who continue participating in sports maintain their muscular strength much better than sedentary adults do, and adults of any age, even very old age, can experience remarkable and dramatics gains in strength following a resistance training program. Resistance training programs increase muscle mass in old adults as well as in young adults, with individual muscle fibers increasing in size and protein content. Even daily strength training, however, cannot postpone indefinitely the inevitable deterioration in muscle mass.

More recently the focus shifted to examine muscle power losses with age. Power refers to the rapid generation of force and appears to decline with age even more than strength. Generating peak power requires timing and coordination and also requires that participants move at their maximum velocity. The causes for a loss in muscle power with age are similar to those reported for strength. Studies using resistance training programs to improve power in older adults are few, but they have been successful. Perhaps the most important reasons for including resistance training for strength and power as one ages are to maintain physical function and mobility, such as walking and stair climbing, and to decrease the risk for disability later in life.

REVIEW QUESTIONS

1. What changes in strength occur with aging? How are these changes affected by gender, type of muscle contraction, upper versus lower body musculature, and cross-sectional versus longitudinal study design?
2. List and describe possible causes of the loss in strength with aging.
3. What is the difference between absolute and relative loss of strength?
4. What are the effects of resistance training on neuromuscular function?
5. Are changes in power different from changes in strength with age? Explain.
6. Describe the relationship between power and physical function.

SUGGESTED READINGS

Fiatarone Singh, M.A. (2002). Exercise comes of age: Rationale and recommendations for a geriatric exercise prescription. *Journal of Gerontology: Medical Sciences, 57A*(5), M262-M282.

Rantanen, T. (2003). Muscle strength, disability, and mortality. *Scandinavian Journal of Medicine and Science in Sports, 13*, 3-8.

Vandervoort, A.A. (Ed). (2000). Strength training for older persons: Benefits and guidelines. *Topics in Geriatric Rehabilitation, 15*, 1-98.

Vandervoort, A.A. (2002). Aging of the human neuromuscular system. *Muscle and Nerve, 25*, 17-25.

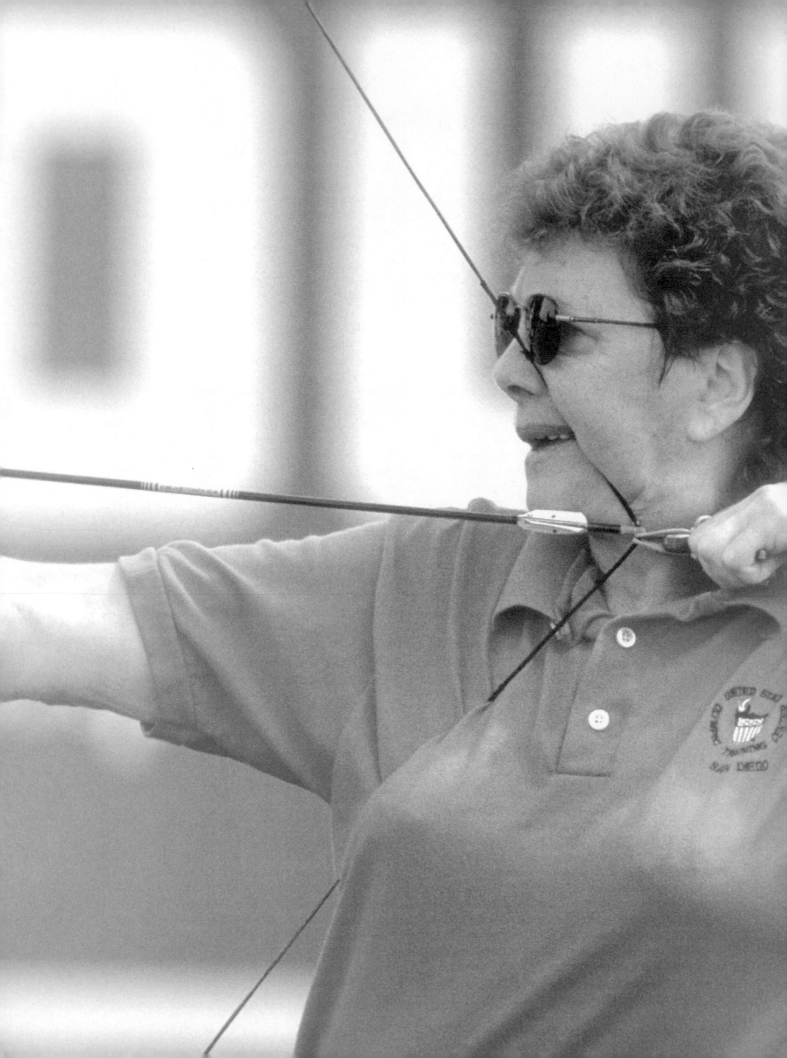

PART III

Motor Coordination, Motor Control, and Skill

Balance, Posture, and Locomotion

Debra J. Rose, PhD
California State University, Fullerton

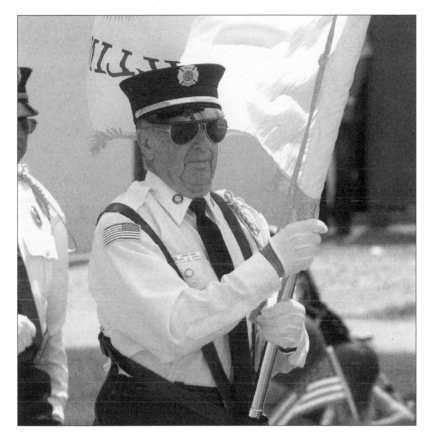

The objectives of this chapter are

- to identify the ways in which the multiple systems in the body contribute to balance and mobility;

- to describe the important age-associated changes in posture, balance, and locomotion;

- to describe how balance and gait are measured in laboratory and field settings;

- to identify the extrinsic and intrinsic risk factors that contribute to falls in the elderly; and

- to become familiar with the various types of intervention strategies used to lower the risk for falls among older adults.

Our ability to perform a number of basic and intermediate activities of daily living or engage in a number of different recreational or sporting pursuits is contingent on our ability to control the multiple dimensions of **posture**, balance, and locomotion. Unfortunately, advancing age is all too often associated with an observable decline in each of these dimensions. Although some older adults experience only modest changes in function, others experience more profound changes that place them at high risk for loss of independence attributable to fall-related injuries. This chapter describes the multiple dimensions of posture, balance, and locomotion and the effect that aging has on each of these dimensions. Ways to measure the multiple dimensions of balance and gait in both a laboratory and a clinical or field setting are then described. Finally, the risk factors that contribute to falling among the elderly are identified as well as how to prevent or reduce the incidence of falling among older adults by using a variety of different intervention strategies.

Defining the Multiple Dimensions of Balance

This chapter will introduce a number of new terms that are used in the literature to describe the multiple dimensions of posture, balance, and locomotion (or gait). Some of the more important terms are introduced in this first section; others are described in later sections.

Balance, Stability Limits, and Mobility

Balance can be defined as the process by which we control the body's **center of mass (COM)** with respect to the base of support (BOS), whether it is stationary or moving. For example, when a person is standing upright in space, the primary goal is to maintain the COM within the confines of the BOS, whereas when that person is walking the COM continuously moves beyond the base of support. A new BOS must be established with each step taken. Although standing upright on a stable surface is usually categorized as a static balance task and leaning through space, transferring, or walking are categorized as dynamic balance tasks, maintaining a stable upright position also involves the active contraction of various muscle groups to control the position of the COM against the destabilizing forces of gravity.

How far older adults are able to lean in any direction without having to change their base of support constitutes their **stability limits.** It has been estimated that for adults able to align their COM directly above their BOS during quiet standing, it is possible to sway as far as $12°$ in a forward and backward direction and $16°$ laterally before it is necessary to take a step because the limits of their stability have been exceeded (Nashner, 1990). Reduced or asymmetrical limits of stability (LOS) may be the result of such things as musculoskeletal abnormalities caused by weakness in the muscles of the ankle joint or reduced range of motion about the ankles, neurological trauma that adversely affects weight bearing or weight shifting in a particular direction (e.g., stroke, Parkinson's disease, multiple sclerosis), or a fear of falling. The boundaries of the stability limits will also vary according to an individual's inherent biomechanical limitations, the task being performed, and the constraints of the environment.

Mobility has been defined as the ability to move independently and safely from one place to another (Shumway-Cook & Woollacott, 2001). Adequate levels of mobility are required for many different types of activities that are performed during daily life. Mobility activities include transfers (e.g., rising from a chair, climbing or descending stairs), walking or running, and other types of recreational activities (e.g., gardening, sport, dancing).

Anticipatory and Reactive Postural Control

Although many of the balance- and mobility-related activities that are performed during our daily lives can be consciously planned in advance, there are times when an unexpected event forces us to respond more subconsciously or automatically. Well-learned balance skills also tend to be largely controlled at a subconscious level so we can attend to other elements occurring in the environment or perform a second task simultaneously that requires conscious attention. **Anticipatory postural control** is the term often used to describe actions that can be planned in advance, whereas **reactive postural control** is a term used to describe situations that cannot be planned in advance of the action required. Anticipatory postural control is needed to avoid obstacles in our path as we walk to the store or plan to open what appears to be a heavy door. Anticipatory postural control also assists us in adapting our gait pattern as we move between different types of surfaces (e.g., firm to compliant or moving surfaces, wide to narrow). In contrast, reactive postural control becomes necessary when we have to respond quickly to an event that we did not expect, such as stepping in an unseen hole or being bumped in a crowd.

Postural Control Strategies

Research studies conducted over the years have revealed the existence of at least three distinct postural control strategies that are commonly used either consciously or subconsciously to control the amount of body sway in a forward or backward direction. These strategies are referred to as the ankle, hip, and step strategies (see figure 6.1). In the case of the **ankle strategy**, the body moves as a single entity about the ankle joints as force is exerted against the surface. A person using an ankle strategy moves the upper and lower body in the same direction (in-phase). Because the amount of force that can be generated by the muscles surrounding the ankle joint is relatively small, this strategy is generally used to control sway when we are standing upright in space or swaying slowly through a very small range of motion. The ankle strategy is also used subconsciously to restore balance following a small nudge or push.

In contrast to the ankle strategy, the **hip strategy** involves the activation of the larger hip muscles and is used when the **center of gravity (COG)** must be moved more quickly back over the base of support as the speed or distance of the sway increases. A person using a hip strategy will move the upper body in a

direction that is opposite to the lower body (out-of-phase). The hip strategy becomes increasingly important as the speed and distance of body sway increase or when we are standing on a surface that is narrower than the length of the feet. In this surface condition, the ankle strategy becomes ineffective because there is not enough surface against which to push to generate sufficient force to restore balance using the smaller ankle muscles.

The final postural control strategy that is used to control balance is the **step strategy.** Traditional thinking was that this strategy came into play when the COG was displaced beyond an individual's maximum LOS or the speed of sway was so high that a hip strategy was not sufficient to maintain the center of gravity within the stability limits. In this situation, at least one or more steps must be taken to establish a new base of support and avoid a fall. More recently, however, researchers have found that when the behavior of the individual being tested is not constrained (i.e., individual is not instructed to maintain feet in place during the surface perturbation) or attention is allocated to a secondary task, the step strategy often occurs before the LOS have actually been exceeded (Brown et al., 1999; McIlroy & Maki, 1996). Maki and McIlroy (1996) argued that stepping actually appears to be the preferred strategy, even when the perturbation is small, and the individual is free to respond naturally. Although each of the postural control strategies discussed in this section is described as if it were a distinct pattern of postural control, various combinations of these strategies are also used to control sway in a standing position under different experimental conditions (Horak & Nashner, 1986; Jensen et al., 1996; Runge et al., 1999).

What factors are likely to limit a person's ability to use each of these three postural control strategies? In the case of the ankle strategy, adequate range of motion and strength within the muscles surrounding the ankle joint are needed. The surface below the feet must also be firm and broad, and the individual must have adequate sensation in the feet to be able to feel the surface. Older adults experiencing a significant decline in sensation in the feet or ankles will find it particularly difficult to employ this strategy.

Unlike the ankle strategy, the ability to use a hip strategy to control postural sway is determined more by

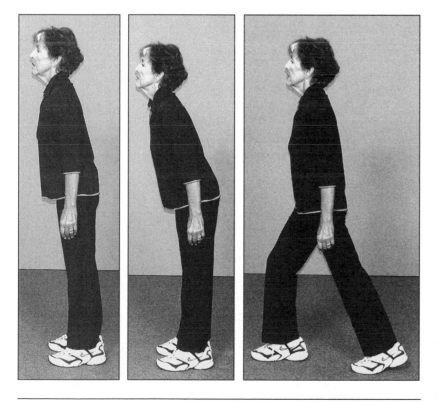

Figure 6.1 Three distinct postural control strategies have been identified. These include the (a) ankle, (b) hip, and (c) step.

Reprinted, by permission, from D.J. Rose, 2003, *FallProof!* (Champaign, IL: Human Kinetics), 6.

the amount of muscle strength and range of motion available in the hip region as opposed to the ankle. Sway in the lateral direction is also controlled by the hip, particularly the **adductor** and **abductor** muscle groups. Any weakness in these muscles will adversely affect lateral stability, an important requirement when walking.

As mentioned earlier in this section, the stepping strategy is used to establish a new BOS when the perceived or actual LOS are exceeded. The ability to use this particular postural control strategy effectively will be very much affected by both the amount of lower limb strength available and the speed with which it can be generated for rapid initiation of the step (i.e., muscle power). Slowed central processing is also likely to adversely affect an older adult's ability to use this strategy effectively. Reduced somatosensation in the feet and below-normal range of motion at the hip joints are also factors in determining how quickly the step is initiated and the length of the step or steps taken after a loss of balance.

Theoretical Framework of Balance and Mobility

In contrast to the more traditional theoretical approaches used to study posture, balance, and locomotion (e.g., reflex or hierarchical), contemporary approaches assume that multiple systems collaborate to control bodily orientation and locomotion. Although certain systems provide the sensorimotor processes that constitute the physiological basis of postural control, other systems (e.g., musculoskeletal, cognitive) constrain an individual's capability for achieving a particular goal-directed action. This contemporary approach to the study of human postural control is generally known as the **"systems theory"** (see Shumway-Cook & Woollacott, 2001, for a more detailed description of this theoretical approach). In addition to the intrinsic subsystems that both shape and on occasion constrain an individual's movements, two additional constraints on action also play an important role in shaping the action that emerges. According to the systems theory, these include the goals of the action being attempted and the properties of the environment in which the action is to take place.

Given that we currently reside on earth, gravitational and inertial forces are always acting upon the upright body in any given environmental context. Although the influence of these external forces is minimal when an individual is performing a relatively simple task such as standing quietly on a broad, firm surface, these forces are magnified as the person begins to perform more difficult tasks in changing environmental conditions.

As the number of intrinsic systems declines toward a critical threshold of function, manifesting in balance-related impairments (e.g., muscle weakness, reduced range of motion, sensory loss), an individual's ability to accomplish a single daily task such as rising from a chair or climbing and descending stairs becomes compromised. The added challenge of performing a second task simultaneously with the first (e.g., carrying a bag of groceries and talking to someone at the same time) further compromises action because of the need to divide attention between the two tasks. The existing environmental conditions (e.g., reduced lighting conditions, the absence of handrails on the stairs) contribute one more element of complexity to the task situation and constitute another important variable likely to affect overall fall risk. An illustration of how the different goals associated with an action and the properties of the environment interact with an individual's intrinsic capabilities to shape action is provided in figure 6.2.

In recognition of their compromised abilities, older adults either cease to perform certain daily tasks or cease participating in social activities that they think will place them at high risk for falling. Or, they begin to limit the types of environments in which they are prepared to engage in those activities. Although these self-imposed restrictions on activity will decrease falls in the short term by reducing expo-

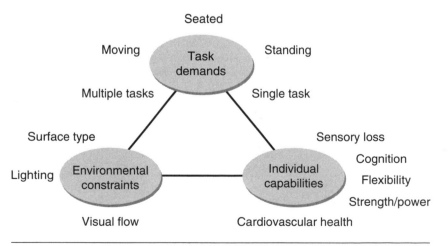

Figure 6.2 Action is shaped by the interaction that occurs between the individual, the task demands, and the constraints of the environment.

sure, over the long term diminished self-confidence and severe physical deconditioning will only hasten the onset of physical frailty and increase the risk for falls (Tinetti et al., 1988).

Action is shaped by the interaction that occurs between the individual, the task, and the environment.

Intrinsic Systems Contributing to Balance and Mobility

In this section, three important intrinsic systems that contribute to a person's ability to maintain balance in standing and moving environments are described. These systems include the sensory, motor, and cognitive systems. First, the various sensory systems (i.e., vision, somatosensory, and vestibular) provide information arising from the surrounding environment and as a result of our own actions. This information is critical for successful goal-directed action planning as well as subconscious or automatic adjustments that are needed to maintain a given position in space or respond rapidly to a change in task or environmental demands. Each of the three sensory systems provides the information needed to anticipate changes that will affect action, as well as respond to changes that have already occurred. Second, the many structures and pathways within the nervous system that comprise the motor system are critical for action.

The motor system acts on the sensory information arising from the external environment as well as other sensory areas within the nervous system. Action is accomplished as a result of the nervous system constraining groups of muscles throughout the body to act together. These are referred to as **muscle response synergies** and are responsible for the many coordinated actions we are able to produce during the course of our daily lives. Third, the cognitive system plays an important assistive role so that we can appropriately interpret the incoming sensations and plan the ensuing motor response. This system, which encompasses the processes of attention, memory storage, and intelligence, provides us with the collective ability to anticipate and adapt our actions in response to changing task demands and the environment.

Sensory Systems

As indicated earlier, three sensory systems are particularly important for good postural control and largely determine how well we perceive what needs to be done based on the information presented to us. These are the visual, somatosensory, and vestibular systems. Although no individual system provides all the sensory information we need for determining our position in space, each system contributes its own unique and important kind of information about body position and movement to the central nervous system (CNS). Vision responds to light, the somatosensory system is sensitive to touch, vibration, and pain, and the **vestibular system** responds to movements of the head. The individual contributions of each sensory system to balance and mobility are summarized in table 6.1.

We depend most heavily on the visual system for information about our movements and where we are in space. This system not only provides a visual layout of the environment around us but also provides critical information that informs us about our spatial location relative to objects within the environment. Once we begin moving through space, vision also helps us to navigate safely, anticipate changes in surfaces we encounter, and avoid obstacles in our path. It is therefore a very important source of mobility information.

The somatosensory system provides us with information about the spatial location and movement of our body relative to the support surface and the position and movement of body segments relative to each other. This latter information is provided by

Table 6.1　Sensory System Contributions to Balance and Locomotion

Vision	Layout of surrounding environment; position of limbs relative to other limbs; position of body relative to objects in space; navigation during locomotion; anticipation of surface changes; avoidance of obstacles during locomotion
Somatosensation	Spatial position and movement of body relative to support surface; position and movement of body segments relative to each other (proprioceptors). Assists with maintenance of balance and navigation when vision is absent.
Vestibular	Position and movement of head in space; assists in resolving sensory conflict

proprioceptors located in the muscles and joints throughout the body (e.g., muscle spindles, joint receptors). In the absence of vision, the somatosensory system becomes the primary source of sensory information for maintaining upright balance and moving about in dark environments.

In contrast to the visual and somatosensory systems, the vestibular system does not refer to external objects in space or the horizontal surface, but rather internally measures the gravitational, linear, and angular accelerations of the head in relation to inertial space (Nashner, 1997). The efficient functioning of the vestibular system is critical in situations where the visual and somatosensory inputs are absent or distorted. For example, we rely heavily on the vestibular system to maintain our balance when standing or moving across a compliant or unstable surface in the dark.

The vestibular system also helps to resolve the conflict that arises between the sensory systems in complex visual environments such as freeway traffic or crowded malls. Sensory conflict occurs when the information provided by the visual or somatosensory system is not in agreement. One common situation in which sensory conflict arises is when you are sitting in a vehicle at a stoplight and are fooled into thinking that your vehicle is moving when really the vehicle next to you is rolling. In this particular situation, the visual system is signaling movement while the somatosensory and vestibular systems are signaling no movement.

Once the sensory information derived from each of the three sensory systems has been organized and integrated by the central nervous system and we have determined where we are in space and what we wish to do, the various structures comprising the motor system are responsible for generating the appropriate action plan. As we act, the sensory systems continue to receive additional information from the environment and our movement response so we can quickly modify our current plan of action or begin planning the one that will follow. This intricate and continuous interplay between the sensory and motor systems is often referred to as the **perception–action cycle**. While the sensory systems give rise to a perception that is used to guide initial action, the results of that initial action generated by the motor system are then used to alter or confirm the accuracy of the original perception. This perception–action cycle is illustrated in figure 6.3.

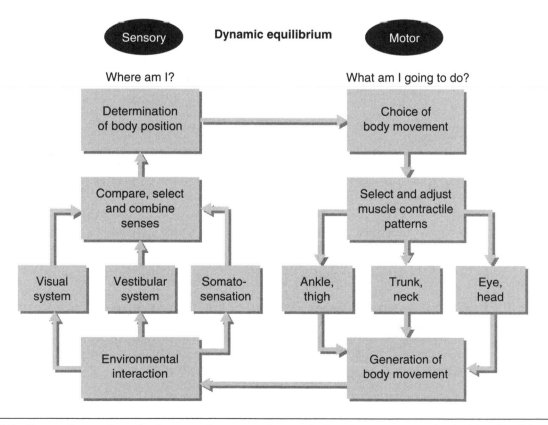

Figure 6.3 The continuous interplay between the sensory (perception) and motor systems (action) is critical for the successful control of balance, posture, and locomotion.

Reprinted, by permission, from L.M. Nasher, NeuroCom International, Dynamic Equilibrium Model.

This dynamic equilibrium model, as it is called, was developed by Nashner (1990) and nicely illustrates the processes occurring in both the peripheral and central components of the sensory and motor systems that characterize the perception–action cycle. The visual, vestibular, and somatosensory receptors comprise the **peripheral component** of the sensory system, whereas the transmission pathways and specialized areas within the CNS comprise the **central components** of the sensory system. In the central component, the information received from the environment via visual, vestibular, and or somatosensory receptors is compared, selected, and then combined so that we can finally determine the position of our body in space. The formulation of different context-specific sensory strategies occurs at this level.

Rather than use a fixed combination of input from the three sensory systems to guide action, we select and weight incoming sensory inputs as the context requires. The sensory strategies formulated then guide the action. Although in most contexts, inputs from the somatosensory and visual systems will dominate the control of body orientation and balance because they are more sensitive to subtle displacements of the COM, in certain situations (i.e., sensory conflict) these inputs provide erroneous sensory information and must be suppressed in favor of more accurate sensory inputs. When one is standing on a compliant or moving surface, for example, the somatosensory inputs can no longer provide accurate information and should therefore be suppressed. The same is true in situations where we erroneously perceive that we are moving on the basis of visual information that is not accurate. In the first situation, the strategy must shift to one of relying on visual and vestibular inputs, whereas in the second situation, somatosensory inputs should be weighted more heavily.

The CNS selects and weights incoming sensory information according to the specific movement context.

Motor System

Once we have determined where we are in space, we begin the process of determining what we are going to do on the basis of the information received. This action planning process begins within the central component of the motor system with the selection of the various muscles groups needed to carry out the plan of action. The movement may be as simple as standing quietly in space or as complicated as running over uneven terrain. The many different groups of muscles throughout the body that comprise the peripheral

component of the motor system will ultimately be responsible for generating the desired movement.

Cognitive System

Both the speed and accuracy of the movement that is generated in response to incoming sensory information will also be influenced by how well we initially evaluate the environment, remember what we are supposed to do in a given situation, and efficiently allocate our attentional resources, particularly when we are required to perform more than one task at a time. Any impairments in cognition or attention will severely compromise our ability to perceive accurately the type of response needed and then effectively implement the response, or responses.

Age-Associated Changes in the Systems Contributing to Balance and Mobility

Changes in each of the intrinsic systems that contribute to good balance and mobility are inevitable with aging. Even older adults who lead physically active lifestyles or have no observable pathology experience declines in the functioning of one or more systems contributing to balance.

Individual Sensory System Changes

Although individual system changes do not necessarily result in observable or adverse effects on function, when multiple systems fall below a minimum threshold of function, their cumulative effects will almost certainly produce significant and observable changes in postural control. At a behavioral level, these cumulative changes occurring in the sensory, motor, and cognitive systems, in particular, manifest themselves in a reduced ability to perceive quickly and accurately where the body is in space, which, in turn, compromises the older adult's performance of a wide variety of complex movements that require speed, accuracy, balance, strength, and coordination. These changes also appear to affect adversely older adults' ability to adapt their movement patterns quickly to accommodate changing task and environmental demands. In this section of the chapter we consider some of the common age-related changes that occur in each of the three sensory systems known to contribute to balance (vision, somatosensory, vestibular), as well as the motor and cognitive systems.

Vision

Common age-associated changes in the peripheral component of vision include reduced acuity, contrast sensitivity, and depth perception, and a narrowing of the visual field, particularly in the peripheral region. These changes can be expected to alter the quality of the information received in the central component of the system and result in slower processing of the sensory information, less efficient integration of visual inputs with those received from the other sensory systems, and possibly an altered perception of the body's vertical orientation. Age-related diseases of the visual system are also common and include cataracts, glaucoma, and macular degeneration.

Despite age-associated negative changes in the visual system, a number of researchers have demonstrated that older adults continue to be strongly influenced by visual inputs for the control of balance. To demonstrate how vision influences balance, researchers have manipulated the visual flow to create the illusion of postural sway. This illusion is created with the help of an experimental room in which the walls and ceiling move but the floor remains fixed. In these experimental conditions, healthy older adults, compared with younger adults, are significantly more sensitive to visual flow, as indicated by their increased postural sway (Wade et al., 1995). When unstable older adults, particularly those who have experienced a recent fall, are subjected to the same visual flow conditions, the amount of sway exhibited is even greater (Ring et al., 1998; Sundermeier et al., 1996). The collective findings indicate that both unstable older adults and, to a lesser degree, stable older adults are unable to suppress the inaccurate visual information in preference for the more accurate somatosensory information. This over-reliance on vision is thought to be attributable to the increasing prevalence of **peripheral neuropathy** among older adults but may also stem from a preference for visual inputs as the primary source of body orientation information at a more central level.

Despite age-associated changes in vision, older adults continue to be strongly influenced by visual inputs to control balance.

Somatosensation

With advancing age, the sensitivity of the cutaneous receptors to different levels of touch and pressure declines as do the number of sensory pathways innervating these receptors (Bruce, 1980). In fact, older adults experience a two to tenfold increase in the vibration threshold needed to detect sensations of touch, resulting in a reduced ability to feel the quality of contact between the feet and the surface below (Perret & Reglis, 1970). Age-associated declines in both the number and sensitivity of muscle and joint receptors also contribute to a less accurate knowledge of limb position, particularly when the body is moving. In some cases, a partial to complete loss of sensation occurs because of a condition known as peripheral neuropathy. Reduced sensation is particularly problematic in situations that require rapid postural adjustments as a result of an unexpected threat to balance. It has been suggested by some researchers that cutaneous receptors on the **plantar surface** of the feet provide information about the quality of the support surface below and limb loading. They may also help the CNS determine how close the COM is to the individual's stability limits (Maki & McIlroy, 1998). This idea is supported by research demonstrating that plantar sensations are important for controlling the initiation of forward-step reactions (Do et al., 1990; Do & Roby-Brami, 1991). Older adults with severe somatosensory deficits also exhibit delayed muscle response onset latencies and an inability to scale the motor response appropriately to the size of the perturbation delivered (Horak, 1994). At a functional level, impairments of the somatosensory system require the older adult to rely more on the other two sensory systems for postural control.

Vestibular

Changes in the vestibular system begin as early as age 30 with a gradual decline in the density of hair cells that serve as the biological sensors of head motion. This decline continues progressively through adulthood and results in reduced sensitivity to head movements. It has been estimated that by the age of 70 years, the number of vestibular hair and nerve cells have declined by as much as 40% (Rosenhall & Rubin, 1975). A moderate reduction in the gain of the **vestibulo-ocular reflex** (VOR) has also been reported with advancing age (Paige, 1991; Wolfson, 1997). Because this reflex is responsible for stabilizing vision when the head moves quickly through space, any reduction in the gain of the VOR will adversely affect older adults' ability to determine accurately whether it is the world or themselves who are moving in certain situations. Older adults who are experiencing vestibular problems often comment on how much they dislike going into crowded malls or grocery stores because they feel increasingly unsteady in complex visual environments. They may also report sensations of dizziness or vertigo (spinning sensation) that add to their perception of instability. In fact, it has been reported that dizziness is the number one reason for a visit to the primary care physician in the over 75 age group (Sloane, 1989).

Motor System Changes

Changes in both the voluntary and involuntary or automatic control of movements as a function of age have been well documented in the literature. Specific age-related changes observed in the motor system include the loss of large motor neurons within the motor cortex and other areas of the motor system, a decline in important neurotransmitters such as dopamine, and a significant decline in nerve conduction velocity. **Chronometric measures** (i.e., simple and choice reaction time, movement time, and response time) used to quantify the time required to plan and execute actions have revealed that the most significant age-related declines are in the action-planning phase (i.e., the time taken to process incoming sensory information and formulate an appropriate motor response) (Spirduso, 1995). Age-related changes in the motor system were discussed in more detail in chapter 3 and 5, but those relevant to balance and mobility are reviewed here.

Electromyographic studies have further revealed significant age-related differences in the quality of the movements generated. Unlike the stereotypical and symmetrical responses exhibited by young adults, apparently healthy older adults exhibit considerably more variable muscle activation patterns and a reduced ability to inhibit inappropriate responses (Stelmach et al., 1989) following unexpected perturbations of the support surface. Inappropriate postural responses are evident when the functional base of support is reduced, the support surface is compliant or unstable, visual input is altered, and a rapid response must be made to a loss of balance (Alexander, 1994; Thelen et al., 2000). The selective loss of fast-twitch motor units also adversely affects older adults' ability to quickly execute movements. Recently, researchers have demonstrated that age-related changes in the firing behavior of motor units also occurs (Erim et al., 1999). This change in the neuromuscular component of the motor system, coupled with the loss of anticipatory postural control abilities attributable to slower central processing speeds, places the older adult at a greater risk for falling when balance is unexpectedly perturbed.

Age-associated changes in the musculoskeletal component of the motor system result in longer movement execution times. Decreases in muscular

Multiple Systems Contribute to Good Balance

Many systems within the central and peripheral nervous system contribute to the effective control of posture, balance, and locomotion. How these multiple systems interact is further influenced by the demands of the task being performed and the constraints associated with the environment in which it is performed. Sensory systems are particularly sensitive to changes in the environmental constraints (e.g., visual flow, surface characteristics), the motor system is responsive to different task demands, and the cognitive system is influenced by changing task demands and environmental constraints. Age-associated changes in a single system may have little observable effect on balance and locomotion whereas changes in multiple systems are associated with observable and adverse effects on balance and locomotion.

strength, power, and endurance have been well documented (chapters 5 and 12). Between the ages of 50 and 70 years, muscle strength, particularly in the lower body, has been shown to decline as much as 30%, with even larger decreases noted after age 80 (Lindle et al., 1997). This is thought to be attributable, in large part, to a decrease in both the size and number of muscle fibers. Physical inactivity exacerbates the loss of muscle strength, particularly in the antigravity or postural muscles required for upright posture. A decline in muscle power probably has the greatest consequence for the performance of basic activities such as walking, climbing stairs, or rising from a chair because these activities require muscle power for their successful completion. Loss of muscle power may be one of the most important contributing factors to an older adult's inability to respond quickly and effectively to an unexpected loss of balance. Loss of muscular endurance also decreases with age resulting in an earlier onset of fatigue during activity that places an older adult at heightened risk for a loss of balance or a fall.

Cognitive System Changes

Age-associated changes in the cognitive system adversely affect the older adult's balance and mobility. In fact, at least 10% of all persons over the age of

65 years and 50% of those older than 80 have some form of cognitive impairment, ranging from mild deficits to dementia (Yaffe et al., 2001). Cognitive impairment has been identified as an important intrinsic risk factor associated with increased fall risk among older adults. Adverse changes occurring in the processes of attention, memory, and intelligence are most likely to affect the older adult's ability to anticipate and adapt to changes occurring in the environment.

Older adults find it particularly difficult to store and manipulate information in working memory simultaneously when a second task that demands cognition is presented. The requirement to divide attention between tasks, particularly when one of the tasks involves balance, is more problematic for healthy older adults than it is for younger adults (Brown et al., 1999; Shumway-Cook et al., 1997) and even more so for older adults with known balance impairments (Brauer et al., 2001; Shumway-Cook et al., 1997). In a recent study, Brauer and colleagues (2001) compared the ability to recover balance after a mild postural disturbance between a group of healthy older adults and a group of balance-impaired older adults. The researchers found that the ability to recover balance was more attentionally demanding for the balance-impaired older adults than for their healthy counterparts. Moreover, when a second cognitive task was performed simultaneously, the balance-impaired older adult group experienced greater difficulty restoring their balance. Their responses to the postural disturbances in this dual-task situation were not only slower but less efficient compared with the healthy older adults whose responses were not influenced by the addition of a second task. Drawing on their findings, the authors suggested that the performance of a second task might contribute to postural instability and subsequent falls in balance-impaired older adults.

> Cognitive impairment has been identified as an important intrinsic risk factor for falls among older adults.

Posture

Good posture refers to the biomechanical alignment of each body part as well as the orientation of the body as a whole to the environment and is critical to good balance (Shumway-Cook & Woollacott, 2001). When one is standing quietly in space, the goal is to align each body part vertically and thereby expend the smallest amount of internal energy necessary to maintain an upright and stable position relative to gravity. To counteract the forces of gravity, a number of muscles are tonically active during quiet stand-

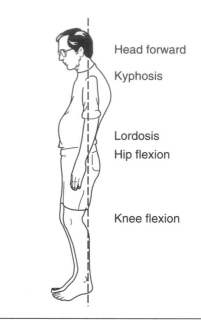

Figure 6.4 Significant age-associated declines in pelvic and spinal flexibility can result in a flexed or stooped posture.

Reprinted, by permission, from D.J. Rose, 2003, *FallProof!* (Champaign, IL: Human Kinetics), 92.

ing. These include the soleus and gastrocnemius muscles, the tibialis anterior (when the body sways in a backward direction), the gluteus medius and tensor fasciae latae, the iliopsoas, the erector spinae muscles in the thoracic region of the trunk, and the abdominal muscles, somewhat more intermittently (Basmajian & De Luca, 1985).

Any significant age-associated decline in pelvic and spinal flexibility in particular, can result in a flexed or stooped posture (Elble, 1997; Studenski et al., 1991) (see figure 6.4). Changes in postural alignment may also occur as a result of a muscular impairment or as a means of compensating for other impairments (e.g., arthritis, hemiplegia resulting from a stroke). The often-observed forward-flexed head and **kyphotic posture** (increased posterior curve of the spine) among older adults will greatly restrict movement and, in more severe cases, place the older adult at greater risk for backward falls. Physical inactivity and prolonged sitting can also contribute to faulty postural alignment in older adults.

Evaluating the Multiple Dimensions of Balance

Because of the multidimensional nature of balance, any evaluation of the balance system requires the use of multiple tests. At least four important dimensions of balance should be evaluated. These include (a) voluntary postural control in static and dynamic environments (i.e., standing quietly and leaning or moving through space), (b) anticipatory postural control (i.e., stabilizing the body in preparation for making a voluntary movement), (c) reactive postural control (i.e., responding to an unexpected threat to balance), and (d) sensory reception and integration. Some of these tests require sophisticated equipment and are usually conducted in laboratory settings, but in some cases equivalent tests are available that require little equipment and are therefore well suited to clinical or field settings. Examples of tests for both laboratory and clinical or field settings are described in this section.

Laboratory Settings

The primary tools used to evaluate the multiple dimensions of balance in laboratory settings include **force plate** systems that are designed to measure the changing pressures under the feet as the body maintains a static posture or moves through space. Electromyography and high-speed filming systems are also used to capture the spatial and temporal aspects of muscle activation patterns as well as the coordination of the various limb segments in response to the goal of the task. Computerized dynamic posturography (CDP) systems have also been developed and provide a very precise evaluation of both the sensory and motor system contributions to balance across changing task and environmental contexts. The various tests used to measure the multiple dimensions of balance in laboratory settings are briefly described next.

Voluntary Postural Control in Static and Dynamic Environments

One of the most common tests currently used in laboratory settings to measure static balance abilities is to ask an individual to stand quietly on a force plate for a given period of time while the amount of sway (as measured by center of pressure excursion) is recorded. The general assumption is that the smaller the amount of sway observed, the better the standing balance. Although this assumption has generally been supported by a number of investigators who have shown sway amplitude to increase with age and pathology, some exceptions to the rule exist. For example, individuals with certain pathologies such as Parkinson's disease or vestibular dysfunction do not sway more during quiet standing than persons who are asymptomatic (Horak, 1992). Patla and colleagues (1990) also challenged the interpretation

that the larger sway excursions often observed among older adult subjects are indicative of a malfunctioning postural control system. These authors speculate that swaying more may actually assist the older adult in obtaining more information about body orientation from the sensory systems.

These same authors also criticized the use of static balance tests, particularly when conducted with the feet in a normal standing position, because these tests do not sufficiently challenge the postural control system, even in healthy older adult populations. Patla and colleagues recommend that these tests be performed with the feet in an altered base of support (**tandem stance** or one-legged stance) and with the eyes open and closed. The recording of a second measure, sway velocity, has also been recommended, particularly when measuring certain populations (i.e., institutionalized elderly). Researchers have shown that sway velocity, as opposed to sway excursion, better identified residents of nursing homes who had fallen one or more times in the previous year. At least for this population, sway velocity appears to be the more sensitive measure of postural stability (Fernie et al., 1982).

> Multiple dimensions of balance must be assessed to better understand why certain older adults are at greater risk for falls.

In contrast to assessments of static balance, dynamic balance is often measured in laboratory settings by asking the person standing on a force plate to lean away from a midline position in multiple directions without losing balance. In addition to being able to quantify an individual's ability to control the movement of the body through space, a test such as this can be used to determine an individual's maximum stability limits. Musculoskeletal limitations (e.g., muscle weakness or reduced range of motion about the ankles), neurological diseases (e.g., stroke, Parkinson's disease), or even psychological impairments such as fear of falling have been shown to affect an individual's maximal limits of stability adversely.

Anticipatory Postural Control

Daily activities such as retrieving a set of plates from a cupboard, opening a door, or stepping over obstacles all require anticipatory postural control. This dimension of balance is usually measured in laboratory settings by requiring an individual, who is once again standing on a force plate, to maintain a stable upright position while performing a pull–push or lifting task with the upper extremities (Cordo & Nashner, 1982;

Inglin & Woollacott, 1988). Electromyography has been used to show that muscle response synergies in the lower body are activated before the muscles of the upper extremities are required to perform the task. This preactivation of the postural muscles in the legs is intended to stabilize the body while the upper body task is being performed.

Anticipatory postural control also has been measured using reactive balance control tests. In this scenario, the person being tested attempts to anticipate the size of the upcoming perturbation by scaling the amplitude of the postural response in advance. Repeated practice responding to the same size perturbation results in a reduced postural response but not at the speed with which the response is activated. If the size of the perturbation changes from trial to trial, however, no such advance scaling is observed (Horak et al., 1989). In studies investigating age-associated changes in anticipatory postural control, older adults, on average, exhibit slower and less efficient anticipatory postural adjustments when compared with younger adults (Frank et al., 1987; Inglin & Woollacott, 1988). Researchers have further speculated that changes in this dimension of balance may be a major contributor to heightened fall risk among older adults (Shumway-Cook & Woollacott, 2001).

Reactive Postural Control

Unexpectedly moving the force plate surface on which the person is standing in different directions is the most commonly used test to quantify an individual's level of reactive postural control. The surface can be either translated to simulate a slip or trip or tilted up or down at different speeds and degrees of tilt to simulate a more severe loss of balance (e.g., bus in which you are standing stops suddenly, or you step in a hole while walking). In addition to measuring the time taken to respond reflexively to the unexpected balance threat following these types of surface perturbations, electromyography is often used to study the pattern of muscle activation in the various muscle response synergies used to restore upright balance. Collectively, these tests have revealed that older adults respond more slowly to surface translations, sometimes adopt different movement strategies (e.g., hip vs. ankle strategy), and exhibit different muscle activation patterns in response to perturbations of progressively higher magnitudes. These differences are even more pronounced in posturally unstable older adults (Horak, et al., 1989; Lin, 1998).

A second method for assessing reactive postural control abilities in laboratory settings is to use a horizontal lean-control cable device to measure an individual's ability to recover from an unexpected loss of balance. Releasing the lean-control cable at different magnitudes of release force and at different time-delay intervals induces loss of balance in a forward direction. The person being tested is instructed to adopt progressively greater forward lean angles until he or she can no longer regain balance by taking a single recovery step. Researchers who have used this apparatus to compare age-associated differences in reactive postural control have found that healthy, physically active older adults experience much more difficulty recovering balance when the available time decreases (i.e., greater forward lean angles). What is perhaps most interesting, however, is that the differences between older and younger adult males appear to be attributable to decreases in the speed with which the older adult is able to execute the recovery step and not in the time required to plan and initiate the response (Thelen et al., 1997). Clear gender differences have also been found, with older females being slower to execute the recovery step compared with an older male group. The older females also were less successful in recovering their balance as the lean angle increased (Wocjik et al., 1999).

Sensory Organization

Computerized dynamic posturography (CDP) is used to examine the contributions of each of the three sensory systems in isolation and in combination. Specifically, the Sensory Organization Test (SOT) measures

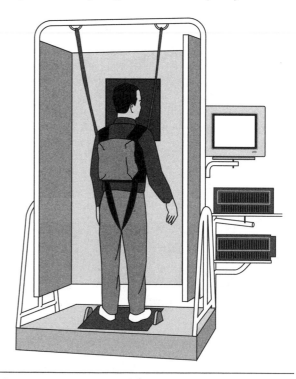

Figure 6.5 Computerized dynamic posturography (CDP) is used to measure multiple dimensions of balance, including sensory organization and integration abilities.

Balance, Posture, and Locomotion

an individual's ability to (a) individually use visual, vestibular, and somatosensory inputs to control upright stance, and (b) suppress each of the systems when they provide inaccurate information about the body's orientation in certain sensory conditions. To measure these abilities, the person is required to stand on a moveable dual force plate facing into a three-sided enclosure (figure 6.5) that can also be moved using a "sway-referencing" technique. This technique involves programming the force plate or visual surround to follow the movement of the individual's center of gravity sway in a forward and backward direction. As is depicted in figure 6.6, neither the force plate nor visual surround moves in conditions 1 or 2, the visual surround alone is moved in condition 3, and only the force plate moves in conditions 4 and 5. In the final test condition, both the floor and visual surround are sway-referenced. By systematically manipulating the movement of the force plate or surround, the researcher can test the functioning of the three sensory systems in isolation or in combination. The sensory systems available in each of the six test conditions are also illustrated in figure 6.6.

In addition to identification of impairments in the various sensory systems resulting from different pathologies, the SOT has also been used to investigate

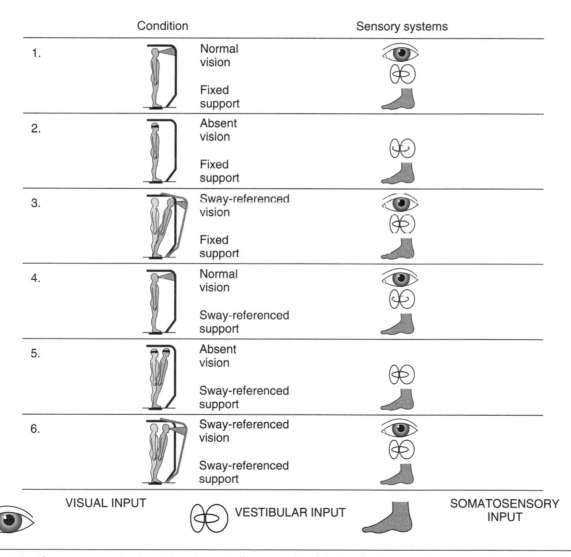

Condition		Sensory systems
1.	Normal vision / Fixed support	
2.	Absent vision / Fixed support	
3.	Sway-referenced vision / Fixed support	
4.	Normal vision / Sway-referenced support	
5.	Absent vision / Sway-referenced support	
6.	Sway-referenced vision / Sway-referenced support	

VISUAL INPUT   VESTIBULAR INPUT   SOMATOSENSORY INPUT

Figure 6.6 The sensory environment is systematically manipulated during the Sensory Organization Test (SOT) so that the contributions of the visual, somatosensory, and/or vestibular systems to balance can be quantified.

Adapted, by permission, from NeuroCom International, The Six Conditions of the Sensory Organization Text. [Online]. Available at http://www.onbalance.com/neurocom.protocols/sensoryImpairment?SOT.aspx

143

Table 6.2 Tests for Dimensions of Balance

Dimension of balance	Laboratory test	Clinical or field test
Voluntary postural control in static and dynamic environments	Static: quiet standing on force plate with eyes open—record amount and velocity of sway. Dynamic: limits of stability—measure distance leaned (in degrees) in four or more directions.	Quiet standing (observe amount of sway for given time period). Multidirectional reach test—measure distance leaned (in inches) in four directions.
Anticipatory postural control	Maintain stability while performing upper body task or minimize response to expected perturbation of force plate—record timing of muscle activation patterns.	Observe fluidity of movement while negotiating obstacles or resisting anticipated perturbation delivered manually.
Reactive postural control	Feet-in-place response to unpredictable translation or tilt of force plate surface at different speeds and amplitudes—measure muscle onset latencies and amplitudes.	Postural stress test—use visual scale (0-9) to grade response or describe behavior observed. Manual push or nudge maneuver—qualitatively grade response using 0, 1, or 2 scale.
Sensory organization	Sensory organization test—measure sway excursion and velocity.	Clinical test of sensory interaction in balance—measure time in balance and balance losses.

whether age-associated changes occur with respect to sensory organization. Researchers have shown that when young adults are compared with healthy older adults, little difference in the amount of postural sway is observed between the groups in the sensory conditions in which only one sensory system is being manipulated. However, significant differences emerge when two of the three sensory systems are being manipulated. In conditions 5 and 6 in figure 6.7, for example, when both the somatosensory and visual inputs are manipulated, older adults exhibit significantly more postural sway with at least half of the older adult subjects losing balance during the early trials. With repeated exposure to the same set of sensory conditions, however, most of the older adults are able to remain standing during the later trials (Woollacott et al., 1986).

Significantly higher levels of postural instability are observed in older adults when two of the three sensory systems are manipulated.

Clinical and Field Settings

In clinical or field settings, many of the same dimensions of balance and mobility can be measured using similar tests that require less sophisticated equipment (table 6.2). Although these tests do not provide the same quality of information, they can be used to identify average or below-average behavior in most cases. To measure static balance abilities, for example, clinicians ask the older adult to stand quietly for a given period of time while the amount of postural sway is qualitatively described. To make the task more challenging, older adults are required to maintain a quiet standing position in an altered base of support (e.g., feet together, tandem stance, one-leg stance). In some cases, differences in the amount of postural sway are noted between eyes-open and eyes-closed test conditions. The amount of time the older adult is able to maintain standing balance in each experimental condition is also recorded.

Similar to laboratory methods, dynamic balance is evaluated in clinical and field settings by asking older adults to voluntarily lean toward their maximum stability limits. The most commonly used test to measure this dimension of balance is the Multidirectional Reach Test (MDRT) developed by Newton (1997, 2001). This test is an expanded version of the forward functional reach test (Duncan et al., 1990) that was used to measure forward reach only. The MDRT measures how far an individual is able to lean through his or her region of stability without altering the base of support in a forward, backward, and lateral direction. The distance leaned in each direction is recorded in inches. Although the distance leaned is affected by the participant's age and height, the test provides useful information about each individual's maximum limits of stability.

Although it is much more difficult to quantify changes in anticipatory postural control in clinical or field settings, it is possible to evaluate anticipatory capabilities qualitatively by asking older adults to negotiate an obstacle course or resist a push or nudge that they know is going to be applied in advance of the action. Older adults who walk up to an obstacle they need to step onto or over but then hesitate before doing so are considered to be experiencing adverse changes in anticipatory postural control. Similarly, individuals who are unable to resist or are slow to respond to a push or nudge are experiencing a decline in their anticipatory control abilities. A person with good anticipatory abilities will negotiate obstacles with little discernible slowing in her movements or will quickly respond to an expected perturbation by stabilizing the body in advance of the push or nudge and then resist it once applied by quickly moving the center of mass in a direction that is equal and opposite to the direction of the nudge. The Dynamic Gait Index is also a useful clinical test that incorporates multiple test items designed to measure anticipatory control abilities (e.g., turn and stop quickly, step over an obstacle, negotiate a course of cones) as well as other dimensions of gait (Shumway-Cook & Woollacott, 2001).

One clinical test that has been developed to measure reactive postural control in clinical settings is the Postural Stress Test (PST) (Whipple & Wolfson, 1990). Unlike the laboratory-based tests of reactive postural control, the PST unexpectedly perturbs the subject in a backward direction only by using a weighted pulley system connected to a spotting belt worn around the pelvis. Small weights representing 1.5, 3.0, and 4.5% of total body weight are used to simulate a small, medium, and large perturbation. These percentages were selected to replicate the different perturbation levels applied during the Motor Control Test performed on a CDP system. The videotaped responses are then numerically scored using a visual scale (i.e., 0-9) that hierarchically illustrates the different movement responses. This test has been successfully used to investigate reactive postural control abilities in groups of older adults with and without a history of falls (Whipple & Wolfson, 1990). Clinicians also have tested reactive postural control abilities in older adults using the nudge test developed by Tinetti

(1986). An unexpected nudge against the sternum is delivered lightly with the palm of the hand three times, and the quality of the movement response is scored using a scale of zero, one, or two.

In an effort to construct a clinical equivalent of the Sensory Organization Test, the Clinical Test of Sensory Interaction in Balance was developed (Shumway-Cook & Horak, 1986). The six test conditions that originally comprised the clinical version of the SOT were altered, with a foam surface being substituted for the sway-referenced force plate surface used in Conditions 4, 5, and 6 and a headpiece fashioned from a Japanese lantern replacing the sway-referenced visual surround used in Conditions 3 and 6. The six-condition test has since been modified to a four-condition version that eliminates the use of the headpiece, because it did not serve as a reliable substitute for the visual surround. Although unable to distinguish between the different sensory system impairments, this clinical test is useful for determining whether the use of sensory information in different sensory environments is normal or abnormal.

Clinical tests that consist of multiple test items can also be used to evaluate the various dimensions of balance as well as an individual's ability to perform functional activities likely to be associated with daily living. Tests such as the Berg Balance Scale (BBS) and Fullerton Advanced Balance (FAB) scale are two examples of valid and reliable clinical tests that are appropriate for use with older adults (Berg et al., 1992; Rose, 2003). The FAB scale is intended for use with higher functioning older adults, and the BBS can be used with more frail older adult populations. Older adults who score less than 45 points out

No One Test Can Measure the Multiple Dimensions of Balance

Practitioners often want to know if there is one single test that they can use to evaluate an older adult's balance. The answer to that question is NO! Multiple tests are needed to understand why an older adult may be at higher risk for falls and/or loss of functional independence as a result of poor balance. At least four dimensions of balance must be evaluated before an effective intervention can be implemented. These dimensions include: (a) volitional postural control, (b) anticipatory postural control, (c) reactive postural control, and (d) sensory organization and integration skills.

of a possible 56 points on the BBS are considered to be at high risk for falls. No cut-off score for fall risk has been developed for the FAB scale. The individual items associated with each test and the dimensions of balance they measure are described in tables 6.3, and 6.4, respectively. A comparison of the different test items used in these two tests should quickly confirm why the FAB scale is better suited for use with higher functioning older adults. In general, the majority of the activities performed on this test are considerably more challenging than the test items associated with the BBS. You will also notice that more dimensions of balance are evaluated with the FAB scale.

Locomotion

The ability to move about successfully in a variety of different environmental contexts that impose different timing (e.g., stepping on and off escalators, crossing busy streets) or spatial demands (e.g., stepping over obstacles, walking in crowded malls) requires a gait pattern that is both flexible and adaptable. At its most fundamental level, successful locomotion is contingent on a person's ability to integrate the control of posture with upper and lower body limb movements. For example, initiating gait, walking, stopping, and turning are all movements that also require a change in our postural orientation.

Overview of the Gait Cycle

Because the act of walking is cyclical, the **gait cycle** is arbitrarily defined as the time between the first contact the heel of one foot makes with the ground to the next heel–floor contact made with the same foot. The gait cycle is measured in seconds. One single limb cycle usually requires approximately 1 s to complete and consists of two phases: stance and swing. The stance phase begins when the foot first contacts the ground and the swing phase begins as the foot leaves the ground. When walking at a preferred speed, adults usually spend as much as 60% of the gait cycle in stance phase and 40% in the swing phase (see figure 6.7 for an illustration of the complete gait cycle). As is apparent in the illustration, both feet are in contact with the ground from the time the right heel

Table 6.3 Test Items of the Berg Balance Scale (BBS) That Measure Multiple Dimensions of Balance

Test item	Dimensions of balance measured
1. Rise from a chair	Dynamic balance
2. Stand unsupported, eyes open	Static balance
3. Sit unsupported with feet on floor	Static balance in seated position
4. Stand to sit	Dynamic balance
5. Transfers	Dynamic balance
6. Stand unsupported, eyes closed	Sensory organization (use of somatosensory inputs)
7. Stand unsupported, feet together	Static balance in reduced base of support
8. Reach forward with extended arm	Forward limits of stability
9. Pick up object from floor	Dynamic balance
10. Turn to look behind each shoulder	Dynamic balance
11. Turn in full circle to right and left	Dynamic balance, sensory organization
12. Alternate toe touches up onto bench	Dynamic balance
13. Maintain tandem stance	Static balance in reduced base of support
14. Stand on one leg	Static balance in reduced base of support

Note: Each test item is scored using a 0-4 ordinal scale. The maximum score possible is 56 points.

Table 6.4 Ten Test Items of the Fullerton Advanced Balance (FAB) Scale

Test item	Dimension of balance measured
1. Stand with feet together, eyes closed	Sensory organization (use of somatosensory inputs)
2. Reach forward to retrieve object	Forward limits of stability
3. Turn in a full circle to right and left	Sensory organization, dynamic balance
4. Step up and over bench	Anticipatory postural control, dynamic balance
5. Tandem walk	Dynamic balance in reduced base of support
6. Stand on one leg, eyes open	Static balance in reduced base of support
7. Stand on foam, eyes closed	Sensory organization (use of vestibular inputs)
8. Two-footed jump for distance	Dynamic balance, whole body motor coordination
9. Walk with head turns	Sensory organization (visual–vestibular inputs)
10. Unexpected backward release	Reactive postural control

Note: Each test item is scored using a 0-4 ordinal scale. The maximum test score is 40 points.

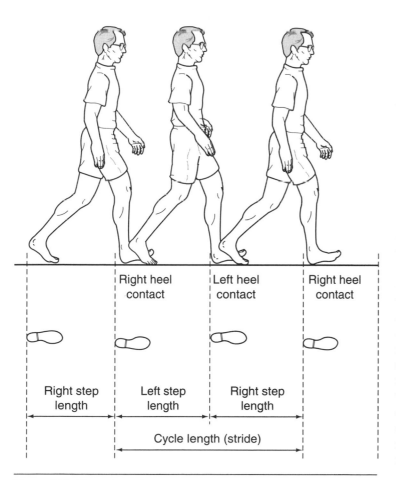

Right heel contact | Left heel contact | Right heel contact

Right step length | Left step length | Right step length

Cycle length (stride)

Figure 6.7 The gait cycle.

Reprinted, by permission, from D.J. Rose, 2003, *FallProof!* (Champaign, IL: Human Kinetics), 179.

contacts the ground until the left toe leaves the ground (lasting approximately 10% of the gait cycle) and then again when the left heel contacts the ground until the right toe leaves the ground (approximately 10% of gait cycle). When both feet are in contact with the ground during gait, this is referred to as **double-support time.**

During the gait cycle, three major tasks must be achieved. These include weight acceptance, single limb support, and limb advancement. Weight acceptance (initial contact and loading) is perhaps the most demanding task that must be accomplished during walking. Successful completion of this task requires adequate knee flexion (approximately 15°) so that the shock associated with accepting the body's full weight on impact is absorbed, good limb stability as the foot contacts the ground, and the ability to keep the center of gravity moving forward in preparation for the swing phase of gait. The key muscle groups involved in completing this task include the hip extensors (provide limb stability), quadriceps (constrain knee flexion), and dorsiflexor muscle groups (heel strike, foot contact with floor, and preparation for limb loading).

During the task of single limb support that occurs during midstance and terminal stance, one limb must assume the dual responsibility of supporting total body weight and simultaneously progress forward in preparation for the swing phase. The key muscle groups that are activated during the completion of this task include the hip abductor (stabilize the hip), trunk (maintain an upright position), quadriceps (assist forward progression of the center of gravity), and plantar flexor (control the forward movement of the tibia during midstance and terminal stance) groups.

The final task that must be completed during each gait cycle is that of advancing the limb (pre-swing and swing). This task begins during pre-swing as the knee begins to flex (approximately 35°) in preparation for the limb being lifted off the floor. During the swing phase, the limb will be advanced. The knee will continue to flex to approximately 60° to allow for toe clearance (approximately 1 cm above the floor) before reaching full extension in preparation for heel contact. How far the limb is advanced during this phase will determine step length. The key muscle groups involved in the completion of this final task include the hip flexors, knee flexors, dorsiflexors, quadriceps, and hamstrings (during terminal swing). Each of the muscle groups involved in completing these tasks must remain strong to preserve the quality of the gait pattern and minimize the risk of falls.

> Three major tasks must be completed during the gait cycle: weight acceptance, single limb support, and limb advancement.

Achieving a normal gait pattern requires that individuals possess an adequate range of joint mobility, appropriate timing of muscle activation across the gait cycle, sufficient muscle strength to meet the demands involved in each phase of the gait cycle, and unimpaired sensory input from the visual, somatosensory, and vestibular systems. Particularly important muscles groups for gait include the hip extensor, knee extensor, plantar flexor, and dorsiflexor groups. Any significant weakness in any of these muscle groups will adversely affect the quality of the gait pattern. In terms of lateral stability during the initiation and control of the walking pattern, it is also important that the hip abductor muscle groups remain strong.

Contributions of the Sensory and Motor Systems to Locomotion

Walking is one of the most complex activities in which we engage as humans. Elements of the locomotor pattern contribute to the successful completion of a number of different mobility activities performed during daily life (e.g., stair climbing and descending, transfers between chairs, turning). Locomotion is accomplished through the interplay of higher centers in the brain that are responsible for initiating and adapting goal-directed gait and lower centers in the spinal cord that control the rhythmic and subconscious coordination of the major muscle groups involved in locomotion. In this section, the more specific contributions of the sensory and motor systems (including musculoskeletal component) to locomotion will be described.

• Vision. Vision plays a particularly important role during locomotion, particularly when individuals move about in complex environments. Patla (1997) identified two important roles played by vision during locomotion. First, vision serves an avoidance role by assisting us to momentarily modify our gait pattern to avoid a barrier within the environment. For example, vision helps us place the foot during gait, avoid obstacles by signaling the need to lift the limb higher above the ground so we can successfully step over the obstacle, or change the direction of the walking pattern if the obstacle is perceived to be too high to clear successfully. Vision is also used to help us stop. On the other hand, vision helps us to accommodate to a changing environment by signaling when to adapt the gait pattern in response to a change in the physical environment (e.g., slope of the ground, type of walking terrain). Characteristics of the gait pattern will be altered in this latter scenario. For example, vision helps us accommodate to changes in the physical environment by signaling the need to alter stride length (e.g., decrease stride length when walking across an icy surface) or increase the contractile power of certain muscle groups as the task demands change (e.g., when climbing stairs).

• Somatosensation. Just as the somatosensory system is critical for controlling standing balance and signaling a pending loss of balance, it also serves an important reactive role during locomotion. Sensory input received from proprioceptors in the muscles and joints as well as the cutaneous receptors contribute to the reflexive control and modulation of gait by providing limb position information during critical phases of the gait cycle. The proprioceptors also inform us about the position of the limb in space during the various phases of the gait cycle.

• Vestibular system. Finally, the vestibular system, in conjunction with vision, plays an important role in stabilizing the head during walking through the **vestibulo-ocular reflex (VOR)**. This important reflex allows us to generate eye movements that ensure clear vision even though the head is moving during locomotion. Specific impairments within the vestibular system lead to increased instability during gait because it becomes more difficult to stabilize the head (Berthoz & Pozzo, 1994).

• Motor system. Locomotion is accomplished at multiple levels within the CNS. As described earlier in this section, specific areas of the brain (e.g., cerebral cortex, basal ganglia, cerebellum, brainstem) are largely responsible for the overall control, variation, and adaptation of the locomotor pattern, whereas complex networks of neurons located in the spinal cord, often referred to as **central pattern generators,** are believed to be responsible for the rhythmic and subconscious coordination of the major muscle groups involved in walking. The musculoskeletal component of the motor system also plays an important role in locomotion by providing the muscular force necessary to support the body during the stance phase of gait and move it forward during the swing phase. Because gravity is acting against the body, adequate levels of muscle strength are necessary to minimize the energy expended during gait while maximizing biomechanical efficiency. Adequate range of motion is also necessary in the joints of the trunk and lower limbs.

Age-Associated Changes in Gait

Although it is difficult to know whether the changes observed in the gait pattern of healthy older adults are attributable to the aging process alone or some underlying disease process, clear differences exist when healthy, older adults are compared with younger adults. The most significant change is in the variable of gait speed. Even healthy older adults with no history of falling walk at a preferred speed that is, on average, 20% slower than the speed exhibited by younger adults. Conversely, when walking at a fast speed, the two groups demonstrate a 17% difference in gait speed (Elble et al., 1991). What is most interesting is that the slowing in gait speed that accompanies age is largely attributable to a decrease in stride length as opposed to stride frequency. Unfortunately, this reduction in stride length also has negative consequences for other aspects of gait, including reduced arm swing, reduced rotation of the hips, knees, and ankles, increased double-support time, and a more flat-footed contact with the ground during the stance phase prior to toe-off (Elble, 1997). These changes will, over time, affect an older adult's ability to remain an independent community ambulator and also will increase the older adult's risk for falls in time-constrained situations (e.g., crossing a street before the light changes, getting onto and off

Doing Two Things at Once: A Challenge for Older Adult Gait Control

Obstacle negotiation skills have been shown to be further compromised when older adults are required to perform a second task. Chen and colleagues (1996) performed an experiment that required older and younger adults to avoid a virtual obstacle (band of light) projected on a walkway in front of them. The researchers compared the number of times the obstacle was contacted during a walking-only condition with a second experimental condition that required the subjects to verbally respond as soon as a red light appeared at the end of the walkway. Although the younger adults studied contacted the obstacle more often when a second task was introduced, the older adults showed significantly higher decrements in performance when their attention was divided between the task of walking and locating a visual object in space. These results may help us better understand why many older adults experience falls while walking in the community.

moving walkways) and obstacle avoidance situations that require rapid modifications of the gait cycle.

Common adaptations observed in the gait patterns of older adults include the tendency to more cautiously load the limb during the weight acceptance task of gait, a tendency to exhibit a flatter foot-to-floor contact pattern, less forward progression of the limb during single-limb support, and reduced knee flexion during the pre-swing and swing phases of gait. A summary of the changes commonly observed in the temporal and distance variables in the gait pattern of older adults is presented in table 6.5.

In addition to the changes that are observed when older adults walk across a level surface that is free of any physical barriers, when approaching obstacles older adults further reduce their gait speed and clear the obstacle using a slower, shorter step. Although this decreases the likelihood of tripping, it often results in the heel or sole of the foot contacting the obstacle before it returns to the ground on the other side of the obstacle (Chen et al., 1991).

Age-related changes in each of the sensory systems previously described are also likely to affect gait speed adversely. In addition to providing continuous feed-

Table 6.5 Summary of Age-Associated Changes in the Gait Pattern

Temporal and distance variables	Decreased velocity
	Decreased step length
	Decreased step frequency (i.e., cadence)
	Decreased stride length
	Increased stride width
	Increased stance phase
	Increased time in double support
	Decreased time in swing phase
Kinematic variables	Flatter foot–floor pattern
	Reduced arm swing

back that is essential for adapting the gait pattern to changes in terrain and a changing visual display, vision also serves a very important **feedforward** role by helping us to anticipate changes in the environment and thereby preserve a smooth and continuous walking pattern (Rose, 1997). Age-related decreases that occur in the visual perception of motion are also likely to affect the gait pattern adversely, leading to inaccurate responses in some cases or slower movement responses in other situations.

Measuring Gait

Laboratory-based analyses of gait usually require sophisticated equipment such as high-speed digital video recording systems, floor-mounted force plates, and electromyography. High-speed video captures the **kinematic** qualities (i.e., motion of the body) whereas force plates capture the **kinetic** qualities (i.e., forces) of the gait pattern. Finally, electromyography is used to quantify the spatial and temporal qualities of the muscle activation patterns throughout the gait cycle. The results of research studies that use these sophisticated measurement tools have provided us with a significantly better understanding of the characteristics of gait and how they are influenced by age and pathology (Winter et al., 1990; Wolfson et al., 1995). Unfortunately, because of the high cost of equipment, the space needed to conduct the testing, and the amount of time needed to complete a comprehensive evaluation of gait, the use of this type of equipment is limited to research laboratories and rehabilitation settings where a more comprehensive evaluation of gait is warranted.

In a field setting, certain gait variables such as stride length, frequency or cadence, and gait velocity can be easily and inexpensively measured using a stopwatch and walkway as short as 10 m. Gait velocity can be determined by timing how long the person takes to walk the required distance, whereas stride length can be calculated by counting the number of steps taken over the same distance. Gait velocity values are often then normalized to height (i.e., recorded gait speed in centimeters per second divided by height centimeters) so that values can be compared among a group of individuals (Bohannon, 1997). Clinicians often supplement these temporal measures of gait with visual gait analysis forms of varying complexity to evaluate the quality of the movement observed in each body segment (i.e., head, trunk, and upper and lower extremity) during each phase of the gait cycle. Examples of standardized visual gait analysis forms include the Gait Assessment Rating Scale (Wolfson et al., 1990), which also has a modified version (Van Swearingen et al., 1996), the Rivermead Visual Gait Assessment (Lord et al., 1998), and the Essential Components of Gait Form (Carr & Shephard, 1998). The Essential Components of Gait Form is considered to be the gait analysis form that is easiest to use.

Falling— When Balance Fails

For many older adults, the age- and pathology-associated changes occurring in the multiple systems that control balance, locomotion, and mobility become so profound that the older adults begin to fall. In fact, more than 30% of adults over the age of 65 years will experience at least one fall per year (American Academy of Orthopedic Surgeons, 1998), a percentage that increases to 50% in adults over 75. Although falls occur at all ages, it is considerably more likely that they will result in serious injury in old age. Even when falls do not result in serious injury or death, they are often associated with a heightened fear of falling that can often lead to restrictions in physical and social activities, increased dependence, and greater need for long-term care (Howland et al., 1993, 1998).

| Falls are not a normal part of the aging process.

Falls are more often than not attributable to factors that are amenable to intervention. These include such factors as muscle weakness, impaired balance and gait, environmental hazards, and the misuse of medications and alcohol. In the next section of this chapter, the risk factors that have been most strongly associated with increased falls are identified as well

Common Risk Factors Associated With Falls Among Older Adults

- Muscle weakness
- History of falls
- Gait deficit
- Balance deficit
- Use of assistive device
- Visual deficit
- Arthritis
- Impaired activities of daily living
- Depression
- Cognitive Impairment
- Age (> 80 years)

From: "Guideline for the prevention of falls in older persons" by American Geriatrics Society, British Geriatrics Society, and American Academy of Orthopaedic Surgeons Panel on Falls Prevention. *Journal of the American Geriatrics Society, 49,* p. 665. Adapted with permission.

as the types of intervention strategies that have been effective in reducing the prevalence of these risk factors.

Risk Factors That Contribute to Falls

In addition to understanding that falls are not a normal part of the aging process, researchers have shown that when older adults do fall, it is rarely for the same reason. In fact, a multitude of reasons and factors contribute to the increased fall rates observed among older adults. These factors may be attributable to age- or disease-related changes occurring within the older adult (intrinsic risk factors) or to factors that are more external in nature such as the presence of environmental hazards in the home or community that elevate the risk for falls during the performance of routine activities associated with daily living (extrinsic risk factors). In a recent examination of several fall–risk factor studies, Rubenstein and Josephson (2002) identified the most common risk factors for falls. These are presented above. Nevitt and colleagues (1989) demonstrated that an older adult's risk for falls increases as the number of risk factors increase. For example, the authors showed that the percentage of community-residing older adults experiencing multiple falls increased from 10% when only one risk factor was

evident to 69% when four or more risk factors were identified.

Medication and Falling

In addition to the risk factors identified previously, certain medications often prescribed for older adults have been associated with an increased risk for falls. Psychotropic medications (i.e., sedatives and hypnotics, antidepressants, benzodiazepines, neuroleptics), class 1a antiarrhythmic medications, digoxin, and diuretics have all been found to increase the risk for falls significantly (Liepzig et al., 1999a, 1999b). It remains to be determined, however, whether the positive associations are caused by the side effects of the particular drug (i.e., sedation, confusion, cognitive dysfunction, psychomotor impairment, or orthostatic hypotension) or the medical indications for its use.

Can Falling of the Elderly Be Prevented?

In response to the serious public health problem associated with falling among the elderly, representatives from three national organizations (i.e., the American Geriatrics Society, the British Geriatrics Society, and the American Academy of Orthopaedic Surgeons) collaborated in developing a set of written guidelines intended to assist health care professionals more effectively assess and treat older adults at different levels of fall risk. The guidelines constitute the first attempt to provide recommendations for screening and treating older adults at different levels of fall risk.

Routine Fall Risk Assessments

Brief fall risk assessments as part of the routine primary health care visit are recommended for relatively low-risk older adults, whereas those identified at high risk for falls (i.e., persons who have sustained multiple falls, are prone to injurious falls, reside in a nursing home, or are seeking medical treatment immediately following a fall) should receive a comprehensive and detailed fall risk assessment. This more comprehensive assessment would include obtaining the circumstances surrounding the fall, identifying existing risk factors for falls, documenting any medical conditions, noting functional status, and assessing the immediate home environment. The specific assessment recommendations for each level of fall risk are provided in the final published document that appeared in the *Journal of the Geriatrics Society* (American Geriatrics Society, British Geriatrics

Society, and American Academy of Orthopaedic Surgeons Panel on Falls Prevention, 2001).

> Brief fall risk assessments as part of the routine primary health care visit are recommended for low-risk older adults, whereas older adults identified at high risk for falls should receive a comprehensive and detailed fall risk assessment.

Interventions to Prevent Falling

Over the past few years, a number of reports have been published in different regions of the world describing **best practice approaches** to the prevention of falls among the older adult population (Gillespie et al., 2002; Hill et al., 2000; Rubenstein & Powers, 1999; Scott et al., 2001). The evidence for these best practice approaches was based on a careful examination of the many research studies in which the central focus was on different intervention strategies. Intervention strategies that have been investigated include (a) exercise, (b) environmental modifications, (c) multifactorial risk factor assessments and interventions, (d) health promotion and education, (e) medication withdrawal, and (f) hip pad protector garments.

Exercise

Although much is still to be learned about the role of exercise in reducing falls among older adults, the current research findings indicate that intervention strategies that include exercise have the potential to reduce significantly many of the risk factors that contribute to falls and, in the case of community-residing older adults, the actual number and rate at which falls are sustained (Buchner et al., 1997; Campbell et al., 1997; Day et al., 2002; Wolf et al., 1996).

A number of different exercise interventions have been described and range from single exercise (e.g., resistance exercises, walking, t'ai chi) to multiple-component exercise programs (e.g., aerobic endurance training, flexibility, strength training, or balance). Moreover, although a more general or non-targeted approach has been adopted in some exercise studies, others have included exercises that specifically target balance and gait impairments or other physical factors known to be associated with heightened fall risk (e.g., muscle weakness, reduced flexibility) (Buchner et al., 1997; Fiatarone et al., 1994; Lord et al., 1995; MacRae et al., 1994; Means et al., 1996; Mulrow et al., 1994; Rubenstein et al., 2000; Wolf et al., 1996).

The multiple-center FICSIT (Frailty and Injuries: Cooperative Studies on Intervention Techniques)

randomized, controlled trials represented the first systematic and large-scale attempt to investigate the role of exercise in reducing frailty and fall incidence rates among older adults. Researchers at seven of the eight intervention sites located in different regions of the United States investigated the efficacy of an exercise intervention strategy, while researchers at the final intervention site studied the effectiveness of hip pad protector garments in reducing fall-related fractures among high-risk nursing home residents. Although the exercise interventions varied with respect to the type of exercise used and the intensity, frequency, and duration of the intervention, the results of a pre-planned meta-analysis that combined the multiple-site outcomes demonstrated a significant reduction in the risk of falling for the seven interventions that included exercise as a component of the intervention. Fall risk was further reduced, however, if the exercise intervention was more targeted by including specific balance activities (Province et al., 1995). In recent years, individualized exercise programs that have targeted specific physical impairments identified during an initial assessment have been shown to significantly lower fall incidence rates. These programs are generally designed and supervised by physical or occupational therapists in the home setting (Campbell et al., 1997, 1999).

In contrast to the significant findings emerging from a number of studies conducted with community-residing older adults relative to fall incidence rates, the interventions used in a smaller number of studies conducted in long-term care settings have not been successful in reducing the incidence of falls among the older adult residents (Fiatarone et al., 1994; Mulrow et al., 1994; Nowalk et al., 2001). The interventions have, however, resulted in significant improvements in overall function of the exercise groups. For example, a number of researchers focusing on resistance exercise training have reported significant improvements in physical function (e.g., improved sit-to-stand performance, increase in absolute strength) or mobility (e.g., change in ambulation status, improved gait speed) (Brill et al., 1998; Meuleman et al., 2000; Sullivan et al., 2001).

> One problem that pervades all exercise intervention studies conducted with the frail, older adult is that the functional gains achieved are lost very quickly once the intervention ends. This suggests that every effort must be made to institute long-term exercise interventions for the frail, older adult that foster sustained adherence.

Environmental Modifications

Researchers have shown that fall incidence rates can also be significantly reduced as a result of making modest safety modifications to an older adult's immediate home environment (Cumming et al., 1999; Hornbrook et al., 1994; Plautz et al., 1996; Thompson, 1996). The three key areas of the home that create the biggest problems for older adults include outside steps to the home's entrance, inside stairs to a second floor, and unsafe bathroom areas (Pynoos et al., 2003). Examples of the types of modifications commonly made include installing grab bars in the bathroom, adding night-lights to dark corridors, adding safety markings and handrails to stairs inside and outside the home, and removing loose floor rugs. Recent studies have documented the widespread prevalence of home hazards, particularly in the homes of frail older adults (Gill et al., 1999). These findings suggest the need for more home visits by health professionals trained to identify home hazards that are likely to increase the resident's risk for falls. However, studies have shown that for this type of intervention to be successful, the identified home hazards must actually be modified and at little or no cost to the resident. High compliance with environmental recommendations also has been shown to be more likely when it is combined with other intervention strategies such as behavioral counseling and risk factor education by trained professionals (e.g., occupational therapist).

Eliminating hazards in the home lowers fall risk. According to Rubenstein (1999), between 35% and 45% of falls are attributed to home hazards such as inadequate bathroom grab rails and stairway railings, poor lighting, clutter on the floor, exposed electrical cords, and loose throw rugs.

Multifactorial Risk Factor Assessment and Intervention

Given that not all older adults fall for the same reason, and are in fact most likely to fall as a result of the presence of multiple fall risk factors, multifactorial intervention strategies designed first to identify and then minimize the intrinsic and extrinsic risk factors contributing to heightened fall risk are likely to produce the most successful outcomes. The most common fall risk factors targeted in these studies include gait and balance impairments, muscle weakness, transfer difficulties, number and type of medications, cardiovascular risk factors, and environmental hazards in the home.

Multifactorial fall risk assessments and follow-up have been conducted with older adults identified at high risk for falls both before and immediately after falls. This type of intervention strategy generally requires a multidisciplinary team of providers consisting of emergency room physicians and nurses, general practitioners, physical and occupational therapists, pharmacists, psychiatrists, and social workers. Once medical personnel identify the risk factors, the individual is then referred to the appropriate services for specific treatment and follow-up.

The results of a meta-analysis of a small number of randomized controlled trials using this multifactorial approach with community-residing older adults at high risk for falls demonstrated a significant reduction in fall risk as well as fall incidence rates (Gillespie et al., 2002). A frequently cited study conducted by Tinetti and colleagues (1994) reported that a smaller proportion of the study participants who received the multifactorial intervention fell during the 1-year follow-up period (31%), and the time to the first fall was also significantly longer. More recently, Close and colleagues (1999) demonstrated a significant reduction in falls in the year after discharge in a group of older adults who received a multifactorial fall risk assessment and appropriate referral and follow-up when compared to a control group who received usual care in a hospital emergency department after a fall (only 32% of the intervention group vs. 52% in the control group reported at least one fall).

Ray et al. (1997) also investigated the efficacy of a multifactorial approach to reducing fall rates in multiple nursing home settings. Four specific safety domains were targeted in their study: environmental and personal safety, wheelchairs, psychotropic medication use, and transferring and ambulation abilities. Based on the outcome of the initial assessment, an individualized treatment plan was implemented by trained personnel. At follow-up, the mean proportion of recurrent fallers was significantly lower in the intervention facilities (19%). A lower, albeit non-significant, mean rate of injurious falls was observed among residents in the intervention facilities. The authors speculated that a greater reduction in fall incidence rates may have been demonstrated had more of the safety recommendations made by the consultation team actually been implemented. The researchers reported that less than one third of the safety recommendations had been completed at 3 months after the initial risk factor assessment.

Health Promotion and Education

Although many of the successful multifactorial intervention strategies described have generally included an educational component that targets either the older adult participant or the providers of the intervention (staff, family members, community health care workers), little evidence currently exists that supports the efficacy of educational programs in and of themselves as a medium for reducing fall-incidence rates among older adults. In one of the few randomized controlled trials that have been conducted to address the issue, Reinsch and colleagues (1992) found no significant differences in any measures, including fall incidence rates, after 1 year among the groups receiving an education and relaxation program, exercise alone, a combination of the two strategies, or no intervention. It has been previously argued that for these programs to be successful, older adults must perceive that they are at risk for falls and that they can actually lower their risk. Although one might intuitively think this would be the case, a survey conducted by Braun (1998) to assess older adults' perceptions and level of knowledge related to fall risk factors actually found the perceptions of healthy, community-residing respondents to be incongruent with their objective risks.

Medication Withdrawal

Growing evidence exists that medication review and reduction can positively influence fall risk and actual fall incidence rates among older adults. Using a multifactorial intervention approach that included medication reduction and the use of other non-pharmacological strategies (e.g., physical therapy for gait and balance impairments, home modification), Tinetti and colleagues (1994) demonstrated a 23% decrease in the number of study participants (who received the multifactorial intervention) taking four or more prescription medications at the end of the 1-year follow-up period. A significant reduction in the proportion of intervention subjects who fell during the same period was also reported. Unfortunately, because of the multifactorial nature of the intervention, it was not possible to determine the contribution of medication reduction alone to

the reduced fall rates reported for the intervention group.

More recently, Campbell and colleagues (1999) investigated the effect of gradually withdrawing psychotropic medications on fall risk in a group of community-residing older adults who were currently taking this type of medication. At follow-up, some 44 weeks later, a 66% reduction in fall risk was evident for the medication withdrawal group compared with a control group. Unfortunately, 47% of the study participants who had successfully ceased taking psychotropic medications during the study had resumed taking their medication 1 month after the study ended. It has been suggested that additional support services and perhaps hospitalization may be needed to assist older adults in successfully curtailing the use of psychotropic medications because they are at the greatest risk for severe withdrawal reactions (Foy, 1993).

Hip Protector Garments

One promising new intervention strategy for reducing fall incidence rates and fall-related injuries among high-risk older adults, in particular, involves the wearing of hip protector garments. Although hip protector garments were not designed to reduce falls, the results of a small number of studies have demonstrated a significant reduction in fall-related fractures when these protective garments were worn by nursing home residents with a history of falls. Lauritzen and colleagues (1993) reported a 50 % reduction in fall-related hip fractures in a group of nursing home residents who wore hip pad protector garments. An even higher reduction in hip fractures was reported by Kannus and colleagues (2000) two years after hip pad protector garments were prescribed to residents in 22 geriatric care programs in Finland. The number of hip fractures declined by 84% among residents who wore the hip protectors. Although these results are promising, issues related to compliance (with wearing the protector) remain an important limiting factor in the adoption of hip pad protectors.

SUMMARY

According to the systems theory of human postural control, multiple systems within the body collaborate to control bodily orientation and locomotion. Important systems include the sensory, motor, and cognitive systems. The type of movement response produced is further influenced by two additional constraints on action. These include the goals of the task being performed and the properties of the environment in which it is being performed.

With advancing age, a number of changes occurring within the sensory, motor, and cognitive systems have the potential to compromise the older adult's ability to successfully perform a number of daily and recreational activities that require balance and mobility. Because of the heterogeneous nature of the older adult population, age-associated changes may have little observable impact on overall function in some adults, but may lead to the loss of functional independence for many other older adults.

The multiple dimensions of balance can be evaluated using sophisticated instrumentation available only in laboratory settings or with less expensive clinical or field tests. These tests can be used to quantify changes in static and dynamic balance, anticipatory and reactive postural control, and sensory reception and integration. Age-associated changes in locomotion also can be evaluated using laboratory and field-based tests.

For many older adults, age- and pathology-associated changes occurring in the multiple systems that control balance and locomotion are so profound that these people fall. Common risk factors that contribute to increased falling rates among older adults include muscle weakness, impairments in balance and gait, a history of previous falls, visual deficits, restricted activities of daily living, depression, and cognitive impairment. A number of intervention strategies have been developed with the goal of reducing fall risk and fall incidence rates among older adults. Intervention strategies that have been investigated include exercise, environmental modifications, multifactorial risk assessments and interventions, health promotion and education, and medication withdrawal. Hip protector garments have also been shown to significantly reduce the number of fall-related hip fractures when worn by older adults who experience multiple falls.

REVIEW QUESTIONS

1. Briefly describe the roles of the sensory, motor, and cognitive systems in the control of balance.

2. Identify each of the major changes occurring in the multiple dimensions of balance with advancing age.

3. Briefly describe the three distinct postural control strategies used to control the amount of body sway in a forward and backward direction. What factors limit the effective use of each of these strategies?

4. Identify the various factors that influence good posture.

5. Briefly describe how an individual's ability to receive and integrate sensory inputs for balance is measured in (a) a laboratory setting and (b) a clinical or field setting.

6. Identify the three major tasks that must be accomplished during every gait cycle.

7. Identify the major age-associated changes in locomotion.

8. Identify the primary risk factors that contribute to heightened fall risk in older adults.

9. What types of prescription medications have been positively associated with increased fall rates?

10. Identify four best-practice approaches used to reduce falling rates among the elderly.

SUGGESTED READINGS

Skelton, D. (2001). Effects of physical activity on postural stability. *Age and Aging,* 30(Suppl. 4), 33-39.

Tennstedt, S.L. (2003). Falls and fall-related injuries. (Ed.). *Generations* 26(4), 1-100. (Journal published by the American Society on Aging)

Rose, D.J. (2003). *FallProof!* A comprehensive balance and mobility training program. Champaign, IL: Human Kinetics.

Behavioral Speed

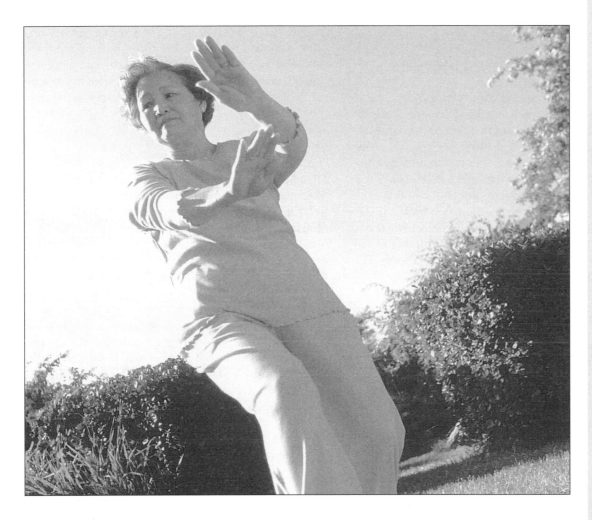

The objectives of this chapter are

- to describe how aging affects the speed with which older adults react and move about in their environment,

- to show how reactivity and movement speed are measured in old adults,

- to clarify the various factors that influence reactivity speed,

- to describe the mechanisms proposed to explain why aging slows reactivity and movement, and

- to explore the implications of age-related slowing in the daily lives of old adults.

One of the most visible landmarks of aging is the slowing of behavior, especially physical movements. Although this occurs in a very individualistic manner, the speed with which individuals initiate, execute, and complete physical movements gradually and inexorably decreases with advancing years. This age-related change in physical movement speed is so profound that actors portraying older characters capitalize on this common phenomenon by exaggerating the slowness of individual movements.

Response Speed

A reduction in the speed with which older people can react and move has substantial significance for all aspects of their life. It takes longer to complete physical tasks, which means that fewer tasks can be accomplished in a day. It takes longer to dress, groom, and complete daily home management chores. Slowing modifies performance of older automobile drivers, and it contributes to an increased accident rate at home, in the yard, at work, and in other aspects of life. Behavioral slowing affects performance across a wide variety of tasks and situations. Clearly, the importance of completing a task in a finite amount of time has varied consequences. On one end of the continuum, the societal pressure to respond and move quickly—to write out a check in the grocery line or to provide a credit card as quickly as possible to the salesperson—is rampant in our society. This societal pressure to hurry can be socially intimidating to older people, discouraging them from active involvement in community activities outside the home. In addition, employers are less likely to be satisfied if older workers produce fewer units within a specified period of time or cannot keep up with externally paced industrial tasks. If "time is money," then older individuals may make less of it. Although the ability to move as quickly as possible may be important to the individual in some circumstances, the inability to do so is not associated with drastic physical consequences. At the extreme other end of the continuum, failing to walk across the street in a finite amount of time may have severe physical consequences. Thus, in some tasks the individual sets a demand for speed with which he or she is comfortable (preferred or natural speed), particularly when the physical consequences are absent or minimal. However, some tasks have inherent speed-related demands that if not realized lead to unsuccessful performance and may be associated with severe physical consequences.

Behavioral speed consists of two major components: speed with which individuals can react to environmental stimuli and the speed with which they can move their limbs. The focus of this chapter is on the reactivity and speed of limb movements that occur in psychomotor laboratory tasks and some types of functional movements, such as playing the piano. These are voluntary responses and are different from involuntary reactions, such as recovering from a stumble, discussed in chapter 5, and in postural perturbation paradigms in chapter 6. Examples of speed-of-performance changes are also discussed chapter 8. Health and physical fitness are thought to influence the maintenance of response speed, but because this influence is widely debated and of great importance, it is discussed separately in chapter 9.

Reaction Time

Reaction time is the time interval from the onset of a stimulus to the initiation of a volitional response. When an obstacle suddenly appears in the road and the driver must stop as quickly as possible, the time that passes from the driver's first sight of the obstacle to the lifting of the foot from the accelerator is called simple reaction time. When the situation involves only one stimulus (the obstacle) and one response (to stop), the response is called a **simple reaction time (SRT).** The fastest possible reactions occur when the driver is told that an obstacle will appear, but he or she does not know when. If a driver is told that an obstacle may appear, just the uncertainty as to whether it will increases his or her reaction time. This is called a **discrimination reaction time.** If the driver has to choose between stepping on the brake pedal or further depressing the accelerator, then the interval between the perception and the reaction is called a **choice reaction time (CRT).**

In the laboratory, reaction time is a type of psychomotor task that is frequently used to determine the effects of aging on response speed. Almost any factor that enhances or disrupts central nervous system (CNS) function is reflected by a change in reaction time. Drugs, sleep deprivation, arousal level, disease, and maturation are factors that affect CNS function and also cause changes in reaction time. For this reason, reaction time may be thought of as a behavioral window through which scientists can study CNS function. Gerontologists have used reaction time for many years as an index of the effects of aging on the integrity of the CNS.

The **reaction time stimulus** may be visual, auditory, or tactile and may be simple or complex. For example, in a visual display, the complexity can be manipulated by degrading the stimulus as in adding various nonrelated stimuli that the subject must ignore to make the correct response. The **reaction time response** may also be simple or complex and in this case is made with the musculoskeletal system. The stimulus–response relationship can be manipulated by changing the compatibility, and the response can be manipulated by increasing the number of choices or by changing the response–response compatibility. In both SRT and CRT, the time between the stimulus onset and the first response of the muscle is assumed to represent the CNS processing time that is necessary to complete the task. When the response is initiated and the movement begins, other central mechanisms are responsible for controlling and monitoring the movement.

To understand more fully the effects of age on central versus peripheral response speed, reaction time has been divided into several components by electroencephalographic (EEG) and electromyographic (EMG) analyses to determine when specific mechanisms of the response become active. If EEG electrodes are placed on the scalp overlying the cerebral visual cortex (for a visual stimulus) and motor cortex of the brain (for a motor potential

response), and an EMG electrode is placed over the belly of the muscle to be used, the combination of records from the electrodes and the chronoscope microswitches (or computer keys) provides a more detailed analysis of the response. The fractionation process is shown in figure 7.1. As soon as the stimulus light is activated, the subject lifts the forearm to the shoulder as quickly as possible. The stimulus light initiates five traces across the oscilloscope. Lifting the forearm releases the switch attached to the subject's arm and causes an offset on the trace labeled RT key, an indication of reaction time (RT). Passing the wrist through the beam emitted by the light-emitting diode activates the movement time (MT) switch, causing an offset of the total response time trace. The motor potential (MP), which is the time when the activity of the motor cortex controlling the movement is coupled with the stimulus, is recorded on an EEG trace. The visual evoked potential (VEP) is an EEG record of activity in the cortical occipital lobe that is coupled to the stimulus. It reflects the receipt of the visual stimulus in the brain. The beginning of electrical activity in the muscle (before the arm moves) signals the arrival of the movement command to the muscle. The time between the stimulus and this arrival is called the premotor time (PMT).

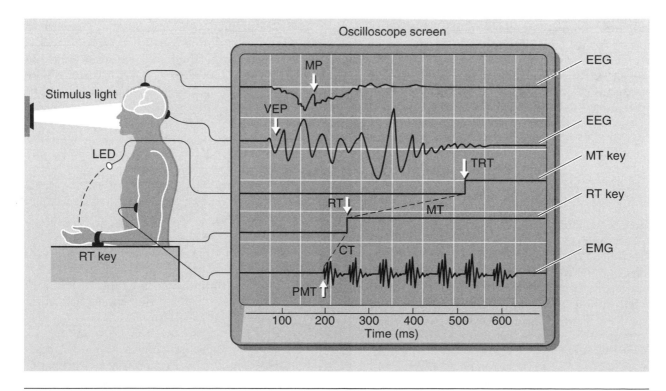

Figure 7.1 Fractionation of reaction time. RT = reaction time; LED = light-emitting diode; TRT = total response time; MT = movement time; MP = motor potential; EEG = electroencephalographic trace; VEP = visual evoked potential; PMT = premotor time.

From these observed values, it is possible to calculate the other variables:

Information processing time = MP – VEP

Nerve conduction velocity = PMT – MP

Contraction time = RT – PMT
(time required to contract the muscle sufficiently
to move the wrist off the RT key)

MT = TRT – RT
(movement speed independent of reaction)

Researchers have also distinguished between central and peripheral processing by manipulating factors (i.e., task complexity) that influence stimulus and response processing (central) but not the speed with which information is relayed to the muscles (peripheral) (Cerella et al., 1980).

Understanding the phenomenon of attention has also been enhanced by SRT paradigms. Even when one stimulus and one response are used, the length of the interval of time between the warning signal and the stimulus onset (preparatory interval) greatly affects the SRT. If the time period between the warning signal and stimulus onset is always the same, then subjects can anticipate when to respond after a period of practice and hence the reaction time is no longer a measure of processing speed. Thus researchers vary the length of the preparation interval in their paradigms in order to minimize anticipation of the response. Results from these studies reveal that long preparatory intervals produce the greatest age deficits (Wilkinson & Allison, 1989), perhaps because long preparatory intervals require an individual to attend to the task for a longer period of time and attention deteriorates with increased age in many older people. Some researchers have suggested that young adults can better sustain attention and make use of a longer period in which to prepare to respond.

Simple Reaction Time

SRT is so named because it requires a very simple behavior, usually lifting one finger from a switch or button, in response to the activation of a stimulus. SRT requires relatively low-level CNS processing: perception of the stimulus (such as seeing a light or hearing a buzzer), remembering its significance and the behavior to be associated with it, and programming and executing a movement response. SRT represents speed of response, that is, the speed with which a person can move a finger or limb when almost no calculation, integration, or decision making is required. It is thought to represent the general responsiveness of the central nervous system and has been described

as "a general primary response mechanism of the CNS" (Gottsdanker, 1982, p. 342).

Although SRT is less complicated than many other behaviors, it contains several components that enable researchers to study CNS function. For example, it has been used as a measure of basic central control mechanisms. Increases in latency of response that are associated with an increase in the complexity of the movement to be made (e.g., a smaller target or a longer distance to be moved) are taken to indicate that a more complex processing is necessary to activate the movement.

The slowing of SRT with aging has been observed so many times that it is considered one of the most measurable and recognizable behavioral changes that occurs with aging. Francis Galton, an English scientist who between 1884 and 1890 measured the SRTs of thousands of people of all ages, was the first to report that 60-year-olds were approximately 13% slower than 20-year-olds (Galton, 1899). Later, his data were reanalyzed and confirmed using more advanced statistical techniques (Johnson et al., 1985; Koga & Morant, 1923). Since then, almost every researcher who has measured reaction time has found it to be slower in older people by approximately 25% (i.e., Amrhein et al., 1991). Age-related slowing is apparent even as soon as the late 30s and early 40s (Myerson et al., 1989). Galton's work was later replicated by Wilkinson and Allison (1989). Their measurement of 5,325 visitors to the Science Museum in London showed, like Galton's results, that the average, median, and fastest SRTs are significantly slower in older people (figure 7.2). One of the most important points in figure 7.2, however, is that use of the fastest reaction time is not indicative of usual performance. Although age differences cannot be eliminated entirely (even by using the fastest RT), the magnitude of the age differences seen in most SRT studies is attributable partially to the fact that many investigators use a single test session in which only a few trials are provided. If experimental factors such as novelty, practice, stimulus quality, and performance expectations are held constant, age differences in simple reaction time can be substantially reduced.

The simplest auditory reaction time slows linearly and approximately 0.5 ms a year between ages 20 and 96 (Fozard et al., 1994). Requiring additional decisions prior to reacting further increases the slowing effect. For example, adding one decision to be made about the stimulus, as occurs in a discrimination reaction time, increases the slowing to 1.6 ms a year (figure 7.3). Males were faster than females for both simple and discrimination reaction time.

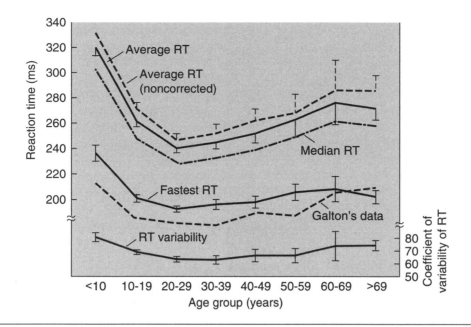

Figure 7.2 Population simple reaction times: average reaction time (RT), median RT, and fastest RT as a function of age.

Reprinted, by permission, from R. T. Wilkinson and S. Allison, 1989, "Age and simple relation time: Decade differences for 5,325 subjects," *Journal of Gerontology: Psychological Sciences* 44: 31.

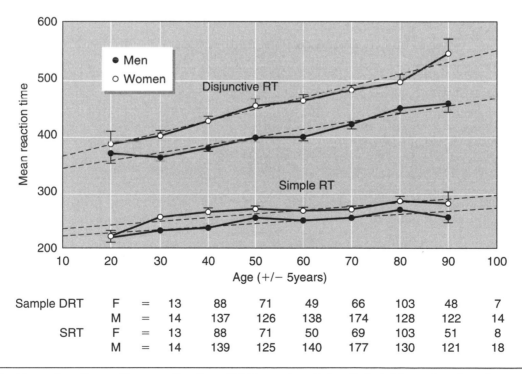

Sample DRT	F =	13	88	71	49	66	103	48	7
	M =	14	137	126	138	174	128	122	14
SRT	F =	13	88	71	50	69	103	51	8
	M =	14	139	125	140	177	130	121	18

Figure 7.3 Mean of median auditory reaction times (RTs) for each participant's first visit as a function of age, gender, and task type expressed with standard error bars, spline fitting, and first-order regression lines. Age intervals are by decade, ±5 years (e.g., the 6th decade contains participants 55-64 years of age). Sample sizes for the 2nd through 9th decades were 27, 227, 197, 190, 246, 233, 172, and 26. DRT = discrimination reaction time; SRT = simple reaction time.

Data from Fozard et al. (1994).

The longitudinal analysis revealed similar results, in that slowing (mean of median SRTs) from age 20 to 90 increased with age by 27% (from 229 to 292 ms). The slowing was gradual and linear until the 80+ age range. Errors in responding (both failure to respond and incorrect responses) also increased with age. These results do not support the hypothesis that older adults use a speed–accuracy trade-off strategy in their performance.

Choice Reaction Time

In a CRT paradigm, more than one stimulus is presented and a specific movement must be paired with each stimulus. The subject must choose the movement that is associated with the stimulus presented. For instance, in a driving simulator, if a red light is activated the subject applies pressure to the brake pedal to stop, whereas if the green light is activated the subject applies pressure to the gas pedal to accelerate. CRT paradigms can become very complicated when several possible stimuli are paired with specific responses of varying degrees of complexity.

CRT has at least three components: the perceptual process of identifying the stimulus; the decision process, in which the stimulus–response code is retrieved and the response is selected; and the motor process required to initiate the response. The perceptual process and the motor process are relatively stable and represent the base level of response in an SRT paradigm. However, the middle component, the processing of the stimulus–response code and the selection of the motor response, varies with the complexity of the choices to be made in the CRT paradigm. The choices relate to the number and type of stimuli to be selected, although the nature and difficulty of the response movement to be made also affect the response latency. Both the difficulty of the decisions to be made and the difficulty of the movement response contribute to the response complexity.

A review and analysis of nine studies revealed that as the task difficulty increases, the reaction latencies of old subjects are disproportionately slower than those of the young (Hale et al., 1987). In other words, advancing age has a greater impact on the central processing components than on the perceptual and motor output components of the CRT response. These results further confirm those of Fozard and colleagues mentioned earlier and shown in figure 7.3. As can be seen in figure 7.4, both latency and variability increase with age (Hultsch et al., 2002); as we will discuss in a later section, age-related changes in variability are also extremely important when considering the reaction time performance of older adults.

Age-Sensitive Factors That Affect Response Speed

Several factors affect the stimulus, response, or both and can therefore alter the speed of response. Experimentally manipulating various stimulus and response factors enables researchers to determine the manner in which slowing affects performance. Understanding how these factors affect the individual and hence influence response speed is important for understanding the general aging process and for developing programs for older adults in both learning and relearning paradigms.

Stimulus Discrimination and Stimulus–Response Compatibility

The complexity of a task is defined by the number of stimuli or response choices or by other task con-

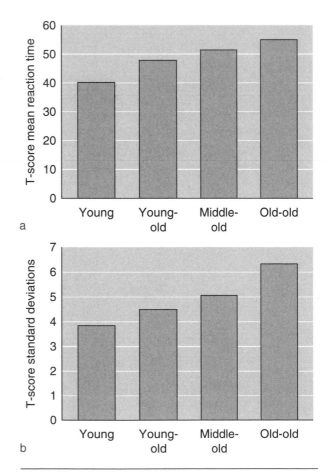

Figure 7.4 T-scores of mean reaction time *(a)* and standard deviations *(b)* for choice reaction time performance. Significant group differences were found for both measures ($p < .001$).

Data from Hultsch et al. (2002).

ditions such as the discriminability of the stimulus and the stimulus–response (S–R) compatibility. If a stimulus is easy to detect and clearly different from another one, people can discriminate between them and respond much more quickly than if a stimulus is degraded (e.g., faint or blurry) or is very similar to another stimulus. One of many examples of real-world tasks where degraded stimuli make it especially difficult for older adults to respond easily and quickly is seen in the design of many ATM machines. These machines are often located outside so that the glare of the sun during the day or outside lighting in the evening reduces the contrast between text and background dramatically. The font resolution and size are often small, and the curvature of the screen frequently makes it difficult to read the text. In addition, the choices are often linked to the response button by a dashed line that does not exactly correspond to a particular button; often the dashed line terminates between two buttons, not pointing at one or the other. Our technologically advanced society seems to increase the complexity of stimulus and response conditions annually.

Another factor that influences task complexity is stimulus–response compatibility. If the response seems compatible to the stimulus, such as reacting with the right arm to a stimulus on the right side of the stimulus panel and the left arm to a stimulus on the left side, then the reaction is quicker than if the stimuli and responses seem incompatible. A substantial portion of the age-related slowing of reaction time observed by Smulders and colleagues (1999) was attributable to processing the stimulus and not to the compatibility of the response to the stimulus. In their study, RT, which includes both stimulus processing and response selection and therefore would reflect both stimulus degradation and S–R compatibility, was slower in the older adults (figure 7.5a). But the P300 latency, which is the approximate latency associated with stimulus evaluation, was differentially slower in the older adults only for P300, indicating that stimulus degradation slowed their responses, but S–R compatibility did not (figure 7.5b).

Response Complexity and Response–Response Compatibility

Besides the reactive latency delay induced by a complicated stimulus display, can the delay also be attributed to the difficulty of the response? Response complexity is another factor that contributes to the complexity of the task, delays response speed, and makes age differences more pronounced. Regardless of how simple the stimulus is, a response that

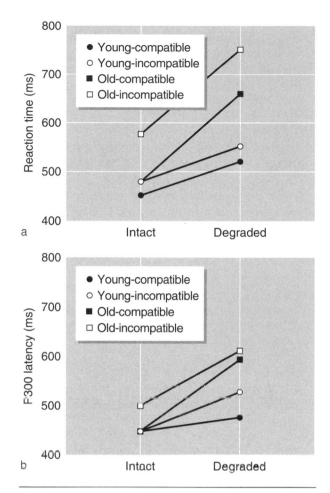

Figure 7.5 Reaction time (a) and P300 latency (b) in milliseconds for compatible and incompatible stimulus–response pairings for intact and degraded stimuli for young (mean age = 21) and old (mean age = 71).

Data from Smulders et al. (1999).

is more complex in terms of its duration, timing, rhythm, number of component parts, compatibility, and accuracy requirements increases the amount of time necessary to program and initiate the movement within both the SRT and the CRT response.

Differentially slower responses are made by older individuals when they have to choose between making movements that are simple because they are partially reflexively controlled and highly practiced, such as the pinching movement used to pick up some objects, and movements that are rarely made together and have to be voluntarily controlled, such as doing a task with two index fingers. Light and Spirduso (1990) required subjects to respond to a visual stimulus with either the index finger, the index finger and thumb (pinching movement), both index fingers, or both index fingers and thumbs (pinching movements; figure 7.6). Of those four movements, only the pairing of the index finger and thumb in

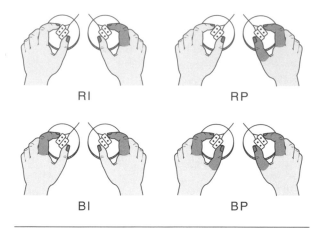

RI   RP

BI   BP

Figure 7.6 Movements used to initiate a reaction. Choice reaction time responses were made to a light stimulus by closing a reaction time switch with either the right index finger (RI), the right index finger and the thumb in a pinching motion (RP), both index fingers simultaneously in a bilateral response (BI), or a bilateral pinch (BP).

the pinching movement is part of our daily repertoire; the **bimanual** (both hands) and **unimanual** (one hand) index finger responses are infrequently made. In each of the testing conditions, two of these four movements were paired and subjects reacted to whichever movement was signaled. Figure 7.7a is a typical monitor display that signals the two possible choices to be made in figure 7.6 (right index finger and thumb or right index finger), and figure 7.7b is a monitor display with the visual stimulus indicating the appropriate response, which in this case is the right index finger.

The pairing in this case is within the right hand, and hence only the decision of digit combination needs to be made. Each time the stimulus was activated, the subjects had to choose one of two movements. Throughout the testing session, every movement was paired with every other movement, and the CRT for each movement was an average of the response latencies for that movement when paired with every other movement. Because the subjects had to make a binary choice of movements in every response, the major difference between the reac-

tion latencies for different movements was attributed to the complexity of the movement. Older subjects were significantly slower than young adults on the two more complex movements (involved two sides of the body), the bilateral pinch and the bilateral index response (figure 7.8). However, only in the oldest group (70-80 years) were the differences in the speed with which they could initiate the two bilateral movements significant. Light and Spirduso (1990) concluded that the response programming capability of older women was sensitive to changes in movement complexity.

Response–response (R–R) compatibility refers to the ease with which responses are performed simultaneously or individually when paired with another alternative response.

An example of a compatible response would be raising both hands over the head at the same time, where an incompatible response would be raising one hand over the head while tapping the table with the other hand. Spatial and temporal characteristics are more similar for compatible than for incompatible tasks. In the Light and Spirduso (1990) paradigm (figure 7.6), the movement response pairs varied

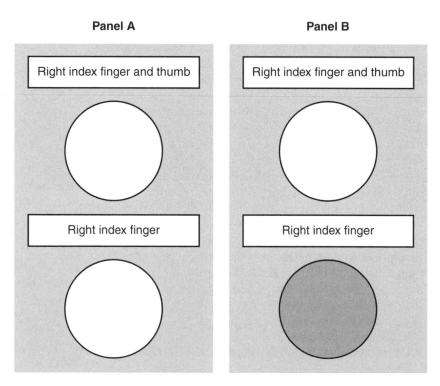

Panel A   **Panel B**

Right index finger and thumb   Right index finger and thumb

Right index finger   Right index finger

Figure 7.7 Monitor display for a pairing of the right index finger and thumb movement with the right index finger movement. (a) The monitor screen before the stimulus; (b) indicates that the subject should respond by pressing the button with the index finger.

Reprinted, by permission, from K.E. Light and W.W. Spirduso, 1996, "Age factors influencing response–response compatibility in relation time tasks," *Journal of Aging and Physical Activity* 4: 179-193.

Differential Effects of Aging on Stimuli, Responses, and Stimulus–Response Compatibility

Smulders and colleagues (1999) provide an excellent example of partitioning stimulus reception and response execution, in combination with using behavioral responses (RT) and psychophysiological measures (P300) to determine age effects. The subjects responded to visual stimuli, the word *right* or *left*, presented on a computer monitor screen. If the stimulus was intact, the word *right* or *left* would appear on the computer screen enclosed in a rectangular frame. In the stimulus degradation condition, the word stimuli were degraded by a series of dots surrounding the stimuli. The S–R compatibility condition was manipulated by pairing the *right* visual stimulus with a right index finger response and a *left* visual stimulus with a left index finger response. The S–R incompatibility condition was pairing of the *left* visual stimulus with a right response or the *right* visual stimulus with a left response. The easiest task condition pairing would be intact and compatible (i.e., visual stimulus *left* paired with a left index finger response) and the most difficult would be degraded and incompatible (i.e., visual stimulus *left* degraded by dots paired with a right index finger response).

The authors used the P300 latency to indicate whether aging influenced the subjects' ability to react to stimulus characteristics (i.e., intact or degraded) and the RT latency to indicate whether aging affected the response selection part of the reaction. Thus, if aging affected the subjects' ability to detect a degraded stimulus and also their ability to cope with a response that was incompatible with the stimulus, both the P300 and RT latencies would be differentially longer than those of the young subjects.

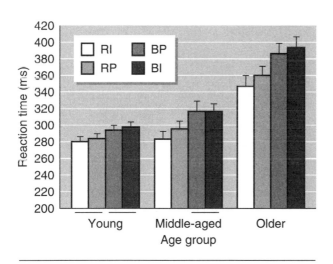

Figure 7.8 Age differences in initiating movements of varying complexity. Reaction time means and standard errors for young (*M* = 22), middle-aged (*M* = 43), and older (*M* = 63) subjects for right index (RI), right pinch (RP), bilateral pinch (BP), and bilateral index (BI) movements. Age effect and movement-type effect were both significant (*p* < .001). The interaction between age and movement was also highly significant (p < .001). Nonsignificant differences among the movements for each age group are depicted by connecting lines under the abscissa.

Reprinted, by permission, from K. Light and W. Spirduso, 1990, "Effects of adult aging on the movement complexity factor of response programming," *Journal of Gerontology: Psychological Sciences* 45: 108.

from very compatible to very incompatible. A closer examination of the most and least compatible mean RTs revealed that RT latency increased with age particularly for the older group (figure 7.9). To determine the contribution of R–R compatibility independent of task complexity, the authors subtracted the overall mean of the response choice from the mean of the same movement when paired with another response. For example, a mean RT response of 270 ms for the right index finger and thumb when paired with the right index finger compared to an overall mean of RT response of 250 ms for the right index finger and thumb over all conditions reveals that older adults are differentially affected when there is a possibility of activating the index finger alone. The results of this analysis further support the added effect that R–R compatibility has on older adults (figure 7.10).

Reaction Time and Variability

Throughout the following discussions of reaction time and aging, many references are made to observations that reaction times are slower in older people. However, most of the data reported are average or median reaction times from many individuals at different ages (i.e., cross-sectional sampling) rather than reflections of change within individuals over a series of years (i.e., longitudinal analysis). Very wide

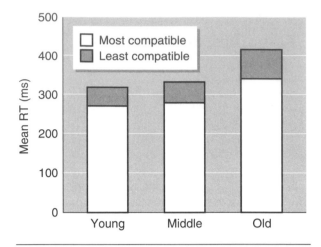

Figure 7.9 Means of reaction times (RTs, milliseconds) for the most compatible (right index finger and thumb response when paired with bilateral index finger and thumb) and least compatible movement (bilateral index finger response when paired with the right pinch). The gray area of the bar is the mean RT for the most compatible response (fastest), and the black area of the bar indicates the additional time taken to respond in the least compatible response condition. The black area accentuates the age-related effects of response–response compatibility.

Data from Light et al. (1996).

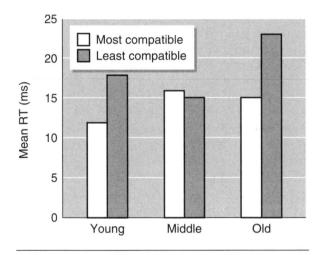

Figure 7.10 Absolute value of the mean difference in the reaction time (RT) for the response and the response paired with another response. Before converting to the absolute value, the mean RTs for the most compatible condition were less than the mean of the movement without pairing. This type of computation provides an analysis of R–R compatibility independent of task complexity.

Data from Light et al. (1996).

individual variation exists in reaction time at all ages, and some people in their 50s who are almost as fast as the fastest 20-year-olds are considerably faster than many of their cohorts. Aging rates also vary, so

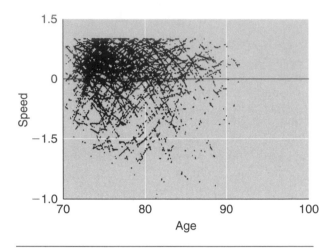

Figure 7.11 Each line represents an individual's speed of processing score on the first occasion and second occasion (3.5 years later) of testing.

From H. Christiansen et al., 1999, "An analysis of diversity in the cognitive performance of elderly community dwellers: Individual differences in change scores as a function of age," *Psychology and Aging* 14(3): 365-379.

that some individuals may lose very little behavioral speed over a long period, whereas others may slow significantly each decade or precipitously before death. Thus, when discussions mention reaction times of 20-year-olds or 40-year-olds, bear in mind the discussion of individual differences in chapter 2 (see figure 2.4, p. 37): These are averages of many individuals within each age category.

In addition to the general responsivity (speed) of the CNS, another indicator of neurological integrity is variability of performance. The majority of researchers provide group means and standard deviations as indicators of performance capabilities, and from these it is indeed clear that latency and variability of RT increase with age (figure 7.4, p. 162). Even after researchers control for the potential association between latency of response and variability, **diversity** increases with age (Hultsch et al., 2002). Thus, adults become more heterogeneous with increasing age.

As individuals age, performance changes are not uniform in that some individuals may experience drastic rates of decline whereas other individuals may maintain performance. Figure 7.11 displays scores from 426 elderly individuals who were measured systematically for 3.5 years. The lines represent each individual's score for the first and second testing sessions. What a variety of trajectories! Some individuals decline quite rapidly, and others maintain their initial level of performance.

Deterioration in performance does not seem to be inevitable, at least for this relatively short period of time. A second interesting finding from this study was that interindividual variability in **change scores** was present even after individuals with dementia or "probable" dementia were excluded.

Variability within an individual may be a valuable indicator of neurobiological changes with age. Not only do aging people exhibit different rates of slowing in their response speed (individual differences; **dispersion**), but they also exhibit different rates of increasing variability of response speed (within-individual consistency of performance). Both of these contribute to the increasing heterogeneity in CNS function of older adults.

Hultsch and colleagues (2002) conducted one of the first studies to examine age changes in all three types of variability—diversity, dispersion, and **inconsistency**—and the results of their study emphasize the importance of sources of variability as indicators of age-related changes in behavioral speed. Furthermore, stable levels of intraindividual variability across measures and within a task across occasions, as were observed in their study, support the hypothesis that CNS slowing is best explained by neurobiological mechanisms.

The specific mechanisms that explain increased variability with age have not yet been identified. It has been suggested that both age-related declines in performance and increases in interindividual differences in performance may be a function of the increasing intraindividual variability in neurobiological mechanisms in the brain (Li & Lindenberger, 1999). Thus, within-individual consistency might be the best behavioral indicator of age-related decline of neurobiological mechanisms that support the integrity of the brain across a wide range of functions. As neurobiological inconsistency increases in older brains, additional resources may be recruited to manage executive functions of otherwise relatively simple tasks (Dixon & Backman, 1999). The brain is highly interconnected, so that even small localized neural deficits affect the function of other brain areas. If these deficits affect the function of a managerial component, such as frontal lobe executive function, then this small, localized deficit may appear as a generalized impairment (Raz, 2000).

Older adults are more heterogeneous in CNS function than young adults in three ways:

- Diversity—individual differences; individuals decline at different rates.

- Dispersion—the rate of decline is not the same across multiple tasks; older individuals age more in some tasks than in others.

- Inconsistency—older individuals are more inconsistent than young, and their inconsistency across tasks is greater than in young individuals.

Other Factors Influencing Speed of Processing

Several factors may contribute to age-related behavioral slowing. Health status as an indicator of changes in behavioral speed has received a lot of attention. It seems plausible that because of differential declines in various systems as well as an increase in the prevalence of disease processes in older adults, less healthy individuals would not perform as well as healthy individuals on speeded tasks. Salthouse (2000), on the basis of single-item self-report scores, argued that minimal support exists for a direct influence of health status on behavioral speed. However, it is quite common to observe that adults with hypertension, cardiovascular disease, diabetes, depression, coronary obstruction and pulmonary disease, psychosocial stress, and other chronic diseases are slower at responding than adults who have none of these symptoms. This issue is discussed in much more detail in chapter 9.

The second potential factor that may influence processing speed is experience. Krampe and Ericsson (1996) found that task-specific slowing (speeded music-related tasks) was not evident for amateur and expert pianists who had a certain amount of deliberate practice, particularly later in life. A third factor that may influence speeded performance is task characteristics. For example, age may influence processing speed differentially for tasks that represent different cognitive domains (e.g., lexical vs. nonlexical) (Lima et al., 1991).

Theories of Response Slowing

Age-related behavioral slowing has been observed so long and so consistently across a range of speeded tasks that many theories have been developed to explain the phenomenon. These theories can be categorized into two broad groups that explain behavioral slowing as general or global and process-specific or unique. The major tenets of the general slowing model are that slowing occurs in all components of processing from stimulus encoding to response selection, that the amount of slowing is proportional in older relative to younger adults, and that as task complexity increases slowing becomes increasingly apparent. The process-specific view suggests that slowing may occur to a differential extent in one part of the processing (i.e., stimulus encoding) versus another part (i.e., response processing) and that the specificity of slowing may vary from task to task. Theoretical debates over whether behavioral slowing with age is general or process-specific are ongoing. The purpose of the following section is not to resolve the theoretical debate but to describe it by presenting findings from representative studies that support and challenge the general slowing theory.

General Slowing Hypothesis

The definition of general slowing is slowing of the speed of processing that affects all components of a stimulus response approximately the same, whether the comparison is of different levels of complexity within the same task (process independent) or of similar components across several different types of tasks (task independent).

The structure of processing (e.g., stimulus encoding, stimulus identification, decision making, response selection, response execution) is viewed to be unaffected by aging. It is the speed of processing, or the timing of the structural components, that is thought to be degraded by aging. Proponents of the generalized slowing theory note that large proportions of age effects on individual variables are shared across many variables; in fact, unique age-related impacts on individual variables are rarely seen (Salthouse, 2000). The effect of age is the same throughout an individual's distribution of reaction latencies; that is, the fastest and slowest reactions slow at the same rate.

Brinley plots in which older adults' responses are plotted against younger adults' responses generally reveal a high linear relationship with an intercept of 0 and a slope of 1.4 to 2.0. This systematic relationship is generally taken to support the idea of a general speed factor. Brinley plots also reveal a similar relationship in accuracy tasks, so if these plots are used to support the idea of a general speed factor, they would also have to be used to support a general accuracy factor.

Brinley Plots

A graphing technique called a Brinley plot expresses the response speed of one category of respondent to the other (e.g., old vs. young, male vs. female, diseased vs. healthy, experimental vs. control) to determine whether the effect of another variable (such as complexity of task) has a differential effect on one of the groups above and beyond the effects of the variable on the other. If a claim is made that increasing task complexity slows older adults more than it does younger adults, it has to be shown that the increases in delay as the task gets harder are significantly greater in the old than in the young. This is generally revealed by an age-by-task interaction term in analyses of variance.

Cerella and colleagues (1980) analyzed numerous studies that included several different tasks and conditions to examine the relationship of reactions of older adults to those of younger adults. In figure 7.12, mean RT values are plotted for the older group relative to the younger group. Note that each data point in the figure represents the mean RT for one task in one study and that the collection of points

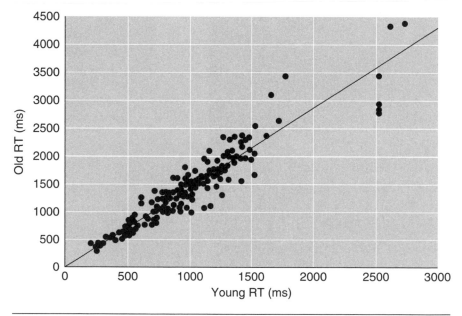

Figure 7.12 Scatter plot, with regression line, of an imaginary set of data points generated to resemble the set of reaction time (RT) data used in the meta-analyses by Cerella and colleagues (1980).

Reprinted, by permission, from T.R. Bahore et al., 1997, "The decline of cognitive processing speed in old age," *Current Directions in Psychological Science* 6(6): 163-169.

can be described by a linear function with a slope of 1.36 and an intercept at 0. This graph shows that age differences increase in magnitude as the task increases in complexity and requires more central processing time and that age-related slowing can be estimated by multiplying the mean of young RT by the slope of the line. However, the type of task contributed almost nothing to the prediction of age effects. These results are compelling and provide enormous support for the general slowing hypothesis in that information processing is slowed to the same degree with age regardless of the task or condition. This graph shows that age differences increase in magnitude as the task increases in complexity and requires more central processing time.

Challenges to the Generalized Slowing Theory

Using different analyses, some researchers observe that aging does differentially influence components of the stimulus response, and it differentially influences certain variables and not others (Bashore et al., 1997).

Physiological Evidence of Process-Specific Slowing

Bashore and colleagues' (1997) review, which included several of his own studies, provides a

comprehensive description of how researchers have challenged the general slowing theory by using both typical RT measures and the P300 component of the event-related potential to separate early elements of stimulus processing (perhaps stimulus encoding) from later processes, especially those related to selecting and executing the correct responses to the stimulus. This process was described earlier as a means of determining the extent of aging effects on stimulus processing versus stimulus compatibility (see figure 7.5b and accompanying text, p. 163). Because P300 also is not sensitive to speed–accuracy tradeoffs and is linearly related to age, Bashore et al. (1997) could apply Brinley plots and statistical analyses and replicate the same RT results as the general slowing theorists (i.e., Cerella et al., 1980), that is, an intercept of about 0.0 and slope (function) of about 1.27 (figure 7.13a). However, the results of the analysis of P300 latency were different (figure 7.13b). The slope was approximately 1.0, as was true for RT, but the intercept was elevated, indicating that early stimulus encoding was affected by age, but response selection processes were not. Bashore et al. (1997) used several other strategies to find differential effects in different components of processing. By comparing the quality of stimuli (degraded vs. intact), stimulus–response compatibility, P300 latencies (stimulus sensitive) to EEG measures that are thought to reflect response system activation, interactions among contextually

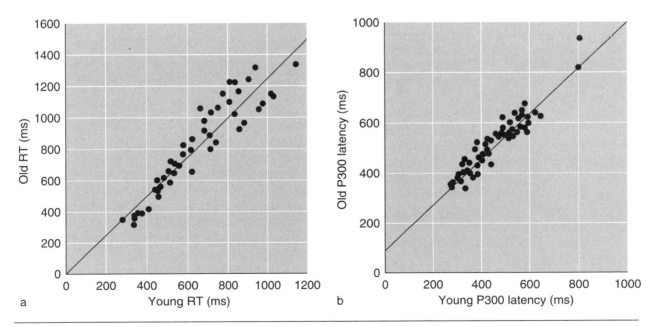

Figure 7.13 Scatter plots, with regression lines, of the reaction time (RT) and P300 latency data used in a meta-analysis by Bashore and colleagues (1989).

Reprinted, by permission, from T.R. Bashore et al., 1997, "The decline of cognitive processing speed in old age," *Current Directions in Psychological Science* 6(6): 163-169.

distracted stimuli and response compatibility, and different types of task (lexical vs. math), the authors concluded that some age-related slowing is process specific and task dependent. However, some generalized slowing exists.

Sequential Effects of Process-Specific Slowing

Two-choice serial reaction time tasks are influenced by the preceding stimulus or by previous stimuli. The length of time between the response and the next stimulus (interresponse interval) is critical in defining the dominating mechanisms underlying sequential effects in serial reaction time tasks. Shorter interresponse intervals are typically influenced by the preceding stimulus and are referred to as automatic facilitation, which suggests that previous levels of activation can be used for the next response and hence faster responses are typically found. If the interval is longer, activation levels from the previous response are decayed and subjective expectancy tends to dominate. The longer interresponse interval provides the subject with time to anticipate and prepare for an upcoming response. This period of time could be advantageous if the upcoming stimulus meets the participants' expectations or costly if the stimulus is different from that expected by the subject. Melis, Soetens, and van der Molen (2002) examined sequential effects in a serial reaction time task to determine if their findings could be explained by the general

slowing hypothesis. They used interresponse intervals of 50 ms (short) and 100 ms (long) and manipulated the conditions such that the upcoming stimulus was either repeated or alternated with respect to the previous stimulus. In addition to constructing Brinley plots to examine the data, the authors used an analytical strategy (analysis of variance, or ANOVA) to control for generalized slowing in an effort to determine whether the results were process-specific or generalized. Figure 7.13 shows the data expressed by Brinley plots where the old RT data are expressed relative to the young RT data. A shorter response to stimulus interval as depicted in figure 7.14*a* has a large distribution that cannot be explained by a linear function. However, it is clear that a longer response to stimulus interval can be explained by a linear function, suggesting that older adults need a longer period of time to anticipate and prepare for an upcoming response (figure 7.14*b*). These data confirm the analyses from an ANOVA. These results suggest that age has a differential influence on reaction time for a two-choice serial reaction time task and can be explained by process-specific mechanisms when the interresponse interval is short; however, generalized slowing accounts for the effects of a long interresponse interval. The authors suggested that aging alters the information processing mechanisms that underpin automatic facilitation and that this cannot be explained by generalized slowing alone.

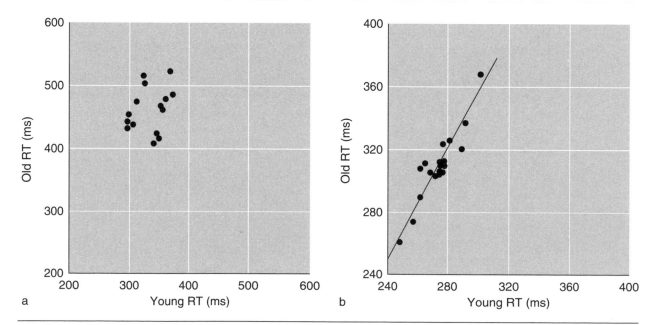

Figure 7.14 Reaction time (RT) of the old subjects expressed relative to the young subjects for *(a)* short response–stimulus intervals and *(b)* long response–stimulus intervals.

Reprinted from *Brain and Cognition*, 49, A. Melis et al., Process-specific slowing with advancing age: Evidence derived from the analysis of sequential effects, pp. 420-435. Copyright 2002, with permission from Elsevier.

Selective Slowing in Cognitive–Motor Experts

A second challenge to the general slowing theory comes from those who study older experts in activities that require fine motor skill coordination and speeded movements, for example, piano and violin virtuosos or expert typists. These individuals have a specific cognitive–motor expertise that is clearly superior to nonmusicians and nontypists, and they have preserved their performance capabilities throughout many years by constant practice and performance. Krampe and colleagues (2002) cited many examples where the experts have aged at a typical rate in many other types of movements but have maintained their performance capabilities on their instrument. In addition, music passages that were played at varying tempos, moving from slower to faster, were studied across tasks, with the result that some processes specific to their domain of expertise were preserved and some others not related to their domain were degraded, as is typically seen in older adults. One explanation is that the constant practice maintained their expertise and protected them from the general slowing observed in others. A second explanation is that these experts have acquired mechanisms that allowed them to adapt to specific task constraints in their area of expertise. One example of this is advance preparation, which means that the combination of years of experience, familiarity, and practice enables them to plan movements well in advance, reducing the time between individual finger movements, and therefore enabling them to play a fast passage in the same amount of time as young individuals would play it.

Thus, older experts express normal age-related decline in general processing speed but little or no decline in speed measures that are specific to their domain of expertise. In summary, research on experts

has shown that cognitive processes that are specific to rapid, complex cognitive–manual skill performances, processes such as timing, sequencing, and executive control, do not follow the trajectory that general slowing hypothesis would predict. Either these experts have found a way to rely on mechanisms that are not sensitive to slowing, or they have maintained their speed of processing selectively by their activities.

Some theorists believe that age-related slowing of responses is better explained by viewing processing as a limited capacity system as opposed to a structural explanation that views a stimulus as the trigger that initiates a series of processes designed to produce an overt response. General slowing theorists explain the age-complexity effect as higher levels of complexity placing greater demands on processing resources, resulting in poorer performance by older adults than young adults because the older adults have smaller amounts of resources available. However, process-specific theorists suggest that the efficiency of processing is based on multiple resources that are fixed, process-specific, and broadly task-specific. From their perspective, aging may reduce the capacity of response or the capacity of the individual to transfer resources from one processing resource to the another.

Older Expert Pianists Can Maintain Skill With Deliberate Practice

Wilhelm Kempff was one of the greatest pianists of the 20th century. His career as a concert pianist spanned 65 years from his first concert in Germany at the age of 15 to his final concert in Paris at the age of 80. Throughout his career he continued to enchant audiences around the world with his expertise and talent (Krampe & Ericsson, 1996).

Neurobiological Explanations of Age-Related Slowing

Our discussions of age-related slowing to this point have been from a psychological perspective, using behavioral data and statistical analyses to develop hypotheses. However, many researchers have focused on neurobiological changes to explain changes in processing speed.

Diffuse cell loss results in the transmission of neural impulses across longer and more mazelike pathways to reach the same end state. Thinning of dendritic branching, loss of active synapses, and reduced myelin lead to slower propagation of neural impulses. In addition, loss of synchronization of neural impulses may be the result of a reduction in the number of neurotransmitters or changes in neurotransmitter turnover. Finally, increased levels of neural "noise" result in the deterioration of the signal-to-noise ratio.

Some biological evidence suggests that brain plasticity is maintained with practice, which provides a mechanism to explain the retention of high levels of

Why Older Adults Respond More Slowly Than Young Adults

1. The general slowing hypothesis (Birren hypothesis) states that speed of processing is correlated with aging, and most speeded performances are correlated with other speeded performances. Slowing is seen within individuals' slowest, average, and fastest reaction times, across tasks, and, in most cases, in all processes of the responses. General slowing is attributed to many biological changes that occur in the brain that, taken together, suggest mechanisms by which slowing occurs.

2. Physiological evidence exists, however, that process-specific slowing occurs; age-related slowing tends to be more pronounced in response-related processes than in stimulus-related processes. This type of evidence also indicates that speeded processes in some variables but not others may be slowed.

3. Older adults need a longer period of time to anticipate and prepare for an upcoming response; thus, the process-specific mechanism hypothesis predicts this age differential better than the general slowing hypothesis does.

4. Cognitive–motor experts, such as violinists, pianists, and expert typists, reveal age-related general slowing in many aspects of cognition but either selectively maintain processes that are specific to performing their cognitive skill or learn to rely on mechanisms that can circumvent slowing in those processes crucial to their domain.

5. Age-related slowing may be explained as age-related losses of resources (biological changes) in a limited capacity system. High-complexity demands place greater demands on aged resources that are reduced; thus, older adults exhaust their energy resources in the early phases of responses (stimulus-related elements) so that they are slower in the later phases of a response (response-related elements). Cognitive-skill experts may be able to shift energy resources that allow them to maintain processes critical to their domain but not other general cognitive functions.

---

speeded performance in older musicians. The cortical representation of the hand and single fingers was larger in older violinists and was related to their years of training (Elbert et al., 1995), and plasticity intensified in those who increased their training regimen later in life (Elbert et al., 1996).

It has always been difficult to link specific neurobiological events with CNS control mechanisms or specific movements. For years researchers have been observing and documenting behavior and behavioral changes and inferring the underlying brain activity. The recent development of neuroimaging techniques has great promise for enhancing our understanding of brain changes that underlie the aging process in the absence and presence of disease. In addition, neuroimaging techniques can help us to understand how brain activity changes during the learning process, a development that has important implications for rehabilitative techniques.

Two promising analytical methods include positron emission tomography (PET) and functional magnetic resonance imaging (fMRI). These techniques may further define cortical activation level as

a potential underlying factor influencing information processing speed. The pattern of brain activation appears to be task dependent for both activity level and region. One of the major challenges with neuroimaging techniques is to identify the relation between cortical activation and behavioral measures, particularly to identify whether specific changes in neural structures exist.

"As in investigations based entirely on behavioral measures, it is likely that there are both general and specific neural influences on behavioral slowing. The reduction in volume of both gray and white matter occur throughout the brain, as well as age-related increases in cerebrovascular lesions, potentially contribute to age-related slowing independently of specific task demands. These general changes may lead to the compensatory recruitment of specific neural regions." (Madden, 2001, p. 304)

It is well established that not all older adults experience the same rate of decline within a given system, and in fact some older adults may perform as well as younger adults. Cabeza and colleagues (2002) examined prefrontal cortex activity using PET scans during recall and source memory of recently studied words. The authors separated the groups into a high- and low-performing group based on a composite memory score. Compared with young adults, low-performing older adults recruited neural activity from the same region as young adults (right prefrontal cortex); however, high-performing adults recruited not only from the right prefrontal regions but also from the left prefrontal region. These results suggest that older high-functioning adults can use a compensatory strategy to counter age-related neural decline, whereas low-functioning adults engage the same area as young adults but are not as efficient as young adults.

Provocative results have been reported through the advent of neuroimaging techniques suggesting that adult brains are much more "plastic" (malleable) and more capable than has ever been imagined. Karni and colleagues (1995) investigated motor skill learning in a complex finger sequencing task that required speed and accuracy. Underlying neural activity was assessed using an fMRI of local blood oxygenation level–dependent signals evoked in the primary cortex. The authors found improvement in behavioral measures of speed and accuracy and evidence for adult motor cortex plasticity in level of activation. These changes were retained across several months. These results suggest that older adults can learn new tasks and that plasticity is a life span phenomenon, thus providing a neurobiological rationale to support the concept of "life-long learning" classes and programs for older adults.

Movement Time

The degree to which age-related slowing occurs with movement depends on task parameters. Highly complex movements are performed more slowly than simple movements, and MT is affected to a greater extent compared with RT when a complex movement is initiated by a simple decision. Conversely, when simple movements are initiated by a complex stimulus array, more age differences are seen in reaction time. The greatest effects occur in the cumulative condition, where the decision process is complicated and the movement to be made is complex.

Fast Repetitive Movements

Making repetitive movements as quickly as possible exaggerates age differences in movement speed. Almost all investigators who have studied repetitive

measures have found large age differences. A common laboratory measurement of repetitive movements is tapping speed, in which the subject taps a finger or a pencil-like stylus in one place as many times as possible within a specified period of time, usually 10 or 15 s. The stationary tapping test involves only the activation and control of the appropriate muscles with minimal monitoring required. Because the task requires only that the individual repeat the process of starting and terminating a movement as rapidly as possible, repetitive tapping is thought to measure motor processing speed, which in turn provides an estimate of motor outflow integrity. This assumption is based on the premise that tapping the finger or a pencil-like stylus for such a short period of time requires almost no muscle strength, endurance, flexibility, or accuracy, so the delimiting factor has to be the speed with which the CNS can issue the repeated start and stop motor command. Stationary tapping is so sensitive to age differences that it has been used frequently in neuropsychological test batteries. Often it represents a so-called pure motor component in psychomotor or perceptual motor test batteries.

Another measure of movement speed is reciprocal (target) tapping; the subject moves the finger or stylus from one target to another as rapidly as possible within a specified period of time. This type of task requires not only initiating and terminating movements but also, depending on the accuracy requirements (size of targets and distance between targets), the monitoring of movements. The speed with which reciprocal target tapping is accomplished as a function of the relationship between speed and accuracy in an aiming action is expressed by Fitts' law:

$$MT = a + b[\log 2(2A/W)],$$

where MT = movement time, a = the movement speed that would occur in a movement of zero accuracy (as in repetitive tapping), and b = the added time to move caused by increasing the index of difficulty of the movement slope. The index of difficulty is defined as $\log 2(2A/W)$ for one unit, where A = the amplitude of the target (distance between targets) and W = the width of the target (Fitts, 1954). Fitts' law applies to older adults as well as young, except that adding the components of age and gender to the equation slightly improves the prediction of MT for older people (Vercruyssen, 1991). The slope of the Fitts' law equation increases with aging, implying that as individuals age they take a disproportionately longer amount of time on difficult rapid hand-movement tasks (Brogmus, 1991). This topic will be discussed in greater detail in chapter 8 (see "Aiming Movements" on page 184).

Functional Significance of Behavioral Speed

Age-related changes in behavioral speed have great significance for the elderly both in slowing of reactions and mental functions and in the execution of movements. The effects that slow reactions and movements have on activities of daily living such as grooming, eating, and home management chores were mentioned at the beginning of this chapter, as were the detrimental effects of slowing of behavioral speed on automobile driving or crossing the street in the limited amount of time provided by some traffic lights. These effects, in combination with the age-related changes in coordination that occur, are so important that they are discussed in much greater detail in chapter 8. But behavioral speed is also significant to researchers who study cognitive processing in the elderly because measures of speed tend to share about 75% of the age-related variance with other cognitive variables (Salthouse, 2000).

Because RT serves as a behavioral window through which the integrity of the CNS may be assessed, it has also been used to identify possible pathological conditions. For example, a slow SRT recorded in an experimental protocol in which the regularity of the preparatory interval is manipulated has long been recognized as being associated with schizophrenic disorders. Similar to unimpaired individuals, schizophrenics benefit from short regular preparatory intervals (<2 s); however, they fail to take advantage of information from regular stimulus intervals that are greater than 4 s in length. In fact, the reaction times are lengthened more than if the stimulus intervals are irregular. This characteristic of schizophrenics is known as the crossover phenomenon.

Reaction time also has been used as an indicator of dysfunction to differentiate normal aging from path-
ological conditions. Another example of the use of RT to identify cognitive impairment is that discrimination RT has correctly identified 86% of senile patients from controls in one study (Ferris et al., 1976). Also, CRT is sensitive to mild stages of Alzheimer's disease and deteriorates with the progression of the disease (Pirozzolo & Hansch, 1981). Within-age comparisons reveal that the generalized slowing seen with aging is accelerated by Alzheimer's disease (Madden et al., 1999; Nebes & Madden, 1988). Kraiuhin and colleagues (1989) examined reaction time and P300 event-related potentials in an effort to determine if the processing modes of Alzheimer's patients were similar to those of normal subjects. The authors found that three of the Alzheimer's patients had an abnormally delayed P300 component, whereas seven had an abnormally delayed RT component.

Selective prolongation (impairment) of SRT was initially thought to be a universal phenomenon for persons with Parkinson's disease. However, a comprehensive review of 16 studies revealed that impairment was not specific to SRT but in some cases was specific to CRT, and in some cases both SRT and CRT and other cases neither SRT or CRT was impaired (Jahanshahi et al., 1993). It seems difficult to generalize with these types of conclusions, but the authors suggest that there is a "tendency" toward impairment in both types of reaction time tasks. In a case study of an individual with Parkinson's disease and frontal complications, SRT was prolonged and in fact CRT was faster than SRT (Henderson et al., 2001).

The results discussed here solidify the increased heterogeneity associated with pathological conditions and draw attention not only to the interaction between aging and pathology but also to various pathologies and complications thereof. This makes generalizations across populations difficult and emphasizes the need to consider the individual.

SUMMARY

Behavioral speed, indicated by age-group means, slows with aging. The correlations of age to reaction time are generally moderate to high. Considering that these correlations occur across several research studies in which the variables are measured differently, and age ranges differ, the magnitude of the correlations is remarkable.

Slowing is functionally significant to individuals, because it affects the way they perform daily functional tasks, such as automobile driving, and increases the risk of accidents. The functional significance of a slowed behavioral speed for many older citizens is
increased accident rates and health insurance rates, age discrimination, job loss in externally paced environments and in professions such as piloting airplanes, and reduced sport participation. However, as emphasized in chapter 2, a very wide degree of individual variation exists in speeded responses at all ages. Some 50-year-olds are considerably faster than many 20-year-olds, so although chronological age is correlated with speed of response, it is a poor indicator of individual response speed. Generally, more complex stimulus displays, less compatible stimulus response pairings, and a greater number

of decisions to be made result in greater differences in RT of young and old persons. Similarly, the more complex the movement to be made, the slower the response of older people. The effects of a complicated stimulus display combined with a complex movement are cumulative and reveal the greatest age differences.

Theories of age-related slowing in response speed fall into two broad categories: those that explain slowing as general or global and those that attribute the slowing process to specific or unique processes. General slowing theorists support the view that all components of processing decline at approximately the same rate, independent of task complexity and task types. Other theorists challenge this view, suggesting that slowing may occur to a greater extent in one component of processing versus another and may influence certain variables more than others. At present, the evidence suggests that adopting an all-or-none position, general or process-specific, when explaining the changes in behavioral speed should be approached with caution.

Another compelling explanation for age-related changes in response speed is based on neurobiological deterioration. New analytic techniques may enable researchers to further define cortical activation as a factor underlying processing speed.

REVIEW QUESTIONS

1. How does aging affect response speed in older adults? What age-sensitive factors affect response speed?
2. Describe how reaction time is measured in the laboratory. What are the general conclusions from these research paradigms?
3. Do all older adults experience similar rates of slowing in their response speed? Explain.
4. List three factors that may influence speed of processing in older adults.
5. Describe conceptually the two major behavioral theories that have been proposed to account for age-related behavioral slowing.
6. Can age-related slowing be explained through neurobiological changes?
7. What is the functional significance of age-related changes in behavioral speed?

SUGGESTED READINGS

Madden, D.J. (2001). Speed and timing of behavioral processes. In J.E. Birren & K.W. Schaie (Eds.), *Handbook of the psychology of aging* (pp. 313-348). New York: Academic Press.

Visi, V., Michalopoulou, G., Tzetzis, G., & Ioumourtzoglou, E. (2001). Effects of a short-term exercise program on motor function and whole body reaction time in the elderly. *Journal of Human Movement Studies, 40,* 145-160.

Wielgos, C.M., & Cunningham, W.R. (1999). Age-related slowing on the digit symbol task: Longitudinal and cross-sectional analyses. *Experimental Aging Research, 25,* 109-120.

Motor Coordination and Control

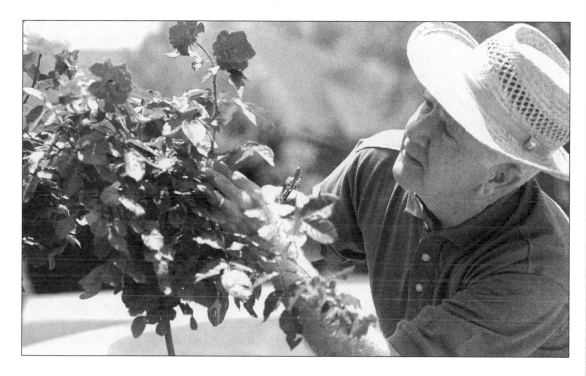

The objectives of this chapter are

- to describe how changes in the sensorimotor system affect basic mechanisms of motor coordination and skill;

- to explain the age-related changes in basic eye-hand coordination movements such as aiming, reaching and grasping, and precision gripping movements;

- to explain the age-related changes in bimanual coordination;

- to describe the extent of age-related changes in functional tasks such as driving an automobile and handwriting;

- to describe the extent to which aging affects the learning of new motor skills, and how neural plasticity occurs with practice;

- to discuss strategies used by older adults to compensate for the sensorimotor losses and declines in coordination and skill; and

- to show how attention, motivation, and anxiety influence coordination and learning.

In previous chapters we have discussed the physical abilities of aerobic capacity, muscular strength and endurance, flexibility, agility, and response speed of older adults. In this chapter we address the effects of age on older people's ability to coordinate muscular activity into useful and functional movements. When people describe others as being "coordinated" or "having a lot of coordination," they really are referring to the person's ability to coordinate the eyes, hands, and feet so that a particular movement can be made to accomplish a goal. Throwing and catching a ball, hitting a golf ball, and bowling are examples of this type of coordination. When a physical task requires primarily the integration of vision and hands to manipulate objects, the task is said to require eye–hand coordination. Eye–hand coordination is defined as the "skillful, integrated use of the eyes, arms, hands, and fingers in fine, precision movement" (Williams, 1983). Sewing, using the computer, slicing a carrot, and turning a knob to change a radio station all have to be learned, and all require eye–hand coordination. In chapter 6, the focus was on coordination and control of the lower extremities to balance and to walk. The majority of information in this chapter concerns upper extremity function, which is important to grasp, reach, and manipulate objects.

Definitions of Coordination, Control, and Learning

Two terms are used, often interchangeably, to describe the skillful execution of movements to accomplish a goal. These terms are **coordination** and **control**. The process of developing smooth and skillful execution of a movement is called **motor learning.**

Coordination

If an activation pattern of muscles is complex, this pattern must be practiced many times before it becomes a skill. Even simple forms of movement such as reaching and grasping must be practiced and learned. More complex forms of movement, such as writing and crocheting, require additional learning and even more complex coordination.

For the purposes of this chapter we will define coordination as "the patterning of body and limb motions relative to the patterning of the environmental objects and events" (Magill, 2001, p. 43). This definition stresses the importance of the relationship between the individual and the context in which the skill is performed. For example, the pattern of our walking movements would be quite different if we were rushing to get to class on time, carrying a hot cup of coffee and a laptop versus heading toward a park bench with the intention of sitting by a pond and watching the ducks.

Coordination of joints and segments can be observed and quantified either within the same limb (intralimb coordination) or between limbs (interlimb coordination). Handwriting is an example of a complex task that requires intralimb coordination of the arm, wrist, and fingers for effective stroke execution, whereas crocheting is an example of an interlimb coordination task that requires the ability to integrate the limbs into a functional movement.

The ability to execute daily tasks with ease is compromised with increasing age. However, the reason for this decline is not clear. Is coordination compromised because of deterioration of the underlying components of movements, such as muscular strength, or because the central nervous system function of sensory integration is impaired?

Motor Control and Motor Learning

Control is the process by which the movement pattern is constrained. Progression toward an optimal solution of a movement problem involves condensing or constraining the available degrees of freedom (represented by muscles and joints) into the smallest number necessary to achieve a goal (Rose, 1997). "**Motor control** is the study of movements and postures and the processes that underlie them" (Rose, 1997, p. 4). Everyday tasks such as eating, dancing, and shopping are expressions of motor control. To determine how movement changes throughout the life span, we must understand how movement is controlled.

When complicated movements, such as throwing balls, shuffling playing cards, tying shoelaces, or typing letters, are first attempted, the result is a jerky, poorly timed movement that requires a substantial amount of energy. However, these complicated physical skills, which require an ongoing integration of visual input and motor output, can become very fluid and reliable as a result of consistent practice and experience. For the purposes of this text, motor learning will be defined as "a change in the capability of a person to perform a skill that must be inferred from a relatively permanent improvement in performance as a result of practice or experience" (Magill, 2001, p. 169).

Even very young children can develop extremely complex eye–hand coordination. Wolfgang Mozart (possibly the greatest child musical prodigy the world has ever known) was said to have been an accomplished pianist by the age of 5, and Tracy Austin had the exquisitely sophisticated eye–hand coordination necessary to win a world championship in tennis by 14 years of age. But what happens to eye–hand coordination as people age? Daily observations of adults' motor skills suggest that these skills that have been so painstakingly developed and maintained over many years begin to deteriorate. The 70-year-old golfer does not make the putts he did in his 30s. The 78-year-old embroidery expert's stitches are not as uniform and tiny as they once were. The 85-year-old finds buttoning a blouse, formerly accomplished without conscious thought, to be a challenging task that requires full attention and considerable energy.

Age-Related Sensorimotor Changes That Affect Coordination and Control

Once a goal has been defined, information is collected from the visual and somatosensory system to define the relationship between the individual and the environment. The visual system contributes information about the location, direction, and speed of movement, whereas the somatosensory system provides information regarding cutaneous contributions and proprioceptive information about changes in pressure, head position, muscle length, tension, and joint position.

Sensorimotor information is critical to performing even simple movements such as picking up a glass of water, putting on a pair of eyeglasses, removing a credit card from a wallet, or filling a tea kettle with water. It is well documented that changes in the visual and somatosensory systems occur with increasing age. However, these systems have a built-in level of plasticity in that the type of information provided by these systems overlaps, providing redundant information. Thus, initial decrements in a system may not be observed until the loss of information is severe enough that redundancy is no longer present. Researchers often use testing paradigms that remove or restrict the use of sensory information to identify deficits in particular types of sensory information. For example, removing or restricting vision as a source of information could be used to determine if underlying changes in somatosensory information are present. If vision is removed or restricted and older partici-

pants perform differentially worse under these conditions, then it might be assumed that somatosensory changes have occurred.

Vision

The visual system is a major contributor to movement, providing information about the environment and the location, direction, and speed of the individual. The vision of most older adults is degraded and provides decreased or distorted information. With aging, people often lose the ability to detect spatial information that would assist in movement control. On average, they need three times more contrast to see some stimuli at slow frequencies (Sekuler et al., 1980), and their depth perception is poorer. They also progressively lose peripheral vision (Manchester et al., 1989). Almost all elderly people use bifocal eyeglasses, which requires the processing of dual information systems, especially for those with extreme corrective lenses. Trying to operate within a dual mode of information processing (i.e., with and without glasses) has the potential to create conflicting peripheral versus central vision information, which could be confusing and maladaptive.

Despite the various changes that occur with age in the visual system, older adults tend to rely more on vision to control movement. Is the increased reliance on vision a result of deterioration in other types of sensory input? Seidler-Dobrin and Stelmach (1998) examined the effects of practice on a discrete aiming task under both normal and obstructed visual conditions in order to determine whether increased visual monitoring during task execution was a result of changes in other types of sensory information. Both young and old subjects found the aiming task to be more difficult when vision was obstructed. Following a period of practice, the young adults learned to restructure their movement by increasing the amount of time spent in the initial ballistic phase of the movement and less time in the secondary phase in which visual feedback is needed to guide the hand to the target. Older adults did not restructure their movement following practice and hence continued to be more reliant on visual input even when it was obstructed. The reason for increased reliance on visual input with age was not clear, but the authors suggested that decrements in other types of information such as cutaneous, muscle, or joint information may play a role.

Somatosensation

The somatosensory system is also critical to movement control and provides information related to body contact and position. It includes cutaneous receptors that provide information about touch and vibration (tactile sensitivity), muscle receptors, and joint receptors that provide information about position of the limbs and body. The vestibular apparatus is also considered a form of proprioceptive input and is discussed in chapter 6.

Cutaneous Contributions

Cutaneous receptors in the skin signal when any mechanical stimulus is applied to the body surface. Thus, when the skin is contacted and changes in pressure on the skin occur, neural impulses are directed centrally. The importance of this information is fully appreciated when one experiences the difficulty of balancing or walking when this information is absent. Normal individuals often experience the loss of these receptors when they sit in one position for a long time, restricting the blood supply to the lower limbs. This causes a temporary loss of the function of cutaneous receptors; the feet and lower legs feel numb, and we say, "my foot has gone to sleep." Clearly, the contact of the skin with the shoes and the changes in pressure that result as the body weight shifts from heel to toe are important sources of information in the maintenance of balance.

Cutaneous sensation decreases with aging. One way to measure cutaneous sensation is to determine how accurately individuals can detect vibration of the skin. In this technique, a vibrator is placed on the skin surface, displacing the skin slightly with each vibration. Persons with a keen sense of vibration can detect very low levels of vibration, but those with less sensory acuity may be able to detect only very fast vibrations. Although the ability to detect cutaneous and vibratory stimuli is greatly influenced by disease and nutrition, it declines significantly with aging (Skinner et al., 1988; Whanger & Wang, 1974). The speed with which vibration information reaches central control centers and the amplitude of this information also decrease. Another test of cutaneous sensitivity that clearly indicates this decline with age is the two-point discrimination test. In this test, the skin is touched lightly with an instrument that has two prongs. The subject's task is to determine whether the prongs are separated or together. If the prongs are far apart, as much as a half an inch, it is very easy to detect the two points of touch. However, as the separation distance of the two prongs decreases, it is more difficult to determine whether the touch is by one or two prongs. The smaller the separation distance that the subject can still detect as two touches, the more sensitive the sense of touch. Older adults cannot detect two points of touch at separation distances as small as

younger individuals can. Thus, sensitivity of touch is compromised with age (Bolton et al., 1966).

Muscle Receptors and Joint Information

Muscle proprioceptors provide information about mechanical displacements of muscles and joints. When muscles are stretched (e.g., the calf muscles when the body leans forward), stretch receptors in the muscle signal the change in muscle length to central mechanisms. Reflexively, the muscle is contracted so that the desired muscle length and tension are obtained. Similarly, when a joint angle is changed, information is provided from muscle and joint receptors. Joint position sense at the knee and ankle is measured either by moving the subject's knee and asking what the new angle of the joint is or by moving the subject's limb to a new position and asking the subject to duplicate that position in the next trial.

The ability of older people to detect motion of their limbs is significantly impaired when these manipulations are done at a slow speed, but when fast rates of joint extension are used, the age differences are minimal (Skinner et al., 1988). Because fast rates of joint extension are required for many dynamic balance needs, these investigators concluded that age-related differences in position sense are not functionally important. Age differences that may exist in the ability to perceive motion of the joints appear only when the extremes of age groups are compared with each other. Thus, joint position sense in the joints of the arms and legs does not markedly decline with aging (Kokmen et al., 1978). A gradual loss of cervical articular mechanoreceptor functions occurs (Wyke, 1979), indicating that perceptions about the position of the neck and head may grow less accurate with aging.

> Visual and somatosensory systems deteriorate with aging, and this affects coordination and control. However, these effects vary drastically across individuals, depending on the rate of aging within and between systems and also on the integrity of the compensatory strategies.

Sensorimotor Integration

In addition to receiving input from individual sensory systems, the central nervous system must integrate input from multiple sensory systems for successful task execution. As previously mentioned, there is redundancy in the sensory systems. Thus, it is possible to have decline in one or more systems and still have the coordination and control that is necessary to perform a task. In chapter 6 we discussed the results from studies that have assessed sensory integration and posture. The findings from these studies reveal that presenting older adults with either conflicting sensory information or removing one or more of the sources of sensory input result in declines in postural stability.

The research that supports the information in this chapter is framed within one of these two theoretical approaches. It is beyond the scope of this chapter to provide a comprehensive discussion of these theories, but both of these theories have contributed significant insights to the understanding of coordination.

Theoretical Strategies to Explain Coordination, Control, and Learning

Two dominant theoretical approaches have been used to describe movement capabilities of older adults: information processing and dynamic systems. Both of these theories have had a valuable impact on the study and understanding of motor behavior.

The **information processing theory** is a multi-stage approach that relies on environmental input into the system. The information is transmitted through a series of stages in a sequential or parallel fashion. Each step is assumed to take a finite amount of time and hence lends itself to temporal measures such as reaction and movement time. This model was the basis of most of the information presented in chapter 7.

In contrast to the information processing approach, **the dynamic system theory** states that movement is not solely attributed to centrally driven commands, but rather movement emerges from the interaction of many body systems. One of the major tenets of this approach is that movement emerges from the interaction of the organism, environment, and task. In addition, behavior is constrained or shaped by these three components. For example, the organismic constraints are properties of the individual, such as the physical characteristics or the emotional state (anxiety); environmental constraints are the physical factors such as gravity, surface area, lighting, and sociocultural factors such as opportunity, access, reinforcement, and acceptance; task constraints include rules or demands of the performance (Clark, 1994). Although this is not a new theoretical approach, the application of this approach to the aging process, particularly upper extremity function, is relatively new.

How Coordination and Control Are Accomplished

Age-related changes in coordination are problems for the elderly. Writing, typing, and sorting papers are important to older adults who wish to continue their employment. The ability to turn the dials of radios and televisions, use a paintbrush, or manipulate a camera is essential for some types of entertainment. In the oldest-old, the ability to dial a telephone,

Motor Coordination Test

Lee Calvert, a subject in a study at Pepperdine University, takes a test designed to assess coordination.

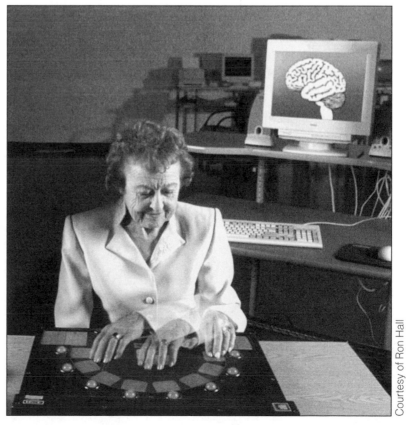

Courtesy of Ron Hall

remove a jar lid, and grasp, carry, and place objects is necessary for independent living.

Psychologists, motor behavior experts, and ergonomics experts who study eye–hand coordination try to use laboratory tasks that simulate daily physical activities. But motor coordination is so complex that most researchers have used a strategy of either studying very simple movements or breaking complex skills into components and studying each component in isolation. Furthermore, to reduce variability, measure more accurately, and place less stress on older subjects, the movements studied have generally been small movements that operate through a small range of motion.

Although many of these studies of coordination and control are analyses of movements that only resemble real-life physical tasks, the studies nevertheless provide valid answers about the components of more complex real-life tasks. This strategy will eventually lead to a better understanding of complex motor skills.

A more direct approach is to study functional skills directly by developing rating scales or timed tests of the ability to use eating utensils, button buttons, cut with scissors, and accomplish other manipulative tasks. Research information on this type of coordination is meager and somewhat unsatisfactory in terms of understanding the mechanisms of age-related changes in coordination. However, there is evidence to suggest that performance of "real-life" skills is related to performance on laboratory tests (Potvin et al., 1980). Potvin and colleagues developed laboratory tests that simulated both functional tasks performed on a daily basis and components of more complex tasks. The top portion of table 8.1 shows that the decline in the ability to coordinate the two hands in several tasks

of daily living increases from a low of 21% in the manipulation of safety pins to a high of 43% in cutting with a knife. In the coordination tests shown in the bottom portion of the table, the decline was least (14%) in the ability to perform interfinger manipulations and greatest (27%) in finger grasping and placing with the right hand. These findings suggest that laboratory tasks, although not direct measures of daily tasks, are indicators of age-related changes in function.

Motor skill performance can be assessed by both performance outcome and performance production (Magill, 2001). **Performance outcome** measures describe the result of the performance: how long it takes an individual to walk up a flight of stairs, or how far an individual can throw a ball. Movement time, the time interval from the initiation to the completion of the movement, is a commonly used outcome measure. Although these measures are useful indications of performance, they do not tell us how a person performed a movement in relationship to spatial and temporal patterning of movement or the forces involved in producing the movement. **Performance production** measures quantify the behavior that produced the outcome. **Kinematics** is the branch of mechanics that describes movement without regard to force or mass. These measures—displacement, velocity, and acceleration—are derived from video analysis of a person performing a movement. **Displacement** is a descriptor of the body moving through space and time; **velocity** is the rate of change in position over the change in time; and **acceleration** is the rate of change of velocity. Examples of displacement, velocity and acceleration of a person using an instrumented pen to move a computer cursor to a computer target as fast as possible are displayed in figure 8.1. **Kinetics**

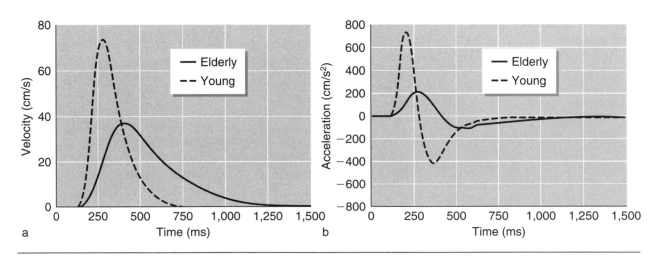

Figure 8.1 (a) Velocity and (b) acceleration profiles of young and older adults.

Reprinted, by permission, from N.L. Goggin and G.E. Stelmach, 1990, Age-related deficits in cognitive-motor skills. In *Aging and cognition: Mental processes, self awareness and interventions*, edited by E.A. Lovelace (New York: Elsevier Science), 146.

Table 8.1 **Reliability and Decline in Function in Coordination and Functional Tasks**

Test name[a]	Reliability coefficient (r)	Decline in function from age 20 to 80 years (%)
Rising from chair with support	.55	31
Putting on shirt	.63	40
Managing large button	.65	27
Managing small button	.70	22
Manipulating safety pins	.47	21
Zipping garment	.54	34
Tying bow	.66	24
Rotating large peg	.78	27
Speed of handwriting	.84	30
Cutting with knife	.62	43

Coordination tests	Units of measure	r	Decline (%)
Finger grasping, placing R[b]	No. pegs/30 s	.88	27
Finger grasping, placing L	No. pegs/30 s	.80	25
Interfinger manipulation R	Rotations/10 s	.84	23
Interfinger manipulation L	Rotations/10 s	.70	14
Lateral finger reach, tapping R	Bits/s	.64	—
Lateral finger reach, tapping L	Bits/s	.56	—
Random arm tracking	Degree · s/s	.51	17
Progressive arm tracking R	Radians/s	.84	15
Progressive arm tracking L	Radians/s	.78	15

[a]For all tests, the measure is tasks completed in 100 s; [b]R denotes right body side, L denotes left body side.

Adapted, by permission, from A.T. Potvin et al., "Human neurologic function and the aging process," *Journal of the American Geriatrics Society* 28: 5.

is the branch of mechanics that explains the cause of motion and is based on Newton's laws of motion. Joint torque is an example of a kinetic measure that describes the forces involved in rotation of body segments about their joint axis. Another performance production measure, electromyography, assesses the electrical activity in the muscle via electrodes.

As noted in chapter 7, age-related slowing in movement speed makes a robust difference in some movement outcomes. It is important, however, to determine whether older adults' movement patterns are different primarily because they are moving more slowly or because aging has actually changed the kinematics of the pattern (coordination). The general rule to follow is that when age group differences exist in the time taken to complete a task, then the dependent measure should be expressed relative to the total time taken to complete the task. However, if no differences exist in the time taken to complete a movement, then absolute timing measures are adequate.

Upper Limb and Hand Control

The majority of information regarding coordination comes from laboratory-developed tasks. Because almost all laboratory tests are unique and unfamiliar to subjects, however, and because older adults especially have more difficulty with unfamiliar environments and task novelty than young people do, most researchers provide ample practice trials for these tasks.

Movements of the upper extremities can be categorized as **unimanual** or **bimanual**. Unimanual tasks require just one limb or hand and the focus is on eye–hand coordination within one side of the body. Bimanual tasks require coordination of both limbs, and the focus is sometimes on the mechanisms by which the brain integrates sensory and motor information between the two sides of the body.

Unimanual Tasks

Two types of unimanual tasks are considered in the following sections: aiming movements and prehension. Factors of interest in aiming movements are the components of the movement and the speed–accuracy trade-off. Prehension, which is the use of the arm and hand to reach out and close the fingers around an object, involves the reach and grasp and the precision grip.

Aiming Movements

A host of coordinated movements that are used every day require not only relatively fast movements but also accurate movements. One way to study accuracy is to analyze the ability of a person to make a discrete movement and reach a small target with the hand or finger or with a hand-held object (e.g., stylus). Fitts' law, a well-known law of movement control, specifies that the more difficult the movement to be made, the slower it is made. That is, movements to hit small targets that are far away from each other take longer to execute than movements to hit larger targets close to each other. An aiming movement is made more difficult by making the target smaller or by increasing the amplitude of the movement (distance to the target; figure 8.2). Thus, the effects of aging on accuracy of fast movements can be analyzed by varying the size of the target, the distance between the targets, or both. End point accuracy is determined by the distance the subjects overshoot or undershoot the target.

The kinematics of the movements are also analyzed. Even when older adults appear to perform the same motor task at the same speed, they may use a different movement pattern to accomplish the task. Many of the age-related changes that have been discussed in previous chapters (e.g., loss of strength, balance, and flexibility) may cause the elderly to move in ways that are subtly different from the movement of young people.

Components of the Movement The movement pattern in a discrete aiming task contains a primary and a secondary submovement. The primary submovement is the initial ballistic portion of movement in which the limb is propelled toward the target. The primary movement is based on central processing, such as specifications of force–time relationships of agonist–antagonist muscle contractions, and is not reliant on sensory feedback. Movements that are predominantly executed in the primary submovement are considered more efficient and often are regarded as a reflection of the efficiency of central processing (Meyer et al., 1988). The primary submovement, however, particularly in complex movements, may not be precise enough to reach the target and a secondary submovement is needed to guide the limb to the target. The secondary submovement involves online processing of sensory feedback regarding the position of the limb with respect to the target, which results in slower movements that are embedded with movement-related error (Von Donkelaar & Franks, 1991).

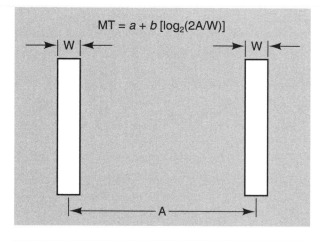

Figure 8.2 The Fitts paradigm. The performer taps a stylus alternately between two targets of width W separated by a distance A. The formula MT = a + b[log2(2A/W)] indicates that if the targets are made smaller (a decrease in W) or the distance is increased between the targets (an increase in A) or both, then the movement becomes slower. The subject must sacrifice speed because the accuracy demands are greater.

Reprinted, by permission, from R.A. Schmidt, 1988, *A behavioral emphasis*, 2nd ed. (Champaign, IL: Human Kinetics), 173.

The greater the accuracy demands in a timed target test, the more aging slows the performance. Different components of the movement are differentially affected, depending on the nature of the task. For example, if the aiming movement is made more difficult by decreasing the size of the target, older adults take more time in the secondary submovement to hone in on the target than in the primary submovement. In fact, the time that they spend in the secondary submovement accounts for 76% of the variance of movement duration for older adults and only 23% in younger adults (figure 8.3; Ketcham et al., 2002). The smaller the target, the greater their time in the secondary submovement. If, on the other hand, the task is made more difficult by increasing the distance to be moved but keeping the targets the same size, older adults take longer to complete the high-amplitude movements and they are less able to

scale peak velocity with increasing movement amplitudes. Thus, the source of slowing in the kinematics of older adults in these simple aiming tasks depends on the task demands.

Overall, older adults are slower, take longer to reach peak velocity, produce shorter primary and longer secondary submovements, and are less smooth in their movements.

Many of these age-related differences in rapid arm aiming movements are also seen in children, which indicates that the ability to control rapid aiming movements changes across the life span. Velocity profiles of four age groups, young children (mean = 6.4 years), older children (mean = 9.2 years), young adults (mean = 24.4 years), and old adults (mean = 73.5 years) are shown in figure 8.4 (Yan et al.,

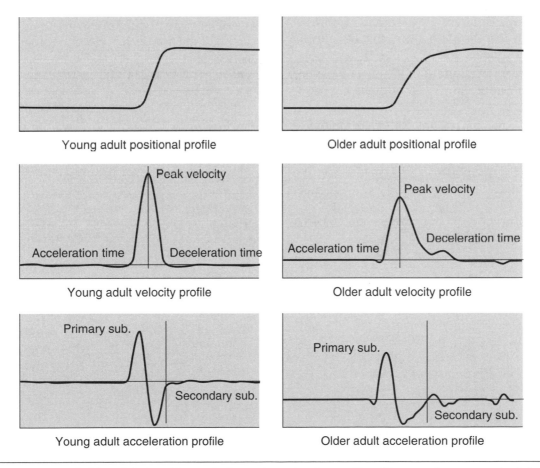

Figure 8.3 Young and older adults' position, velocity, and acceleration profiles. Primary submovement is defined as the time up to the second zero crossing of the acceleration profile, and the secondary submovement encompasses the remaining acceleration and deceleration. Young adult is on the left, older adult is on the right, position is on the top, velocity is in the middle, and acceleration is on the bottom. Vel = velocity; Accel = acceleration; Decel = deceleration; Prim Sub = primary submovement; Sec Sub = secondary submovement.

Journal of Gerontology. Series A, Biological Sciences and Medical Sciences by C.J. Ketchem, R.D. Seidler, A.W.A. Van Gemmert, and G.E. Stelmach. Copyright 2002 by Gerontological Society of America in the format textbook via Copyright Clearance Center..

2000). These profiles were collected under conditions of varying movement complexity (increase in the number of movement components or the accuracy of the movement), response uncertainty (choice reaction time), and availability of precues. The young children and older adults performed similarly, taking longer to reach peak velocity, generating smaller amplitude movements, and varying more in the time to reach peak velocity. In general, older adults and young children exhibited longer movement times and greater movement variation. The smoothness and efficiency of movement of the older adults and younger children were not different from those of the young adults during the response uncertainty or precue conditions. This suggests that older adults and young children program a very small part of the movement in advance, and the majority of movement is monitored online by comparing and adjusting for the difference between the location of the hand and the target. These behavioral similarities between young children and older adults, however, do not imply that the mechanisms that underlie the behavior are similar.

Speed–Accuracy Trade-Off When a task requires both speed and accuracy, individuals choose to emphasize one or the other. The speed–accuracy trade-off is a phenomenon commonly observed in tasks that require both speed and accuracy. If an individual chooses to emphasize accuracy, speed is reduced, and if an individual chooses speed, accuracy is reduced. Older adults typically choose to emphasize accuracy over speed. When older adults execute a fast aiming movement, the smaller the target the slower they move. Young adults do that too, but they do not slow their movements as much as older adults. In six different combinations where the movement distance and the target width were manipulated, older adults were slower but made fewer errors than young adults (Goggin & Meeuwsen, 1992). The older adults produced lower peak velocity and acceleration, required a longer time to reach peak velocity and acceleration, and spent a longer amount of time decelerating.

Why are older adults slower and more accurate than younger adults? Morgan and colleagues (1994) used a clever research design to determine whether slower more accurate movements could be attributed to differences in strategy or declines in central and peripheral mechanisms. They asked, If older adults are pushed, can they move at a faster speed in an aiming task with the same degree of accuracy as younger adults? If they can, then the observed slowing may just be their choice or strategy; however, if errors increase when they are forced to move at a higher speed, then the slowing may be attributable to deterioration of central and peripheral processes. Both groups executed the task at a fast speed (mean of the young group's preferred time) and slow speed (mean of the older group's preferred time). Behaviorally, the older adults were able to move at the same speed as young adults and were just as accurate. However, a closer analysis of the kinematic structure of the movement revealed that at higher

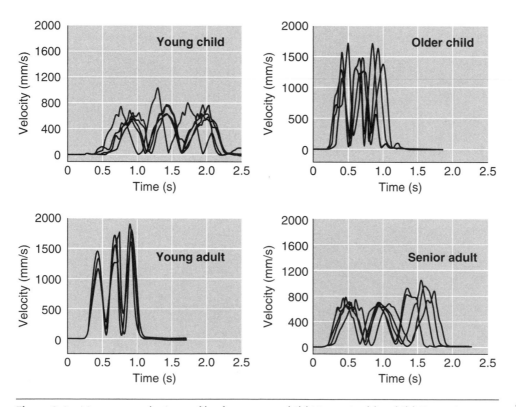

Figure 8.4 Movement velocity profiles for a young child (6 years), older child (9 years), young adult (24 years), and older adult (74 years).

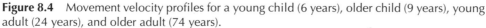

Journal of Motor Behavior, 32: 126, 2000. Reprinted with permission of the Helen Dwight Reid Educational Foundation. Published by Heldref Publication, 1319 Eighteenth St., NW, Washington, DC 20036-1802. Copyright © 2000.

speeds, older adults required more submovements to reach the target, particularly small targets, compared with young adults. In addition, the older group had longer pauses between movements at both movement speeds. Thus, age-related slowing in an aiming task is not solely attributed to a preference for accuracy but probably reflects declines in the central and peripheral systems.

In aiming tasks, older adults, when compared with young adults, produced lower peak velocity and acceleration, required a longer time to reach peak velocity and acceleration, and spent a longer amount of time decelerating.

Prehension

The literature on aiming movements provides a basic foundation for understanding age differences in the control of limb movements, but aiming is just one component of many functional movements, such as picking up a glass of water, brushing teeth, and eating. Other basic components of functional movements are reaching, grasping, and transporting objects.

Reach and Grasp Reach, grasp, and transport research protocols require subjects to initiate a movement and grasp small or large objects (e.g., Bennett & Castiello, 1994). Small objects are grasped (naturally) by all subjects with a precision grip (index finger and thumb) and larger objects with a whole hand grasp. The subjects can perform these tasks at their preferred (natural) speed or at their maximum speed. The kinematics of movement position, acceleration, velocity, and deceleration are analyzed throughout the movement pattern as the subject initiates the movement, accelerates the limb, reaches peak velocity in approaching the target, begins to decelerate as the limb draws close to the target, and then closes the hand on the object. The kinematics of the lift and transport of the object from one place to another is also analyzed (Weir et al., 1998).

At *preferred* speeds, older adults reach, grasp, and transport objects in a similar manner, with about the same relative timing (Bennett & Castillo, 1994). That is, if they are asked to pick up different types of objects at their own speed, they select the same types of movements and carry them out with about the same timing characteristics as young adults. Under these conditions, accuracy is the same for young and old adults. However, old adults accelerate their limbs less rapidly and the overall movement speed is slower than that of young adults. The velocity differences are amplified if the grasping requires precision, such as in a precision pinch. Older adults spend more time in the deceleration phase of the reaching movement

because they are using feedback to guide the reach and the processes of receiving, interpreting, and correcting the movement (Weir et al., 1998). Their hand-closing times (on the object) are slower, and they are more variable in their performance. If maximum speed is a requirement to complete the task, these age differences are exaggerated.

In reaching, grasping, and transporting objects, older adults

- are similar in the type, accuracy, and relative timing of the movement components at preferred speeds;
- accelerate the movement more slowly;
- spend a higher percentage of time in the deceleration phase;
- spend more time in hand-closing as they grasp the object;
- transport objects more slowly;
- are differentially slower the higher the accuracy demands of the task; and
- display these differences even more when the task requires maximum speed.

Precision Grip The ability to control fingertip forces is necessary to execute many daily tasks. For example, fastening buttons, taking change out of a purse, picking coins up off a table, and sewing require the modulation of fingertip forces for efficient force control. These common tasks, done so subconsciously and easily in youth, become a struggle in old age. Eventually many of them become insurmountable, and the inability to perform these tasks may lead to loss of independence and hence reduced quality of life.

What mechanisms underlie the age-related decline in fingertip force control? In chapter 5 we discussed one possibility, the loss of absolute strength. However, very few daily tasks that require manipulation of fingertip forces require maximum strength output. A second mechanism discussed in chapter 7 is the loss of behavioral speed that occurs with increasing age. Both of these mechanisms may contribute to age-related changes in manual dexterity, particularly behavioral speed. In the first part of the following section we will discuss a typical paradigm used to assess fingertip force control and describe the results of several behavioral studies suggesting that other mechanisms may contribute to observed impairments in manual function.

Several researchers (Cole & Rotella, 2002; Cole et al., 1999; Lowe, 2001) performed well-controlled experiments designed to investigate the loss of fingertip force control and to determine the potential mechanisms underlying these changes. They used a "grip and lift" paradigm in which subjects grip an object between their thumb and index finger (or any other combination of fingers) and lift it to a predetermined height (figure 8.5).

Older adults apply grip forces that are twice those of younger adults, and older adults modulate their grip and lift forces less smoothly (Cole, 1991; Kinoshita & Francis, 1996). Excessive grip force is thought to be a compensatory strategy used to counteract age-related compromises to underlying

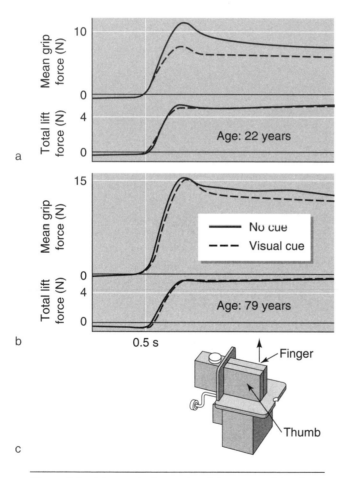

a

b

c

Figure 8.5 Mean grip force signal (average of the force normal to the gripped surfaces) and total lift force signal (sum of the vertical tangential force at each surface) from a 22-year-old subject (a) and a 79-year-old subject (b). Each trace is the mean of 10 lifts, aligned at the onset of gripping. The trials comprising each mean were for lifts of the object with sandpaper grip surfaces that were preceded by a lift with the acetate gripping surfaces. (c) The test object: Gripped surfaces (black) are indicated for the thumb and finger of a right-handed subject.

Reprinted, by permission, from K.J. Cole and D.L. Rotella, 2002, "Old age impairs the use of arbitrary visual cues for predictive control of fingertip forces during grasp," *Experimental Brain Research* 143: 35-41. Copyright 1988 Springer-Verlag.

mechanisms essential for fingertip force control. These changes could be attributable to degradation of tactile sensitivity or skin properties. It is likely that increasing skin slipperiness explains excessive grip force in adults younger than 60 years, and further decline may be attributable to the capacity of the encoding capabilities of a select group of cutaneous mechanoreceptors (Cole et al., 1999). However, in a grip, lift, and place task in which the subjects had to rely only on their tactile sensitivity (no vision), the older subjects performed as well as the young subjects. These results suggest that the observed behavioral changes are task-specific. It is possible, however, that the observed differences could be partially attributed to the researchers' subject pool. For example, Lowe (2001) found no age differences in grip force control, using a similar paradigm. Her participants were part of subject pool that was rigorously screened for visuomotor deficits and neurological function. In addition, several of the participants were involved in a resistance training program. Lowe's subjects may have been healthier, had stronger hands and fingers, or had more experience producing grip and finger forces than subjects in other studies who do not have to go through a rigorous screening or enroll in a training program.

Older adults also have more difficulty coordinating the thumb and index finger forces independently on an instrument with two spring levers in which the thumb force moved a cursor on a computer screen horizontally and the index finger force moved the cursor vertically (Spirduso & Choi, 1993). The task was to coordinate the force input and output of the thumb and finger so that the cursor would travel along a 45° diagonal line. Both time and errors were measured. The older adults were differentially less accurate in controlling the force of the index finger and thumb independently. In particular, the older adults had more difficulty in controlling the release of force than they did in controlling the application of force.

Bimanual Coordination

Bimanual movements can be simple, as in lifting a box with both hands and placing it on a shelf or complex as in knitting, dealing cards, or playing the piano. These tasks all share the requirement that the two hands and arms must operate together, coordinating their movements so that the goals of the task are achieved. But knitting or playing the piano are very complex and difficult to analyze, and so more quantifiable and controllable laboratory tasks have been devised to study the effects of aging on biman-

Studying Force Control of the Fingers in a Pinch Grip

An excellent example of a research study of grip force control was that by Cole and colleagues (1999), who studied differences in fingertip force control in four groups whose average age was 33, 54, 66, and 77. The subjects lifted an object, held it at a predetermined height for approximately 4 s, and returned it to the table. The friction or slipperiness (sandpaper, acetate) and weight (2 or 4 N) of the object were varied. To determine "slip force," the subjects were instructed to lift the object to a predetermined position and then to release the force applied by the thumb and index finger to allow the object to slip from their grasp (estimated slip force). The results of this experiment confirmed earlier reports of age-related increases in grip force in that the three older groups used relative safety margins (grip force that exceeds the minimum force needed to prevent an object from slipping) that were twice those of the young group.

To determine whether tactile impairments might explain these excessive grip forces in older adults, Cole and colleagues (1998) set up an experiment in which the subjects had to rely only on their tactile sensitivity. The authors removed vision in one condition by blindfolding their subjects, reasoning that if age-related changes in the ability to control fingertip force are attributable to changes in tactile sensitivity, then removing visual information should result in a disproportionate impairment in the older group. Subjects gripped (thumb and index finger), lifted, and transported a metal sphere to a receptacle as quickly as they could. The duration for both the grasp and transport component was compared both with and without vision (blindfolded) in young and older adults. The older group was slower in both phases of the task regardless of the visual condition. In the no-vision condition, it took both groups twice as long to complete each phase. However, older adults were not disproportionately slower in the no-vision condition. Therefore, mechanisms other than tactile sensitivity must be responsible for the age differences in performance in this particular grip, lift, and transport task.

---

ual coordination. Thus, much of the research on age-related changes in upper extremity performance has been limited to unimanual or single-joint movements.

One way to analyze bimanual coordination is to measure the time required to initiate and terminate movements of both hands simultaneously in a discrete movement, bimanual reaction time task. If subjects place each index finger on a home key and then, with each hand, initiate a response to a target key that is displaced a specified distance from the home keys, a bilateral reaction time is obtained for each hand. If both hands leave the home keys at the same time, then it is assumed that they have been programmed together as one unit of movement. If the two hands land simultaneously on their respective targets, then subjects have controlled execution of the two arms' movements as one movement. By measuring the reaction and movement time of both hands, researchers can determine the degree of bimanual coordination between the two hands. When young people are asked to use both hands to leave a home key and contact a target key, they tend to "yoke" the hands together. That is, they program the two hands together into one movement. If the movements are asymmetrical (one hand has to move 6 in. while the other hand moves 18 in.), these subjects still yoke the movements together even though the hand that only has to move 6 in. theoretically could arrive much sooner on its target than the hand that has to travel 18 in. However, the hands tend to compensate. The hand that moves a short distance slows down as if to wait for the hand that travels a longer distance. They arrive on the two targets almost simultaneously, even though the subjects have not been instructed to do so.

Do older people maintain the ability to initiate and terminate their movements simultaneously in complex tasks requiring bimanual coordination? If older adults lose the ability to coordinate their limbs in a coupled fashion, then simple daily tasks such as picking up a large vase from a table would be a challenge. Imagine trying to pick up a large vase when one of your hands starts the action before the other hand. Further imagine that one hand terminates the action before the other. In both cases the movement would probably result in a broken vase. The answer to this question is not completely clear. In one study, older subjects (aged 67-75) did not initiate bimanual movements as simultaneously as younger subjects (aged 21-25) and were not able to compensate during the movement. The result was an asynchronous termination of the movements (Stelmach et al., 1988a). The researchers suggested that as people age, they prepare short movements less well than they prepare long movements, whereas young people prepare long and short movements in the same way. In another study, however, the bimanual coordination of two groups of healthy older adults (average age 66.5 and 78.1 years) was not different from that of younger subjects (19.7 years), but the older adults took longer overall to complete the movement (Rothstein et al., 1989).

Another way to examine age-related differences in coordination is to determine the stability of movement patterns. Researchers who view motor control from a **dynamic systems perspective** have suggested that natural tendencies exist in our movement patterns (Wishart et al., 2002). These preferred and stable modes of coordination are referred to as in-phase (symmetrical) movements when limb movement results from simultaneous activation of homologous muscle groups and antiphase (asymmetrical) movements when limb movement occurs from simultaneous contraction of nonhomologous muscle groups. An example of an in-phase pattern of movement would be to extend or flex the elbow joint simultaneously, whereas an antiphase pattern of coordination would be to flex one elbow joint while extending the other. An illustration of a laboratory in-phase, antiphase, and 90° bimanual coordination

task is shown in figure 8.6. A measure commonly used to reflect coordination at the behavioral level is **relative phase.** This measure reflects the difference in phase between the limbs. The relative phase of an in-phase pattern is 0°; the relative phase of an antiphase pattern is 180°. The difference between the intended goal, 0° or 180°, and the produced pattern provides a measure of temporal coordination accuracy. The standard deviation (variability) of these scores provides a measure of the stability of the pattern.

Older adults retain the ability to perform both in-phase and antiphase patterns of movement at their preferred speed with the same relative degree of accuracy and consistency as their younger counterparts (Greene & Williams, 1996; Wishardt, 2001). However, if temporal demands are placed on the system that exceed those of the preferred speed, age-related differences emerge. In these bimanual tasks, older adults' preferred speed is sometimes 35% slower and their maximum speed 40% slower (Greene & Williams, 1996). In Greene and Williams' study, the difference between the preferred speed and the maximum speed was also greater in the young group (1.9 Hz) than in the older group (1.0 Hz). Despite the age differences in speed, the right and left hands of both groups performed the same way, suggesting

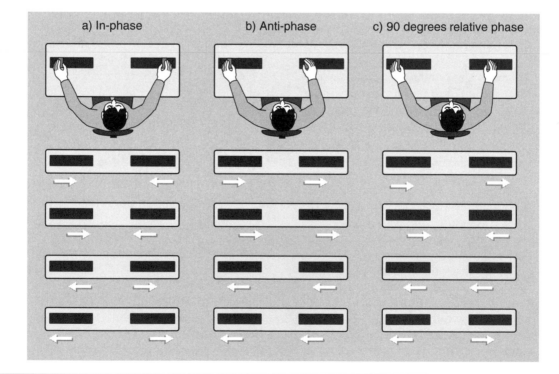

Figure 8.6   Bimanual coordination patterns. An in-phase or symmetrical pattern *(a)*, an antiphase or asymmetrical pattern *(b)*, and a 90° relative phase pattern in which one limb follows the other a quarter of the way through the cycle *(c)*.

Reprinted, by permission, from L.R. Wishart et al., 2002, "Age-related differences and the role of augmented visual feedback in learning a bimanual coordination pattern," *Acta Psychologica* 110: 247-263.

that the hands were temporally coupled. To control for the effect of speed differences, Green and Williams (1996) used a measure of relative speed so that both groups were compared at different speeds relative to their maximum. The goal was to maintain an antiphase pattern of movement as the speed was increased from 80% to 120% of the individuals' maximum speed. Older adults shifted from an antiphase to an in-phase pattern of movement at a lower speed compared with the young adults. The antiphase pattern of older adults' movement became less stable as the movement speed increased, which could explain the earlier shift to a more stable in-phase pattern. Age differences were minimal for the in-phase pattern of coordination, suggesting that this is a more stable pattern of coordination for both groups.

In general, older adults require more time to change modes of coordination, regardless of whether the transition is from in-phase to antiphase or antiphase to in-phase, compared with young adults (Greene & Williams, 1996). In addition, older adults take a differentially longer time to switch from an in-phase to an antiphase pattern of movement compared with antiphase to in-phase. These results suggest that it is more difficult for older adults to switch to a less stable mode of coordination, particularly when they are operating in a stable and hence efficient mode of coordination.

Older adults seem to have more difficulty with asymmetrical movements than symmetrical movements. In general, the oldest-old experience greater spatial decoupling between the hands. Fortunately, many daily tasks that require coordinating two or more movements at once are so well learned and practiced that they are controlled subconsciously. These tasks include clerical typing, cutting with a knife, using a fork, dialing a telephone, picking up coins, inserting a coin into a vending machine slot, squeezing toothpaste and placing it on a toothbrush, unwrapping a Band-Aid, and zipping a skirt or slacks. Other functions that may be more recreational, such as dealing cards, knitting, crocheting, or playing the piano, also require complex coordination but are carried out at an almost subconscious level. Yet, aging presents some difficulties in the coordination of these tasks for some individuals.

Older adults

- prepare short movements less well than long movements,
- terminate bimanual tasks more asynchronously,
- move more slowly,

- can maintain stability in bimanual performance at preferred speeds but not at higher movement speeds,
- have less difference between their preferred and maximum speeds,
- have greater difficulty shifting from preferred to new bimanual coordination patterns, and
- take longer to switch from in-phase to antiphase patterns.

Multilimb Coordination

Can older adults control multijoint movements as proficiently as single-joint movements? Seidler and colleagues (2002) studied age-related differences in the ability to perform multijoint movements. The task required the subjects to point to one of four predetermined target locations: Target 1 required elbow extension only (single-joint movement) and Targets 2 through 4 required elbow extension and increasing contribution of shoulder flexion to reach the target (multijoint movements). Older subjects' movements were less smooth and accurate than those of young adults. In addition, these performance differences were exacerbated in multijoint movements. Older subjects also had higher coactivation levels in the single-joint task; however, the level of coactivation was reduced for multijoint movements (figure 8.7). The authors suggested that younger adults may be using coactivation as a strategy to gain control when the task is more complex. The older adults did not appear to do that.

Aging Effects on Two Important Functional Tasks: Driving and Handwriting

Although functional tasks are much harder to quantify, driving vehicles and handwriting have attracted considerable research interest because they are important to maintaining normal lives for most people.

Automobile Driving

Driving an automobile is a psychomotor skill that is learned by almost all adults in the United States and executed daily by a great many people throughout the world. It is a skill that most adolescents passionately desire to learn and that almost all aging adults dread

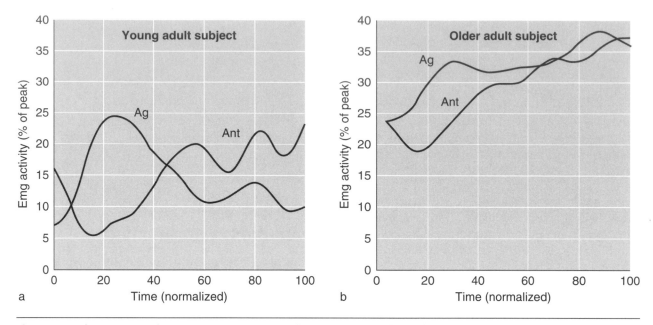

Figure 8.7 Electromyographic (EMG) activity expressed as a percentage of peak for a young and older subject. AG = agonist; ANT = antagonist. The older adult demonstrates a different activation pattern (greater coactivation) than the young.

Reprinted, by permission, from R.D. Seidler-Dobrin, J. He, and G.E. Stelmach, 1998, "Coactivation to reduce variability in the elderly," *Motor Control* 2(4): 323.

to lose for the same reason—because it affords independence, personal freedom, status, mobility, and self-esteem. Nevertheless, a time eventually arrives when the question has to be raised: Are the perceptual motor skills and judgment of an individual adequate to drive an automobile safely (Persson, 1993; Walser, 1991)? The question of safety is an important one, because it has been estimated that by the year 2030, more than 20.7% of the population will be over age 65 (Donatelle et al., 1991).

Aging Effects on Physical and Behavioral Attributes Necessary for Driving

Driving an automobile requires vision and eye–hand–foot coordination to execute the correct sequencing of accelerator, brake, and steering wheel. Vision is extremely important in driving (table 8.2). An estimated 90% of the information used in driving a car is visual (Kline et al., 1992). The visual functions important to driving (from the most to the least important) are dynamic acuity, **saccadic fixation** (the ballistic movement of the eyeball that directs the eye to a target of interest), acuity, size of the useful visual field, detection of motion in depth, and detection of angular motion (Henderson & Burg, 1974). The visual functions important to driving that decline with increasing age are visual acuity, size of useful visual field, and changes in motion perception (Klavora & Heslegrave, 2002). According to Owsley and colleagues (1998), glaucoma and changes in the useful field of view are

significant risk factors for accidents. A recent report from The Blue Mountain Eye Study found that 51% of the individuals more than 70 years of age stopped driving because of visual problems (Gilhotra et al., 2001). Specific visual factors associated with driving cessation were visual acuity, difficulty seeing in the dark, sensitivity to glare, and glaucoma. Other factors included chronic disease such as stroke, cardiovascular disease, diabetes, self-rated health, severe hearing problems, and use of benzodiazepines.

Driving a vehicle is a psychomotor skill because it requires perceptual acuity, vigilance, short- and long-term memory, and motor programming. All of these functions decline with age. Particularly important in driving is the ability to attend selectively to specific task-relevant stimuli. Selective attention, which is related to driving performance in any vehicle, deteriorates with aging. Yet for successful driving, attention must be continuously allocated to different areas of a very complex visual field. Thus, driving requires the ability to divide attention between the perceptual–motor task of manipulating the controls of the vehicle and the active visual search for information in unpredictable locations. The ability to divide attention (Ponds et al., 1988) and visually search (Plude & Hoyer, 1985) is impaired in many adults over age 60.

Driving situations often require the ability to attend to several tasks simultaneously. Understanding the age-related changes in divided attention is important in understanding the difficulty older

On the Record . . . Traffic Fatalities of Older Adults

Motor vehicle crash rates are higher per mile driven for older drivers, particularly for those over 75 years of age (Retchin & Anapolle, 1993). Data from the National Highway Traffic Safety Administration (2001) show that the number of older adult licensed drivers has increased 39% since 1989 (from 11.5 to 18.5 million; figure 8.8). Fatality rates (fatalities per annual miles driven) are highest for young adults (age 16) and older adults (ages 85+).

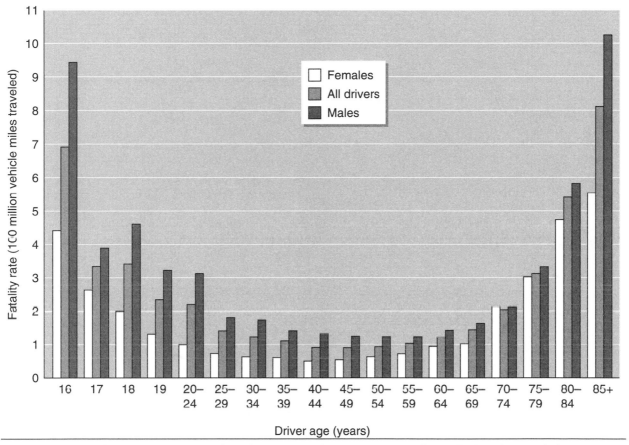

Figure 8.8 Driver fatality rates by age and gender, 1996. Fatality rate per 100 million vehicle miles traveled.

Data from National Center for Statistics.

adults have with particularly complex situations such as making a left-hand turn. Brouwer and colleagues (1991) investigated the ability of young and old drivers to perform a simultaneous task of lane tracking and visual analysis at the same time. The lane-tracking task required the subjects to stay in the right lane despite perturbations simulating wind. At the same time they were required to respond to the appearance of dots on the screen by either pressing a button indicating whether the number of the dots were equivalent to 9 or by saying yes or no. Older adults were differentially worse than younger adults when they performed the lane-tracking and dot-counting tasks simultaneously.

As people age they become more field dependent, which means they are less likely to detect signs and symbols in the "background" field of vision while driving (Panek et al., 1978). Old drivers tend to neglect some of the information from road signs, traffic lights, and traffic, particularly if it is overwhelming (McFarland et al., 1964). It has been fairly well established that it is not a loss of muscular strength or simple reaction time that causes old people to have accidents, but rather the slowness with which they make decisions and their inability to rapidly discriminate relevant information from irrelevant information (Birren, 1974).

Table 8.2 Age-Related Declines in Visual Functions That Relate to Driving Problems for the Elderly

Visual difficulties	Driving outcomes

Reading signs in time to turn
  Visual processing speed
  Dynamic vision
  Near vision
  Visual search
	Failing to heed signs

Self-report
  Difficulty judging one's own speed
  Surprised by other vehicles when merging
  Other vehicles appearing unexpectedly in peripheral vision
  Believe other vehicles are moving too quickly
	Failing to yield right-of-way
	Failing to turn appropriately

Laboratory test results
  Shrinking of visual field
  Estimating velocity
  Visual search for peripheral targets
	Failing to yield right-of-way
	Failing to turn appropriately

Reduction of useful field of view	Failing to respond to information from many different sources

Decline in
  Retinal illumination
  Acuity in low illumination
  Accommodation reserve
  Resistance to glare
	Difficulty seeing instrument panel at night
	Haze and sun glare on windshield

Binocular field losses	Higher rate of accidents

Data from Kline et al. (1992).

Differences in perceptual style, selective attention, and the time it takes to make complex decisions affect aging drivers in particular ways. A driver must scan the environment, retain in memory what was seen at the beginning of the scan, determine relevant information, and make a decision. Older drivers may take a long time to interpret traffic conditions. By the time they look one way and then determine what is happening in the other direction, the information from the first observation will no longer be valid. Because the decisions take longer, corrections also take longer. Older people are more easily distracted by irrelevant information, shifting their attention from one object in the visual field to another, thus making poor decisions. Moreover, their ability to estimate vehicle velocity is less efficient (Cremer et al., 1990; Scialfa et al., 1991).

Driving a vehicle requires perceptual acuity, vigilance, short- and long-term memory, motor programming, and attention (selected and divided), all of which decline with age.

Compensatory Changes in Behaviors of Older Drivers

In light of all these age-related deficits that affect driving, we might predict that older drivers in general must be involved in many more accidents than younger drivers. Exactly the opposite is true, however, for drivers under the age of 70. In terms of traffic fatalities, the driving record of adults between the ages of 40 and 65 is the safest record of any age. Senior drivers are the least likely citizens to be involved in traffic accidents, whereas teenage drivers are the most likely. Moreover, if the major automobile crash statistics are examined, the evidence is overwhelming that far more 20-year-old males are involved in traffic fatalities than either males or females over 60 years old. Figure 8.8 (p 193) shows that adults between the ages of 35 and 65 are involved in relatively few traffic fatalities. Furthermore, the probability of dying in a traffic accident is at least 10 times higher for 20-year-old men than for either males or females between the

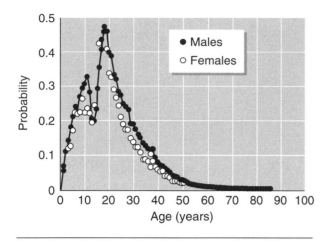

Figure 8.9 The probability of death attributable to a motor vehicle crash. From FARS (1983-1985) and National Center for Health Statistics (1984).

Reprinted, by permission, from L. Evans, 1988, "Older driver involvement in fatal and severe traffic crashes," *Journal of Gerontology: Social Science* 43: 190.

ages of 50 and 80 (figure 8.9) (Evans, 1988). Twenty-year-olds are also involved in many more pedestrian fatalities, so older individuals between the ages of 50 and 70 apparently pose no more significant risk to the health and safety of pedestrians than drivers of other ages.

What is the explanation? If so many sensory-motor functions critical to driving are compromised with aging, why is the driving record of older adults so much better than that of young adults? A major reason is that they drive substantially less than younger adults. For example, male drivers over the age of 70 travel about 5,775 miles (9,293 km) a year, compared with 19,251 miles (30,981 km) a year for 35- to 39-year-old drivers (Evans, 1988). Thus, younger men drive distances that are more than three times those driven by older drivers every year. The driving fatalities shown in figure 8.8 accounted for travel distance, and yet younger drivers still were involved in a greater number of traffic fatalities than were older adults. If the average distance driven is not taken into account, the number of driver fatalities of 20-year-olds is almost five times higher than that of 70-year-olds. Another interesting phenomenon is that females between the ages of 15 and 18 have as many fatal accidents as males of the same age, but between the ages of 18 and 40, they have substantially fewer fatal accidents than males. At age 50 and older, no gender differences are observed.

Other reasons why older drivers between the ages of 50 and 80 have a better safety record than young males is that they take advantage of their experience and wisdom to take fewer risks when they drive, and they also trade off speed for accuracy to compensate

for declining psychomotor abilities. The speed–accuracy trade-off phenomenon that is exhibited by elderly persons was discussed in chapter 8. Older individuals drive more slowly to compensate for slower reaction time and visual problems. They avoid driving at night so that their deficit in dark adaptation is not a factor. They avoid driving in bad weather and driving while intoxicated, and they generally drive with more caution. In addition, older adults tend to travel during less frequently traveled times and avoid highway driving (Tasca, 1992). These compensatory strategies result in many older persons being safer drivers than many young people. The incorporation of these strategies is also why psychomotor measures, psychological tests, and personality tests alone cannot predict the probability of an individual being in an automobile accident (Barrett et al., 1977).

An Emotional Debate: When to Take Away the Keys?

Compensatory changes in driving behavior cannot compensate forever for the inevitable effects of aging. The driving-related fatalities of adults over age 80 are much higher than all other age groups. At about age 85, older drivers' crash rates are exponentially higher. Also, these older adults are more likely to be involved in more than two vehicle accidents and are four times more likely to be injured or killed (National Highway Traffic Safety Administration, 2000).

Several factors account for an age-related loss of driving competence, including an increase in the number of medical problems and continued loss of visual and perceptual motor abilities in the oldest age categories. Other diseases, such as Parkinson's and osteoarthritis, restrict head and neck movements. Symptoms of epilepsy and other seizure disorders increase in the elderly. Many also suffer lapses of consciousness from cardiovascular disease or microstrokes; some cardiologists recommend against driving up to 7 months after a heart attack or ventricular arrhythmia. Lapses of consciousness can also occur from uncontrolled diabetes and narcolepsy. Many of the oldest-old suffer from fainting spells or dizziness. In addition, visual difficulties may be further exacerbated by diseases such as glaucoma and cataracts. Despite these daunting health problems, most elderly adults cling to their right to drive as ferociously as teenagers harass their parents to let them begin to drive. The reason? In most communities in the United States, driving equals freedom and independence.

Officials in some states have attempted to mandate an age ceiling above which individuals may not drive, or to develop and enforce laws requiring frequent

Pain of Hanging Up the Keys

Ruth watched the charitable organization's tow truck pull her car farther and farther down the road until it became a speck on the horizon. At 88, after more than seven decades of a perfect driving record (almost), she had just made the painful decision she knew she had to make—to quit driving. "I got my first set of wheels, a beat-up old convertible with a rumble seat, when I was 18. What a sense of freedom it brought. That car, and all my ensuing ones, left me with very vivid memories—of taking my daughter to her wedding, of racing my nephew to the hospital after he fell out of a tree. And now, as I watched my car dancing along behind the tow truck, I knew part of me was leaving forever. As the taillight disappeared, I found myself whispering, 'Goodbye, sweet freedom.' It hurt to see it go" (Nedbor, 2003, p. 21).

physical and mental examinations for older individuals. Legal requirements such as these are extremely difficult to pass, however, because they evoke issues of age discrimination, lessened mobility, social isolation, and possible loss of job and income. Very few states even have laws requiring regular vision testing after a specific age. Almost none require physical examinations, yet Nelson and colleagues (1992) showed that if visual testing is mandated for renewal of a driver's license, the number of fatal crashes involving older drivers is significantly reduced. Underwood (1992) recommended that physicians assume some responsibility for screening older citizens to assess their driving ability and counseling them in terms of safety procedures. His recommendations, some of which could be implemented effectively if state legislative bodies would provide legal support, are shown in table 8.3. He also suggests that physicians support and work with the families of extremely old adults who refuse to quit driving voluntarily to assist them in making the hard decision to take away the keys.

Some civic leaders, in an effort to avoid age discrimination laws, have recommended innovative changes in the driving environment, the adoption of technological aids for older drivers, and educational programs for those who may have difficulty passing a driving test. For example, the driving environment can be improved for the elderly by using larger highway signs, designing intersections for safer turns, providing better lighting for roads, painting wider stripes on the road shoulders, and using icons rather than text for road signs. Staplin and Fisk (1991) found that older adults could improve their left-turn error and decision response time if provided with precues (e.g., posting of a sign to wait for the signal before turning) about the upcoming turn. Automobiles can be made more functional with pivoting seats, a brightly colored dashboard, clear, untinted windshields, and simplified car interiors. Some impressive technology that will be available in the future includes cars with collision warning devices, lane-keeping systems that tug gently at the wheel when the car drifts out of the lane, signals that advise the driver about upcoming turns or road hazards, and navigation systems that suggest a route to the destination and give the driver turn-by-turn instructions (Sheldrick, 1992). Until such advanced technology is on the market, older adults can be encouraged to drive larger cars, wear seatbelts, take annual night vision tests, and use certain compensatory driving behaviors, such as going around the block to avoid left turns and avoiding rush-hour traffic and freeways.

Intervention programs may provide older adults with the opportunity to maintain and enhance their driving ability. However, a limited amount of attention has been allocated to potential intervention programs. Margolis and colleagues (2002) identified several risk factors that were associated with motor vehicle crashes such as fall history (for sedentary individuals who do not walk for exercise), decrease in orthostatic blood pressure, and foot reaction time. It is not known whether intervention programs designed to target these various risk factors actually improve driving ability. One promising intervention approach is useful field of view (UFOV) training. UFOV is defined as the useful visual field out of which relevant information can be extracted. The ability to extract relevant information from the periphery is an essential parameter of driving performance (Sekuler & Bennett, 2000). The extent of the UFOV is reduced with increasing age and was found to be a significant predictor of motor vehicle crashes (Ball et al., 1993). Ball and colleagues (1988) found that following 5 days of training, the UFOV was extended by 133%. This increase persisted across a 6-month period. These results suggest that implementation of intervention programs is an important factor in maintaining the ability to drive.

Handwriting

Handwriting is one of the most important functional continuous movements that all adults must control.

Table 8.3 Recommendations for Office-Based Assessment of Risk of Motor Vehicle Injury in Older Drivers

Driving record
  Past crashes or near-crashes, violations, insurability, getting lost while driving, observations of family and friends
  Use of safety belts
  Driving habits
  Importance of continued driving to patient; availability of alternative methods of transportation if driving not advisable

Visual screening
  Evaluation of static visual acuity (near and distant) and visual fields (by automated perimetry in selected cases), intraocular pressure measurement, examination for eyelid abnormalities limiting visual field

Auditory screening
  Otoscopic examination and use of audioscope for detection of clinically significant hearing loss

Cognitive screening
  Detailed history from patient and family member
  Systematic, objective testing for cognitive impairment (using instruments of known validity and reliability, such as Mini-Mental State Examination)

Psychological screening
  Assessment for signs and symptoms of depression or behavioral disorders

Assessment of functional status
  Basic activities of daily living: feeding, bathing, dressing, toileting, transferring, mobility, and continence
  Instrumental activities of daily living: use of transportation, shopping, housework, handling finances, using telephone, administering medications

Musculoskeletal screening
  Evaluation for signs of neuromuscular impairment, including testing of cervical mobility, gait, and balance

Screening for sleep disorders
  Inquire about sleep habits, assess for daytime somnolence or other evidence of sleep apnea

Alcohol screening
  History of present or past use and relationship to driving habits

Review of medication list
  Review use of drugs with possible sedative or cognitive effects (including over-the-counter medications)
  Assess for problems attributable to polypharmacy or drug interactions

Reprinted, by permission, from M. Underwood, 1992, "The older driver: Clinical assessment and injury prevention," *Archives of Internal Medicine* 152: 738.

Birren and Botwinick (1951) recognized long ago that handwriting speed of adults, beginning in the middle to late 50s, slows with aging. These authors reported a moderately high curvilinear relationship between age and handwriting both for digits and for words, even after accounting for education. Writing speed for both words and digits was relatively stable until the 40s, and then it slowed considerably (figure 8.10). (These results once again reveal the increased effect of aging on complex tasks.) After age 60, the speed at which words can be written slows more than the speed at which digits can be written. The handwriting speed of individuals who held jobs that required a substantial amount of daily writing was affected less than the speed of persons who did little daily writing (Smith & Greene, 1962). Similarly, no age differences were found in the handwriting speed of clerical workers whose jobs required extensive handwriting, compared with skilled laborers or executives who presumably wrote comparatively little (LaRiviere & Simonson, 1965). Age differences are also magnified for tasks that are unfamiliar to individuals, whereas minimal differences occur in familiar tasks (Dixon et al., 1993).

Highly related to studies of handwriting speed are those that measure the time taken to copy numbers, letters, or symbols. Welford (1977) presented a classic case of age effects on number tracing (figure 8.11). In this figure it is clear that people approximately 20 to 40 years old exhibit little difference in the time required to trace numbers. After age 40, however, the age groups separate. Each increasingly older group traces the numbers more slowly. Adults 70 to 79 years old traced substantially slower than the other groups. Of particular interest was the decreased copying speed, especially in the older groups, when the numbers were reversed. The reversal condition was no longer routine and highly overpracticed and had to be consciously controlled and reversed. The younger age groups adapted to this change very well, but the oldest groups slowed considerably.

The perception that older adults' handwriting is less fluent and hence not as legible as young adults' handwriting is quite prevalent in our society, but one study showed that untrained observers of handwriting samples found it difficult to differentiate between writing samples of old and young adults (Lovelace et al., 1993). However, more quantitative studies using kinematic analyses of handwriting performance reveal that older adults do indeed produce movements that are more variable in comparison to young adults. Older adults take longer to stop the movement from peak velocity, have higher force inefficiency values, and have a greater number of acceleration and deceleration cycles (Salvin et al., 1996) (see figure 8.12). The smoothness with which older adults produce force in their handwriting is about the same as that of the young adults, but older adults have more spatial coordination impairments (higher normalized straightness error scores) (Contraras-Vidal et al., 1998). Thus, the age differences in movement variability appear to result from impaired spatial coordination of the wrist and fingers, not from an inability to control force.

Older adults take longer to sign their name on a check or write a letter to a friend.

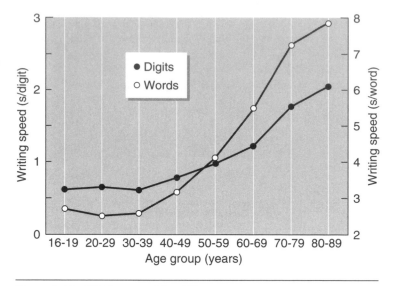

Figure 8.10 Writing speed for different age groups.

Adapted from J.E. Birren and J. Botwinick, 1951, "The relation of writing speed to age and to the senile psychoses," *Journal of Consulting Psychology* 15: 243-249.

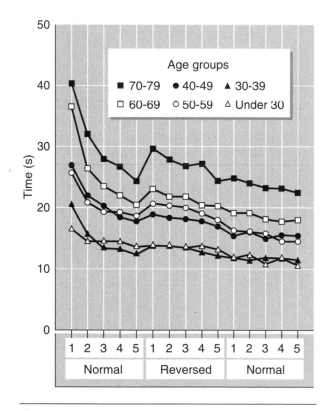

Figure 8.11 Figure-tracing times.

Reprinted, by permission, from A.T. Welford, 1977, Motor performance. In *Handbook of the psychology of aging*, edited by J.E. Birren and K.W. Schaie (New York: Van Nostrand Reinhold), 460.

Learning Physical Skills

Can an old dog learn new tricks? Age-related changes in performance are obvious, but how does aging affect the learning of motor skills? Conventional wisdom has always implied that older adults cannot learn skills as readily as young adults can, but is this really true? Older adults are slower, are less accurate, and display more intertrial variability, but can these age-related differences be negated with practice? If

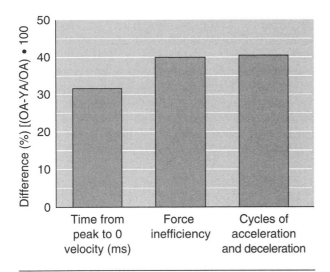

Figure 8.12 The effects of age on three measures of handwriting performance: time from peak to zero velocity, force inefficiency, and cycles of acceleration and deceleration or number of submovements. OA = older adults; YA = young adults.

Data from M.J. Slavin, J.G. Phillips, and J.L. Bradshaw, 1996, "Visual cues and the handwriting of older adults: A kinematic analysis," *Psychology and Aging*, 11(3): 524)

older adults learn new skills more slowly, it may affect their willingness to try something new. More importantly, the ability to learn or relearn motor skills has important implications for maintaining contact with the "real world" and for rehabilitation when the need arises. This section addresses the concept of motor skill learning, the effects of age on older adults' ability to learn a new skill, age-related differences in the rate of skill acquisition, and the manner in which older adults learn new skills. Implementation of strategies for facilitating learning and consideration of the heterogeneity of the older adult group are also addressed.

Learning and Older Adults

Many factors influence motor learning and make it more difficult to determine how aging affects motor learning. The nature and complexity of the task, in addition to the amount of previous practice that subjects have had, influences the outcomes of motor learning studies and modifies age differences that are observed. In general, complex tasks are learned more slowly than simple tasks. Older adults learn the simple tasks as fast as young adults but are slower at learning complex tasks. Skills in which individuals have a lifetime of experience, such as handwriting, are at a maximum level where additional learning is hard to achieve. Also, because of age and experience, it is difficult to start an experiment in which the amount

of practice that young and old have had on a functional task is equal before the study begins. In laboratories, tasks that are complex and conducted in an unfamiliar environment may discourage participants. Frustrated or poorly motivated old adults drop out leaving only the successful ones, who may be poor representatives of the age group as a whole.

Quantifying Learning

Two common methods of assessing motor learning are retention and transfer tests. A retention test assesses an individual's ability to retain a skill over a period of time, whereas a transfer test assesses the individual's ability to adapt a movement pattern learned in one context to a similar but related skill. Learning is inferred if there is retention or transfer. For example, a student enrolls in 10 lessons of golf. As a pretest, the instructor records the number of 30-in. (76 cm) putts that the student can make out of 20 tries. Following each of the 10 golf lessons, the student also records the number of successful putts out of 20 that she made. Then, a week later, following a period of no practice, the student again records the number of putts made out of 20. A large improvement occurs with practice (10 golf lessons), but the real evidence that learning has occurred is that little change occurs from the posttest (10th golf lesson) to the retention test 1 week later (figure 8.13).

Another way to infer learning is to see whether the individual can adapt the skill to a different but similar problem. For example, instead of just performing well

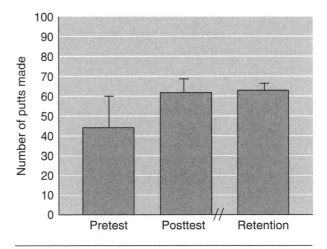

Figure 8.13 Number of putts out of 20 were recorded on 10 separate occasions. The first bar displays the mean and standard deviation of the number of putts made for the first five sessions, and the second bar displays the mean and standard deviation of the putts made for the second five sessions. The retention test is the number of successful putts out of 20 following a week with no practice.

on a retention test that mimics the practice test, can the individual putt from different distances from the hole (change in condition) or on different surfaces (change in context; location on the course or a different course)? If the success rate is similar on the transfer test to the average performance on the posttest following practice, then learning has occurred.

Ability to Learn a Novel Skill

Older adults learn novel motor tasks well, but age-related differences in performance prevail following a period of practice (Lazarus & Haynes, 1997; Seidler-Dobrin & Stelmach, 1998). Lazarus and Haynes (1997) distinguished some of these differences by using an isometric visuomotor tracking paradigm, which is a novel, complex, continuous task with the goal being to track a computer-generated pattern. The location of the cursor on the screen was controlled by the participant who applied or released force on a **dynamometer** in an attempt to match the computer-generated pattern. Both the computer-generated pattern and the ongoing self-generated cursor path were visible to the subject (concurrent visual feedback). Of interest was the subject's ability to anticipate the location of the upcoming computer-generated pattern (predictive strategy) as opposed to reacting to the pattern after it appeared on the screen (feedback strategy). Both young and old participants improved their performance over a 2-day practice session (110 trials), retained the skill 1 week later, and were able to adapt (transfer) to a new tracking pattern. In particular, both groups increased their accuracy of force production and the strength of the relationship between the produced pattern (self-generated) and the target pattern (computer-generated). One week later, both groups' performances were similar to those of the second day of practice and both groups transferred the skill to a new computer-generated pattern. However, the older adults exhibited less smooth force trajectories, a weaker relationship between the self- and computer-generated pattern, and higher lag scores (an indication of ability to predict the movement of the computer-generated pattern). Thus, older adults can learn a novel, complex task, but the quality of the performance may be compromised, perhaps by poorer peripheral reorganization, slowing of processing, or changes in tactile sensitivity.

Can older adults learn a new pattern of bimanual coordination that requires inhibition of the preferred modes of coordination? Older adults practiced a new pattern of bimanual coordination that had a phase offset of 90° and hence was between their two previously identified preferred modes of coordination

(in phase and antiphase, Wishart, 2002). They could see the computer-generated real-time display of their limb movements on the screen after every trial (concurrent augmented feedback) and the result of the performance (terminal feedback) every fifth trial. **Transfer** (the ability to adapt a movement pattern learned in one context to a similar but related skill or context) tests were given before and at the middle and end of each practice day. Transfer trials were repeated after 5 min and 1 week following the acquisition. Transfer conditions included blindfolded, normal vision, and augmented vision trials. Initially both groups had difficulty producing the new pattern of movement. However, the older adults experienced greater difficulty learning the new movement. Younger adults became more accurate across days, but older adults actually became less accurate and therefore age-group differences increased. Thus, the rate of improvement, despite feedback, was lower for the older group. The older group grew more consistent across days and trials, but it was because they were remaining with a movement that resembled the preferred coordination modes rather than shifting to the pattern to be learned. However, both groups seemed to use the feedback in a similar fashion, and both performed better when they had augmented visual feedback. Although the older adults used feedback in the same ways that the young did, the older adults' performance was differentially better when they had visual feedback than when they were blindfolded, and it was even higher when the feedback was augmented. This suggests that the older group relied more on additional information to increase their performance.

Use of Feedback

Do older adults use feedback in the same manner as young adults? We have already seen that older adults perform a greater proportion of their movement under feedback control (Pratt et al., 1994). Can they learn to restructure their movement such that a greater proportion of the total movement is planned before the movement (program control) rather than using feedback (online control; visual, proprioceptive) to guide the movement toward the target? Seidler-Dobrin and Stelmach (1998) investigated reliance on visual feedback in a discrete aiming task. The subjects moved a lever as quickly and accurately as possible to a target. In the visual condition, they could see both the target and the cursor (representing arm movement) on a computer screen, but in the no-vision trials, which were randomly inserted into the practice trials, the cursor was removed so the subjects had no feedback regarding limb position. For the purposes of analysis, the movement was divided into a primary submovement, indicative of the acceleration phase (program control), and a secondary submovement, indicative of the deceleration phase (feedback control). Before practice, both groups performed similarly when vision was present and both groups were equally affected by the removal of vision. Following practice with vision, both groups decreased the distance covered in the secondary submovement (less reliance on feedback control), decreased the number of corrections, and reduced the total movement time. The young adults extended their primary submovement and the elderly adults increased their endpoint accuracy. Following practice without vision, both groups decreased the total movement time. The young group also increased the primary submovement distance and increased the target hit rate, but the elderly group did not. Without visual feedback, then, the older adults were unable to develop a program to control the majority of the movement without needed feedback. This failure may be attributable to an impaired programming ability, increased inconsistency of performance, which makes it difficult to predict endpoint location, or impaired sensory processes. Performing more of the movement under feedback control may explain some of the observed age-related slowing.

Strategies to Facilitate Learning in Older Adults

One way to facilitate learning of a novel skill is to provide augmented feedback, externally provided information about the movement process (knowledge of performance) or the movement outcome (knowledge of results). This type of information can be presented concurrently, at the same time the movement is being performed, or terminally, after the movement is completed and before the next movement. The information can be delivered as visual, auditory, or verbal, but it is known that feedback should not be given after every trial (100% of the time) because the learner uses the feedback as a crutch or guide instead of actively engaging in the problem-solving process. The best results (most learning) come from initially giving feedback 100% of the time and then gradually withdrawing it so that the overall feedback rate is 50% (Winstein & Schmidt, 1990).

For example, younger adults learned a new bimanual coordination movement using visual augmented feedback provided every fifth trial over a 3-day practice period and retained the skill 1 week and 1 month later. On the same task with the same type of feed-

back, older adults did not improve (Wishardt et al., 2002). In a following study in which visual, augmented feedback was provided after every trial, the young group benefited from concurrent feedback on the first day of practice but did not improve more on the second or third day. In contrast, the older group did not benefit from concurrent feedback on the first day of practice, but by the end of the third practice day they were as accurate and able to move at the same frequency as young adults. The only difference that remained was that old adults were not as consistent as young adults. For this type of bimanual coordination pattern, then, feedback following every trial facilitated learning in older adults, but providing feedback following every fifth trial did not facilitate learning.

Another strategy to enhance learning, called content-dependent feedback, is to provide information specific to the task. If the task is to learn the underarm throw, content-dependent information would describe strategies for underarm throw: the ready position, grip, arm swing down, arm wing forward, release, and follow-through. A content-independent strategy would be to provide information that is not specific to the movement, such as information about the performance in general, that would be relevant to any self-paced gross motor skill with a predictable environment. The learner would be told to be ready, to imagine the movement, to focus, and then to execute the movement and evaluate it. Older adults who learned three closed-motor skills, the dart throw, lawn dart throw (jart), and ball toss, did improve more when they were provided with cognitive strategies, but it did not matter whether the strategies were content dependent or independent (Greenwood et al., 1993).

A third type of learning strategy is to provide extensive practice. In one study of older adults, the baseline level of performance on several physical variables was measured: hand grip strength, maximum pinch force, steadiness of pinch force, hand steadiness, pegboard test, and the Hoffman reflex (Ranganathan et al., 2001). The subjects then practiced a ball-rolling exercise during two 10-min training sessions per day for 6 days each week across an 8-week period. The authors found that the extensive manual training on ball rolling improved submaximal pinch force, hand steadiness, speed of peg placement (pegboard test), and motor neuron excitability.

Individual Differences

At this point we should remember that old adults are more heterogeneous as a group than young adults (chapter 2). Thus, older adults' performances range from those who perform as well as young adults to those who perform much worse. For example, although older adults as a group are slower than younger adults in handwriting ability, both in familiar and unfamiliar tasks, before and after practice, a few older adults will perform as well as the younger ones (Dixon et al., 1993). There is a substantial overlap in the two groups' performances, because individuals age at different rates and chronological age is not the best indicator of motor performance.

Mechanisms of Learning: Neural Plasticity

Even though older adults cannot, by extensive practice, eliminate age differences in many coordinated motor performances, they can improve their performances dramatically. Beginning as early as the 30s, the brain undergoes morphological and biochemical changes with increased aging, but no matter how old, the brain possesses a remarkable capacity to adapt to new stimuli and new conditions. Both brain morphology and neurochemistry, which are most adaptable in youth and during maturation, maintain a substantial amount of plasticity in aging. Brain plasticity means that the brain has the capacity to make positive changes morphologically and functionally, in either repair or growth processes. For example, significant changes in brain neurotransmitter function have been associated with learned behaviors. The full range of

models that have been proposed as explanations for brain plasticity are beyond the scope of this text, but a few examples of morphological changes that occur as a result of aging, practice, and physical activity can illustrate the mechanisms by which learning and improvement occur in the aging brain (see also Cerella, 1990).

Morphological Changes With Age

Morphological changes abound in the aging brain. Many neurons die with advancing age, and of those that survive, changes occur in the axons, dendrites, and cell bodies. Brain weight decreases. One of the most striking changes is that the dendritic branches, the primary path by which neurons communicate with each other, thin and lose interneuronal contact. It is possible that the losses of dendrites and synaptic contacts are the source of the interruptions in neuronal networks described in chapter 7 as a likely basis for the generalized slowing phenomenon.

Morphological Changes With Practice

Unlike the losses that occur in aging, morphological changes that represent new contacts and neurochemical changes that facilitate specific pathways are developed by repetitions (practice) of neuronal circuit activity. Morphological changes such as the number, cell structure, and density of neurons

Motor Learning in Older Adults

Older adults

- can learn novel motor skills and perform very similarly to young adults, except that subtle qualitative differences can be seen in the smoothness of force trajectories, the speed of performance, and abilities to predict movements that will be necessary for success;
- learn at a slower rate, particularly if they have to inhibit a preferred or well-learned coordination and replace it with a new one;
- depend more on feedback to hone their fast movements to a target, and, unlike young adults, they seem unable through practice to restructure their movement so that this feedback period is shorter;
- perform better if they have concurrent, visual feedback after every trial, whereas young adults can learn as well if feedback is provided on an intermittent basis; and
- perform better if they are provided with some type of cognitive strategy, such as content-dependent or content-independent information during the learning .

Extensive practice on some types of manual skill can transfer to and improve older adults' performance on other types of manual skills, physical function, and neuromuscular integrity, but practice does not generally raise their performance to levels accomplished by young adults.

accompany repeated physical activity in animals. Large differences in dendritic branching have been seen in young monkeys, rats, and mice that were provided opportunities to experiment and play with toys, compared with animals that were raised in confined cages and allowed few opportunities for physical experimentation and movement (Floeter & Greenough, 1979; Pysh & Weiss, 1979). In the brains of young rats that learned to perform a task with only one paw, the neuronal morphology of the cortical hemisphere that controlled the practiced paw was substantially different from the hemisphere that controlled the nonpracticed paw. Similar physical activity and practice-related morphological changes have also been observed in the brains of very old rats, so that neural mechanisms that support learning in young animals are also present in old animals.

Another example of experience-dependent plasticity in the anatomy of neurons is the plasticity that accompanies enriched physical activity in recovery of brain function. In these studies, unilateral and bilateral sensorimotor lesions were made in the brains of rats, and then the rats were allowed to recover in either a movement-enriched environment (a cage with toys and climbing apparatus) or a movement-impoverished environment (a standard, small holding cage). In these studies, the rats in the movement-enriched environments recovered function to higher levels than did the rats in the movement-impoverished environments (Gentile et al., 1987; Held et al., 1985). In another study, rats housed in a movement-enriched environment coupled with social interaction improved more on a series of behavioral tests after focal brain ischemia than rats that were housed with a movement-enriched environment with and without social interaction (Johansson & Ohlsson, 1996). These studies support the hypothesis that the aged brain is capable of morphological and functional change and that chronic physical activity assists in maintaining certain types of brain function.

Compensatory Strategies for Losses of Coordination

Although systematic practice can contribute to the maintenance of some types of motor function for a great many years, eventually efficiency and speed of performance decline in the latter part of life. As the passage of time blunts efficiency and reduces the speed of processing, individuals inevitably develop strategies to cope with these losses; thus, for many years the loss of function in a highly practiced,

healthy individual is so slight it is unnoticeable. Such compensatory strategies include anticipation, simplification, and the speed–accuracy trade-off.

Anticipation

For some types of tasks, older people develop ways to anticipate movements that they will have to make, so that when the time comes, these movements can be made quickly and efficiently. They learn over a lifetime of experience that certain movements will be needed at certain times, and knowing this, they can begin their movement planning sooner.

One of the best examples of the use of anticipation to accomplish a task with the same efficiency as young people is the anticipation older typists use to enable them to type as fast as younger typists. Older typists learn to preview letters and words farther ahead, while continuing to type, so that they can type almost as quickly as young typists (Salthouse, 1984). Figure 8.14 shows the correlation of reaction time with age in two studies. On the x-axis of the figure are the conditions of preview that were provided for the typists. At the extreme left of the x-axis, no preview at all was provided about the words to be typed. Under this condition, the typists had to type words as they were presented; therefore, the task was basically a pure reaction time task with a predictable stimulus. On the extreme right is the condition of normal typing, in which the typists could read far ahead of the words being typed and thus anticipate the words

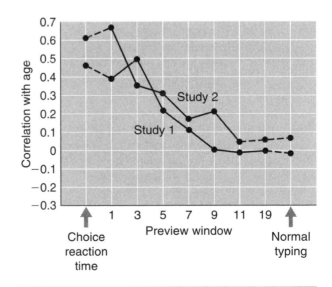

Figure 8.14 Correlation coefficients between interkey interval and typist age across preview window conditions and the choice reaction time and normal typing tasks.

From T.A. Salthouse, 1984, "Effect of age and skill on typing," *Journal of Experimental Psychology: General* 113: 357. Copyright © 1984 by the American Psychological Association. Reprinted with permission.

to be typed. The correlation between age and preview condition decreases so that the correlation between age and typing speed is essentially zero under conditions of normal typing. These results are evidence that the opportunity to preview stimuli before needing to react to them is important to older adults.

A real-world example of anticipation would be retrieving a piece of luggage from a slowly revolving baggage claim at the airport. If a young man is blocked by the crowd from viewing any of the approaching luggage until the moment at which it is immediately in front of him, he can still quickly plan the movements necessary to lean out and retrieve his suitcase. But by the time an older man sees his luggage and begins planning the retrieval movement, the luggage has passed by and he must wait until it comes around the baggage claim again. However, if the older man can see the luggage coming for several feet, he can plan his movements, be ready when the bag arrives, and successfully retrieve it from the baggage claim. Because he uses anticipation, his performance looks exactly like that of the young man's.

Simplification

An effective way to compensate for losses in coordination is to make simpler, less complicated movements, so that less complex movements have to be coordinated. When adults find their coordination decreasing, they begin to search for simpler, smaller, or slower movements that accomplish the same goals that were previously met by more complicated coordinated movements. Young adults jump off a low wall instead of bothering to descend by using the steps. Older adults may sit on a small stool to weed the garden, whereas young adults bend over and stand up many times while doing the same chore. A young person may open the refrigerator door with an elbow while holding the newspaper under an arm and a dish in both hands. The older adult places the newspaper and one plate on the table before opening the door. In all cases, the goal is accomplished, but older people find ways to involve fewer muscles and use movements that are less complex. This process is repeated in hundreds of ways during everyday activities, and the simplification process increases with increasing age.

> George Burns, the nonagenarian comedian who was famous not only for achieving advanced age but for continuing to be humorous about it, said, "You know you are old when, while leaning down to tie your shoelace you think, what else can I do while I'm down here?"

Speed–Accuracy Trade-Off

As discussed in the section on "Aiming Movements" in this chapter, it is well known that older people often trade speed for accuracy, because they generally choose to be more accurate than faster.

Psychological and Emotional Factors That Influence Coordination and Learning

Anyone who has tried to sink a free throw in the last seconds to win a basketball game, or has been graded by the teacher while he or she learned a new skill, understands that psychological and emotional factors influence both performance and learning. Three of these factors that are particularly relevant are attention, motivation, and anxiety.

Attention

To execute a complex motor task, and certainly to learn it, an individual has to pay attention to it. Attention is the mechanism by which the central nervous system prepares to process stimuli and determines what to process and to what depth it should be processed. Attention is like a flashlight beam: When the beam is focused on some object, the object becomes visible. The beam of conscious awareness—attention—can be diffused, so that nearby objects are also visible, or it can be intensely focused, so that the viewer is aware of only one object. Attention is limited by the amount of information that can be held in consciousness at a given time; therefore, the individual directing the beam of attention has to be selective about which objects are illuminated. Selective attention is the filtering of information to focus only on information that is interesting or relevant to a goal. Because attention is limited, to see other objects the person must move the beam from object to object. Attention switching occurs not only when the focus moves from object to object but also when attention is turned from objects in the external environment to objects or operations in memory. The ability to sustain attention in the search for expected short-term stimuli is called vigilance. To be vigilant, the perceiver must maintain attention on a specific goal. A stargazer watching for the appearance of an anticipated comet has to be vigilant not to miss the event.

Can Older Adults Coordinate Movements As Quickly As Young Adults?

Morgan and colleagues (1994) performed an experiment to determine whether older adults could move at a speed faster than their preferred speed with the same degree of accuracy as young adults. Two speed conditions, fast and slow, were set based on the mean young adult performance and the mean old adult performance, respectively, for each of four target sizes. The task required the subjects to draw a line from target to each of nine target circles in a zigzag pattern (figure 8.15). Older adults were able to move at the same speed and as accurately as young adults. However, older adults were less efficient when moving at a faster speed than their preferred speed, as was exhibited by an increase in the number of submovements.

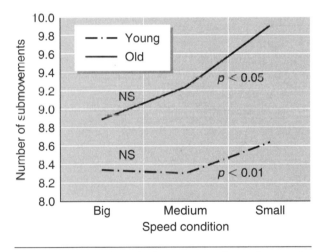

Figure 8.15 Number of submovements for each group for the three target sizes. The task is done with a minimum of eight movements. NS = nonsignificant.

Journals of Gerontology, Series A, Biological Sciences and Medical Science by M. Morgan. Copyright 1994 by Gerontological Society of America. Reproduced with permission of Gerontological Society of America in the format textbook via Copyright Clearance Center.

Although the ability to switch attention to task-relevant stimuli is critical to do the task, attention switching can greatly disrupt performance if attention is inadvertently switched from relevant to irrelevant stimuli. One of the most significant changes that occur with aging is that older adults find it increasingly difficult to keep their attention fixed on a task. Events in their environment, intentions, or memories

that are irrelevant to the task interject themselves into their thoughts. Controlled and purposeful inhibition of neurophysiological responses to irrelevant information is absolutely essential in controlling movement and learning. Thus, one of the functions of the attention process is the inhibition of unwanted neurological excitation. Infants, small children, and older adults have a difficult time attending only to important stimuli relevant to the task (Philips et al., 1989; Prinz et al., 1990). These age differences are depicted graphically in figure 8.16.

Backman and Molander (1991) provided a good example of the effects of attention on performance in their study of golfers' putting capabilities. The older golfers were not able to perform as well when a meaningful noise, such as an informational broadcast, was played as background noise during the putting competition. Older golfers found themselves listening to the broadcast, whereas the younger golfers were more able to block the irrelevant stimuli from their thoughts and concentrate on their putting. The researchers suggested that the background noise increased the cognitive demands of the motor coordination task, placing high demands on memory and on the ability to attend selectively to the task.

In some fine motor skills, the performer must divide attention between the actions of the two hands, because each must perform a different action that is not easily synchronized with the other hand. In these dual tasks, the person must control each hand in a time-shared fashion. In general, older adults have

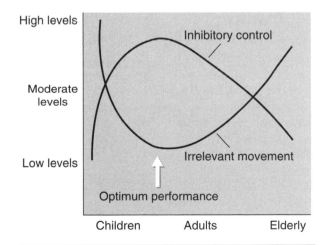

Figure 8.16 Proposed relationship between central nervous system inhibitory control and the initiation of irrelevant movements. Children and older adults exhibit less inhibitory control and make more irrelevant movements than young adults. The ordinate is only a gross scale of the levels of inhibitory control and the number of irrelevant movements made.

more difficulty dividing attention between two tasks than younger adults do (McDowd & Craik, 1988; McDowd et al., 1991). Driving is a good example of a task that requires the parallel use of a number of different controls (i.e., turn signal, steering wheel, accelerator, brake). When older adults are faced with a situation where they must attend to several factors or controls at once, they tend to switch from a parallel to a serial mode of control (Hakamies-Blomqvist et al. 1999). In general, older adults choose to use fewer controls in a serial manner, whereas young adults use a greater number of controls in a parallel manner. Even though they executed the task somewhat differently, older adults with more driving experience were able drive the car as well as young adults.

Older adults tend to allocate attention and maximize performance on tasks that are associated with high risk. Imagine walking with a group of friends on a paved surface versus a dirt trail that is overrun by tree roots, rocks, and an uneven surface. Also imagine that while you are walking you engage in a lively conversation. Will the conversation be affected to a greater extent when you are walking on a dirt trail compared with a paved trail? Yes, if a primary task (walking) becomes more attention demanding (as in the dirt trail condition), then performance on a secondary task might be compromised. Older adults might choose to prioritize walking to an even greater extent than young adults if they feel threatened or are afraid of falling. Older adults who are asked to walk while performing a memory task choose to allocate attention to walking and hence prioritize walking (Li et al., 2001).

Motivation

One hypothesis about learning and the aged is that older adults have little incentive to perform well on psychomotor laboratory tasks and so they do not improve as much as young subjects do. Would a special incentive or reward make older subjects learn any faster than young subjects? The answer is probably no (Hertzog et al., 1976; Surburg, 1976). Grant and colleagues (1978) provided two groups of women (aged 19-27 and 64-76) with monetary rewards for fast performance on 20 trials of the Digit-Symbol Substitution test. Neither age group improved substantially more than the other (figure 8.17), and although it appeared that the older women improved more with monetary incentive, this improvement was not statistically significant. The monetary incentive did not improve either age group's performance appreciably more than did practice alone. However, high motivation and appropriately provided reinforcement are important for older individuals to reach their optimum performance, and researchers

or professional workers may have to attend more to the motivation levels of older adults than they do to those of younger adults to ensure that both are functioning at optimum levels.

Anxiety

Anxiety is a state in which high levels of arousal occur from concerns about performance and the outcome of performance. We know almost nothing about how aging affects performance anxiety. The results from the few studies of anxiety effects on cognitive performance are equivocal (Kausler, 1990). However, Lars Backman of Sweden (i.e., Molander & Backman, 1990, 1994) conducted an interesting series of studies of the interaction of age and anxiety on aiming and coordinating the hands and arms to sink a golf putt. These studies compared the putting performance of young and old adults under relaxed or highly competitive conditions. The older competitors performed as well as the younger competitors under the relaxed conditions but were not able to coordinate the putting stroke movement as well during competition. Thus, experience might maintain a highly complex skill throughout aging only under conditions that are relatively relaxed, nonthreatening, and low in risk. It was particularly noteworthy that the ability to perform a highly coordinated skill, such as putting, was negatively affected by the stress of competition even in subjects as young as 46 years of age.

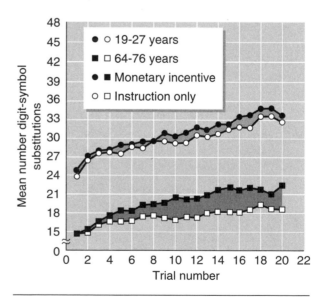

Figure 8.17 Digit-Symbol Substitution performance as a function of age, incentive, and number of practice trials.

Reprinted, by permission, from E.A. Grant, M. Storandt, and J. Botwinick, 1978, "Incentive and practice in the psychomotor performance of the elderly," *Journal of Gerontology* 33: 414.

SUMMARY

Coordination and skill deteriorate with age. The loss of the ability to perform simple and more complex movements has been observed in laboratory tasks designed to represent daily tasks and other functional tasks such as driving and handwriting. It is evident that changes in sensorimotor mechanisms contribute to these decrements; however, the nature of the age deterioration in terms of the extent, rate, and types is not well established.

Older adults take longer to perform simple tasks such as aiming, reaching and grasping, and precision gripping. Even when speed-related differences are minimal, older adults may be using different movement patterns to accomplish tasks. In tasks that require both speed and accuracy, older people tend to emphasize accuracy over speed.

Many functional types of movements such as buttoning buttons, manipulating safety pins, cutting with a knife, and dialing a telephone are impaired in the elderly, and these deficits have particular significance because they affect the ability to live independently. Handwriting and driving are two functional tasks that are significant to the elderly. Driving represents freedom, mobility, and autonomy. Older people have deficits in almost all requirements for driving, but they also develop many compensatory behaviors. The number of adults over the age of 65 with a driver's license has markedly increased. Policy makers should consider testing programs that ensure that adults who drive well may continue to drive, but those with poorer vision and driving skills may not. These programs should include the development of technological aids, more comprehensive and individual performance screening, increased alternatives for transportation, and better counseling of those elderly who may be at risk for traffic accidents.

Even though large decrements are seen in many types of coordination and skills, practice can greatly attenuate these losses. However, the rate that older adults learn a skill is slower, particularly when the new skill requires them to inhibit a previously learned skill. Not only do older adults take longer to learn tasks, but the manner in which they learn is different. Older adults may not benefit from feedback initially, but with repeated exposure to feedback performance gradually increases.

Older adults, no matter their age, make substantial improvements in physical skill with practice. Research on animals has shown that the brain remains extremely plastic and remarkable changes occur in the structure and function of the brain as a result of practice.

One of the most significant changes that occur with aging is the increasing difficulty to keep attention focused on the task at hand. Older adults also have difficulty dividing their attention between tasks that must be carried out simultaneously. The more complex these tasks are, the greater the age deficit in dividing attention.

Most older individuals maintain for most of their lives the coordinated skills necessary to function socially by practicing and developing compensatory moves for age-related losses of coordination. Some of these strategies involve anticipation, in which older adults preview or plan ahead for movements that young adults might successfully achieve by reacting spontaneously to them. Another strategy involves simplification, in which older adults divide a task into components and execute one part at a time. A third strategy involves trading off speed for accuracy.

REVIEW QUESTIONS

1. Describe the changes in the visual and somatosensory system that occur with increasing age.
2. Can older adults learn or re-learn previously acquired skill at a similar rate and manner as young adults?
3. What strategies do older adults employ to compensate for changes in sensorimotor control?
4. Describe how psychological and emotional factors influence coordination and learning.
5. Describe two laboratory-based experiments that assess upper limb and hand control.
6. What factors should be considered when determining whether it is safe for an older adult to continue to drive?

SUGGESTED READINGS

Klavora, P., & Heslegrave, R.J. (2002). Senior drivers: An overview of problems and intervention strategies. *Journal of Aging and Physical Activity, 10,* 322-335.

Yan, J.H., Thomas, J. R., Stelmach, G.E., & Thomas, K. T. (2000). Developmental features of rapid aiming arm movements across the lifespan. *Journal of Motor Behavior, 32,* 126.

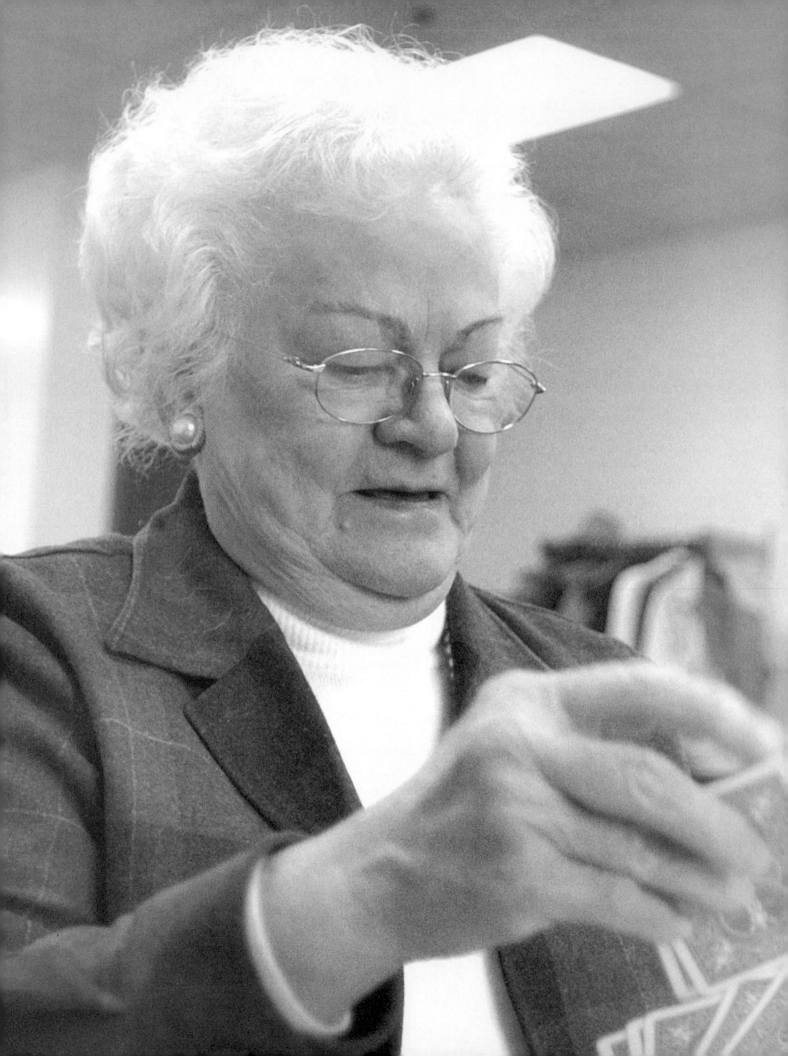

PART IV

Physical–Psychosocial Relationships

Health, Exercise, and Cognitive Function

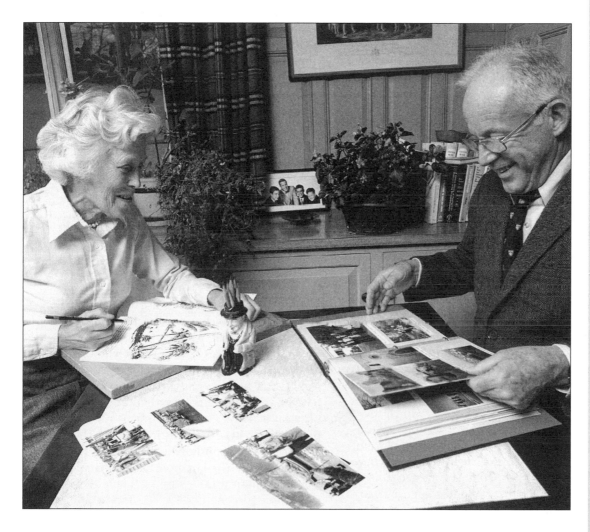

The objectives of this chapter are

- to explain the extent to which health and physical fitness may postpone age-related declines in cognitive functions such as processing speed, attention, and memory in aging adults;

- to discuss the primary physiological and psychosocial mechanisms by which health and fitness influences cognitive function; and

- to describe the importance and implications of health and fitness in terms of maintaining an optimum cerebral environment for cognitive function.

A question of major importance to society as well as to individuals concerns the extent to which cognitive efficiency and speed of processing are associated with physical health throughout life. Everyone has experienced the difficulty of thinking clearly and focusing on cognitive problems when in poor health or in pain. Episodes of sickness, disease, and poor health are more frequent with increasing age, and occurrences of chronic disease and physical disability increase in the population as a whole.

Most people assume that a decrease in cognitive abilities is an inevitable consequence of growing old, especially in the very aged. In the last 30 years, however, many researchers in the field of aging have disassociated the aging process itself (primary aging) from the declines caused by pathological conditions and poor health behaviors (secondary aging). Pathological conditions such as Alzheimer's disease have been linked to declines in cognitive function. How much of the age-related cognitive decline that is seen in older populations is attributable, not to primary aging of the brain, but to secondary aging that accompanies cerebrovascular disease or diabetes? To what extent is cognitive dysfunction related to asymptomatic yet low levels of physical fitness? If age-related cognitive decline could be prevented by improving individual health and physical fitness, health care costs, health insurance, and human suffering might be substantially reduced. Thus, understanding the types and extent of cognitive decline that can be attributed to secondary aging could lead to behavioral interventions and preventive behaviors that would enhance the quality of life for many elderly.

This chapter explores the relationships of health, fitness, and cognitive function in the aging adult and describes the possible mechanisms by which these constructs are related to each other. The proposed relationship of health and fitness is extremely complex and in some cases is not clear. Still, many researchers have proposed biological and psychosocial mechanisms by which health and fitness might influence cognition, in terms of both primary and secondary aging. The chapter concludes with a discussion of how health and fitness may affect cognitive function and the implications of this relationship for society.

Concepts of Physical Activity, Health and Fitness, and Cognitive Function

The terms *health, physical activity, fitness,* and *cognitive function* are used loosely and many times erroneously by people. These concepts are not interchangeable; they have specific meanings. The definitions used in this text were adopted from Casperson, Powell, and Christenson (1985), three researchers from the Centers for Disease Control who differentiated these terms for epidemiological research.

Health and Fitness

Health is an attribute of people that is related to many factors such as genetics, nutrition, sleep, psychological stress, and abstinence from smoking and drugs. Health professionals define health as physical, psychological, and social well-being, but in gerontological studies of health and cognitive function, objective health is defined as the absence of symptoms of disease, particularly those that are age-related, such as cardiovascular disease, adult-onset diabetes, and arthritis. Objective health is usually determined based on the outcomes of a physical examination administered by a physician. In some studies the definitions are further specified as **subjective health,** which is the perception of individuals of their own health (self-reports), and **functional health,** which is the way individuals function within the constraints of their objective health. The interpretation of functional health varies quite drastically between individuals with the same disease. For example, one person with diabetes may use it as an excuse to be very sedentary and socially isolated, whereas another person with the same level of diabetes may control it with medication and live a lifestyle of a person who has a higher objective level of health.

Physical fitness is a set of attributes that people have or achieve that relates to the ability to perform physical activity. Physical fitness is an outcome of physical activity, usually from exercise. The components of cardiorespiratory fitness and the factors that affect it are discussed in more detail in chapter 4. The way that physical fitness impacts elite performance is discussed in chapter 12. The fitness component thought to be related to cognition is aerobic fitness. Aerobic fitness is defined as the maximum level of physical work of which an individual is capable. When directly assessed, the "gold standard" of physical work capacity is maximal oxygen consumption ($\dot{V}O_2$max), a measure of aerobic capacity reported in milliliters of oxygen consumption per kilogram of body mass per minute ($ml \cdot kg^{-1} \cdot min^{-1}$). $\dot{V}O_2$max has been analyzed or estimated along with behavioral response speed measures. Individuals who are physically fit have high $\dot{V}O_2$max levels for their age group, and they can sustain physical work (walking, running, cycling, swimming) longer than

Inferring Health and Fitness From Behaviors, Activities, and Assessments

We use self-reported health habits, physical activity levels, and exercise activities to infer levels of health and fitness. The most reliable assessment of aerobic fitness is the $\dot{V}O_2$max test.

Components of Health and Fitness

Behaviors and activities	Attributes and status
Health habits Diet Sleep Stress control Drug use	→Inferred health
Physical activity level Sedentary Moderate High	→Inferred fitness
Exercise Self-report Observed	→Inferred fitness
$\dot{V}O_2$max	→Quantified fitness

less fit individuals. Because the measurement of $\dot{V}O_2$max is time consuming and expensive in older adults, few studies include direct measures of oxygen consumption. Far less accurate, but used by many of the studies discussed in this chapter, is to estimate the aerobic capacity of subjects from their self-reports of the amount of aerobic-type physical activities in which they participate each week.

Physical Activity and Exercise

Physical activity is any bodily movement produced by skeletal muscles that results in energy expenditure (measured in kilocalories). It is nearly always obtained by having people report on a questionnaire the type and amount of physical activities that they do in work and leisure (e.g., sport, exercise, yard work, home repair, cleaning). These activities are then categorized along a scale such as "active," "moderately

active," "moderately sedentary," or "sedentary," and the person's physical activity lifestyle can also be described by these categories. Another technique is to estimate the kilocalories spent per day or week on the basis of these self-reports of activity. Thus, self-reported physical activity level is frequently used as a marker or a surrogate for fitness, but it is not a measure of fitness.

Exercise, a subset of physical activity, is physical activity that is planned, structured, repetitive, and purposive in the sense that improvement or maintenance of one or more components of physical fitness is an objective. Self-reported levels of exercise are also used frequently as a surrogate for fitness, but they are notoriously inaccurate compared with laboratory assessments of fitness.

Cognition

Cognition can be thought of in terms of functions of the brain, such as memory, association, comparison, abstract reasoning (verbal and quantitative), spatial ability and manipulation, and synthesis. Executive control plans actions and coordinates many of these functions. The processes of cognition—attention (mental energy), working memory, information processing speed, psychomotor ability, and perception—support the cognitive functions. Together, cognitive functions and processes interact to enable individuals to make decisions and behave intelligently. Intelligence tests have been developed with the hope of assessing the application of brain functions to psychological and social function. Besides testing cognitive functions, intelligence tests also test verbal abilities, word fluency, arithmetic reasoning, and general information. However, as Salthouse (1991) pointed out, the tests used to assess cognition of adults rarely include functions such as wisdom, sagacity, judgment, insight, social cognition, and long-range planning.

Effects of Health and Physical Activity on Cognitive Function

Since 1975, a substantial amount of research attention has been focused on potential relationships among health, fitness, and cognition. In figure 9.1, areas of research are shown and their relationships indicated by arrows. The left column describes the area of studies in which physical activity lifestyle (PA) and exercise lifestyle have been related to their

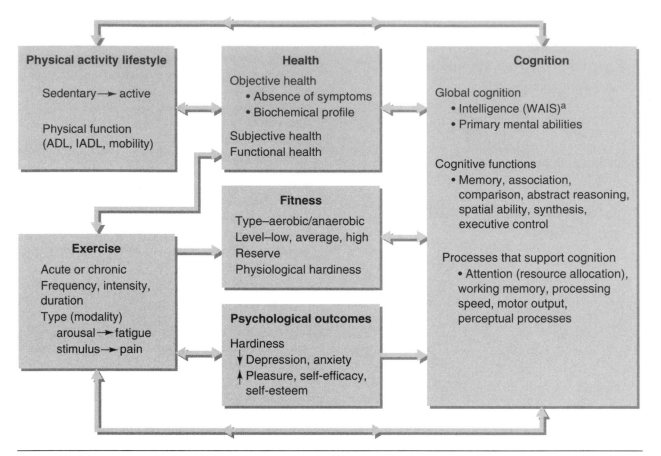

Figure 9.1 Proposed relationships among various components of cognition, health, and fitness. The following references refer only to the development of intelligence scales or proposed cognitive constructs, not to the proposed relationships among components in the figure: [a]Wechsler (1981). ADL = activities of daily living; IADL = Instrumental Activities of Daily Living; WAIS = Wechsler Adult Intelligence Scale.

outcomes and to cognition. Thus, in many PA studies, people who report that they are "very active," or score high on an instrumental activities of daily living (IADL) scale, also have higher objective health and perform better on cognitive tests. Similarly, people who exercise regularly seem to have higher levels of health and fitness, lower anxiety and depression, and higher cognitive scores. From the large number of bidirectional arrows, it is clear that these relationships are "two-way streets." That is, PA influences cognition, but cognitive competency also influences the nature and amount of PA. Similarly, exercise is thought to directly influence cognition through biochemical changes and indirectly affect it by affecting health, fitness, and psychological outcomes, but a certain amount of cognition is necessary to maintain motivation to exercise and to organize the workout sessions.

The first half of this chapter describes the evidence to support each of the areas and the relationships shown in figure 9.1. The second half describes possible mechanisms by which these relationships might exist.

Health and Cognitive Function

It seems intuitive that disease would take a toll on cognitive capability and judgment. Many years ago, Botwinick and Birren (1963) pointed out that the factors of health and sickness play a large role in determining age differences in cognitive function. Van Boxtel and colleagues (1998) calculated the effects of both insulin-dependent and non-insulin-dependent diabetes on "cognitive age" (ratio of the regression coefficients associated with disease state and those associated with age) and found that active diabetes added 21 years to the cognitive age on memory function and 19 years on cognitive flexibility.

Evidence from several studies has supported the hypothesis that in aging populations, hypertension, coronary heart disease, cerebrovascular disease, and atherosclerosis impair neuropsychological function (Ylikoski et al., 2000). One of the effects of disease is to slow basic mechanisms of sensory-motor speed, which in turn slows perceptual processing speed. The most robust relationship between disease and cog-

Objective and Subjective Health, Information Processing Speed, and Serial Learning

Objective health and subjective health are related to information processing speed and serial learning. A study by Milligan and colleagues (1984) is an example in which better cognitive performance was associated with both a composite objective health rating score, made by a medical professional, and the subjective perception of an individual's own health. Individuals answered questions about their physical and mental health, activities of daily living, and the economic and social supports available to them. Reaction time (RT) measures correlated higher with objective health than any other dependent variable. In fact, the only consistent predictors of reaction time and serial learning were both the subjective and objective measures of health.

nition is that between hypertension and cognitive function.

Most investigators have found that elevated diastolic blood pressure is associated with poor performance on several types of neuropsychological tests. From comparisons of clinically derived health examinations, magnetic resonance brain images, and neuropsychological performance in 113 neurologically healthy subjects from 55 to 85 years of age, the strongest contribution to a decline in cognitive function was hypertension (Ylikoski et al., 2000). Anstey and Smith (1999) used a very comprehensive health status test battery and found that health status was directly and positively related to cognitive performance.

The strong relationship between hypertension and cognitive performance has also been supported by longitudinal evidence (Sands & Meredith, 1992). Even in a study of animal discrimination learning, mice selected for high blood pressure performed worse than mice selected for low blood pressure (Elias & Schlager, 1974).

An effect of cerebrovascular and coronary heart disease as well as atherosclerosis on sensory-motor speed is generally seen, although Earles and Salthouse (1995), finding a negative relationship between self-reported health and processing speed, indicated that this effect was weak.

Although the relationships between health and different types of cognition are not yet clearly understood, several conclusions can be drawn from information about health and cognition. First, studying health and cognition is extremely difficult. Researchers do not ask the same questions, use the same measurements and instruments, or even review the same literature. The effect of health may be relatively modest compared with the overall cognitive decline that is seen with aging; thus, investigators and reviewers can interpret these modest effects in different ways. Third, there is most certainly a survival effect (Stewart et al., 2000) operating in most studies of this nature. Even considering these problems, however, almost all studies, including the meta-analysis of Thomas and colleagues (1994), provide evidence that suggests a relationship between health and cognition. These positive findings and trends of relationship, not just intuition or wishful thinking, drive the continued interest and federal research funding in this area of study.

Physical Activity and Cognitive Function

Self-reported levels of physical activity, such as "high," "moderate," or "sedentary," have been used by some epidemiologists studying large samples to determine in older adults whether different levels of physical activity are related to cognitive function and psychological well-being. Not many of these large studies included cognition as a variable, however. Of the small number of them that did include cognition, little support was found for moderate or highly active older adults also having higher cognitive function.

Fitness and Cognitive Function

Hundreds of research studies have been conducted since 1975 in which the researchers sought answers to these questions: Do older adults who are physically fit maintain their cognitive function better than those who are sedentary? Can cognitive function of older adults be improved by participating in endurance training or other types of exercise programs? What types of exercise would improve cognition? What types of cognitive function benefit the most? In the first edition of this book (1995), the answer to the question of a general benefit was "perhaps," but the types of exercise that are beneficial and the types of cognition most benefited were far from clear. Results from studies were quite mixed, with cross-sectional studies generally supporting a relationship between fitness and cognition and intervention studies sometimes not supporting the relationship. Some thought that the largest effect was on tasks that relied on processes that support cognition, particularly information processing speed (reaction time). Others proposed that the greatest effects were on tasks that required attention and working memory. Still others thought that cognitive tasks that were complex might benefit the most, regardless of the type of cognition required.

Studies of Relationships of Fitness to Cognition

For the most part, the cross-sectional studies have supported a relationship between fitness levels and some type of cognitive function. Spirduso (1975) was the first to use an age-by–physical activity cross-sectional design to compare the reaction times of young and old exercisers and nonexercisers. In this design, people both young (~20) and old (≥60) who reported that they participated in vigorous physical exercise at least three times a week for at least 3 years were compared with young and old sedentary individuals. Spirduso concluded that the old exercisers were significantly and substantially faster at both simple and choice reaction tasks than the old nonexercisers but not significantly different from the 20-year-old participants. This general design was repeated several times with similar results (Emery et al., 1995; MacRae et al., 1995; Sherwood & Selder, 1979; Spirduso & Clifford, 1978), except in some cases the exercise groups of both age groups (old and young) were superior to the nonexercisers. In the only animal study of physical fitness and reaction time, a group of old rats that exercised aerobically for 6 months at high levels of intensity were able to maintain their fastest reaction times, whereas the reaction times of the old, sedentary rat group deteriorated over the 6 months (equivalent to about 18 human years). In this study, the exercised rats increased their oxidative capacity 100%, which is a much higher increase in fitness than has been recorded in studies of humans (Spirduso & Farrar, 1981). Botwinick and Storandt (1974) were the only research team that failed to find a positive relationship between habitual exercise participation and response speed.

The results from correlational studies also tend to support the fitness–cognitive relationship. Researchers of three different studies found that physiological measures such as pulmonary, hemodynamic, and blood chemistry variables and oxygen consumption were correlated with different types of choice reaction time (Chodzko-Zajko & Ringel, 1987; Clarkson-Smith & Hartley, 1989; Era, 1988) at low to moder-

ate levels, even when age, education, and vocabulary were statistically controlled.

One of the weaknesses in studies of relationships is that the research design does not provide a way to determine whether exercise caused faster reaction time or whether having a fast reaction time occurs more frequently in active than in inactive people. Also, the physical fitness of the participants in most of those studies was inferred from self-reports of their weekly exercise patterns. Those who claimed to have exercised consistently at a criterion-level intensity were assumed to be more fit than those who said they never exercised.

Exercise Intervention Studies

The results from cross-sectional and correlational studies were modestly supportive of the fitness–cognitive relationship, but the outcomes were mixed from the intervention studies. Colcombe and Kramer (2003) hypothesized that the reason the outcome was not clear was that the benefits of fitness are specific to the cognitive process required to complete a task, and that researchers were approaching the questions from four different conceptual frameworks and, consequently, were using four different categories of cognitive tasks. Although acknowledging that cognition is a very complex function and that substantial overlap might be present among some types, Colcombe and Kramer identified these categories as **processing speed, visuospatial processing, controlled processing,** and **executive control.** Therefore, the following evidence from intervention studies is organized according to these four categories.

Processing Speed The results from exercise intervention studies of processing speed were equivocal. Some investigators found exercisers to perform better on tests of reaction time (Clarkson-Smith & Hartley, 1989; Dustman et al., 1984; Rikli & Edwards, 1991). Also, Etnier and colleagues (1999) reported that in a sample of approximately 60 patients with chronic obstructive pulmonary disease, aerobic fitness level and pulmonary function were significant and substantial predictors of speed of processing. The authors concluded that aerobic fitness may lessen age-related declines in cognition even in a sample of participants with pulmonary limitations. But other investigators, such as Barry and colleagues (1966) and Blumenthal and Madden (1988), failed to find changes in reaction time accompanying improvements in aerobic capacity.

Visuospatial Processing This type of cognition requires multiple allocations of resources, that is, a considerable focus of attention to complete

Conceptual Frameworks of the Fitness–Cognition Relationship

In the first column, the conceptual category of information processing is listed. In the second column, the type of processing that is necessary to execute the psychomotor task is described. In the third column, example test items are described.

Category	Type of cognitive processing	Examples
Processing speed	Low-level neurological functioning; cognitive support system	React quickly to a stimulus Tap finger as rapidly as possible for 20 s Recognition memory
Visuospatial processing	Transformation or recall of visual and spatial information Requirement of effort	View three line drawings and later replicate them from memory Geometric shape rotation
Controlled processes	Use of cognitive control to complete a task	React to one of two or more stimuli (CRT)
Executive function	Planning, inhibition, and scheduling of mental procedures	Respond to a central cue but simultaneously suppress conflicting or irrelevant cues presented next to target stimulus item

Note: CRT – choice reaction time.

From Colcombe and Kramer (2003).

(Chodzko-Zajko, 1991; Chodzko-Zajko & Moore, 1994; Stones & Kozma, 1988). These authors proposed that tasks requiring focusing and refocusing, and especially those that require attention sharing, require more effort, and that it is this **effortful processing** that is most influenced by aging and by health and fitness levels. Tasks that require effortful processing may decline at a faster rate than noneffortful tasks and also may be more affected by the beneficial effects of a regular exercise program (Chodzko-Zajko et al., 1992; Stones & Kozma, 1988). But not all of the results of studies supported the resource allocation hypothesis, and Kramer and colleagues (2002) presented a vigorous dissent to the resource allocation hypothesis in favor of a fitness effect on executive control.

Controlled Processing Cognitive tasks that begin by requiring controlled, effortful processing but through practice can be processed automatically require controlled processing (Kramer et al., 1999). This category of cognitive function is based on the research of Schneider and Shiffrin (1977). An example task to tap this category of cognitive processing is a two-choice reaction time task (choice reaction time, or CRT) in which the subject reacts with the left hand to the letter C but with the right hand if the letter M appears. Rikli and Edwards (1991) reported a longitudinal intervention study in which CRT improved

after a 1-year exercise program and then remained stable through 2 more years of the exercise program. Their subjects ranged from 59 to 81 years, and the reaction times of the nonexercising subjects were significantly slower at the end of 3 years than they were at the beginning of the research project. Dustman and his group (1984), however, failed to find an exercise benefit on controlled processing (CRT). They did report an exercise effect on processing speed (simple reaction time, or SRT).

Executive Control A promising line of research in understanding the role of exercise in brain function is the link between executive control and fitness. Executive control includes the planning, scheduling, coordination, inhibition, and working memory functions of the brain. Advances in magnetic resonance imaging have provided evidence that executive control is served by the prefrontal and frontal lobes of the brain. Two links make this an important area of study. First, executive control seems particularly sensitive to aging, and neuroimaging indicates that age-related decline appears to be faster in the prefrontal and frontal lobes of the brain. Second, in earlier studies, circulatory decline, which could result in chronic, mild hypoxia, was disproportionately faster in these brain areas (Gur et al., 1987; Shaw et al., 1984; Warren et al., 1985).

Kramer et al. (1999) were the first to predict that an exercise intervention would influence cognitive tasks requiring executive control more than it would affect single operation tasks that stressed functions such as visual search, spatial attention, tracking (pursuit rotor), working memory, or perceptual comparisons. Older adults participated in either a 6-month walking program or a toning and stretching program. Numerous attention and memory tasks were administered before and after the intervention. The authors found significant improvements in the walking group on those aspects of the attention tasks that required executive control. Furthermore, the fitness changes that occurred in the walking group, as measured by $\dot{V}O_2$max tests, indicated that a change in fitness was related to increases in executive control.

Two other studies, although not recognized at the time for using tasks that required executive control to complete, also supported the proposal that executive control is a major brain function that is influenced by both aging and fitness level (Abourezk & Toole, 1995; Hawkins et al., 1992). Hillman and colleagues (2002) extended these findings to show that both age and fitness affected the electroencephalographic **motor preparation period** preceding a movement to be made in response to an executive control task. Good reviews of the fitness–executive function rationale are provided by Hall and colleagues (2001) and Hawkins and colleagues (1992).

Do Exercise Interventions Affect the Four Categories of Cognitive Function Differently? Colcombe and Kramer (2003) concluded from their meta-analysis of previous intervention studies that aerobic fitness training has a beneficial effect on the cognition of sedentary adults. The effect appeared to be most beneficial for executive control but also very beneficial for controlled processing and visuospatial processing (figure 9.2). A combination of endurance and strength training had more effect than an endurance program alone, and a short training program was as effective as a moderate length program. Longer periods of training were even more effective.

Electrophysiological Evidence of a Fitness–Cognition Relationship

An issue concerning the use of behavioral reaction time as a measure of processing speed (SRT, CRT) is that behavioral reaction time also includes noncognitive components such as the time necessary for the impulse to travel to the muscle and the time taken by the muscle to contract. Accordingly, several investigators fractionated reaction time into its components

and analyzed premotor time, which reflects primarily central processing time. The same experimental paradigm used by Spirduso (1975)—groups of young and old exercised and nonexercised subjects—was used in three studies in which the responses were fractionated. Two of these studies (Clarkson, 1978; MacRae et al., 1995) confirmed earlier findings that the simple and choice reaction times of old exercisers were faster than those of sedentary individuals, but the fractionation technique also revealed that the major contributor to the significant differences was an exercise difference in the component that best represents the beginning of the response, the **premotor time (PMT)**. This can be seen in figure 9.3, where the PMT, which in this protocol accounts for 70% of the SRT, is substantially shorter in the exercisers. The contractile time is also shorter, but it contributes only 30% to the SRT. Only one group of investigators (Panton et al., 1990), who analyzed six reaction time trials before and after an exercise program, failed to find a robust relationship between premotor time and physical fitness.

The question of the relationship between aerobic fitness and cognitive events can be pursued even further: Can brain function, represented by brain waves, be related to fitness? Event-related potentials (ERPs; measured by electroencephalography, EEG) are electrophysiological responses in the brain to external stimuli such as a flash of light (visual), a sound (audi-

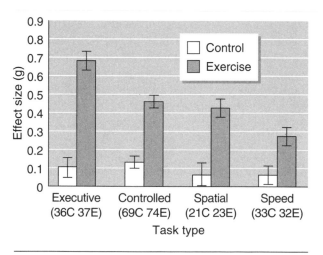

Figure 9.2 Effect sizes for the four different theoretical hypotheses concerning the nature of the process-based specificity of fitness training. Parenthetical notations indicate the number of effect sizes contributing to the point estimates for each category in the exercise (E) and nonexercise (C) groups.

Journals of Gerontology. Series A, Biological Sciences and Medical Sciences by S.J. Colcombe. Copyright 2003 by Gerontological Society of America. Reproduced with permission of Gerontological Society of America in the format textbook via Copyright Clearance Center.

A Meta-Analysis of Fitness Effects on Cognition

Eighteen exercise intervention studies were selected for meta-analysis on the basis of whether (a) groups were randomly assigned, (b) exercise program was supervised, (c) exercise program included aerobic exercise, and (d) participants were 55 years or older. Effect sizes were compared for types of cognitive function, types of training (cardiovascular or cardiovascular plus strength), program duration (short, 1-3 months; medium, 4-6 months; or long, >6 months), exercise session duration (short, 15-30 min; moderate, 31-45 min; or long, 46-60 min), gender (high male, <60% female; high female, ≥60% female), and age (young-old, 55-65; mid-old, 66-70; old-old, 71-75).

Exercise benefits were significant for all types of cognitive processing, especially executive control processing, where fitness training increased cognitive performance more than one half of a standard deviation. Beneficial effects were also significant for controlled processing and visuospatial processing and somewhat less beneficial (although significant) for processing speed. A combination of endurance and strength training had more effect than an endurance program alone, and a short training program (1-3 months) was as effective as a moderate-length program (4-6 months) but not as effective as longer periods of training (>6 months). An exercise session from 31 to 45 min was most effective, but longer sessions were also beneficial (46-60 min). Short exercise sessions of 15 to 30 min were not beneficial. Women benefited more than men, and mid-old (66-70) and old-old (71-75) subjects benefited more than young-old (55-65).

From Colcombe and Kramer (2003).

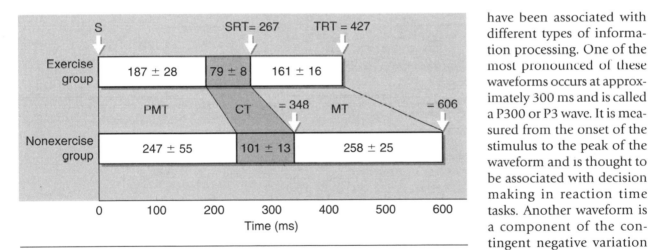

Figure 9.3 Differences between exercised and sedentary subjects' fractionated reaction time components. When a stimulus (S) is presented, the subject reacts by removing the foot from an accelerator pedal and placing it as quickly as possible on a brake pedal. The total response time (TRT) can be fractionated into the simple reaction time (SRT), which in turn is composed of premotor time (PMT) and contractile time (CT). The movement time (MT) is the time (in milliseconds) from the release of the accelerator pedal to the contact of the brake pedal. Exercisers were significantly faster than nonexercisers on all components (Baylor & Spirduso, 1988).

have been associated with different types of information processing. One of the most pronounced of these waveforms occurs at approximately 300 ms and is called a P300 or P3 wave. It is measured from the onset of the stimulus to the peak of the waveform and is thought to be associated with decision making in reaction time tasks. Another waveform is a component of the contingent negative variation (EEG) that is associated with movement preparation. The amplitude of this component was compatible with high preparation ability in older exercisers (Hillman et al., 2002). The amplitude of this component was considerably lower in old sedentary subjects compared with the amplitudes of the old exercisers and the two younger groups.

tory), skin contact (tactile), or movement of a body part (kinesthetic). The ERP technique is described in more detail in chapter 7. In studies where ERPs are obtained in a reaction time paradigm, the ERPs may provide a measure of information processing time that is the least contaminated with the motor aspects of the task. Various waveforms of the ERP

Two research teams independently reported that visual evoked potentials (VEPs) were indeed shorter for physically trained than for untrained men (Carlow et al., 1978; Dustman et al., 1990; Emmerson et al., 1989). Both the P3s and VEP late waves were significantly

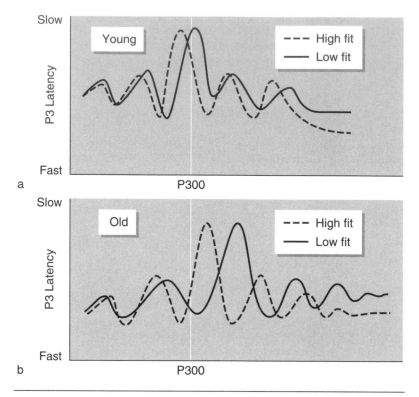

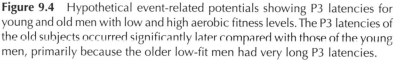

Figure 9.4 Hypothetical event-related potentials showing P3 latencies for young and old men with low and high aerobic fitness levels. The P3 latencies of the old subjects occurred significantly later compared with those of the young men, primarily because the older low-fit men had very long P3 latencies.

Adapted from *Neurobiology of Aging*, Vol. 11, R.E. Dustman et al., Age and fitness effects on EEG, ERPs, visual sensitivity, and cognition, pgs. 193-200, Copyright 1990, with permission from Elsevier.

faster in the young and old highly fit groups than in the low-fit groups, and the relationship between fitness and the EEG variables was stronger in the old subjects than in the young subjects. The P3 latencies of the old unfit men were much slower than those of the old fit men or either of the two younger groups (figure 9.4).

In summary, the results of many behavioral and neurophysiological analyses of processing speed strongly suggest that physical fitness is related to faster processing, and although the results from intervention studies are mixed, more researchers than not have found positive relationships.

Global Intelligence

Studies of the relationships among health, fitness, and intelligence have analyzed scores from the Wechsler Adult Intelligence Scale (WAIS; Wechsler, 1981) or subtests of that scale cross-sectionally either from groups identified as exercisers or nonexercisers or from groups measured before and after an exercise intervention program. The WAIS provides scores of

abilities that are thought to contribute to intelligence. The processing ability of the system (the hardware) is measured by fluid intelligence (problem solving). The ability to perform well on learned material, the database of intelligence, is called crystallized intelligence.

Earlier reports were that fluid intelligence does not seem to be related to health and fitness in normal adults (Blumenthal et al., 1989; Emery & Gatz, 1990; Perlmutter & Nyquist, 1990). Only Elsayed and colleagues (1980) reported an improvement in fluid intelligence following an exercise program. However, in patients with chronic obstructive pulmonary disease, aerobic fitness, as measured by the distance walked in 6 min, was substantially related to fluid intelligence (Etnier et al., 1999). The 6-min mile score predicted 28% of the variance in performance, even after education and depression scores were controlled

Crystallized intelligence, which is not very vulnerable to aging, does not seem to be strongly related to fitness (Elsayed et al., 1980; Perlmutter & Nyquist, 1990). The only positive findings regarding the relationship between fitness and intelligence were reported by Dustman and colleagues (1984), who found that their subjects who participated in an exercise program also improved their scores on the Culture–Fair Intelligence test.

Composite Score of Cognitive Function and Fitness

A composite score, which is created by combining scores from several tests designed to measure a construct, should better represent the construct than does the score of only one test. For example, a composite score combining simple reaction time, stimulus choice reaction time, response choice reaction time, and vocal reaction time should be a better measure of "reactive capacity" than any one of those tests alone, because each requires a unique combination of reactive systems. Therefore, a composite score of cognitive function can be expected to correlate more highly with an aggregate score of physical fitness than any single estimate of either construct, physical fitness or cognition. An example is shown in figure 9.5. Several researchers have found this to be true (e.g., Dustman et al., 1984).

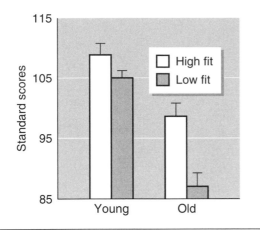

Figure 9.5 Cognitive performance of young and older men with low and high aerobic fitness levels. The cognitive factor measure was derived from scores on the following tests: Sternberg reaction time, Stroop color interference, symbol–digit modalities, and Trails B. Cognitive performance was better for young than older men and better for high-fit than low-fit men. Each mean was based on data for 15 subjects. The error bars are standard errors of the mean.

Adapted from *Neurobiology of Aging*, Vol. 11, R.E. Dustman et al., Age and fitness effects on EEG, ERPs, visual sensitivity, and cognition, pgs. 193-200, Copyright 1990, with permission from Elsevier.

exercise program; and 15 enrollees, who had joined the program after the initial measurements but several months before the final fitness assessments. (The groups were matched for socioeconomic status and intelligence.) Only the stay-ins differed from the other three groups on the aggregate functional fitness score, which was composed of tests of balance, vital capacity, flexibility, and the Digit Symbol Substitution (DSS) test. The stay-ins' aggregate functional fitness score, which included measures of reaction time, sensory function, DSS (WAIS), and anxiety, among others, improved after 1 year of the exercise program.

Psychological Outcomes and Cognitive Function

As depicted in figure 9.1 (p. 214), aerobic fitness plays a role in decreasing depression and anxiety as well as increasing self-efficacy and self-esteem. Research evidence has been accumulating for the past 10 years that these psychological outcomes are linked to enhanced cognitive function. This topic is discussed in more detail in chapter 10.

Stones and Kozma (1988) found that a composite score composed of several neuropsychological tests was related to levels of fitness that differed across five groups: a control group, a group planning to enter an exercise program, exercisers, masters athletes, and Elderhostelers (figure 9.6). Elderhostelers are older adults who participate in continuing education classes sometimes offered in foreign countries. Stones and Kozma (1988) considered Elderhostelers to be physically elite, successfully aging adults. The results of this study were particularly compelling because the groups were equated for socioeconomic status. Still, the groups with higher physical activity levels also tested higher in functional neuropsychological capabilities.

In another study, Stones and Kozma (1989) retested 200 subjects in an exercise intervention study 1 year after initial testing and classified them into four groups: stay-ins, 76 exercise participants who stayed in an exercise program and had a long history of activity; controls, 80 adults who never exercised; dropouts, 29 participants who dropped out of the

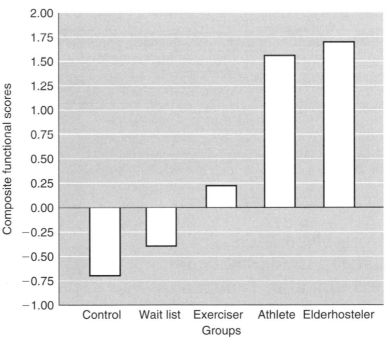

Figure 9.6 Composite functional scores of men varying in habitual exercise. Functional score was developed by combining scores of balance, flexibility, digit–symbol, and vital capacity. Control and wait list groups were men who did not habitually exercise. Exercisers were men who belonged to an exercise program for persons over the age of 50.

Adapted, by permission, from M.J. Stones and A. Kozma, 1988, Physical activity, age, and cognitive/motor performance. In *Cognitive development in adulthood: Progress in cognitive development research*, edited by M.L. Howe and C.J. Brainerd (New York: Springer-Verlag), 321. Copyright 1988 Springer-Verlag.

Bidirectional Relationships

So far the relationships that have been discussed flow from the left to the right of figure 9.1. That is, physical activity and exercise play a role in increasing health, aerobic fitness, and desirable psychological factors that influence cognitive function. However, it is becoming clear that relationships also flow from right to left in figure 9.1. Effective cognition is necessary to organize and maintain beneficial health habits, such as maintaining medical prescription schedules, eating a satisfactory diet, complying with medical appointments, and following other lifestyle behaviors that are conducive to good health. A minimal level of cognitive function is necessary to initiate physical activity, maintain an exercise program, and monitor body signals to regulate the activity. Individuals' levels of health and fitness also affect the types of physical activity that they can do and the frequency, intensity, and duration of exercise that they can tolerate.

> Health and fitness positively influence many types of brain function, but brain function also influences our ability and inclination to exercise.

When cognitive functions occur simultaneously with physical activities, cognitive attention must be shared (see chapter 7). Shumway-Cook and colleagues (1997) found that older adults experienced more difficulty in maintaining their balance on a force plate if at the same time they were trying to follow verbal instructions or do simple math problems. Thus, talking to someone else or listening to a talk show may cause an older adult to fall, drop a pot from the stove, or be unable to finish movement critical to a safe behavior.

Unresolved Issues Related to Health, Fitness, and Cognitive Function

Although correlational and behavioral research findings support some type of relationships among health, fitness, and cognitive function, and some intervention studies support the concept as well, several issues remain to be understood. First, which cognitive functions are influenced by health and fitness? The cognitive functions proposed by Colcombe and Kramer (2003) are a good beginning to answer this question. Second, must an improvement be seen in cognitive function accompanying an exercise program, or would a slower decline in cognitive function

be considered sufficient? Third, what is the minimum **exercise dose** necessary to provide the maximum health and fitness effect? In other words, is there an **exercise threshold effect**? Does exercise affect fitness via an **exercise ceiling effect,** above which greater benefits in cognitive function are not realized? Fourth, what type of physical activity or exercise is effective? Fifth, why does a discrepancy exist between correlational and **cross-sectional research** results and quasi-experimental study results?

Summary of the Fitness– Cognitive Function Relationship

Cross-sectional, correlational, and randomized experimental intervention studies support a relationship between fitness levels and several types of cognition. More research is needed to answer the unresolved issues enumerated previously and to determine the relative contributions that exercise makes directly and indirectly through mediators of cognition. The mechanisms through which exercise enhances cognition are being aggressively studied, and new technologies such as functional magnetic resonance imaging and methods to quantify genetic expression will prove to be rich sources of information about fitness and cognition over the next decade.

Mechanisms by Which Physical Activity May Benefit Cognition

Several mechanisms have been proposed to explain relationships among health, fitness, and cognitive function. This section will primarily focus on physiological mechanisms, but psychosocial explanations also have some validity.

Physiological Mechanisms

Exercise has been proposed to affect four major areas of brain function: cerebrovascular function, cerebral neurotransmitter balance and function, neuroendocrine and autonomic tone, and brain morphology directly. Many reviews of this have been published, the first of which was by Spirduso (1980) and, more recently, Boutcher (2000), Kramer and colleagues (2001), and Hall and colleagues (2001). These areas are illustrated in figure 9.7 as overlapping, interacting areas of primary aging. The proposed impact of exercise is shown by the arrow from exercise to the overlapping areas of aging. Thus, modulations in any

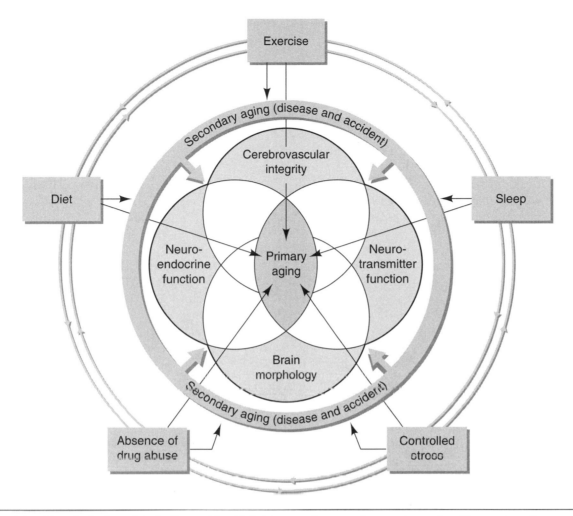

Figure 9.7 Hypothetical model of effects of health habits on primary and secondary aging. The center reflects primary aging of the systems that affect cognitive function: cerebrovascular changes, neurotransmitter depletion or malfunction, brain morphological changes, and neuroendocrine function deterioration. The shaded ring circling the primary aging core depicts factors of secondary aging that can accelerate primary aging: disease, accident, or environmental hazards. The outer ring indicates five health behaviors that may retard the development of both primary and secondary aging (depicted by arrows pointing toward primary and secondary aging). The arrows in the outer ring point in both directions and show that the five health behaviors are interrelated.

of the four major areas of brain function would affect the other three.

Cerebrovascular Integrity

Brain energy requirements, metabolism, and neurotransmitter turnover consume 20% to 25% of the available oxygen and glucose in the body (Friedland, 1990). Aerobic exercise increases the ability of red blood cells to carry more oxygen and to transport it to active cells. The combination of these two facts makes a link between cardiovascular integrity and cognitive function in older adults very attractive. Three mechanisms have been proposed to explain the way that moderate to high levels of physical fitness can maintain cerebrovascular integrity: (a) **angiogenesis,**

which is growth of capillary networks in brain tissue; (b) increased **oxygen transport;** and (c) increased cerebral blood flow and velocity.

Angiogenesis Angiogenesis (the growth of new capillaries) addresses exercise effects on primary aging. It had always been assumed that although exercise clearly increased capillary networks in exercised muscles, it had no effect on capillary beds in brain tissue. However, it has been shown that motor activity does indeed increase capillary networks in the brain, which would ensure an optimal blood supply to all tissue (Black et al., 1989; Jones et al., 1998).

Oxygen Transport The second hypothesized mechanism is that chronic exercise maintains cerebrovascular integrity by increasing oxygen transport, which in turn reduces brain hypoxia (lack of oxygen) in active brain regions. Several types of evidence are suggested to support this theory. First, cerebral hypoxia is common among older people in poor health, and cognitive performance in geriatric patients with chronic obstructive pulmonary disease seems to improve after oxygen administration. Second, cognitive performance is decreased in a high-altitude, oxygen-diminished environment. Third, oxygen is essential for the metabolism of glucose, the brain's fuel, and is a critical ingredient in the metabolism of such neurotransmitters as acetylcholine, dopamine, norepinephrine, and serotonin. Because many old adults exhibit mild hypoxia, an early intuitive remedy was oxygen inhalation (hyperoxia). Beneficial effects of supplemental oxygen on some psychological tests were reported, but the benefits were short term, lasting no more than 3 weeks (Jacobs, 1971). The oxygen transport hypothesis was never accepted, because it was pointed out that in healthy people the hemoglobin in arterial blood leaving the lungs is about 95% to 98% saturated with oxygen and that brain energy levels can be maintained even under moderate hypoxia (Gibson et al., 1961).

Also, oxygen transport may influence brain tissue in other ways. Exercise-induced increases in cytochrome oxidase, an enzyme necessary for a high-energy production compound (adenosine triphosphate) were found in the frontal cortex and striatum (McCloskey et al., 2001). The frontal cortex is associated with executive control functions, which have been linked to tasks that require higher order brain function. Another way that oxygen transport may influence brain tissue is that the synthesis of acetylcholine and the biogenic amines is susceptible to mild hypoxia. Synthesis of some neurotransmitters increases under conditions in which the oxygen level is higher than normal. The results from a substantial number of animal studies make a compelling case that exercise-related increases in oxygen transport and usage affect the metabolism of neurotransmitters, especially acetylcholine, and the biogenic amines, dopamine, norepinephrine, and serotonin.

Finally, in a recent series of four oxygen supplementation studies of young adults, Moss and his colleagues reported that 1 to 3 s of oxygen inhalation before a test battery, and 30 s of oxygen just before each test, improved some types of memory (Moss & Scholey, 1996; Moss et al., 1998; Scholey et al., 1998; Scholey et al., 1999). These studies should be replicated in older adults, because it is known that older adults have lower oxygen saturation levels.

Cerebral Blood Flow Another way that exercise might postpone cognitive aging is by its influence on total cerebral blood flow (CBF) and regional CBF. CBF is thought to be lower in older adults (Slosman et al., 2001), although there is some disagreement (Meltzer et al., 2000). Rogers and colleagues (1990) reported that the CBF of inactive retirees 62 to 70 years old significantly declined after 4 years of retirement, whereas the CBF of retirees who continued to work or who remained physically active during the 4 years was unchanged. These authors proposed several mechanisms (see table 9.1) by which regular physical activity may be beneficial to the brain, most of them related to the maintenance of CBF and the prevention of stroke, which can destroy brain tissue and greatly impair cognition. Even if total CBF does not change with physical activity or exercise, dramatic regional cerebrovascular blood flow shifts are associated not only with a specific movement but also with the ideation associated with that movement. The responsiveness of the regional blood flow shift

Table 9.1 Influence of Regular Physical Activity on Factors That May Retard Age-Related Cerebral Atherogenesis and Sustain Cognitive Functions

Regular physical activity	Beneficial result to brain
Decreases blood pressure	Reduces risk for stroke Assists in maintaining cerebral profusion
Reduces plasma levels of LDL	Reduces risk for atherogenesis Assists in maintaining CBF Reduces risk for stroke
Lowers excessive triglyceride levels	Improves CBF
Inhibits platelet aggregability	Maintains CBF Reduces risk for stroke
Activates the brain	Enhances cerebral metabolic demands, thereby increasing CBF
Improves brain vasculature	Promotes more efficient distribution of CBF[a]

Note: LDL = low-density lipoproteins; CBF = cerebral blood flow.

[a]From Black et al. (1987).

From Rogers et al. (1990).

mechanism to active brain tissue may play a role in maintaining functions related to those regions, and exercise-produced changes in blood chemistry remain a viable area of exploration for mechanisms to explain fitness–cognitive function relationships.

Glucose Utilization

The high metabolic activity of the brain requires 25% of the available glucose in the body. Glucose utilization may be compromised in elderly persons whose glucose tolerance is impaired. Hall and colleagues (1989) found poor glucose tolerance to be related to poorer memory. Glucose supplementation appears to enhance memory, more in old adults than in young (Kennedy & Scholey, 2000). Furthermore, in young adults, effective glucose metabolism influenced tasks that required greater cognitive demands than tasks with lighter cognitive demands (Scholey et al., 2001; Winder & Borrill, 1998). Manning and colleagues (1998) even provided evidence that increased glucose levels enhance specific stages of information processing, specifically memory storage and retrieval. Exercise has been shown to increase local cerebral glucose utilization in the striatum, motor cortex, and hippocampus (Vissing et al., 1996), and this linkage may be one of several different mechanisms by which exercise maintains cognition in older adults.

Neurotransmitter Function

Neurotransmitters are the biochemical messengers used by neurons to send neural impulses and to communicate with each other. Normal aging impairs the brain's ability to synthesize and degrade neurotransmitters, some neurotransmitters more than others. With aging, a gradual linear decline occurs in some neurotransmitters, two of the most notable being dopamine and norepinephrine. Pathological losses of specific neurotransmitters in late middle age and the resultant imbalances that occur in neurotransmitter function cause neurotransmitter-related diseases. For example, drastic losses of dopaminergic neurons and the concurrent imbalance between dopamine and acetylcholine causes Parkinson's disease, which is characterized by the inability to control movements. However, because dopamine synthesis gradually decreases with each year of normal aging, if everyone lived to be more than 100 years old, eventually everyone would display Parkinson-like symptoms. Other neurotransmitter-related diseases include Huntington's disease, which involves, among other losses, an insufficiency of γ-aminobutyric acid, and Alzheimer's disease, which involves a loss of cholinergic neurotransmitters. Other catecholamines also have been associated with

various types of brain function; thus, it is clear that optimal catecholamine function is essential for the performance of psychomotor tasks and many other types of cognitive function.

Several investigators have found that after exercise training, either whole-brain resting catecholamines (Brown et al., 1979) or other characteristics of the catecholamine neurotransmitters in rats changed in a direction counter to the age-associated changes normally seen (Gilliam et al., 1984; MacRae et al., 1987). Fordyce and Farrar (1991b) observed enhancement of brain cholinergic functioning and spatial learning in the same rats after 14 weeks of running training. They also found exercised-induced cholinergic changes only in the brain hippocampus (an area associated with spatial learning) and not in two other areas, the parietal and frontal cortexes, which are responsible for somatosensory and motor functions, respectively (Fordyce & Farrar, 1991a). The evidence from many studies is substantial that exercise training–induced changes in neurotransmitters are relatively long-lasting (Holmes, in press).

Neurohormonal System

Acute exercise bouts increase arousal of the central nervous system and facilitate some types of information processing (for a review, see Tomporowski & Ellis, 1986). Neural activation and stimulation of the ascending reticular activating system (ARAS) influence attention processes, and physical activity activates the ARAS. For example, there is evidence that the CNS of the elderly is underaroused compared with the young and that neuromuscular stimulation of the ARAS via postural changes (lying to sitting to standing) and exercise (to 40% of maximum heart rate) decreases age differences in CNS processing speed (Woods, 1981). Through this mechanism, chronic activity may enhance the ability of individuals to control attention (Woodruff, 1985).

Chronic exercise also may tune neuroendocrine adaptations (figure 9.7, p. 223). The neuroendocrine theory of aging suggests that the neuroendocrine system accelerates aging through hormonal actions on target brain cells (Landfield & Lynch, 1977). For example, aging impairs glucose tolerance and reduces the production of growth hormones and adrenocorticosteroids. Conversely, physical conditioning improves the response to glucose and stimulates growth hormone, thus enhancing the transport of amino acids across cell membranes for protein synthesis. Therefore, staying physically fit may maintain general hormonal regulation such that key enzymatic responses to many different tasks also are maintained.

Physiological Mechanisms: Effect of Fitness on Cognitive Function

The left column of this table describes the physiological mechanisms that are proposed as beneficiaries of exercise that enhance cognition, and the right column describes how the mechanism might work.

Mechanisms	Proposed action of exercise
Cerebrovascular integrity	
Angiogenesis	Develops new blood capillaries
Oxygen transport	Increases oxygen transport; reduces brain hypoxia
Cerebral blood flow	Enhances regional blood flow to active brain areas
Glucose utilization	Increases glucose utilization in brain areas associated with memory
Neurotransmitter (N) function	Increases synthesis and actions of NT that are counter to aging effects on NTs
Neurohormonal function	Maintains hormonal regulation; increases arousal of central nervous system
Neurotrophin function	Enhances maintenance, protection, and growth of neurons
Morphological changes	Changes neuronal structures and dendritic branching Maintains brain tissue volume

Neurotrophins

Neurotrophins, proteins that maintain, protect, and promote growth in neuronal populations, connect with neurons synaptically. Several types of neurotrophins have been identified, and they influence cells in two ways: directly, and by traveling along nerve axons both to and away from the cell body. Two decades ago the most that was known about neurotrophins, aging cognition, and exercise was that they might be related and that they were a promising area to research (Spirduso, 1980). Much evidence is now available that exercise profoundly influences the neurotrophic system. (Holmes, in press). Rats that exercised had higher levels of several types of neurotrophins (e.g., Chen et al., 1998; Russo-Neustadt et al., 2001).

Exercise-Induced Morphological Changes

As the brain ages, many **morphological changes** occur. The volume of brain tissue begins to decline as early as the late 20s and continues to decrease throughout life. Neurons swell, axons (nerve cables) shrink, and dendrites (the projections along which neurons communicate with each other) are lost. The dendritic shape also changes, which affects the neurons' ability to communicate with each other. Old brain tissue, when examined under a microscope, has a very different structure than young brain tissue. Furthermore, the rate of these detrimental age-related morphological changes is different not only for different areas of the brain but for different layers of the brain within an area (Diamond & Connor, 1982).

Animal research provides considerable evidence, however, that morphological brain changes, such as changes in neuronal cell structure, number, and density, are affected by experience, including motor activity. Primates living in movement-enriched environments (i.e., large, room-size cages in which there were toys, ample space to move, and other primates with which to interact) had enhanced morphological changes above and beyond those of primates that were caged alone and also above those of animals that could interact and communicate with other primates but had no opportunity to be physically active (Floeter & Greenough, 1979). Young rats that were forced to use one limb more than the other revealed large morphological changes in the brain areas that controlled the overused limb but not in the brain areas of the underused limb. Also, whole-brain weight is lower in inactive animals compared with active ones (Pysh & Weiss, 1979), although no one has suggested any interesting interpretations of this observation.

Long ago, Vogt and Vogt (1946) proposed that frequent use of neurons postponed nerve cell aging. Nerve cells that are active also have a better chance of retaining their maintenance operations. The brain is very plastic, and several researchers have shown that enhanced movement can produce structural changes. Vigorous exercise also induces new capillary growth in some brain regions of rats (Black et al., 1990; Jones et al., 1998) so that the enhanced metabolic activity of the brain can be supported. An enriched environment that promotes manipulation of objects and encourages physical activity also has been associated with the recovery of brain function in animals that have been brain damaged. For example, rats recovering from sensorimotor lesions of the brain in a movement-enriched environment recovered to greater levels of function than did rats living alone in standard housing (i.e., wire mesh cages; Held et al., 1985; Gentile et al., 1987). The rats that lived in standard housing were movement-impoverished animals, a condition that appears to impair both the rate and the extent of brain function recovery.

Although **brain plasticity** is present in old brain and morphological changes take place in even very old animals (Diamond et al., 1985), the process is not as efficient as in young animals. The plasticity of the brain, as well as activity-induced development of vascular support, begins to decline in middle age (Black et al., 1989). Thus, Black and colleagues (1991) suggested that the major contributions that enriched, complex environments can make to successful aging occur in early youth, when the development of morphological enhancement and vascular support for brain tissue provides a "neural reserve" that can be drawn on in senescence, much as a healthful diet and active lifestyle during youth can develop optimal bone mineral density that later in life can postpone the development of osteoporosis.

A dramatic demonstration of cardiovascular fitness associations with brain tissue volume was recently reported by Colcombe and colleagues (2003). Using high-resolution magnetic resonance imaging scans, these authors showed that the losses of brain tissue that are routinely seen in older frontal, parietal, and temporal cortexes were substantially reduced in adults who were physically fit, even when other factors were controlled statistically.

Results from animal research support the premise that exercise-mediated changes at the cellular level enhance neural transmission, either by structural or chemical modifications, and may explain the effects of exercise on cognition and learning.

Mechanisms That Indirectly Benefit Cognition

Exercise may also indirectly affect brain function by preventing secondary aging. One of several good health habits (which include optimal nutrition, adequate sleep, stress control, and absence of drug use), exercise helps prevent the accelerated aging such as occurs from diabetes or alcoholism. The indirect effect of exercise on aging may operate through the prevention of accidents or disease (such as diabetes) that may produce secondary aging effects. This is illustrated in figure 9.7 (p. 223) by the wide-band arrows directed toward the circle depicting secondary aging. Finally, exercise also may act indirectly by enhancing and supplementing other health habits, such as sleep, diet, and freedom from drug use, to postpone premature aging. This influence is also shown in figure 9.7 by the outer circle of lines that connect all five health habits.

Prevention, Postponement, or Mediation of Disease

Primary aging is normal aging. Secondary aging occurs in the presence of disease and environmental accidents or insults. Cardiovascular disease, adult-onset diabetes, hypokinetic disease, and some types of hypertension accelerate the primary aging process. As discussed previously, these diseases are thought to impair cognitive function. Habitual and moderately intensive exercise dramatically decreases the incidence of cardiovascular disease, atherosclerosis, and hypertension. The absence of these diseases reduces the probability of cerebrovascular plaques, microaneurisms, and ministrokes, which have extremely negative effects on brain tissue function. Cardiovascular conditioning enhances cerebrovascular function by increasing aerobic capacity through increased stroke volume and oxygen extraction in older adults (Boutcher et al., 1998). Exercise helps maintain appropriate body weight, which in turn helps to prevent adult-onset diabetes.

Complementary Health Habits

One relationship that is repeatedly seen in the exercise literature is that people who exercise also tend to have better complementary health habits than nonexercisers. People who exercise have higher socioeconomic and education levels and report higher levels of well-being, all of which are associated with more positive health habits. Usually, habitual exercisers do not smoke or drink excessively, they try to maintain a relatively healthy diet, and they are also at least conscious of the need to control stress. For many, stress control was a motivating factor in beginning an exercise program. As people continue in an exercise program, they may become more and more motivated to improve health habits that counter secondary aging. These beneficial health habits have indirect positive effects on cognition, as shown in figure 9.8. The reduction of cardiovascular disease risk factors, such as increased pulmonary function, lowered blood lipids, controlled adiposity, and low blood pressure, indirectly optimizes the cerebral environment. Exercising enables older adults to eat more calories, which enhances the probability that they will consume at least the minimum dietary components necessary for good health.

Physical fitness may be associated with better cognitive function, because people who are physically fit report that they have fewer sleep problems. If individuals are physically fit, exercise vigorously, and do so at a time not too near bedtime, the exercise may enhance the first sleep cycle of the night (Anch et al., 1988). Sleep provides an energy conservation function, and to the extent that exercise improves the quality of sleep for older individuals, exercise also may contribute to conserving energy necessary for some types of cognitive function.

With regard to the role of complementary health habits in maintaining cognitive function in the elderly, some individuals have a genetic predisposition to greatly reduced cardiovascular risk factors, good sleep patterns, excellent cognition, and behavioral tendencies to eat good diets, so the secondary effects of exercise (or lack of it) would not affect them. This might explain why some people who live totally sedentary lives live a long time and appear to maintain their cognitive function very well.

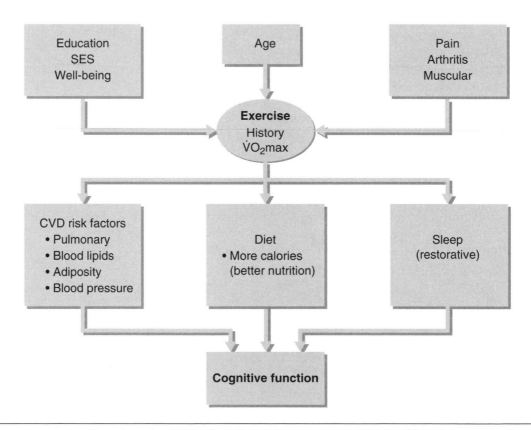

Figure 9.8 The relationships of moderating and mediating factors on cognition in older adults. Age, education level, socioeconomic status (SES), and well-being all are known to influence positively (+) an individual's physical activity pattern. Arthritis and muscular pain also have a negative (–) influence on exercise. Habitual exercise prevents or postpones cardiovascular disease (CVD) and beneficially affects sleep. Also, habitual moderate to intense exercise allows individuals to maintain their weight while eating more calories, which in older adults increases the probability that they will eat enough to obtain all of the minimum daily requirements for good nutrition.

Psychosocial Mechanisms of Exercise Effects on Cognition

The possibility that complementary health habits may counter secondary aging and thus influence cognition in older adults leads some critics to suggest that it is the constellation of health and personality behaviors that exercisers have that produces superior scores on tests of cognitive function.

Psychosocial explanations suggest that none of the proposed biological or neurophysiological mechanisms are valid, because what appears to be a relationship between physical fitness and cognitive function is really an indirect result of a relationship between physical fitness and other factors that are also related to cognitive function. Chronic exercisers differ from nonexercisers in many ways other than just exercise habits. They differ genetically in at least some traits. For example, people self-selected for endurance activity differ from inactive people on the basis of inherited traits relevant to muscle fiber composition (Suominen et al., 1980). Presumably, the same is true of sprinters, for whom having a high proportion of fast-twitch muscle fiber is an advantage. Just as exercisers have genetic differences in physical attributes such as fiber types, they also differ genetically in psychosocial factors. Superior performance in several types of psychosocial behaviors has been associated with people who are in better physical health (Milligan et al., 1984).

People who exercise regularly have less physical impairment; higher life satisfaction, income, educational level, and cognitive ability (Stones & Kozma, 1989); and a more positive attitude (Clarkson-Smith & Hartley, 1989). It is also probable that people who are more mentally capable are more likely to exercise because of their increased awareness of the health benefits of exercise. Cohort differences in combinations of all of these factors make it extremely difficult to tease out a relationship between fitness and cognitive function. Furthermore, lack of education and a low socioeconomic status are correlated with slow psychomotor speed (Era, 1988), a relationship that is more pronounced in longitudinal studies (Lehr & Thomae, 1973). Variables such as socioeconomic status, intelligence, state of anxiety, motivation, and instructional set all interact with the measurement of response speed and have not been well controlled in research studies.

Converging Lines of Evidence

The converging lines of evidence that health and physical fitness benefit cognitive function in older adults are compelling. The results of cross-sectional, correlational, randomized intervention studies as well as animal studies are strong. Behavioral and psychosocial outcomes of exercise are beneficial. Research activity on this topic has increased over the past 10 years, not only in the number of studies funded but in the broad variety of disciplines involved and in the speed with which new technology is applied to the question of fitness and cognition. These factors strongly support the viability of the health, fitness, and cognition relationship.

Process by Which Fitness May Benefit Cognitive Function

If regular aerobic exercise indeed enhances cognitive function, does it do so at all ages or are the effects more beneficial and more apparent in older individuals whose cognitive processing speed is declining? Can the effects be derived from many different acute bouts of exercise, or is a long-term, lifestyle exercise program necessary?

Are Benefits of Exercise the Same for Young and Old?

Does exercise enhance cognitive function at all ages (additive effects) or just in older adults (nonadditive)? If exercise effects are additive, then those who exercise, no matter what age, would simply enjoy an added benefit of better cognition. But if the effects are nonadditive, then the older individuals get, the more they would benefit from exercise-induced health and fitness. Stones and Kozma (1988) articulated these two possible models very well, calling them the tonic and overpractice effect model (TOPE; additive) and the moderator effects model (nonadditive; see figure 9.9). This model proposes that chronological age and lifestyle factors contribute independently to functional age at all ages. Exercise has a generalized (i.e., tonic) effect across physical and psychological domains. It does not postpone or change the rate of aging on respective functions, but it does compensate somewhat for age-related deterioration in functional capability. The possible mechanisms by which this model operates were discussed earlier in this chapter. In the TOPE model, exercise also provides an overpractice effect, like that seen in the skillful execution of familiar movement patterns that are relatively unimpaired in older people who practice systematically. If the TOPE model is correct,

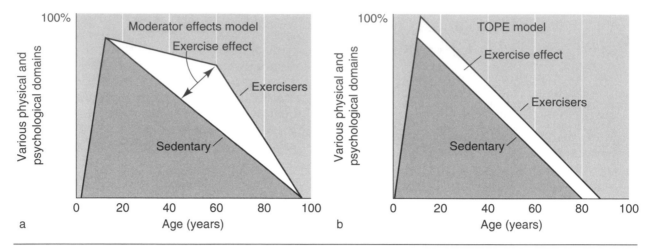

Figure 9.9 Regular exercise may postpone premature mental aging. *(a)* In the moderator effects model, high physical fitness plays an increasingly important role with each increasing age decade in postponing aging symptoms. *(b)* The TOPE, or tonic and overpractice effect, model proposes that exercise produces a tonic physiological effect for all ages and optimizes cognitive function at every age, thus postponing premature cognitive aging.

Adapted, by permission, from M.J. Stones and A. Kozma, 1988, Physical activity, age, and cognitive/motor performance,. In *Cognitive development in adulthood: Progress in cognitive development research*, edited by M.L. Howe and C.J. Brainerd (New York: Springer-Verlag), 321. Copyright 1988 Springer-Verlag.

investigators should find that exercisers at all ages are superior to sedentary individuals on tests of various types of cognitive function, especially those that require information processing speed. The results of several studies support this model (Dustman et al., 1984; Stacey et al., 1985; Stones & Kozma, 1988; Vanfraechem & Vanfraechem, 1977).

The moderator effects model suggests that the more people age (up to a point), the more exercise moderates the natural decline in cognitive function that accompanies aging. This model implies a change in the rate of functional aging and exercise benefits that are greater for the old than for the young. Research supporting this model would have to find differential effects of exercise favoring the elderly; that is, the exercise factor must benefit the older subjects more than the young. Research results supporting this model are mixed, but there are many complicating factors. One is that researchers have for the most part used raw or standard scores for this analysis, and function scores (for old and young) would be a more rigorous test for this interaction. Another factor is that inactive subjects within the older age groups are less active than the inactive 20-year-olds, and the young active subjects are probably more active. Thus, old inactive males who are less active than young inactive males produce a weak interaction between physical activity patterns and age. No investigators have conducted a study in which young and old subjects were matched on the percent of maximum, frequency, and duration that they exercised. Thus, in cross-sectional studies, the exercise factor gets weaker within each additional decade, so it is difficult to compare the interaction of aging and exercise effects when the amount of exercise is not controlled across decades.

Do Benefits Occur From Acute Exercise Bouts or Long-Term Exercise Effects?

A question that requires considerably more research is whether habitual exercise produces long-term physiological changes, acute positive effects following each bout, or both. That is, if beneficial effects occur every time exercise occurs, and if exercise occurs every day, then positive effects could occur even if long-term effects did not. From several reviews, it appears that acute bouts of exercise may enhance attention, working memory, and the ability to time movement patterns (Etnier & Landers, 1997; Tomporowski, 2003; Tomporowski & Ellis, 1986). The hypothesized mechanism is that acute bouts of exercise, as occur with psychostimulant drugs, produce changes in state processes that enhance the allocation of attentional resources (Tomporowski, 2003). That is, moderate exercise produces a physiological state that enables individuals to perform some types of cognitive tasks rapidly and efficiently.

Acute bouts of exercise also can have negative effects on cognitive performance, if the exercise bout is continued to fatigue or results in dehydration. The individual's fitness level plays a role in the extent to which the exercise bout is fatiguing. Very little is known about the interaction between acute and habitual exercise effects, but it promises to be a topic of great interest in the future.

Implications of a Physical Activity–Cognition Relationship for Older Adults

The potential benefit of physical fitness for enhancing the quality of life of the elderly through improved cognition and psychosocial functioning is extremely large, especially if exercise programs, if not a lifelong habit, can be initiated in the 5th or 6th decades. Exercise programs, especially for the elderly who are not yet frail, are so inexpensive and feasible that even small cognitive advantages to be gained by a small percentage of adults would be cost effective. Even if the cognitive benefits of an exercise program are small for some individuals, small benefits over a long number of years can make a large difference in function. Also, for elderly adults who have lost considerable cognitive abilities, small gains, or just maintenance of existing function, are extremely important.

The two primary individual attributes for which elderly individuals are admitted to nursing homes are dysfunction in physical and cognitive functions, both of which may be improved by physical activity (Guralnik et al., 1994; Williams & Hornberger, 1984). Thus, the efforts that are presently underway to enhance the national conscience regarding the benefits of exercise and to increase the numbers of persons who are physically active are likely to result in fewer individuals being admitted to nursing homes on the basis of physical or even cognitive deficiencies. For long-term benefits, exercise programs in public schools and adult educational curricula cost relatively little but have the potential to improve behavioral health habits, which can substantially decrease individuals' health costs as they age.

SUMMARY

It is highly probable that health status and physical fitness have beneficial effects on cognitive functioning in older adults. In cross-sectional and correlational studies, the cognitive function of highly aerobically fit adults is almost always higher in the physically active individuals. The results of exercise intervention studies are mixed, with some researchers finding beneficial effects and others failing to find them. Several reasons have been proposed to explain why exercise interventions may not always result in superior performance. One is that subjects of exercise intervention studies rarely approach the levels of fitness that habitual exercisers have, nor do they have a long history of exercise, which may be necessary for some long-term neural adaptations to take place. Another is that the influences of exercise on cognition may be small and subtle but important in older adults. It is not yet clear what types of cognitive function are influenced by health and fitness. Mixed results have been found in studies of information processing time, working memory, attention, perceptual processes, and psychomotor control. Recently, several researchers have found that **executive function** may be particularly sensitive to health and fitness status.

Several mechanisms by which exercise and physical activity might influence primary aging of cognitive function have been proposed: improvements in cerebrovascular integrity, glucose utilization, neurotransmitter depletion and imbalance, neurohormonal adaptations, neurotrophins, and exercise-induced morphological changes. Exercise also is highly likely to have strong influences on secondary aging, in that exercise plays a role in preventing disease, encouraging complementary health habits, and providing beneficial psychosocial supports for cognition. Although the results of studies have not unanimously confirmed exercise to have a causative positive effect on cognition, so many lines of evidence are converging to support the hypothesis that it is very compelling.

Fitness may benefit cognitive function in older adults more than in young adults. The good news is that research suggests that exercise programs do not have to be of high intensity to have beneficial results. Low to moderate levels of physical activity conducted over longer periods of time may be more effective than shorter, more intense exercise programs.

REVIEW QUESTIONS

1. Following are several indicators of health or fitness. In what order would you rank them to provide the most valid and reliable indicator of the role that exercise may play in the maintenance or improvement of cognitive function, and why? (1 = highest)
   - Health (self-reported)
   - Physical activity levels (observed by a professional)
   - $\dot{V}O_2$max (treadmill test)
   - Health (health professional clinical assessment)
   - $\dot{V}O_2$max + composite scores of cardiac risk factors
   - Physical activity levels (self-reported)

2. What types of cognition seem to be the most related to physical fitness?

3. What is meant by the statement, "The relationship between fitness and cognition is a two-way street?"

4. What are the differences between direct and indirect effects of health and fitness and cognition?

5. What major types of exercise-induced long-term physiological changes might explain a relationship between fitness levels and cognitive function?

SUGGESTED READING

Kramer, A.F., Hahn, S., McAuley, E., Cohen, N.J., Banich, M.T., Harrison, C., Chason, J., Boileau, R.A., Bardell, L., Colcombe, A., & Vakil, E. (2001). Exercise, aging and cognition: Healthy body, healthy mind? In A.D. Fisk & W. Rogers (Eds.), *Human factors interventions for the health care of older adults* (pp. 91-120). Hillsdale, NJ: Erlbaum.

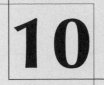

Health-Related Quality of Life

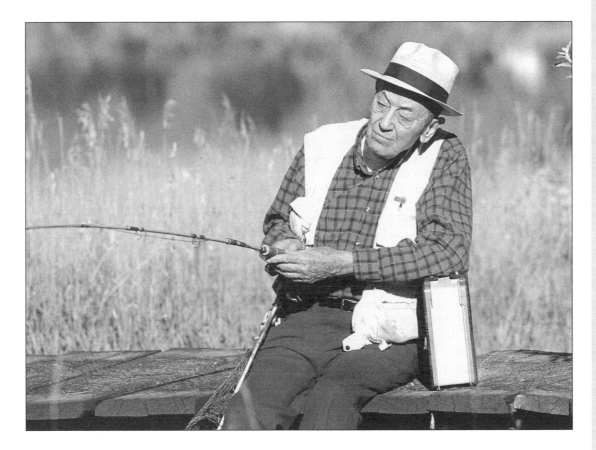

The objectives of this chapter are

- to explore the components of health-related quality of life and their relation-ships,

- to describe the way that subjective well-being is defined and organized for study,

- to show how health and fitness relate to subjective well-being and how enhancing them affects well-being,

- to explain how different characteristics of exercise may or may not influence various components of well-being, and

- to describe various mechanisms that have been proposed to explain relation-ships of health, exercise, and quality of life.

Quality of life in dictionary terms means the goodness, excellence, or fineness of life. But whether life is good or excellent really depends not on an absolute dictionary definition but on how each person defines goodness. In fairy tales, the goal of happiness is achieved by being healthy, wealthy, wise, and loved. In real life, it is a much more complicated matter. Several components of the quality of life for the elderly were introduced in chapter 1 (figure 1.15, p. 27). One of these components is perception of well-being and life satisfaction.

This chapter first describes the theoretical framework used to discuss quality of life and then discusses each component of the framework: emotional well-being, perceptions of self, bodily well-being, global perceptions of well-being, and life satisfaction. Following the description of each component, its relationship to health, physical function, and exercise is discussed. Next, the characteristics of fitness and exercise that seem to moderate well-being are addressed. The chapter concludes with a discussion of potential mechanisms by which physical activity and exercise may influence well-being.

Quality of Life

Physical health has three dimensions that relate to quality of life: physical condition, functional status, and subjective health. **Physical condition** is the presence and number of professionally diagnosed health problems experienced by an individual. A small percentage of older persons are free of chronic diseases, but most individuals over age 70 experience one or more, with hypertension, cardiovascular disease, asthma, diabetes, arthritis, and osteoporosis. Approximately 5.4 million persons over the age of 65 are living with one or more disabilities and require help with personal care and home management (Gill, 2002). Estimates are that the number of persons in the United States with chronic disease will increase 50% by 2040 (Freudenheim, 1996), so actual health conditions are a concern for most elderly adults and will be a greater concern for society in the future.

The second aspect of physical health is **functional health status,** or the degree to which these physical conditions prevent persons from being able to execute activities of daily living (ADLs, i.e., self-care activities), instrumental activities of daily living (IADLs, i.e., preparing meals, doing housework, and having the mobility to go outside), and discretionary activities (hobbies, recreation, and social contacts).

Subjective health status, the personal evaluation that individuals make about their own health, is the third facet of physical health. Subjective health varies greatly among people. For example, a woman who has two serious physical conditions that substantially constrain her activities may believe that her health is average, or even above average for her age, whereas another woman with only one, minimally constraining physical condition may consider her health to be poor or unacceptable. However, many people who live with physical conditions use various coping mechanisms to tolerate the condition, and it is not uncommon to find that most people rate their health as "average" or "better than average," even in groups in which almost everyone has some type of chronic condition. Much of the way people view their health depends on their life experiences, their goals, and the coping mechanisms that they use to deal with failure and disappointments.

Because health is a multifaceted dimension and is interpreted differently by different people, it is very difficult to measure and to relate to other dimensions of life. Some investigators focus on the number and type of physical conditions that people have to assess their health. Others emphasize the functional capacities of the elderly, using the ADL and IADL instruments to measure the degree to which the subjects can perform the basic, instrumental activities of daily living. Others measure subjective health by administering single-item subjective health assessments or by using ordinal scales, such as having subjects rate their own health on the basis of the steps of a ladder. Placing themselves on the bottom step (a score of 1) indicates that subjects believe they have a serious illness, whereas placing themselves on the top step (a score of 9) would indicate their belief that they are in perfect health. These types of tests have relatively low reliability and validity. Nevertheless, despite the type of health or the method of measurement, these indexes of health have generally been found to be significantly related to feelings of well-being and life satisfaction.

Good health is freedom from disease, and although it is a foundation of physical fitness, it is not synonymous with fitness. Some older individuals are relatively free of chronic diseases, or they may be presymptomatic and not yet experiencing the negative functional consequences of their diseases, but they are not physically fit in terms of having acceptable flexibility (chapter 3), aerobic capacity (chapter 4), and strength and endurance (chapter 5) for their age. The definitions of physical fitness, physical activity, and physical function in older adults are discussed in detail in the beginning of chapter 9. Much of what is known about the role of health and quality of life in the elderly is related to the notion of health in the most minimal of definitions, that is, the degree to which the presence of chronic diseases influences the individual's ability to execute minimum survival activities. Therefore, we will emphasize potential relationships between physical function, physical fitness, and quality of life.

In this text, quality of life refers to **health-related quality of life** factors, those that are influenced by health and physical function. Other factors, such as living environment, economic status, availability of resources, and climate, certainly are important aspects of quality of life, but they are not affected much by exercise and physical function. Within this definition, quality of life is determined by how individuals function and how they feel about the way that they function. But researchers vary greatly in how they organize the various constructs of quality of life, and this in turn leads them to select different ways of measuring it and even to measure different aspects of it. Thus, a framework is needed to guide the study process. This text uses a slightly modified framework that was presented by Stewart and King (1991) specifically to guide research and study on health-related quality of life.

The framework to study quality of life is shown in table 10.1. The two major domains that make up quality of life are the functioning domain and the subjective well-being domain. Few would argue that the ability to function well physically, mentally, and socially is the cornerstone of an acceptable quality of life. Similarly, freedom from disease and pain is a strong contributor to quality of life. Physical function, the ability to perform physical tasks necessary to carry out the goals of individuals, the characteristics of disease-related disability, and the independence that it provides are so critical that the entirety of chapter 11 is devoted to them. Effective cognition in terms of self-management, financial management, social interaction, and intellectual and creative fulfillment is also extremely important. The nature of cognition and the interrelationship of health and fitness are the subject of chapter 9.

Well-Being

Well-being is a concept that almost everyone understands but, paradoxically, researchers find it difficult to define operationally. Some researchers focus on specific aspects of well-being, such as bodily well-being, self-concept and esteem, self-efficacy, or sense of control. Others talk about general well-being, a theoretical concept that means a subjective, global evaluation of one's own quality of life. These concepts can be summarized as "a phenomenological, global expression by the individual of the quality of her

Table 10.1 Health-Related Quality of Life Framework

Functioning domains

Physical functioning
- Aerobic fitness, strength, muscular endurance, balance, flexibility
- Physical tasks of daily function (walking, eating, stair-climbing)

Cognitive functioning
- Self-management
- Financial management

Engagement with life (autonomy; independence)
- Social roles
- social activities—social groups, community gatherings
- Hobbies, recreation

Objective health measures (disease symptoms)

Well-being domains (subjective, internal states)

Emotional well-being: positive and negative feeling states (depression, anxiety, anger or irritability, positive affect)

Self-concept: positive and negative perceptions about oneself (self-esteem, sense of mastery and control)

Bodily well-being: feelings about symptoms and bodily states, presence of pain, disease, energy vs. fatigue, sleep disturbance

Global perceptions of well-being: summary ratings and evaluations

Health: personal beliefs and evaluations of health in general "How do you rate your health overall?"

Life satisfaction; contentment with current life; congruence between desired and achieved states

Adapted from Stewart and King 1991.

or his state of existence" (Stathi et al., 2002, p. 77). Well-being generally refers to an individual's feelings at the time they are expressed. It includes the ideas of positive affect (contentment, morale, happiness), personal growth, satisfying social relationships, and autonomy (Kunzmann et al., 2000). It involves most aspects of life, although not all (figure 10.1). When these self-evaluations and judgments about quality of life are made within the perspective of a lifetime, then the term **life satisfaction** is generally used. It implies that quality of life has been good, personal goals have been met, and it has generally been a "good life."

The sense of well-being is intensely personal. Therefore, the feelings of well-being that individuals have must be discovered through self-report. The only

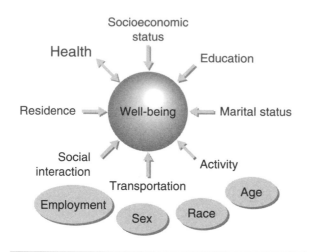

Figure 10.1 Correlates of subjective well-being. The relationships of factors to well-being are shown by arrows, whereas unrelated factors are shown as unconnected to well-being. Health is a somewhat larger correlate, because it was the most strongly related to well-being.

Journal of Gerontology. Series A, Biological Sciences and Medical Sciences by T. Larson. Copyright 1978 by Gerontological Society of America in the format textbook via Copyright Clearance Center.

way to determine how people feel is to ask them. Thus, when well-being is researched, it is sometimes referred to as "expressed well-being" or "subjective well-being." Because well-being is an emotional feeling, it is personal, is relatively transitory, and can be influenced by temporary environmental occurrences. Tests of well-being are difficult to validate and have lower reliabilities than most tests of physical attributes.

Although tests differ in how well-being is described and in the psychological test theory underlying their development, all of them tap a basic conceptual construct. These tests intercorrelate highly, and they also similarly correlate to other constructs. Larson (1978)

> Because sense of well-being is so personal, researchers use the term "subjective well-being."

Subjective Well-Being

Positive factors	Negative factors
Positive affect	Negative affect
Enthusiasm, pride, interest	Anger, anxiety, distress
Self-esteem	Anxiety
Self-efficacy	Stress
Happiness	Depression
Personal growth	
Global well-being and life satisfaction	

emphasized, however, that although the estimates of well-being assessed by tests such as these are useful, several caveats must be kept in mind. These tests cannot measure well-being equivalently across ethnic, cohort, and social classes, because people in these groups have different goals. Also, generalizations from well-being scores cannot be applied to individuals, because individuals might uniquely interpret key words. All of the responses made by subjects in any study of well-being are quick assessments that are made in a social situation. They represent expressed affective experience and thus should not be used to assess complex psychological factors or mental health.

Emotional Well-Being

Learning to understand and control emotion is a cornerstone of well-being. However, in later life, the physical, mental, and social changes that accompany aging bring with them challenges to emotional well-being that are above and beyond those routinely experienced by most younger individuals. As people age, they must adjust continuously to decreasing strength, endurance, physical ability, and health; the deaths of spouses and friends; retirement and reduced income; new social roles; and in advanced age, relocation of physical living arrangements (Schaie & Geiwitz, 1982).

In advanced age, the deaths of friends and loved ones occur more often, so that the elderly may find themselves in a state of unresolved and continual mourning (Billig, 1987). They also find themselves with fewer and fewer relatives and friends their own age who can support them psychologically and socially. Their opportunities for nurturing and being nurtured, for touching and being touched, for expressing feelings, and even for loving decrease with increasing age.

Fears of the Elderly

- The fear of being old and ill
- The fear of being poor and a burden
- The fear of change and uncertainty
- The fear of insanity
- The fear of losing liberty, identity, and human dignity
- The fear of death
- The fear of poor care and abuse

Data from Moss and Halamandaris (1977).

Retirement often may be associated with other types of losses: the self-identity that comes with having a job, financial status, and feelings of independence and worth and of contributing to society. The financial loss itself may be so significant that it imposes a different, often lower standard of living on the retiree. Older individuals also find themselves in new, externally imposed social roles. In advanced age, the elderly may spend hours of anxiety and dread worrying about a potential change in their physical living arrangements. A combination of frequent losses, unresolved mourning, and feelings of increased isolation associated with retirement and changing social roles contributes to a sense of loss of control and helplessness that makes the elderly vulnerable to depression. Also, many elders live in a state of chronic anxiety, sharing the set of fears that are shown in the sidebar "Fears of the Elderly." Given all these losses, it is understandable that one of the greatest challenges that all individuals face in life is coping with age-related events and demands and managing the emotional responses evoked by them.

Although some researchers distinguish between emotional feelings as mood and others as affect (positive or negative), most use the terms interchangeably (Arent et al., 2000). The term **mood** is used to indicate concepts of depression, anxiety, anger, vigor, fatigue, confusion, pleasantness, and euphoria. **Affect** refers to the way a person, situation, or an event makes one feel and is described as positive or negative (figure 10.2; Watson & Tellegen, 1985).

Thus, emotions can be described by two characteristics: valence (positive to negative) and arousal or activation (low to high). In the examples shown in figure 10.2, satisfaction is a positive emotion with relatively low arousal, enthusiasm is a positive emotion with relatively high arousal, sadness is a negative emotion with relatively low arousal, and scorn is a negative emotion with high arousal.

Emotions can be described by two characteristics: valence and arousal or activation.

Positive and negative affect are viewed as distinct and independent dimensions, not just opposite ends of a continuum (Kunzmann et al., 2000). Positive affect, which includes enthusiasm, pride, and interest, declines steadily throughout aging, irrespective of marital status, income, or nationality (Diener & Suh, 1997). Negative affects of anger, anxi-

ety, and distress remain the same or decrease with increased aging. The ability of mentally healthy adults to maintain emotional control in the face of repeated disappointments and losses is described as the stability-despite-loss paradox (Kunzmann et al., 2000). As discussed later, good health and physical fitness contribute positively to the ability to maintain emotional stability.

Health and Emotional Well-Being

It is commonly assumed that because aging is accompanied by declines in function and increased losses and disappointments, declines in positive affect and increases in negative affect also occur. Similarly, people presume that declines in health negatively affect individuals' self-evaluation, limit their interactions with the external world, and thus decrease their quality of life. The Berlin Study (Kunzmann et al., 2000) put these two assumptions to the test. These researchers analyzed the relative effects of aging and health constraints on two emotional dimensions of well-being—positive and negative affect.

The authors used a cross-sectional and longitudinal research design (4 years) to study the contributions of age, functional health (mobility, vision, and hearing), and physical function (ADL and IADLs) on positive and negative affect (scores from Positive and Negative Affect Schedules; Watson et al., 1988). In this scale, positive affect included enthusiasm, pride, and interest, and negative affect was represented by anger, anxiety, and distress. The Berlin Study was relatively large, including 43 men and women in each of

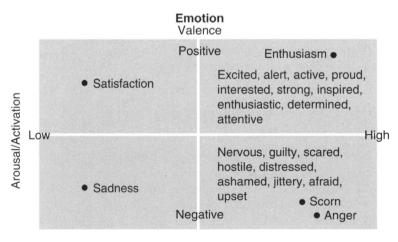

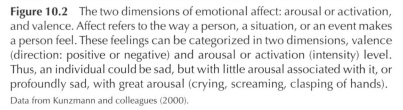

Figure 10.2 The two dimensions of emotional affect: arousal or activation, and valence. Affect refers to the way a person, a situation, or an event makes a person feel. These feelings can be categorized in two dimensions, valence (direction: positive or negative) and arousal or activation (intensity) level. Thus, an individual could be sad, but with little arousal associated with it, or profoundly sad, with great arousal (crying, screaming, clasping of hands).

Data from Kunzmann and colleagues (2000).

six age categories between 70 and 103 years old (N = 258). What did they find?

Negative affect did not change very much over a lifetime. If anything, it may have improved. As people age, it is in their interest to control anger, anxiety, and distress, and they may get better at doing it. They learn that disappointments that appeared as a teenager to be unbearable are, in fact, bearable and even forgotten within a short period of time. One of the positive aspects of aging is that people learn to mute negative outcomes and "protect" themselves against disappointment. Functional health constraints were related to negative affect but not as substantially as they were related to positive affect (Kunzmann et al., 2000)

> Poor functional health, however it is measured, negatively influences the positive affect that contributes to quality of life.

Conversely, positive affect declined over age, especially in the oldest age categories, and functional health impairments had a strong relationship with positive affect. The more functional health constraints people had, the more the constraints affected their positive affect. Thus, age negatively affected positive affect, but not negative affect, and functional health constraints were almost twice as strongly related to positive affect as they were to negative affect. When impairments in ADL and IADLs were used as health constraints in place of the health indicators (mobility, visual, and auditory acuity), the same results occurred. The investigators also found that the more health constraints are viewed as "typical" of their age, the less likely they will negatively affect subjective well-being.

> "Age per se is not a cause of decline in subjective well-being but health constraints are."
>
> From Kunzmann et al. (2000, p. 511).

Fitness, Exercise Interventions, and Positive Affect

Anyone who has watched the gamut of emotions that people exhibit when participating in a competitive sporting event, exercising, or dancing surely recognizes the powerful intertwining of physical exertion and emotion. The competitor may be exhilarated one minute and devastated a few moments later. It makes little difference whether he is competing for a masters national championship or she is participating in a close Sunday afternoon tennis match, or whether they are 25 or 75. Similar though perhaps more muted emotional responses occur during "peak experiences" of all types of exercise experiences such as hiking, bowling, and social dance. The truth is that

participating in physical activities that require attention and have a value to the performer demands total involvement and commitment—physical, mental, and emotional. This strong connection between the emotions and physical activity leads researchers to want to understand the meaning of quality of life, to provide the foundation for the use of physical activity as a moderator of mood and affect, and to study its effectiveness in rehabilitation of psychological disorders.

McAuley and Rudolph (1995) and later Arent and colleagues (2000) observed that the preponderance of literature on the relationship between exercise and emotional well-being is focused on potential changes in negative affect rather than positive affect. That is, the goal is to decrease negative affect (anxiety, stress, depression) rather than to improve positive affect (e.g., happiness, vigor, self-esteem). Indeed, McAuley and Rudolph (1995) pointed out that only one study of 81 in a meta-analysis sample focused on variables other than anxiety, depression, personality, mood, or self-concept. Arent and colleagues suggested that "exercise might be much more appealing to the elderly if they were told it could make them feel 'good' rather than simply 'less poorly'" (2000, p. 422).

Not only is the evidence for effects of exercise on positive affect scant, but it comes primarily from the effects of exercise on the one positive domain tapped by the Profile of Mood States (POMS) test, which is almost exclusively a measure of negative affect. For example, moderate-intensity aerobic dance (50-70% of maximum heart rate) performed 60 min, 3 days a week, for 10 weeks resulted in improved psychological vigor, the one positive mood state on the POMS test (Engels et al., 1998; Kennedy & Newton, 1997). Similarly, moderate- and high-intensity strength training (anaerobic) also improved the vigor item of the POMS. Moderate-intensity strength training was as effective as high-intensity training for the 36 older initially sedentary women (60-86 yrs) who trained 3 days per week for 12 weeks in this study (Tsutsumi et al., 1998).

Another way to determine whether relationships exist among physical health, fitness, and mood is by gathering self-reports of the amount of physical activity that people engage in and comparing the moods of those who exercise to those who do not. Results from most of these studies support a relationship. In a very large population study (N = 39,532) of 18- to 23-, 45- to 50-, and 70- to 75-year-old-women, the older women who were more physically active had higher vitality and mental health scores than the older women who were not active (Brown et al., 2000). Similarly, of 1,324 men and women living in the community independently, the older participants

(65-69 and 70-75 years) who reported that they were exercisers rated meaningfulness of life higher than those who were not exercisers (Ruuskanen & Ruoppila, 1995). But Seeman and colleagues (1995) found in 1,015 community-living men and women 65 to 69 and 70 to 75 years old that groups who were classified as "having some physical activity" were not different from those "having no activity" on personal mastery, life satisfaction, and happiness. However, their sample was drawn from the highest functioning one third cohort in the MacArthur Studies of Successful Aging, and it may have been difficult to raise their life satisfaction and happiness scores much by any single factor.

Fitness and Negative Affect (Anxiety, Stress, Depression)

Many researchers have studied the potential that exercise has for amelioration of symptoms of anxiety and depression. Both of these psychological difficulties are overrepresented in the older population, perhaps because of the difficulty of meeting age-related challenges. Physical illness and disability can be extremely painful and can result in dependency, social isolation, loneliness, and huge financial debts. Aging brings inevitable losses, bereavement, and possibly depression. Osterweis and colleagues (1984) emphasized that 10% to 20% of bereaved persons may display symptoms of clinical depression for 1 year or more following their loss.

Suicide is a growing and serious problem among the elderly. In 1992, persons older than 65 repre-

sented 13% of the population but almost 18% of suicides (National Institute of Mental Health, 2003). As shown in figure 10.3, substantially more men than women take their own lives, and every one-half decade of increased age for men, the suicide rate increases. The rate remains essentially the same for women of all ages over 65. This dramatic gender difference has been attributed to the observation that men find the loss of physical independence more intolerable than women do and also because very old men become more socially isolated (Crandall, 1991).

Suicide also may be underestimated in the older population (Crandall, 1991). Overt suicide is a specific act that terminates life, such as the use of poison, a weapon, or inhalation of carbon monoxide. Covert suicide, the adoption of destructive health habits that slowly erode health and eventually cause death, is a suspected strategy in many cases but is not documented. Examples of destructive habits are abuse of alcohol and other drugs, refusal to take medications, smoking, neglect of diet, ignoring disease symptoms or weight abnormalities, failure to have regular medical examinations, and failure to plan for emergencies. Most elderly people, and many of them may be women, who participate in destructive health habits do not consider them to be suicidal. Suicide is tragic evidence that emotional control has been exhausted.

In correlational studies, a lack of physical activity level is negatively related to depression in nonclinical samples. It is common to find that individuals who report more activity report less depressive symptoms (Moore et al., 1999; Strawbridge, 1996). For exam-

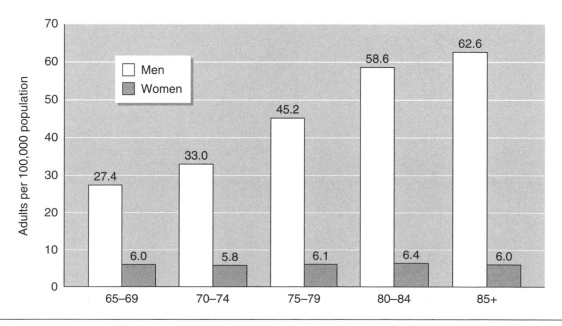

Figure 10.3 Comparison of the rate of suicides of men and women at different ages.

Data from Centers for Disease Control (1996).

Risk Factors for Suicide in the Elderly

A suicidal person may show signs of depression, such as

- changes in eating or sleeping habits
- unexplained fatigue or apathy
- trouble concentrating or being indecisive
- crying for no apparent reason
- inability to feel good about themselves or unable to express joy
- behavior changes or are just "not themselves"
- withdrawal from family, friends or social activities
- loss of interest in hobbies, work, etc.
- loss of interest in personal appearance

A suicidal person also may

- talk about or seem preoccupied with death
- give away prized possessions
- take unnecessary risks
- have had a recent loss or expect one
- increase their use of alcohol, drugs, or other medications
- fail to take prescribed medicines or follow required diets
- acquire a weapon

From HealthyPlace.com (2004). The suicide of older men and women. [Online] http://www.healthyplace.com/communities/depression/related/suicide_3.asp [6.14.04]

ple, a high physical activity group (compared with moderate and inactive groups) reported the lowest depression scores in 3,627 men and women 65 to 74 years old living in the community (Simonsick et al., 1993; for review, see O'Connor et al., 1993). Even in clinical samples, such as that of 146, mostly women, 50 years or older who were diagnosed with major depressive disorder (MDD), lower levels of physical activity were associated with more severe depressive symptoms (Moore et al., 1999). Additionally, in a large sample of 439 persons 60 years and older with knee osteoarthritis and high symptoms of depression, aerobic exercise over 3 months improved their symptoms immediately after the program and after 9 and 18 months of follow-up (Penninx et al., 2002).

Camacho and colleagues (1991) conducted a very large, longitudinal population study of noninstitutionalized men and women, about half of whom were over the age of 40. The investigators collected measures of the extent of physical activity and depression for a baseline in 1965 and then collected test results two more times, in 1974 and 1983. The critical questions asked in this study were whether people who participated in physical activity had a lower or higher risk of developing depression with aging and whether a change in physical activity patterns over time could predict the presence of depression. The authors found that men and women who reported low physical activity at the beginning of the study were at a much higher risk of developing depression 10 or 20 years later than were those adults who reported high physical activity when the study began. This relationship persisted even though the investigators statistically controlled such confounding factors as physical health, socioeconomic status, social supports, life events, and other health habits.

An even stronger relationship existed between physical activity pattern and risk of depression. Those individuals who began the study in 1965 as inactive participants but changed their physical activity habits by 1974 to become active revealed no greater risk for depression in 1983 than those who had been physically active throughout the study. Conversely, those who began the study being active but reported they were inactive in 1974 had a 1.5 times greater risk of being depressed in the 1983 analysis.

An important exception in the study by Camacho and colleagues (1991) was the group of adults who were inactive at all three measurement periods. This group was at a higher risk of developing depression than the active groups, both the chronically active and those who changed from inactive to active, but when the factor of physical health was removed statistically, their risk of developing depression was almost eliminated. In other words, the relationship between depression and physical activity pattern was only an indirect relationship, a result of the direct relationship between depression and their physical health.

Physically active men and women have a much lower risk of developing depression 10 or 20 years later than sedentary men and women. Adults who increase their physical activity level over a period of years decrease their risk for developing depression, and those who decrease or stop their physical activity increase their risk for developing depression symptoms (Camacho et al., 1991).

Several aerobic exercise research programs have been found to reduce symptoms of anxiety and depression in nonclinically depressed adults (Williams & Lord, 1997). Using a very well controlled randomized design, with healthy and initially sedentary subjects, King and colleagues (1993) provided a 1-year aerobic intervention to 357 men and women between 50 and 65 years of age. Several design characteristics made this a particularly strong study. The self-reports of participation were validated, the investigators controlled for possible effects of initial expectations, they used actual rather than estimated measures of functional capacity, and it was a relatively long intervention. Negative affect measures used were depressive symptoms (Beck Depression Inventory), anxiety (Taylor Manifest Anxiety Scale), and stress (Perceived Stress Scale). The researchers also obtained self-reported ratings of perceived change (on a 10-point Likert scale, where 1 = *no change* and 10 = *extreme improvement*) in sleep quality, physical shape and appearance, depression, tension or anxiety, concentration, alertness, confidence and well-being, energy, appetite, physical fitness, stress, coping with stress, mood, weight, and eating habits. The important outcome of this study was that all the exercise groups, whether participants were in organized classes or did exercises at home or whether exercises were performed at low or high intensity, improved on more variables than did the control group.

Strength training (anaerobic exercise) also has been shown to improve mood (Tsutsumi et al., 1998). High and moderate-intensity resistance strength training reduced negative mood (trait anxiety), compared to the control group. Both groups, those who trained three days per week for 12 weeks with moderate intensity and those who trained with high intensity, exhibited decreased tension and state anxiety. Thus, moderate intensity was as effective as high intensity for reducing anxiety in 36 older, sedentary females who ranged in age from 60 to 86 years.

Findings of exercise effects on mood in relatively normal adults are not all positive. Hassmén and Kolvula (1997) reported no change in mood scores (POMS) in 20 men and 20 women with an average age of 66 after low-intensity walking three times a week for 3 months. Both the walking group and the control group improved in mood, but exercise did not seem to contribute to the improvement. The authors suggested that the improvement in mood might have been attributable to the group activity (i.e., walking or social interaction). Their subjects were relatively young, and the sample was small. More likely, however, is that walking at a very low intensity is not an effective intervention.

Several studies of adults suffering from moderate or major depression have found exercise to be an effective treatment. In a study of moderately depressed older adults (mean age 72.5 years), McNeil and colleagues (1991) found that exercise and social contact groups, compared with a wait-list control group, experienced significant reductions in depression, measured by the Beck Depression Inventory (Beck & Beamesderfer, 1974). Furthermore, although the social contact group equally reduced scores in total and psychological depression, only the exercise group experienced decreased somatic symptoms of depression such as poor appetite, increased fatigue, and disturbed sleep. In one study of 156 patients with MDD, the psychiatrists' ratings of depression and the patients' self-reported depressive symptoms scores decreased as much after 16 weeks of walking or jogging (70-85% heart rate reserve) as a group that exercised and took medication and a group that just continued taking their medication (Blumenthal et al., 1999). The participants in this study were only middle-aged (mean age 56 years); nevertheless, these findings are important because they came from a large randomized control study revealing that exercising three times a week was as effective in reducing depressive symptoms as a routinely used medical treatment.

Although exercise did not provide additional benefit in the exercise-plus-medication group over the medication-alone group, a study by Mather and colleagues (2002) that included older participants (mostly female, mean age 68) did find an advantage in decreasing depressive symptoms by combining exercise with medication. Eighty-six moderately depressed patients who had not responded to 6 weeks of antidepressant treatment were randomly assigned to either an exercise program or a health education program. They all continued their medications through 10 weeks of classes, two each week for 45 min. The exercise group reduced its depression scores more than the control group (55% vs. 33%). Singh and colleagues (2001) found that men in their 60s and 70s decreased their symptoms of minor or major depression after 10 weeks of supervised weightlifting classes followed by 10 more weeks of unsupervised weightlifting exercise performed in a group setting.

Therapeutic exercise programs for clinically depressed individuals generally have been beneficial. In addition, those who were the most depressed gained the most benefit from exercise programs (Craft & Landers, 1998). An important conclusion drawn by Martinsen (1990) is that exercise programs have an antidepressive effect on patients with mild to moderate forms of depression, but the exercise program does not necessarily have to result in an increase in

Using Exercise to Control Depression

"For treatment of depression many physicians use exercise as an important adjunct to psychotherapy and antidepressant therapy. Low-intensity exercise and exercise that elicits an increase in $\dot{V}O_2$max are equally effective in lessening depressive symptoms. Evidence has shown that exercise is as effective as psychotherapy and antidepressant therapy in treating mild-to-moderate depression, and even more effective when used in conjunction with the conventional therapies."

From Nicoloff and Schwenk (1995, p. 44).

physical fitness to reduce depression. Other aspects of exercise programs, such as the social support that generally accompanies therapy programs and the changes in self-efficacy that occur, also may contribute to the therapeutic outcomes for some individuals, although several of the studies discussed adequately controlled for social interaction effects.

The finding that exercise is as effective in treating depression as traditional therapies such as group or individual psychotherapy, other behavioral interventions, and some medication protocols for some individuals is significant. Exercise can be very inexpensive, has positive side effects with few negative ones, and will not be limited to a specified time period by health insurance regulations. It is a very attractive alternative to most depression therapies.

Perceptions of Self

In addition to the important contribution that emotional control makes to well-being, the perceptions of self are also important. Perception of self includes self-concept, self-esteem, and self-efficacy. A very important part of the perception of self is body concept and esteem. Especially in older adults, age-related physical changes seem incongruent with the perception of self, because most older adults do not feel that their "self" has changed much over the years—until they look in the mirror. Thus, although bodily well-being is an aspect of self-esteem, in this book, which focuses on physical dimensions of aging, bodily well-being is discussed as a separate subsection of self-perception. This section begins with a discussion of self-concept, self-esteem, and self-effi-

cacy, followed by a discussion on the relationship of health and exercise to these concepts. Subsequent to that is a description of bodily well-being and the way health and physical activity affect it.

Self-Concept, Self-Esteem, and Self-Efficacy

Self-concept is the conscious awareness and perception of self. It is not a unitary construct; rather, it is multidimensional. Shown in figure 10.4, self-concept is the awareness that people have of themselves, including perceptions about their intellectual (or scholastic), social, emotional, and physical functioning (Shavelson et al., 1976). Perception of self in the intellectual or scholastic dimension involves recognition of abilities in literature, mathematics, or science comprehension or of an aptitude for solving problems (e.g., crossword puzzles). The concept of the self as a social identity includes social status, membership in professional or social groups (bridge clubs, teaching), or social labels (e.g., leader, social butterfly, troublemaker). People's perceptions of their personal dispositions include their personality traits, preferences, and predispositions (e.g., anxious, moody, optimistic). Self-concept is developmental in that it changes throughout childhood, throughout adulthood, and with the slow changes that are related to increased aging. In the physical dimension, self-concept includes perceptions about physical appearance and physical skill.

Self-concept is formulated by perception and evaluation, serves as the basis for individuals' beliefs in their competence and capabilities, and is tempered by self-acceptance. That is, it is very difficult to be aware of oneself in specific circumstances without evaluating and comparing oneself with a standard, with others, or with one's own performances at different times. Thus, evaluation of self is ongoing. The results of these evaluations and the feelings about them provide the basis for an individual's self-esteem. Self-esteem is composed of feelings of competence, self-approval, power, and self-worthiness. Some people use the terms *self-concept* and *self-esteem* interchangeably, and in fact, attempts to identify them as separate entities have not been very successful (Sonstroem & Morgan, 1989).

Self-esteem is the respect and appreciation that individuals have for themselves, or the extent to which they feel positive about themselves (Gergen, 1971). Self-esteem includes at least two dimensions: competence and self-acceptance (Tafarodi & Swann, 1995). Self-esteem is clearly a multidimensional construct (Gergen, 1981), because it includes the regard with which people view themselves in all dimensions of their lives—the psychological, social, and philosophical dimensions as well as the physical. A woman may have one feeling of self-esteem regarding her role as mother, another for her job, and yet another as a church member.

Self-efficacy is the belief that one has the capability to organize and execute a course of action necessary to produce a specific level of attainment (Bandura, 1997). It includes two types of expectations: efficacy expectations and outcome expectations. An example of an efficacy expectation is an older adult's judgment that he can successfully walk two miles. Outcome expectations are the estimations of likely consequences: an increased ability to go outside the home and shop, attend recreational activities, and visit friends. Self-efficacy is linked to particular domains, and so it is highly personal (Stidwell & Rimmer, 1995). In the Sonstroem and Morgan model (1989), described subsequently, self-efficacy regarding physical abilities and body awareness is the psychological self-perception that has the most specificity.

Self-efficacy is the most powerful mediator of behavioral performance (Bandura, 1986). When contemplating a course of behavioral action, for example, whether to participate in an exercise program

for older adults, individuals will consider the task attributes, performance conditions, their estimate of their own ability, and the amount of effort that will be required to accomplish the task. If they believe that they cannot perform well enough to complete it, they will not try. If they believe that they can accomplish most of the aspects of the program, they will enroll and participate.

Health, Physical Activity, and Self-Esteem As it relates to physical movement and exercise, self-esteem is based on self-awareness of physical competence, body consciousness, and self-efficacy with regard to physical function or skill. The Exercise and Self-Esteem Model (Sonstroem et al., 1994) is a hierarchical model that specifically proposes that physical worth is one domain of global self-esteem. This model was designed for athletes and young adults, and it includes subdomains of sport, conditioning, body, and strength. However, although it has not been proposed or tested, this model might be modified for older adults, as shown in figure 10.4. In this hypothetical model, the appropriate subdomains for older adults would be physical limitations (e.g., visual, hearing, balance, incontinence), physical condition (strength and endurance), hand function (strength and coordination), and body

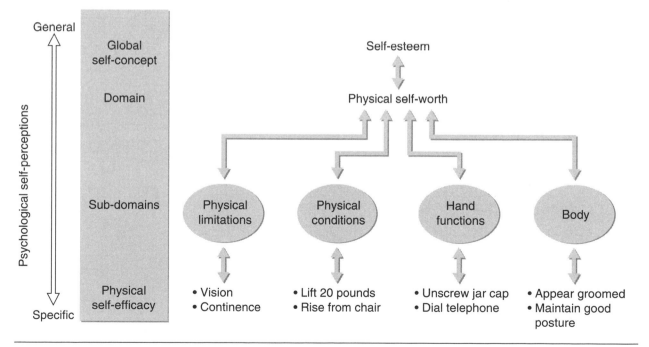

Figure 10.4 Hypothetical hierarchical model proposing how feelings of physical worth are one domain of global self-esteem. Modified for older adults from the Exercise and Self-Esteem Model (EXSEM) proposed by Sonstroem and colleagues, 1994. The EXSEM model was proposed to explain relationships of self-worth in athletes and young adults. In this figure, the basic structures of domains and subdomains are the same, but the specific domains and self-efficacies are changed. This model is proposed and has not been tested.

Adapted from Stidwell and Rimmer (1995).

(appearance, fit of clothes, state of grooming). In this hierarchical model, it is proposed that changes at each level generalize to the level above, so that a change in strength through an exercise program would change the feelings of self-efficacy regarding a person's physical condition, and this in turn would change feelings of self-worth, which finally would affect self-esteem. What is the evidence that health status, physical function, or exercise programs actually affect self-esteem?

From his review of the exercise and self-esteem literature, Sonstroem (1984) concluded that participation in exercise programs is related to subjects' increases in the scores of self-esteem tests. He proposed several possible reasons why exercise participation might enhance self-esteem, the first and most likely being the visible increase in physical fitness. Other reasons are that when program participants see a tangible achievement of their goals, they feel better physically, and they develop a sense of competence, which in turn provides them with feelings of mastery and control. In addition, most exercise participants who stay with an exercise program for an extended period also develop other health habits, such as better nutrition and sleep habits, which in turn make them feel better about themselves. Finally, program participants gain new social experiences with their colleagues in the program and with their exercise leaders, they may receive more attention from their exercise leader than they have had for a while, and they may be praised for continuing the program by their significant others

and friends. All of these factors may contribute to enhanced self-esteem.

Health, Physical Activity, and Self-Efficacy The relationship between health behaviors and self-efficacy is well established (Grembowski et al., 1993), just as the relationship between physical activity and self-efficacy is also well documented (e.g., Clark, 1999; Conn, 1998). Adults who have had good and successful experiences with exercise are more likely to have high self-efficacy with regard to their success in an exercise program (McAuley et al., 1993). People who exercise have high self-efficacy about physical activity, and those who have high self-efficacy are more likely to initiate an exercise program. In older adults, self-efficacy contributes greatly to the maintenance of physical function, particularly for those who are at risk for functional decline (Mendes de Leon et al., 1996). Self-efficacy beliefs with regard to instrumental activities of daily living have substantial impact on the ability of very old adults to complete these activities (Seeman et al., 1999). Thus, self-efficacy status is a predictor of age-related changes in physical function.

> *"High self-efficacy enables older adults to continue carrying out basic self-care activities when their ability to do so is challenged by diminished physical capacity."*
> From Mendes de Leon and colleagues (1996, p. S188).

Resnick (2001) proposed a model explaining how self-efficacy, outcome expectations, age, mental

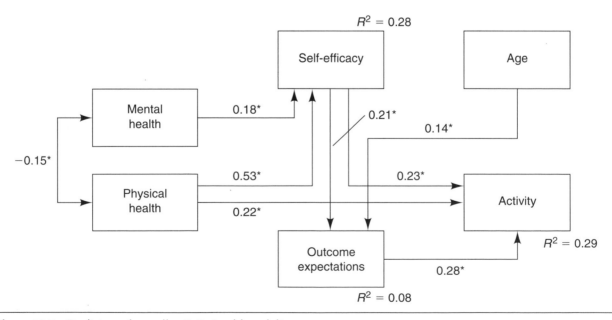

Figure 10.5 Predictors of overall activity in older adults.

Reprinted, by permission, from B. Resnick, 2001, "Testing a model of overall activity in older adults," *Journal of Aging and Physical Activity* 9: 142-160.

health, and physical health might operate together to predict overall activity (figure 10.5). In this model, self-efficacy expectations, outcome expectations, and physical health directly influenced overall activity, even though the overall model accounted for just 29% of the total variance. Still, this model confirms the conceptual ideal that physical activity self-efficacy is one of the most important motivators of physical activity. As such, it can be inferred that older adults who believe that they have the competence to do exercise, and who believe that their exercise will have beneficial results, will be more likely to be active and thus be healthier and more fit.

Physical activity and exercise experiences provide primary information that individuals use in their judgments of self-efficacy. Even short, acute exposures to exercise serve as a source of information on which to make an efficacy evaluation, and longer exercise program experiences make an even larger contribution (McAuley et al., 1993). These contributions occur in asymptomatic, older adults and also in patient populations such as those with osteoarthritis, cardiovascular disease, and chronic obstructive pulmonary disease (Lox & Freehill, 1999). It appears at this early stage of research on efficacy that the effects of an exercise program are curvilinear, greatest at the beginning of the program and then waning somewhat as the program progresses, and are specific to the type of exercise (McAuley & Blissmer, 2000).

Effects of Physical Activity on Self-Efficacy:

- Both acute physical activity and chronic physical activity are primary sources of information to shape self-efficacy.
- The self-efficacy growth pattern is curvilinear, faster at the beginning and then waning.
- Self-efficacy is enhanced by exercise programs in patients with cardiovascular disease, osteoarthritis, and chronic obstructive pulmonary disease (COPD).
- Physical activity has more impact on self-efficacy than do physiological fitness changes.

Bodily Well-Being and Esteem

Bodily well-being is the image and feeling that people have about their bodily states, their energy and fatigue, and the way they perceive themselves to appear to other people. Of all the areas of life that change with aging, declines in physical appearance and function are the most visible.

Obvious losses are those of muscle mass, strength, physical endurance, flexibility, and coordination. Health status becomes more tenuous in old age and, especially in sedentary individuals, may be characterized by sleep disturbances, more frequent disease symptoms and chronic conditions that require longer periods of recuperation, and the presence of pain. Biochemical and electrolyte balances change with age, gastrointestinal and metabolic processes become less efficient, hormonal production decreases, and all of these combine to influence the subtle biochemistry of brain function. Coping with emotional challenges when physical health is compromised is difficult for individuals of any age, but it is even more difficult for older adults who have additional problems and who may have to cope daily with problems such as arthritis, glaucoma, cataracts, congestive heart failure, or osteoporosis.

Even if older individuals are relatively free of symptomatic disease, the loss of physical ability and skills may be emotionally traumatic, especially for those whose main interests throughout their lives have involved activity. Physical ability and strength are an integral part of the self for athletes, workers in physical occupations, and individuals who have hobbies that require strength and endurance (like mountain climbing, rock hunting, hang gliding, sailing). As the physical self begins to erode noticeably, it takes substantial readjustment and psychological coping to maintain self-esteem and emotional well-being. Some individuals deal with the challenge by modifying their expectations. Others may have more difficulty dealing with the decline, abandon their physical hobbies or sports, and either substitute less physically demanding activities in their lives or find other compensations for the loss. Dealing with physical changes in appearance or function is a psychological stressor that all aging people must confront, and, for some, the challenge to emotional well-being is substantial. It involves changing the way the body is perceived and adapting to new constraints.

Body Consciousness: Body Image

The way that individuals perceive their body is called **body consciousness,** and it is an important contributor to self-esteem. Body consciousness has at least three aspects (Miller et al., 1981). The first is public **body image,** which includes the subjective feelings that people have about their physical appearance, for example, wrinkled skin, hair loss, a sagging stomach, and the way that their clothing fits their body. These and other aspects of external appearance are of concern to many older people, because physical appearance is a large part of the general aesthetic impression that people develop of each other.

A second aspect of body consciousness is the private **perception of body function**, that is, the awareness that people have of internal body sensations that are not visible to others. People may have very strong perceptions and concerns about cardiovascular, hypertensive, or genitourinary symptoms and problems that only they know. Whereas they may be perceived by their friends as a person of perfect health who has a body to be envied, these individuals may in private be highly anxious and see themselves as having a weak body that has failed them.

The third aspect of body consciousness is **body competence.** It is the subjective evaluation of the body's ability to accomplish the physical goals that individuals create for themselves. It is also described as self-efficacy.

Body consciousness plays a huge role in the self-esteem of young people, particularly young girls and women. Indeed, McAuley & Rudolph (1995) points out that most of what we know about body dissatisfaction or physique anxiety comes from research on young females, probably because this is thought to be a potential mechanism to explain eating disorders. Little research has been reported on body concepts, satisfaction, or anxiety in older adults.

What is known, though, is that people of all ages have a negative view of the physical changes that accompany aging. In general, men have less dissat-

isfaction with their bodily appearance than women do at all ages, and older women are the least satisfied with their appearance. The over-65 group in Ryff's study (1989) considered the physical changes of their body to be negative and the greatest source of change in their lives over the past 20 years. Both the middle-aged and over-65 age groups listed physical changes in the top four changes (figure 10.6), but the older group indicated that their physical being changed more than any other aspect of their lives. Young and old alike consider the physical appearance of older people to be less attractive (Harris, 1994).

Physically active men and women are more satisfied with their bodily appearance than are sedentary individuals (e.g., Ford et al., 1991). Loland (2000) reported that both the gender and the age effects on self-evaluation of appearance depend on the level of physical activity that individuals experience. In a randomized study of 1,555 male and female Norwegians, she found that inactive older men and women (45-67) were substantially less satisfied with their appearance that younger men and women were, but moderate to highly active older men and women were more satisfied than younger groups (figure 10.7). This was particularly true in active women. Active women aged 45 to 67 were substantially more satisfied with their appearance than women 30 to

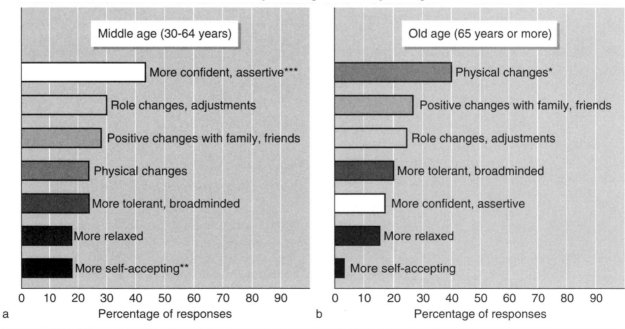

Figure 10.6 The percentage of respondents for each answer to the question, How have you changed from 20 years ago? *$p < .05$, **$p < .001$ indicate a significant difference between what is important to (a) middle-aged and (b) older adults.

Reprinted, by permission, from C.D. Ryff, 1989, "In the eye of the beholder: Views of psychological well-being among middle-aged and older adults," *Psychology and Aging* 4: 206. Copyright © 1989 by the American Psychological Association. Reprinted with permission.

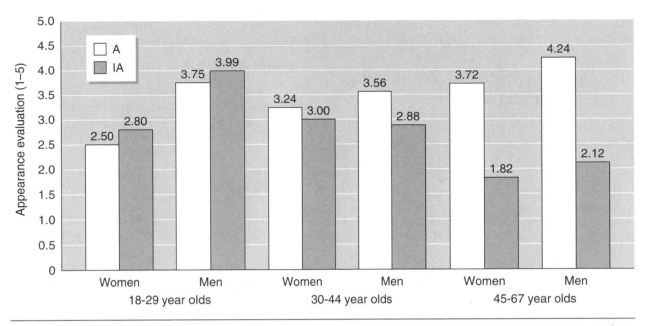

Figure 10.7 Appearance evaluation of active and inactive men and women in three age groups: 18-29, 30-44, and 45-67. A = moderate to high physical activity level, IA = inactive. AE: 1 = *very poor evaluation* and 5 = *very good evaluation*. Data from Loland (2000).

Reprinted, by permission, from N.W. Loland, 2000, "Attitudes toward bodily appearance among physically active and inactive women and men of different ages," *Journal of Aging and Physical Activity* 8: 205.

44 and even more so compared with women 18 to 29. This was attributed to the common observation that young women in North America are under considerable pressure from the media and their peers to be thin and beautiful. Consequently, very few young women are satisfied with the way they look. Although it is somewhat risky to compare research from the two cultures, North America and Norway, the author made a case for the two countries being from the same cultural sphere, particularly regarding ideal norms and values of "the perfect body" as communicated through the mass media and advertisements.

These results suggest that as adults age, they become more realistic and thus more satisfied with their appearance, especially if they maintain their bodily appearance through physical activity. Also, in the Loland (2000) study, as has been shown repeatedly before, men of all ages were more satisfied with their appearance than women were. The only exception in this study was inactive middle-aged adults, whose evaluation of their appearance was about the same for both men and women.

Research generally has supported the notion that organized exercise programs improve the body image of older adults, thus enhancing their self-esteem (Shephard, 1987). Even in nursing home residents, those who participated in rhythmic breathing, slow stretching, and upright exercises twice a week for 8

weeks reported higher body image scores (Olson, 1975).

This section on the contribution that physical activity and exercise make to body concept should not be concluded without a reminder that a major contribution to bodily well-being is enhanced sleep (King et al., 2002; Singh et al., 1997), which blunts some disease symptoms and reduces pain. Studies of the contribution that exercise makes to the reduction of pain in old adults with chronic diseases and conditions are few, but some have been published. Wood and colleagues (1999) reported that aerobic endurance scores were related to pain in a sample of older adults (72-93 years). The faster the participants completed an 880-yd (805-m) walk, the lower their perceived level of chronic pain. The implication was that individuals who exercise at levels high enough to enable them to perform well on endurance tests either prevent physical conditions that are accompanied by pain or do not have painful conditions and thus exercise more.

Perceptions of pain were substantially less in a group of late middle-aged adults (50-65 yrs) who participated in 12 months of aerobic exercise classes. Different levels of exercise intensity were not related to different levels of pain relief, but more of those who participated in more than 100% of their exercise classes, that is, they exercised outside of class requirements, reported reduced pain compared with those who only participated in only 33% of their classes (Stewart et al., 1993).

Global Perceptions of Well-Being and Life Satisfaction

To this point, several components of subjective well-being have been discussed in terms of their relationship to health and exercise: emotional well-being, self-esteem, self-efficacy, and bodily well-being. However, how does health and exercise relate to a global feeling of well-being? Global well-being refers to an individual's feelings of satisfaction about everything in life: oneself, family, social network, and job. Global well-being is highly related to life satisfaction, and both concepts have resisted research attempts at separation. Life satisfaction is really the extent to which an individual is content with how his or her life has developed. It is measured by asking individuals to compare their overall achievements to their lifelong aspirations (George, 1979). Researchers generally believe that life satisfaction tends to be stable in the elderly. Persons who have been satisfied with their lives before old age will most likely continue to be satisfied, and those who have been dissatisfied will probably continue to be dissatisfied. The stability of life satisfaction in the elderly is problematic, however, partly because most of the studies are cross-sectional designs and partly because a large percentage of such studies were conducted in institutions. It is expected that institutionalized people have lower life satisfaction and feelings of well-being than community-dwelling people, and so some of the life satisfaction results may represent more negativity than actually exists in the community-dwelling elderly.

When people consider their lives to be very satisfying, they also have a strong sense of well-being. Thus, life satisfaction scales are many times used as measures of subjective well-being. Both are influenced to some extent by income, race, and employment and to a minor extent by education, marriage, and family (Diener, 1984). Other factors that seem to be related to well-being are friends, a loving relationship with someone, social activity (Okun & Stock, 1987), and the nature of the coping skills people use to deal with negative life events (Matheny et al., 1986). Aging itself does not decrease global perceptions of well-being independently but only indirectly because aging relates to other factors. For example, the decreased health that sometimes accompanies aging has the potential to affect subjective well-being negatively. The question of how health affects well-being and feelings of life satisfaction is

an important one that has substantial ramifications for quality of life.

Health and Global Well-Being

Health and physical capacity are important components of a feeling of well-being. Ryff (1989) asked middle-aged (52.5 ± 8.7 years) and old people (73.5 ± 6.1 years) what they believed was most important in their lives (the results are shown in figure 10.8). Of 12 items, the middle-aged people listed health as the fifth most important, and the old people listed health as second in importance. When asked what they would change if they could, middle-aged people listed their health fourth in importance and old people listed health second. It is clear that health status is of deep concern to both middle-aged and old people. Both age groups indicated that their personality attributes, concern for others, interests and activities, morals and values, and outlook on life had remained relatively stable. Among the biggest changes over the past 20 years, in addition to the physical changes, was their adjustment to role changes, their ability to relax, and their ability to accept themselves. An important point is that both middle-aged and older groups listed physical changes and health events as the most negative of the changes and events that they had experienced over the past 20 years. These findings match those from other studies, revealing more concern in older groups for health, whereas job and career issues are more important to middle-aged people. A subset of older individuals for whom much of their self-identity has been defined by their career can suffer doubly by a loss of health. Their loss of health also leads to the loss of their job. In these cases, the loss of health is a major contributor to a decline in their sense of well-being.

> "Among all the elements of an older person's life situation, health is the most strongly related to subjective well-being. People who are sick or physically disabled are much less likely to express contentment about their lives."
> From Larson (1978, p. 112).

Physical Function, Physical Activity, Fitness, and Exercise

Global well-being or life satisfaction scores of older individuals who have good physical function, who are physically active, or who report that they exercise

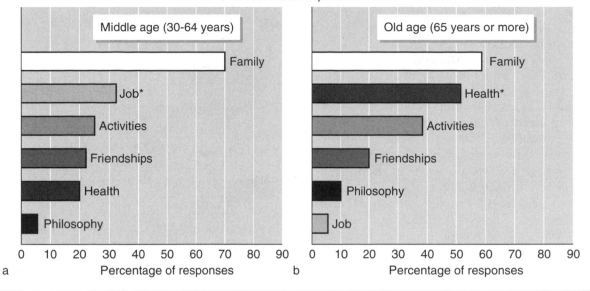

Figure 10.8 The percentage of respondents for each answer to the question, What is most important to you in your life at the present time? *Significant difference (p < .001) between what is important to (a) middle-aged and (b) older adults.

Reprinted, by permission, from C.D. Ryff, 1989, "In the eye of the beholder: Views of psychological well-being among middle-aged and older adults," *Psychology and Aging* 4: 198. Copyright © 1989 by the American Psychological Association. Reprinted with permission.

regularly are almost always as a group higher than those of individuals who are sedentary or disabled (Spirduso & Cronin, 2001). In fact, the relationship of physical status and physical activity to well being has almost reached the level of dogma in this field. Individuals provide passionate testimonials that their activity level is highly related to their well-being. When physical activity levels are compared (high, moderate, low, sedentary) in large population studies, those who report that their activity level is moderate or high generally have higher global well-being scores than those who are sedentary. In fact, in a sample of Finnish people who were interviewed extensively by trained technicians, physical activity level was found to relate not only to the participants' health and physical function but also to their feelings of the meaningfulness of their lives (Takkinen et al., 2001). However, because all of these studies were nonrandomized, correlational, cross-sectional studies, it is not possible to determine whether being physically active with its concomitant fitness benefits enhanced the feelings of global well-being in these adults or whether perceptions of well-being and life satisfaction led to enhanced physical activity.

Similarly, feelings of improvements in well-being following exercise or rehabilitation programs are almost universally expressed by the participants, especially in testimonials. However, hard experimental research evidence for this is either weak or nonexistent (Spirduso & Cronin, 2001). There have

been virtually no randomized, experimental studies of well-being and exercise in adults over the age of 65. A small number of exercise program studies have been published, and they reported improvements in well-being, but they had no control group. The few quasi-experimental studies that have been completed failed to find strong support for an exercise effect on well-being, let alone a dose–response effect of exercise. The strongest evidence for changes in well-being was reported by Stewart and colleagues (1997), who conducted a large physical activity promotion program for older adults. Subjects' ages were 62 to 91 and they participated in existing community-based physical activity classes and programs of their choice. The investigators found enhanced self-esteem in these physical activity groups from the pre- to the posttests but not in a large array of other quality-of-life measures. However, those participants who had learned a new physical activity and who adhered to the classes regularly for more than 6 months, compared with those who were erratic or dropped out, completed the program with higher overall well-being scores.

The research results simply do not match what many individuals believe are positive outcomes. One plausible reason is that most assessments of well-being were not designed for adults over the age of 60, and not many studies have been conducted on this topic. Another potential reason for the failure to quantify a relationship between activity and well-being was adroitly recognized and discussed first by McAuley and Rudolph (1995) and later by Arent and colleagues (2000). Instruments presently used to assess this relationship may not be measuring the correct constructs. Most of these studies use the POMS, which is well known as a multidimensional measure of negative states. McAuley and Rudolph (1995) reviewed complaints from several researchers that these instruments do not have construct validity in the domain of exercise, they are not sufficiently sensitive to exercise-induced change, they tap primarily negative affect although many exercise benefits are positive, and they fail to assess well-known benefits of exercise such as enhanced sleep, social life, sex life, and self-confidence. The investigators suggested two potential tests, the Exercise-Induced Feeling Inventory (Gauvin & Rejeski, 1993) and the Subjective Exercise Experiences Scale (McAuley & Courneya, 1994).

A final problem with exercise experimental studies and global well-being is that it is difficult to obtain groups of participants who have a wide range of well-being scores. Volunteers over the age of 60 for research studies generally feel very good about themselves and their ability to perform physically, or they would not volunteer. Those who agree to participate from a random selection process, and who finish the study, are likely also to have a fairly strong sense of well-being. Thus, it is difficult to observe improvements in older adults who represent the higher levels of well-being.

Influence of Exercise on Well-Being

How might physical activity and the consequent enhanced health and fitness levels affect well-being? This is a very difficult question because the concept of well-being is so broad. It is highly unlikely that any single mechanism could answer this question. In research on humans, correlational relationships have been reported for physical activity and various aspects of positive and negative affect, but the mechanisms are largely assumed. Mechanisms for the beneficial results of exercise with depressed patients in quasi-experimental studies also have relied on presumed physiological processes. Evidence from animal experimental research has supported several mechanisms by which physical activity might change physiological processes related to depressive disorders. But explanations of changes in global well-being and life satisfaction have tended more to be psychosocial. Thus, the proposed mechanisms can be categorized as physiological or psychosocial.

Physiological Effects on Subjective Well-Being

Physiological hypotheses are based on exercise-induced changes in cardiovascular function, neural hormones, endorphins, and body temperature.

Cardiovascular Hypothesis

This hypothesis is that exercise increases the integrity of the cardiovascular system and thus maximizes brain function in areas that control emotional responses. People who are more fit have to spend less energy on physical tasks, and therefore they feel better. Blumenthal and colleagues (1989) proposed that exercise might reduce symptoms of anxiety by reducing heart rate response. One mechanism by which exercise may be linked to emotional change is that it alters regional blood flow in the brain. The circulating blood of the brain is directed to tissue that is metabolically active. Therefore, when individuals exercise, making decisions about what to do and evaluating what is happening, greater quantities of blood are routed to brain areas that are involved in making these decisions and responding emotionally to them. Increased blood flow generally means an increased amount of oxygen to the area, and increased oxygen may influence the central nervous system and initiate mood changes (Oleson, 1971). The support of this hypothesis is weak, however, because a strong relationship between gains in fitness and mood has not been found.

Monoamine Hypothesis

Monoamine neurotransmitters in the brain, which have been linked to anxiety, mood shifts, and depression, are affected by both short-term and long-term exercise. Morgan and O'Connor (1988) call this the monoamine hypothesis. Monoamines, particularly dopamine, serotonin, and norepinephrine (noradrenaline), have been known for many years to be associated with emotion. When people become angry, their epinephrine (adrenaline) levels rise, and people who have higher trait anxiety (measured by trait anxiety scales) also have higher levels of adrenaline both at rest and during exercise bouts. Patients with emotional dysfunction have abnormal levels of norepinephrine. For example, those with paranoia have chronically higher levels of norepinephrine, but norepinephrine is low in clinically depressed persons.

Other evidence that points to the relationship between catecholamines and emotional function comes from drug research. Antidepressants function by increasing the amount of norepinephrine or serotonin in the central nervous system (Forrester, 1987;

Laraia, 1987). Reserpine, which is a drug that induces depression, also depletes brain catecholamines (Ransford, 1982). Electroconvulsive shock therapy, which is used to reduce depression, acts through enhancing aminergic synaptic transmission.

The evidence that these monoamines are influenced by exercise is compelling. In animal studies, brain norepinephrine increases after 15 to 30 min of treadmill running or swimming (e.g., Barchas & Freedman, 1963), and animals that were physically trained for several weeks also had higher levels of brain epinephrine (Brown & Van Huss, 1973; Brown et al., 1979; DeCastro & Duncan, 1985).

Over the past 10 years, substantial progress has been made with animal models in understanding neurobiological responses to exercise. Jacobs (1994) showed that serotonin neurons are preferentially connected to areas controlling body activity, specifically, torso and limbs, and even more specifically, repetitive movements. In addition, serotonin is the major culprit in depressive disorders, and those with depression are listless, finding that even raising themselves out of bed requires enormous effort. Jacobs' work provides a clear mechanism by which exercise may alleviate depressive symptoms.

Reviews by Dishman (1997) and Meeusen and colleagues (2001) provide compelling evidence that long-term exercise training enhances many of the functions of monoamines: adaptations in enzymes involved in the production of monoamines, changes in metabolic activity, and changes in receptor sensitivity. Peptide neurotransmitters that coexist with monoamine transmitters and facilitate locomotor activity are increased and up-regulated by chronic exercise. Neurotrophic factors that maintain, protect, and promote growth in neuronal populations are increased by exercise, particularly those factors that enhance serotonin, a major antidepressant.

Several neurochemical models have been proposed to explain the antidepressant effects of exercise. Even though some of these animal models are based on different systems, the results from them converge to implicate a similar neurochemical mechanism. These models have the potential to provide information as to whether exercise provides *protective* effects against depressive disorders, rather than only to reverse depressive symptoms.

In humans, also, changes have been seen in circulating levels of norepinephrine following short exercise sessions (Dulac et al., 1982; Ransford, 1982) and longer bouts, such as from marathon running (Appenzeller & Schade, 1979). A modification of the monoamine hypothesis, proposed by Siever and Davis (1985), shifts from the notion of circulating levels of monoamines to the idea of monoamine regulation. That is, exercise may assist in regulating monoamines, rather than simply increasing or decreasing their circulation levels. Blumenthal (1989) suggested that in addition to reducing symptoms of anxiety by brain monoamine changes, exercise may also increase central opioid activity (Blumenthal, 1989).

"Our studies suggest that regular motor activity may be important in the treatment of affective disorders. For example, if there is a deficiency of serotonin in some forms of depression, then an increase in tonic motor activity or some form of repetitive motor task, such as riding a bicycle or jogging, may help to relieve the depression."
From Jacobs (1994).

Release of Endorphins

One theory that continues to receive wide publicity is based on the well-documented observations that the brain produces high levels of endogenous opiates in response to acute physical and psychological stress. These high levels of circulating β-endorphins might explain the improvements in mood state, sometimes described as euphoria, that people commonly experience following an exercise bout. Many investigators have suggested that exercise-induced increased secretion of β-endorphins is a viable explanation for feelings of euphoria (acute enhancement of well-being) that follow exercise (Blumenthal et al., 1999). Others have described increases in β-endorphins following vigorous aerobic exercise (e.g., Carr et al., 1981; Hollmann et al., 1986; Lobstein et al., 1989; Rahkila et al., 1987; Risch, 1982), and it is thought that the exercise level must be close to maximum or at least extended for a considerable period of time before any mood change is experienced (Kirkcaldy & Shephard, 1990; Thoren et al., 1990). These studies share a common theme with studies of the relationship between exercise and catecholamines discussed previously: Resting levels in highly fit individuals are lower than those in low-fit individuals, but in response to a physical or psychological stressor, highly fit individuals both increase their levels of endorphins and clear them faster than low-fit people do.

The endorphin hypothesis has some critics, however, and even if true may not apply to older adults. Morgan (1985), after an extensive review of the research to that point, concluded that the arguments for exercise-produced endorphins changing moods were not compelling. He cited one study in particular, by Farrell and colleagues (1986), in which a drug that blocks the effects of endorphins was injected into subjects before they rode a bicycle at 70% $\dot{V}O_2$ for 30 min. If exercise-induced high levels of circulating endorphins are the reason why people feel more relaxed at the end of an exercise period, then these participants should not have felt any beneficial change in their mood, because the injected drug blocked the endorphins before they could act. Yet, these participants also felt significantly more relaxed after their exercise bout. As Morgan emphasized, these results are a serious challenge to the endorphin hypothesis. At best, exercise-produced endorphins may contribute to the feelings of psychological well-being and relaxation that follow an exercise bout, but they may not be considered the primary explanation for the tranquilizing effect of exercise.

Even if the endorphin hypothesis is eventually shown to be valid, it may not be relevant to older adults. To this point, endorphin levels seem to be increased only when exercisers work at high intensities for at least 30 min. Clearly this type of exercise will not be conducted by many people over the age of 70 and certainly not by those over 80 years of age. Thus, it is unlikely that this hypothesis, if it is based on high-intensity exercise, explains the enhanced feeling of well-being that older adults have following exercise programs.

Thermogenic Hypothesis

Increasing body temperature to produce a variety of therapeutic effects has been known for centuries, dating back to at least a.d. 800 in Finland (Morgan & O'Connor, 1988). Hot baths and saunas are one way to achieve this therapeutic effect. For example, Raglin and Morgan (1987) found that a 5-min shower at 38.5°C was associated with a significant decrease in state anxiety.

Body temperature changes during and following exercise may also reduce muscular tension (deVries, 1987). Muscle relaxation following exposure to exercise-induced temperature increases may be the result of changes in the brain stem, leading to decreased muscle feedback and synchronized electrical activity in the cerebral cortex (Von Euler & Soderberg, 1956, 1957). This muscle relaxation, in turn, is associated with reduced anxiety. Indeed, the difficulty of maintaining psychological anxiety in the presence of complete muscular relaxation was the basis for a type of aversion therapy (Wolpe et al., 1964). In this therapy, the patient concentrated on voluntary control of muscular tension while in the presence of a very mild or abstracted version of a stressor (e.g., a line drawing of a snake). Gradually, the stressor was increased in terms of proximity and reality until the

patient could remain physically, and presumably psychologically, relaxed in the presence of a live snake. Wolpe and colleagues' hypothesis was that by controlling muscular tension, the patient could reduce psychological tension, that is, anxiety. This therapy never gained general acceptance, but it was an interesting hypothesis, because it emphasized the strong link between muscular tension and psychological anxiety. The reduction of electrical activity in the muscles and the parallel reduction in anxiety following an exercise bout have been called the tranquilizer effect of exercise (deVries, et al., 1981; Hatfield & Landers, 1987). Moreover, some of the exercise-induced changes in physiological systems last for several hours and therefore may be more effective in reducing psychological anxiety than other psychological techniques (Raglin & Morgan, 1987).

The decreased muscular tension that follows an exercise bout may reduce psychological tension, because muscle tone and the central nervous system are greatly affected by body warming. An increase in body temperature also may influence the functions of some of the brain monoamines and may cause a protein that mediates the increase in body temperature to be released into the blood during body heating. (The internal body temperature of rats was increased just by injecting them with plasma from humans who had been exercising; Cannon & Kluger, 1983.) Thus, the relaxed feeling that people experience following a vigorous, prolonged workout may be partly caused by the increase in body temperature that arises from the workout and may last for several hours.

Psychosocial Hypotheses

Although biological theories certainly contribute to the explanation of the relationship between exercise and emotional function, in and of themselves these theories are probably inadequate for complete understanding of the relationships (Plante & Rodin, 1990). Ekkekakis and Petruzzello (1999) reviewed several complex psychological theories that might explain why and how an acute bout of exercise is related to the affect dimension of well-being: extraversion, sensation seeking, type A behavior pattern and self-evaluative tendencies, theory of psychological reversals, optimal stimulation theory, Thayer's multidimensional activation theory, and the self-efficacy theory. These theories are too complex to be described here, but they provide a powerful guide for those who are studying the impact of physical activity on the way people perceive the world.

Individual perception of events is sometimes more powerful than the objective impact of the event. Habitual exercise is a very different experience from one acute bout of exercise, and lifestyle behaviors have long-term effects on people's perceptions. For example, King and colleagues (1989) found greater psychological improvement based on perceived fitness than on actual fitness improvement. Furthermore, Doyne and colleagues (1987) found that both aerobic and anaerobic exercise produced similar improvements in psychological health. Therefore, psychological effects must also be factored into the equation. Some of the psychosocial hypotheses that have been proposed are mastery, changes in self-efficacy, social interaction, and distraction.

Mastery Hypothesis

This hypothesis is part of the social–cognitive theory of Bandura (1986), which, when applied to an exercise context, suggests that perceptions of improved physical function lead to increased feelings of mastery (self-efficacy), which enhance feelings of well-being. When individuals believe that they have mastery over their environment and their actions, this enhances feelings of power, personal efficacy, and self-directedness. Mastery refers to the extent to which individuals view themselves as personally powerful or influential in affecting their own life outcomes. In adults who have lived without physical constraints, feelings of mastery are greatly affected by age-related losses of sensory and physical ability. But in individuals who have life-long disabilities, feelings of mastery increase substantially as they age into their 50s and older. Thus, age-related losses of mastery are independent of losses attributable to disability (Schieman & Turner, 1998).

Increases in physical strength, endurance, and ability provide individuals with a feeling that they have more control over their environment and, thus, they are less vulnerable (Sime, 1984). Therefore, participation in programs that increase these attributes should also enhance long-term emotional health. Individuals in the large population study, Longitudinal Study on Aging, who had a strong sense of control were more likely to engage in and maintain exercise programs (Wolinsky et al., 1995). However, although mastery experiences that occur in less strenuous activities such as softball, bowling, and golf may contribute to emotional health by providing opportunities for improvement and accomplishment, these types of activities have not shown antidepressant effects comparable to those that occur after aerobic exercise (Ransford, 1982).

Social Interaction and Approval

Many adults who exercise do so in some type of social setting, either with a few friends or in a formal exercise program. Professionals who plan and conduct exercise programs have recognized for many years that the social aspect of the program may be almost as attractive to their older patrons as the health benefits. Because the social interaction that occurs in these settings may substantially improve mood, anxiety, or depression (Hughes et al., 1986), social interaction is another possible mechanism mediating the relationship between exercise and emotional health. However, the need for social interaction is highly individual, and coercing individuals who do not desire much social interaction would be more detrimental than beneficial to their mental health. But for those who perceive a social deficit in their lives, participation in an exercise or sport program with other individuals will certainly improve their emotional well-being. Although the social interaction that occurs in exercise classes contributes significantly to older adults' emotional health, it cannot exclusively account for the psychological benefits observed after exercise programs. In two studies of young subjects, jogging alone produced greater improvements in depression than did participation in group activities of softball, archery, and golf (Brown et al., 1978; Folkins & Sime, 1981). Of course, these latter studies were of young college students, and social interaction needs change with increasing age.

Several researchers (e.g., McAuley & Rudolph, 1995) have suggested that the social interaction that individuals have in supervised classes is a major confounder in trying to determine the relative contributions of physiological responses and social interaction to the amelioration of depressive symptoms. However, Dunn and colleagues (2002) reported that people with depression who exercise alone also experience decreases in depressive symptoms.

Another factor that may contribute to the psychological benefits of exercise classes or programs is the social reinforcement that occurs both during and outside of the class. Class participants encourage each other and praise each other for the accomplishment of different activities within the class. Also, class participants' families and friends outside of the class may praise and congratulate them for their participation. Social approval is a strong form of social reinforcement and can elevate mood states (Ross & Hayes, 1988). This type of social approval also has the potential to enhance long-term emotional health.

Distraction Hypothesis

The distraction hypothesis emerged from the observation that time is a contributing factor to changes of emotional state. Exercise takes time, and whether individuals are exercising or not, time passes. Several authors have suggested that exercise may be considered a diversion from the stresses of daily life, a period in which the individual can legitimately take a "time-out" from occupation and family responsibilities (Bahrke & Morgan, 1978). Thus, an exercise period is a socially condoned activity in which people can "get away from it all." However, a meta-analysis of 32 studies of exercise and mood concluded that the distraction hypothesis was not supported (Arent et al., 2000).

Characteristics of Exercise Related to Well-Being

If exercise and physical activity are related to subjective well-being, what type of exercise should be performed? How frequently should it be done, and for how long? The questions regarding the characteristics of exercise that are related to well-being pertain to the (a) type of exercise—aerobic or anaerobic; (b) characteristics of exercise—intensity, frequency, and duration; and (c) most effective environment in which to exercise. In addition, the interaction of exercise with personality may produce some negative effects.

Type of Exercise

Whether aerobic or anaerobic activity is more effective in improving well-being has not been studied thoroughly in older adults. Most researchers have used aerobic exercise as the intervention, but a few have explored anaerobic activities, such a weightlifting. Both types have been found to enhance components of well-being, and both have been used in some studies that failed to find an influence on well-being (Craft & Landers, 1998; King et al., 1993). Only a few researchers have directly compared the effects of both types of exercise on depression symptoms, and almost all of these included young adults in their samples. However, in the one study of persons over 60, only aerobic exercise significantly improved symptoms in a longitudinal study of 439 persons over the age of 60 who had knee osteoarthritis (Penninx et al., 2002). The improvements occurred in both persons with low and high depressive symptomatology, indicating that exercise is ameliorative and also a buffer against future problems. This is an area that needs much more study.

Characteristics of Exercise

An exercise session or program is described by three characteristics: intensity, duration, and frequency.

Which of these is important to enhance subjective well-being in older adults?

Three meta-analyses (Craft & Landers, 1998; McAuley & Rudolph, 1995; North et al., 1990), and several other studies that focused on this question (Steptoe & Cox, 1988; Tsutsumi et al., 1998) indicated that physical activity and exercise programs do not have to be highly intense to improve well-being. Self-reported tension, depression, fatigue, and anger decreased after a single acute bout of both moderate- and high-intensity step aerobics. Also, vigor increased in both types of exercise (Kennedy & Newton, 1997). In fact, there is some evidence that moderate exercise produces positive psychological changes whereas vigorous activity does not (Arent et al., 2000; Moses et al., 1989). It may be that because most of these adults have not been athletes, and their goals for exercise have changed over the years, moderate-intensity exercise may be viewed as more enjoyable without the high performance demands, excessive fatigue, and fear of injury that some participants report. Conversely, some clinical, experimental trials of exercise with depressive symptoms have found intensity of exercise to be a factor (Singh et al., 1997). Thus, the intensity factor may initiate a mechanism that explains some factors of well-being but not others.

The duration of exercise in terms of individual workout sessions has not been studied. But a longer duration of the exercise program in terms of number of weeks seems to provide more benefits in terms of components of psychological well-being. From their meta-analysis, Craft and Landers (1998) discovered that exercise programs longer than 8 weeks produced more improvements in well-being. Frequency (number of exercise sessions per week) has not been studied extensively enough to determine its effects on well-being.

A factor that influences the effect that all three characteristics of exercise have on almost any outcome is the health and fitness of the person who is exercising. Individuals who are in excellent condition and who embrace physical activity as a lifestyle react physiologically to exercise quite differently, and it is probable that they also have different psychological responses to it. This factor has not been studied in older adults.

Acute or Habitual Exercise Exposure

An important aspect of exercise that was not discussed in terms of mechanisms was whether the exercise exposure was an acute bout (one session or exposure

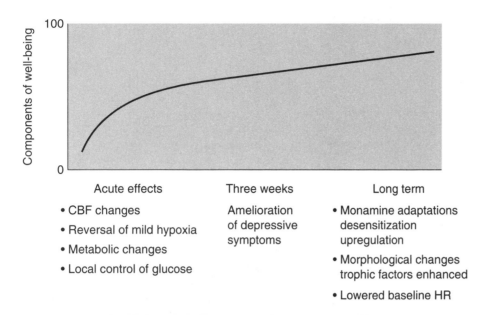

Figure 10.9 Hypothetical time course explaining the relationships of physiological mechanisms to the development of components of well-being. CBF = cerebral blood flow; HR = heart rate.

Finally, many methodological problems will make validating mechanisms and their interactions a difficult and tedious business. The great majority of both human and animal studies of mechanisms have been conducted with young or young to middle-aged subjects, and it is not at all clear how much the findings of these studies apply to human adults over 65 years of age. Neurological and enzymatic changes are extraordinarily difficult to measure in humans, especially older ones. Everyone agrees that studies are needed to sort out acute from habitual effects of exercise, but design problems abound. For example, it is difficult to separate the effects of the last in a series of acute bouts from the habitual effects of an exercise program (Arent et al., 2000).

of exercise) or whether the mechanisms were operative only after habitual exercise sessions over a longer period of time. It is likely that different mechanisms affect different components of well-being after different durations of an exercise program. As can be seen in figure 10.9, some physiological responses, such as increased arousal, occur very early in the onset of exercise, and inasmuch as they affect mood, depression symptoms, or feelings of well-being, then short, acute bouts of exercise would influence those psychological components. In this case, if a component of well-being were affected only by the state of arousal, for example, then well-being would be enhanced each day of exercise, and if exercise occurred every day, it would simply be a matter of daily acute exposures. It would not matter whether the mechanism was acute or chronic. However, other proposed physiological mechanisms, such as morphological changes in neuronal networks or the development of trophic factors, develop only after repeated exposures and as such would only be effective after several weeks of increased physical activity.

It is much too early in the research process to know how physiological mechanisms are affected by acute or habitual exercise behaviors. Although we know that acute versus habitual exposure is a factor in understanding mechanisms, several other factors have been identified: the individual's physiological fitness level, the intensity and frequency of the exercise exposure, and general affect of the individual at the time of activity.

Effects of the Environment

Do environmental surroundings and the situation alter the impact of exercise on well-being? Does it make a difference in well-being whether the activity occurs in supervised exercise classes held in a clinic or research laboratory, exercise classes in a classroom, or unsupervised exercise at home? This question has not been well studied. Primarily, if home and class exercise protocols are adhered to, then there is little difference among the sites. However, if the exercise serves as a therapeutic intervention, such as was a requirement of studies in the meta-analysis of Craft and Landers (1995), the exercise programs were more effective when held in hospital clinics than when conducted at home by patients with MDD.

Negative Effects of Exercise

For most individuals and under most circumstances, exercise yields benefits in many dimensions. However, for a few individuals, exercise can become a compulsive behavior. These individuals become addicted to exercise and are obsessive about their exercise programs, either continuing each session far beyond its scheduled period or repeating a session several times a day. Exercise, like any other addiction, becomes the central focus of their life and they neglect their personal and social obligations, to the detriment of their family and other responsibilities (Dishman, 1985; Veale, 1987). Kirkcaldy and Shephard (1990) reviewed several studies of exercise addiction and concluded that for some individuals, abstinence from exercise leads to feelings of hostility, headache, frustration, and tension (Glasser, 1976) and restlessness, irritability, and guilt (Robbins & Joseph, 1985). It is not unusual to find older adults who, after retirement from work that has been largely sedentary, "discover" running as a pastime and become emotionally dependent on it. Although the effect of age has not been studied in these individuals, older addicted runners probably experience the same negative effects as younger addicted runners do.

SUMMARY

Physical health includes three components: physical condition, functional status, and subjective health status. Although more than 75% of men and women over the age of 70 have one or more chronic physical conditions, they vary greatly in the ways these health conditions affect their functioning and in how they view their health. Health and physical fitness are not synonymous. Health relates to the presence or absence of disease processes, whereas fitness relates to aerobic capacity, muscular strength and endurance, and flexibility. Most researchers who have studied the relationship of health to well-being and life satisfaction have defined health in the most minimal terms—the extent to which physical function enables activities of daily living and instrumental activities of daily living.

The two important categories of health-related quality of life are functioning (physical, cognitive, engagement with life, and objective health status) and subjective well-being (emotional well-being, perceptions of self, bodily well-being, global well-being, and life satisfaction). The relationship of health and well-being is bidirectional. Not only does health status influence perceptions of well-being, but people's feelings of well-being also influence other health-related behaviors. Those who have feelings of well-being and life satisfaction are more likely to take action to maintain their health and prevent disease.

Aging per se does not cause a decline in subjective well-being, but health constraints do. As people grow older, health becomes more important to them because it affects their quality of life. Poor functional health negatively influences the positive affect that contributes to quality of life, self-efficacy, and self-esteem. Similarly, physical activity and exercise may also have beneficial effects on positive affect. However, much more research has been conducted on the effects of physical activity and exercise on negative affect—anxiety and depression. The evidence is very compelling that increased physical function, activity, and exercise have beneficial effects on anxiety and depression. Whether the studies are correlational population studies or experimental studies, or whether the participants are asymptomatic of depression or have depressive disorders, exercise and physical activity appear to reduce anxiety and depression.

The physical dimension of well-being includes the role of the body and its functioning in self-esteem, self-efficacy, and sense of control. Body consciousness, public and private, includes the subjective feelings that individuals have about their bodies. Society in general has a very negative view of age-related physical changes, and it is difficult for aging adults to maintain a healthy body consciousness. Body competence, or self-efficacy, is the confidence that people have about their physical abilities in specific situations. One of the greatest adjustments that all people must make with aging is the adjustment to the loss of physical ability. Exercise programs have been shown to improve self-efficacy and body consciousness in the exercise-related physical activities, and these improvements may generalize to other similar activities.

Physical ability contributes to older adults' sense of control, which is a central component of well-being. The maintenance of health and physical mobility enables older adults to maintain independent living, which is an important contributor to well-being. Even in those older adults who live in long-term care centers, physical health and mobility enhance well-being by providing people with more opportunities to control their own activities and environment and by increasing the variety of activities in their lives.

Several mechanisms have shown promise to explain the relationships among physical activity, exercise, and well-being. Physiological mechanisms include the cardiovascular hypothesis, monoamine hypothesis, endorphins hypothesis, and thermogenic hypothesis. Psychosocial hypotheses include the mastery hypothesis, changes in self-concept hypothesis, and social interaction and approval hypothesis. Many researchers are studying these hypotheses, because understanding the mechanisms underlying relationships among physical activity and well-being will provide methods to optimize the quality of life of older adults.

Optimizing the health and physical fitness of older adults has three major positive outcomes, two of which benefit the individual and one that benefits society. First, and perhaps most important, enhanced health and fitness increase feelings of well-being and life satisfaction, which in turn contribute to high-quality aging. Second, a significant increase in the number of persons who age optimally can have a tremendous impact on reducing the total health care expenditures. The cost of health care for those who experience their terminal years in a state of physical dependency is eight times higher than for those who have aged successfully. Third, the healthy and fit older adult is much more capable of being involved with family, friends, and the community and of interacting in emotionally meaningful ways with people who are important to them and to their well-being.

REVIEW QUESTIONS

1. Describe the different aspects of health and fitness and discuss how they are related.

2. How do age and exercise differentially influence positive and negative affect?

3. What types of evidence support the idea that exercise plays an assistive role in combating age-related depression?

4. How does self-efficacy influence physical function in the frail elderly?

5. Both physiological and psychosocial mechanisms have been proposed to explain how exercise and physical activity may positively affect psychological well-being. Describe them and explain the process by which they work.

SUGGESTED READINGS

Clark, D.O. (1996). Age, socioeconomic status, and exercise self-efficacy. *Gerontologist, 36,* 157-164.

Jacobs, B.L. (1994). Serotonin, motor activity and depression-related disorders. *American Scientist, 82,* 456-463.

Spirduso, W., & Cronin, L. (2001). Exercise dose-response effects on quality of life and independent living in older adults. *Medicine and Science in Sports and Exercise, 33* (Suppl.), S598-S608.

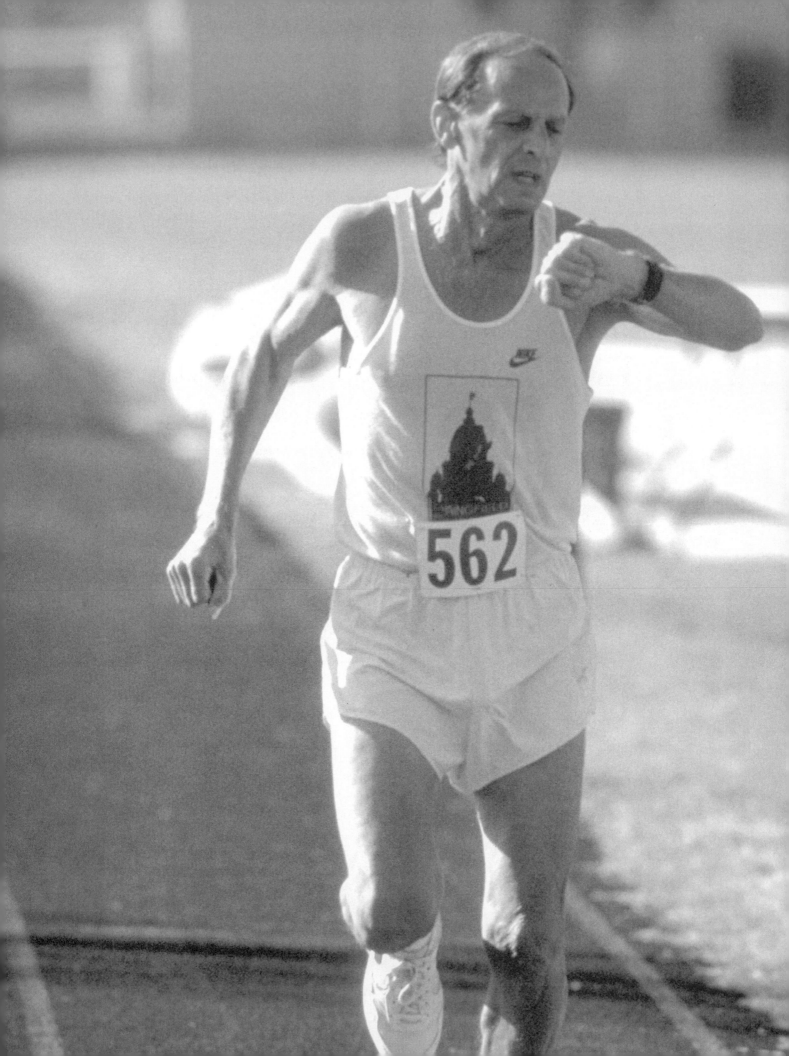

PART V

Physical Performance and Achievement

Physical Function of Older Adults

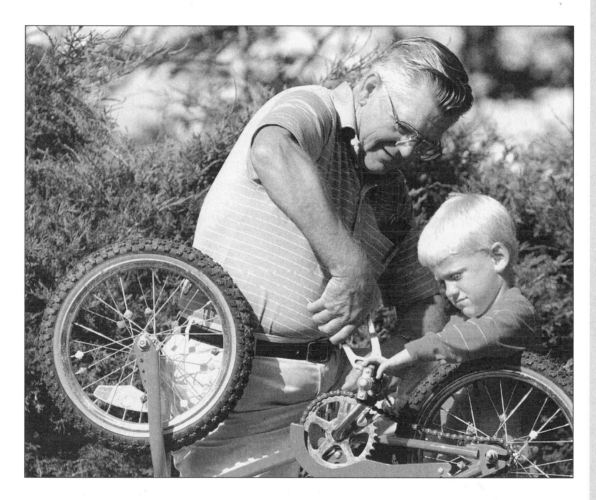

The objectives of this chapter are

- to describe the characteristics and limitations of physical function in the oldest-old,

- to explain the concept of "reserve,"

- to demonstrate how to assess physical function at each level of the hierarchy of physical function,

- to discuss the role of physical activity in postponing disability, and

- to describe the goals and effects of exercise on physical function in the oldest-old.

The individual differences of older adults are nowhere more starkly apparent than in the physical functioning of the old (75-84 years) and the old-old (85-89). In these two age groups, individuals range from those who are extremely mobile, function independently, and can complete a 26.2-mile (42 km) marathon race (see chapter 12) to those who have multiple chronic diseases, are physically disabled, and live in a physically morbid condition. Unfortunately, the number of elderly who are so physically impaired that they cannot live independently is far greater than the small percentage of those who are physically fit or physically elite. Approximately 7 million elderly are presently in long-term care, and the cost of **frailty** in this country is roughly $54 billion a year. By 2030, unless some major improvements are made in **disability** rates of the elderly, 14 million adults will not be able to conduct their daily activities independently (Zedlewski et al., 1990).

This chapter explores the full range of capabilities and assessment of these capabilities of the old and oldest-old. First, a hierarchy of physical function of adults in the oldest age groups is described, with levels ranging from the physically dependent to the physically elite. Several tests that are appropriate for each level of function are described, because in many instances the tests consist of physical tasks that define their abilities. Next, the chapter presents the general methodological issues and corollary problems of testing this group but also discusses the value of testing this group. The chapter concludes with a discussion of the role and effectiveness of physical activity and exercise in postponing disability and a short section on the expectations that health professionals and society in general should have for the physical functioning of the old and old-old.

Definitions of Physical Function

Several terms are used in discussions of elderly function, and sometimes they are incorrectly used interchangeably. **Functional independence** indicates that individuals complete activities of daily living without difficulty, and it implies that these individuals are operating on the basis of at least the minimal levels of physical, cognitive, and mental health. **Functional fitness** refers to the fitness components (strength, power, flexibility, balance, and endurance) necessary to perform normal everyday activities safely and independently without undue fatigue. **Functional performance** is the observable ability to perform tasks

of daily living (walking) or field tests that emulate tasks of daily living (climbing 10 stairs). Those at risk of losing fitness and performance and subsequent independence are designated as frail, and a loss of these abilities is referred to as disability, which will be defined in much more detail under the section on the physically dependent.

Hierarchy of Physical Function in Older Adults

The old and old-old can be categorized broadly into five levels: the physically elite, physically fit, physically independent, physically frail, and physically dependent. Although each level describes individual capabilities, these categories were created to bring some organization to the understanding of physical function in a very old group of adults whose capacities differ widely. Individual differences are profound, and although most people in any one category will be more similar to each other than they are to those in another category, there certainly are many individuals who will be difficult to categorize—for example, those who seem to fit well in a specific category except for one ability. Also, an individual may decline to a lower level (i.e., independent to frail) because of some temporary setback such as sickness or injury but then return to the former level after treatment or rehabilitation.

A hierarchy of the physical function of the old and oldest-old groups is shown in figure 11.1. Table 11.1 lists representative tests of physical function appropriate for persons at each level. Together, they provide a summary of the abilities and the tests available for these abilities at each level of physical functioning, although the table is not a comprehensive list of all available tests, only a representative list. The first column of table 11.1 shows the category of physical function; the second column provides several examples of tests appropriate for that category; and the third column lists the research sources for these tests. Each of the categories of physical function and some of the ways that their function is assessed are discussed in the following sections, beginning with the physically elite and ending with the physically dependent.

Physically Elite

The physically elite elderly are a very unusual group of people in our society. They train physically on a daily basis and compete in tournaments available to individuals their age. Many participate in the Senior

Table 11.1 Tests of Physical Function

Category of physical function (see figure 11.1 Hierarchy of PF)	Sample tests	Sources
Physically elite	$\dot{V}O_2$max; modified Balke treadmill	ACSM (1991)
Physically fit	Bruce treadmill protocol	Bruce et al. (1973)
Physically independent (some AADLs)	Resistance strength tests (dynamometry) Routine flexibility and agility tests	McArdle et al. (2001)
Physically elite	Senior fitness test	Rikli & Jones (2001)
Physically fit	AAHPERD functional fitness test	Osness (1987)
Physically independent (some AADLs)	Fitness tests: • Jumping, hand strength, flexion • Balance, agility, power, flexibility • Jumping, side-step, flexion, reaction time	Kimura et al. (1990) Kuo (1990) Tahara et al. (1990)
Physically independent	AAHPERD field test AADL Continuous-scale physical functional performance test	Osness (1987) Reuben et al. (1990) Cress et al. (1996)
Physically frail	Physical performance test Tinetti's mobility assessment IADL Hierarchical ADL-IADL Classification schema for upper extremity Function & mobility Geri-AIMS Physical impairment scale Functional independence measure	Reuben & Siu (1990) Tinetti (1986) Lawton & Brody (1969) Kempen & Suurmeijer (1990) Williams & Greene (1990) Hughes et al. (1991) Jette, Branch, & Berlin (1990) Granger et al. (1986)
Physically dependent	ADL Mobility test Physical disability index Physical performance and mobility exam Physical function scale of MOS SF-36	Katz et al. (1963) Schnelle et al. (1995) Gerety et al. (1993) Lemsky et al. (1991) Ware & Sherbourne (1992)

Note: ACSM = American College of Sports Medicine; AAHPERD = American Alliance for Health, Physical Activity, Recreation and Dance; AADL = advanced activities of daily living; IADL = instrumental activities of daily living; ADL = activities of daily living; AIMS = arthritis impact measurement scales; MOS SF-36 = Medical Outcomes Study Short Form.

Olympics, in masters tournaments, and in special age-group classifications within a general tournament, such as a 10K running race sponsored by a commercial interest, a city, or a foundation. Another segment of adults in this age group are those who have continued training physically or working in a physically demanding occupation, for example, skiing, scuba-diving, hiking, and mountain-climbing instructors, or forest rangers, firefighters, and police. Not many can continue working in these occupations to very old ages, but a few do. Because these individuals are so unusual, they represent the maximum physical performance capabilities of these oldest age groups and a high physical standard to which many of the old-old should aspire. The physical capacity of the adults in this category, at least in the abilities

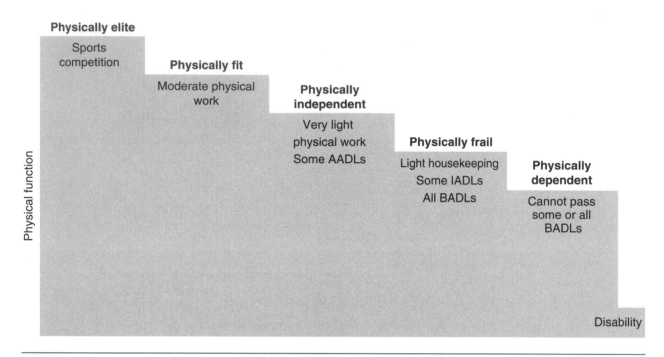

Figure 11.1 Hierarchy of physical function of the old (75-85 years) and oldest-old (86-120 years). AADL = advanced activities of daily living; IADL = instrumental activities of daily living; BADL = basic activities of daily living.

required by their sport or activity, is generally superior to that of untrained adults decades younger. Many of these individuals are genetically predisposed to succeed in physical activities. Their successes and their time investments have paid off for them in old age, as most of them have maintained a considerable amount of function in their last decades. However, maintaining excellent health and physical function in the last third of life, although it requires focus and discipline over a lifetime, also requires some good fortune. Individuals in this category have been lucky enough not to have inherited diseases or to have been in a disastrous accident that either killed them or disabled them, the latter of which would place additional stresses on many physiological systems.

The physically elite are very active, and they can be assessed safely by tests that are routinely used for young adults. Their maximum aerobic capacities can be obtained using a VO_2 treadmill or bicycle ergometer test, their strength can be assessed with cable tensiometers or electromechanical instrumentation, and their muscular endurance can be assessed by multiple trials of submaximal strength production,. Nevertheless, testing individuals over the age of 60 in high-capacity tests such as maximum aerobic capacity or power is still likely to produce more problems than are usually seen when young individuals are tested. Cardiovascular disease is more prevalent in these age groups and must be more seriously considered. The tendency of older adults to dissipate heat less

efficiently presents problems in endurance testing. Interpretations of aerobic capacity are complicated by age-related differences in body composition, which were discussed in chapter 3.

Physically Fit

The physically fit elderly are individuals who exercise two to seven times a week, but they exercise primarily for their health, enjoyment, and well-being. They do not compete, and they do not exercise as long or as intensely as those who do compete. Nevertheless, they are consistent in maintaining their good health habits and their exercise protocol. Because of this consistency, their health status is well above that of individuals who do not attend to their health habits (in terms of nutrition, sleep, alcohol use, drug use, smoking habits, and exercise). The physically fit elderly are generally estimated by their peers to be much younger than their chronological age. Their physiological characteristics are more robust than those of individuals in lower physical function categories. For example, their VO_2 is much higher than that of sedentary adults, although their aerobic capacity does not match that of the physically elite (see the active group in figure 4.4, page 93). They may still be working in their chosen occupation or career and may be participating in many activities with people much younger than themselves. Also, because of the relationship of physical health to emotional control and to feelings of well-being and life satisfaction (chapter 10), these seniors tend to be very active and fully engaged in life.

As is true for the physically elite, most of the physically fit elderly could complete a routine VO_2 treadmill or bicycle ergometer test, and all could complete regular muscle strength and endurance, flexibility, and agility tests. The ACSM recommends that the modified Balke treadmill protocol be used with the elderly, because it uses slow but constant walking speeds and very gradual increases in grade increments every 2 or 3 min.

Several field tests have been developed that do not require extensive and expensive equipment, laboratories, or highly specialized technicians, yet these tests are effective in assessing physical function, and the physically fit elderly would do well on these tests. One of the most recent and best validated tests is the Senior Fitness Test (Rikli & Jones, 2001). The items of this test as well as the physical components tested by the items are shown in table 11.2. This test was administered at 267 test sites in 21 states, including 7,183 men and women between the ages of 60 and 94. Test reliabilities were high, ranging from $r = .80$ to .98 on the items (Rikli & Jones, 2001).

Individuals in the physically fit category could probably do well on Kuo's (1990) physical function test battery. This battery does not measure aerobic capacity, but it enables the test administrator to assess other components of physical fitness: static balance, agility, lower limb power, and flexibility. These data are old, but they are included because it is very rare to obtain physical performance scores from so many older adults, and it is particularly rare to be able to compare functional fitness scores of men and women. The test was administered (first in 1984 and again

in 1985) to 3,562 Japanese participants, the majority of whom were males (64%) between the ages of 45 and 70. Several subjects were over age 75. Their performances on three of the test items are shown in figure 11.2.

Several observations about physical function can be made from these graphs. First, it is clear that as the subjects age, their physical capacities decline. Second, the lower scores among older subjects are exaggerated for women. This was a cross-sectional study, so it is incorrect to say that women's physical function deteriorates faster than men's, although it appears that the physical capacity of older women is much lower than that of older men, except possibly when balancing on one foot with the eyes closed. The greatest difference between men and women is on the test item that measures power, the standing broad jump, where men's scores substantially exceed the scores of women. Not shown in the figure are the scores of trunk flexibility, in which the women were superior to the men. Women older than 55 were only 12% less flexible than the 19- to 25-year-old women, but men over 55 were 39% less flexible than the 25- to 30-year-old men. Third, there were very few scores from persons more than 80 years old, and these were all included in one 80-plus category, a practice typical of many studies.

The physically fit elderly provide 50% to 75% of the upper scores on laboratory strength and muscular endurance tests that are administered to persons in this age group, particularly if their exercise protocol includes some activities that require strength. Because of their habitual physical activity, their performances are also better than those of many much younger but sedentary people.

Physically Independent

The physically independent elderly are those who do not exercise or focus on beneficial health habits but who nevertheless have not been burdened with one or more diseases so debilitating that they lose the ability to function independently. Some of these individuals have no particularly bad health habits and are relatively free of symptomatic disease. Others may be alcoholics or smokers and have several chronic diseases, but they retain the capacity to function. These people are in delicate health and have meager reserves, yet they have few functional limitations. They remain mobile and independent; however, many of them would not have the aerobic endurance to complete a VO_2max test of aerobic capacity. Also, many times they have orthopedic complications or neuropathy in the lower limbs and feet that affect physical performance testing. They terminate the test

Table 11.2 Senior Fitness Test (Rikli & Jones, 2000)

Physical components	Test items
Lower body strength	Chair stand
Upper body strength	Arm curl
Aerobic endurance	6-min walk or 2-min step
Lower body flexibility	Chair sit and reach
Upper body flexibility	Back scratch
Agility and dynamic balance	8 up-and-go

Adapted, by permission, from R.E. Rikli and C.J. Jones, 2001, *Senior fitness test manual* (Champaign, IL: Human Kinetics), 29.

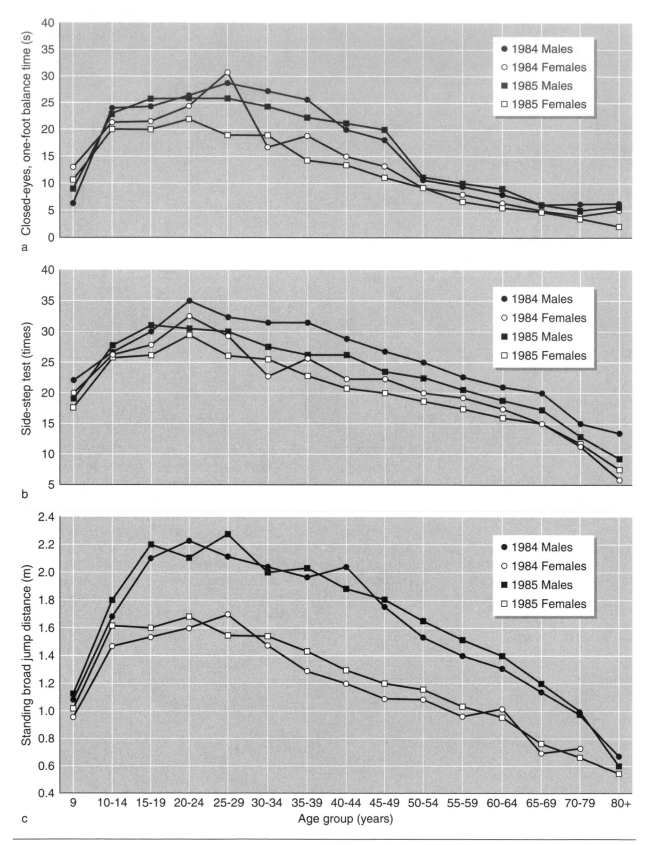

Figure 11.2 Physical fitness levels of people in Taipei in relation to age and gender: *(a)* balance, *(b)* agility, and *(c)* power tests.

Data from G.H. Kuo (1990).

before it is completed, and sometimes it is difficult for the test administrator to determine whether performance is being terminated because participants have reached endurance or strength limitations or because they can no longer tolerate pain in their joints or legs. Most adults in these age groups are also on one or more medications, some of which may influence test results.

These participants have enough physical function to participate in some advanced activities of daily living (AADL), so they can participate in social activities such as vacation travel, golf, or gardening. They can complete successfully most or all of the instrumental activities of daily living (IADLs) and all of the activities of daily living (ADLs), but they are vulnerable to unexpected physical stress or challenge. The ADL–IADL test is explained in more detail in the section titled "Surveys, Inventories, Diaries" (p. 270). Questionnaires and interviews regarding their physical difficulties and abilities are generally used at this level.

More members of the old and oldest-old age group are in this physical function category than in any of the other four. From interviews of 4,463 persons in the 1989 National Long-Term Care Survey (Manton et al., 1993), Spector and Fleishman (1998) determined that only 34% of the subjects had no functional disabilities. Considering that probably less than 5% could be considered physically fit or physically elite, roughly 66% of adults over the age of 65 would be correctly classified as physically independent. From the Older Americans 2000 report (Federal Interagency Forum on Aging Related Statistics, 2000), it appears that 66.8% of men but only 49.7% of women over the age of 70 have no difficulty with basic physical functions (figure 11.3a). This percentage is worse for African Americans over the age of 70, with only 52.6% of men and 37.1% of women reporting that they are able to perform these functions (figure 11.3b).

An Important Target: Reserve

Even though many older adults are physically independent, they are hovering very near the threshold of physical abilities below which they cannot function. A very small setback in health—the incidence of a minor disease, a small accident, or simply the passage of a little time—could change them from being physically independent to being frail and partially dependent. In other words, they have little if any reserve. **Physical reserve** can be defined as "distance from physical frailty," and it incorporates the concept of "margin of safety." Physical assessments should be made to determine older adults' reserve in the

three critical physical components of frailty: musculoskeletal function, aerobic capacity, and motor coordination. Frailty is discussed in more detail in the next section.

Physical reserve is "distance from frailty."

It is particularly ironic, in light of the large number of old adults who are physically independent, that this group falls between the cracks in terms of understanding their physical capabilities. These individuals continue to live in their homes and are somewhat active, yet they do not have enough aerobic capacity or lower leg strength to complete even the least demanding protocol on a treadmill test. Their scores on traditional resistance strength tests would be so low that they would challenge the reliability of some of the tests. Most, however, would make a perfect score on the ADL–IADL tests and on any of the other tests that are appropriate for the next lower level of physical function. And, the ADL–IADL instruments are insensitive to declines in function in physically independent persons other than those on the lower borderline. Nevertheless, functional fitness components such as lower limb strength are exceedingly important to measure, because a decrement in the lower extremity, for example, eventually leads to decrements in IADL (Jette et al., 1990). Leg strength and endurance are necessary for shopping, housekeeping, driving, and food preparation. Thus, it is important to find a more valid way to assess reserve in the physically independent in order to know how far from frailty they may be.

Performance Tests

Self-report inventories have been used successfully to identify the limits of physical function of individuals at the lower extreme of the physical function continuum, but the better the subjects' physical function, the less discriminating self-reports are. Therefore, several efforts have been made to develop performance tests, such as fitness test batteries, to measure adults in this category. One such example is a test battery developed by the Adult Development Council of the American Alliance for Health, Physical Education, Recreation and Dance (AAHPERD).

AAHPERD Functional Fitness Test Described in a test manual by Osness (1996), the AAHPERD Functional Fitness Test includes measures of muscular strength and endurance, coordination, trunk and leg flexibility, and aerobic endurance and was designed specifically for adults over age 60. It was

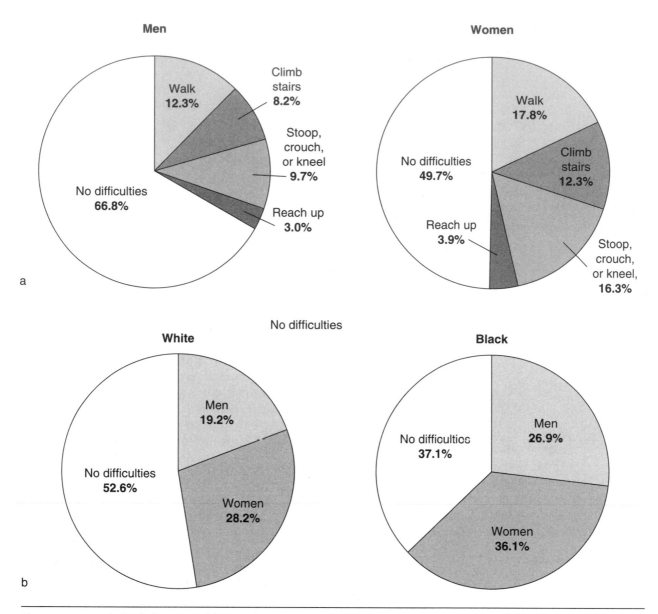

Figure 11.3 Each shaded section of the pie chart shows *(a)* the percentage of older adults who are unable to perform that function and *(b)* the percentages unable to perform in white and African American populations.

From the Older Americans Report (2000).

also designed so that it could be administered by professionals and clinicians in the field who lack measurement equipment, specialized training, and resources. The equipment necessary to administer the test can be made from materials that are readily available in any institution or hospital. The purpose of the test is to provide, through the use of nationally standardized test items appropriate for sedentary, independently living elderly, an estimate of the physical function of those who are not physically fit but also are not yet physically frail. The items are shown in table 11.3, with their respective reliabilities and temporal stabilities, which were obtained

independently by Shaulis and colleagues (1994). The validity of the cardiorespiratory Functional Fitness Test item was $r = -.65$ (Bravo et al., 1994). This test has acceptable reliability and validity and is appropriate for physically dependent and physically frail individuals.

Advanced Activities of Daily Living (AADL) Advanced activities of daily living, a term coined by Reuben and Solomon (1989), are the many nonsurvival functions that people carry out in social, religious, or physical activities that enrich their lives. AADLs are those activities that require abilities well beyond the IADLs. Social AADLs include

Table 11.3 AAHPERD Functional Fitness Test

Component	Test item	Description	Reliability[a] (M,W)
Flexibility	Sit-and-reach test	Sit on floor; reach fingers to or beyond toes.	.97, .98
Agility	Agility test	Rise from chair, walk around one cone, return to chair, rise and walk around another cone, as quickly as possible.	.98, .96
Arm and hand coordination	Soda pop test	Turn six soda pop cans over in a specified order, one at a time, as quickly as possible.	.89, .71
Muscular strength and endurance	Arm curl	Arm curl a 4-lb (1.8 kg) weight with dominant arm; number of repetitions in 30 s.	.94, .81
Aerobic endurance	1/2-mile (0.8-km) walk test	Walk 1/2 mile as quickly as possible.	.99, .96

Note: M = men; W = women

[a]Temporal reliabilities calculated by intraclass correlation.

Adapted from Shaulis, Golding, and Tandy (1994).

employment, traveling, hobbies, and participation in social and religious groups. Physical AADLs include recreational exercise and crafting, such as woodworking and gardening. Because these activities are voluntary and social, the range of activities will vary considerably. Thus, Reuben and colleagues (1990) suggested that a universal measure of AADL probably cannot be developed, but an AADL assessment could be tailored to an individual's particular AADLs so that the individual could be monitored over time. For example, these researchers developed a scale for physical exercise as an AADL in which subjects are categorized on the basis of frequency and intensity of exercise: frequent vigorous exercisers, frequent long walkers, frequent short walkers, or nonexercisers (Reuben et al., 1990). Using this scale, professionals can plot subtle changes in the physical AADL that might signal a larger than expected decline in physical function.

Continuous-Scale Physical Functional Performance Test The continuous-scale physical functional performance test (CS-PFP) was developed by Cress (1996) to assess separate domains of fitness by using performance measures that emulate functional tasks of daily living. It was designed to provide a better indication of abilities to complete instrumental activities of daily living, to provide an indication of which fitness components were weak, and to tap into a broad spectrum of abilities. This test has 15 functional items, such as carrying and then pouring water from a jug of water into a cup, distributing groceries into a paper bag and carrying it 70 m, transferring 7.76 kg of laundry and sandbags from a washer to a dryer and then to a basket, vacuuming a set amount of oats from a prescribed area of carpet, and getting into and out of a bathtub. This test was able to discriminate among three groups of individuals differing in levels of independent living, whereas the traditional instrumental activities of daily living survey was not. The test has high reliabilities and construct validity.

Physically Frail

Frailty is a "condition or syndrome that results from a multi-system reduction in reserve capacity to the extent that a number of physiological systems are close to, or past, the threshold of symptomatic clinical failure. As a consequence the frail person is at increased risk of disability and death from minor external stresses" (Campbell & Buchner, 1997, p. 315). Brown, Sinacore, Binder, & Kohrt (2000) operationally defined frailty as the score on the Physical Performance Test (PPT). The PPT total score is 36, and they identified the following categories: *not frail* = 32 to 36; *mildly frail* = 25 to 31, and *moderately frail* = 17 to 24.

Although frailty and disability frequently coexist, they are different concepts. Frailty indicates instability and risk of loss. Disability indicates loss of function.

The four basic components of frailty are (a) musculoskeletal function, (b) aerobic capacity, (c) cognitive and integrative neurological function, and (d) nutritional reserve (Campbell & Buchner, 1997).

The physically frail elderly can perform the ADLs but have a debilitating disease or condition (such as extreme muscular weakness) that physically challenges them on a daily basis. They may be unable to execute a few of the IADLs, such as shopping, laundering, and mopping, but with some assistance, either human or technological, they can live independently. Many are largely homebound; that is, meals are brought to them by volunteers or city services groups, and their homes may be periodically cleaned by others. Elderly persons in the physically frail category walk a fine line between independent and dependent living, and in many cases their level of physical function is the ultimate determiner of their lifestyle.

Assessment of Frailty

Because this group borders on dependency and it is important to ascertain their risk of disability, several different assessment batteries have been developed to determine the extent of their physical function. These test batteries are used with a variety of populations: hospitalized patients, nursing home residents, those undergoing rehabilitation, and independent members of the community.

Surveys, Inventories, Diaries

The most universally used assessment instrument for this group is the ADL–IADL test. The original ADL test was published by Katz (1963), and an extension of this concept to IADLs was developed by Lawton and Brody (1969). The ADL scale is used to determine the extent to which individuals can carry out activities of daily living that are basic to surviving independently. It is based on six primary tasks that are learned in early life—(in order) feeding, continence, transferring (e.g., from bed to chair), toileting, dressing, and bathing—and lost in the latter years of life in roughly the reverse order. These six functions also have a sociobiological function, even in primitive societies.

The IADL questions relate more to complex physical abilities, such as

preparing meals, light housecleaning activities, heavy housecleaning activities, washing and ironing clothes, making beds, and shopping.

Although many professionals have considered the ADLs and IADLs as separate constructs, Spector and Fleishman (1998) recommended combining them as one scale and administering all items, even if it is thought that some individuals might not pass any IADLs. The items are not completely hierarchical, so that some individuals who fail one or two ADL items may nevertheless pass one or two IADL items (Spector & Fleishman, 1998). These items are shown in table 11.4. In addition, it has been proposed that by adding questions related to whether individuals have (a) modified the way they do ADL–IADLs or (b) decreased the frequency of doing them, a preclinical stage of disability can be detected (Fried et al., 1996); that is, the sensitivity of the ADL–IADL scale may be enhanced.

Table 11.4 Percentage of Functionally Disabled Persons ≥ 65 Years Who Report Difficulty With ADL and IADL Items

Item	ADL-IADL	Percentage
Going outside of walking distance	IADL	73
Shopping	IADL	71
Doing laundry	IADL	51
Bathing	ADL	49
Getting around outside	IADL	46
Preparing meals	IADL	38
Taking medications	IADL	36
Managing money	IADL	34
Getting around inside	ADL	32
Light housework	IADL	32
Dressing	ADL	31
Transferring	ADL	28
Toileting	ADL	28
Using the telephone	IADL	21
Help with incontinence	ADL	14
Feeding	ADL	14

Note: ADL = activities of daily living, that is, basic activities of hygiene and personal care; IADLs = instrumental activities of daily living, that is, basic activities necessary to reside in the community.

Adapted from Spector and Fleishman (1998).

Life inventories include questions about individuals' work (job, house, yard), recreational activities (watching TV, listening to the radio), automobile driving, and participation in social activities (clubs, volunteering, going to church). Sometimes the results from these inventories are just used to categorize individuals as very active, active, moderately active, or sedentary. A few investigators calculate the amount of energy expended during the activities by determining the number of metabolic equivalents expended for each activity.

Self-reported difficulties provide another way to determine frailty. Individuals are given a list of physical tasks necessary to function well and are asked to check those with which they have difficulty. These include items such as bending, lifting, stooping, climbing stairs, lifting, and carrying objects.

The ADL–IADL scale is self-administered or administered by a proxy, a caregiver, or an interviewer. Item responses can also be abstracted from medical records or directly observed by a professional or caregiver.

Williams-Greene Classification Schema for Upper Extremity Function and Mobility

Williams and Greene's (1990) battery of physical function tests is particularly attractive because it is based on theory: a movement classification schema. In this classification schema, which is specifically designed to organize and understand movements that are important to the physical functioning of the elderly, movements are classified as either upper extremity function or mobility movements. Upper extremity function is dependent on strength and steadiness and is composed of simple arm and hand movements and distal extremity control, such as occurs in object manipulation and self-help actions. The movements that enable mobility are strength and flexibility, transferring maneuvers from one posture to another (sitting to standing, lying to sitting), and balance. Gait and mobility functions include simple gait control, precision gait control, maximum gait control, and body agility. For each of these upper extremity functions and mobility movements, tests have been developed by these researchers or drawn from the research literature.

Performance Tests

To avoid the weaknesses of self-report inventories, investigators have developed some batteries of physical tasks that are very similar to tasks of daily living. These performance tests measure primarily gross or large-muscle physical performance of the frail elderly, but tests of this type vary in the kind of assessment made, the setting in which they are appropriate, and the experience that is necessary to administer the tests.

The PPT (Reuben & Siu, 1990) is a good example of a timed performance test. The items were selected to simulate activities of daily living, to vary in difficulty, and to take as little time as possible to complete. Items were also selected to include all components of fitness for older adults: upper body fine motor function, upper body gross motor function, balance, mobility, coordination, and muscular endurance. An additional feature is that for clinical purposes, the test can be administered by untrained assistants. The reliability among different raters is high.

The PPT can be administered as a nine-item or a seven-item battery (the seven-item battery is shown in table 11.5) that includes writing a sentence, simulated eating, putting a book on a shelf, putting on and removing a jacket, picking up a penny, walking 50 ft (15 m), and climbing a flight of stairs. As can be seen, the range of scores is broad, and the test discriminated well among older adults who were members of several clinical practices, a hospital primary care unit, a board-and-care home, and a senior citizens apartment.

Another excellent example of a physical performance test for this level of functioning is Tinetti's Test of Mobility (1986). This test assesses the individual's ability to get around in the environment. The responses of the individual are rated normal, adaptive, or abnormal for a wide variety of movements—from maintaining balance during sitting and while rising from a chair to the much more complex control task of turning while walking. Also included are movements such as bending over from a standing position and picking up a small item, and placing a light object on a high shelf. This test may be administered by physicians, nurses, and other trained personnel, and the reliability of ratings made by different raters is high. In one test of reliability, the testers agreed on 85% of the individual items, the total scores never differing by more than 10%.

The Functional Independence Measure is a test used frequently by physical and occupational therapists for this group. It is used nationally and internationally and has published norms.

Physically Dependent

The lowest level of the hierarchy of physical function includes the physically dependent, shown at the right bottom of figure 11.1 (p. 264). Physically

Table 11.5 Performance on Individual Timed Physical Performance Test (PPT) Items

Timed PPT items	% Able to complete	Average time to complete (sec)	Range (sec)	SD (sec)
Writing a sentence	94	16.7	7.0–49.0	6.5
Simulated eating	100	15.4	7.5–56.5	6.8
Lifting a book and putting it on a shelf	94	4.0	1.5–40.0	4.0
Putting on and removing a jacket	97	15.6	2.0–71.5	8.4
Picking up a penny	98	3.5	1.5–20.5	2.1
Walking 50 ft	98	25.0	10.5–315.5	31.0
Climbing a flight of stairs[a]	91	10.6	4.0–76.0	11.4

Note: Based on six patient populations:
1. Patients in the UCLA Department of Medicine Practice Group's Geriatric Practice
2. Patients of the Rhode Island Hospital's Medical Primary Care Unit
3. Residents of a senior housing unit in Providence, RI, attending a health screening fair in the unit
4. Patients of a community-based geriatrics practice in Los Angeles
5. Patients entering a board-and-care home in Los Angeles
6. Patients with Parkinson's Disease, Brown University

[a]Excluding subjects at Sites 4 and 5.

Reprinted, by permission, from D.B. Reuben and A.L. Siu, 1990, "An objective measure of physical function of elderly outpatients: The physical performance test," *Journal of the American Geriatrics Society* 38: 1108.

dependent individuals cannot execute some or all of the ADLs and are dependent on others for food and other basic functions of living. The extent of physical disability suffered by these older adults is measured by the degree of their inability to perform activities of daily living, such as dressing, getting into and out of bed, rising from a chair, washing their face and hands, eating and drinking, washing themselves completely, using the toilet, moving around inside the house, going up and down stairs, moving around outdoors on flat ground, and taking care of their feet, fingernails, and toenails. Difficulty with bathing is the most commonly reported problem. Women are more disabled than men, with the difference increasing with each additional one half decade (Anderson-Ranberg et al., 1999). The highest levels of disability are among the centenarians. Individuals overrepresented in this disability are older, female, African American, and poor.

Physical disability can result from a history of chronic or acute diseases, accidents, or certain lifestyle habits, but common observation indicates that not all people who have chronic diseases or who live unhealthy lifestyles become physically disabled. Potential predictors of physical disability are shown in table 11.6. Two of these, hypertension and arthritis, are consistent predictors of disability, whereas the other diseases and lifestyle habits are sometimes considered significant predictors. The potential for many elderly people to become physically frail is very high, because the incidence of chronic disease among the elderly is also very high (see figure 1.8, page 14).

Age-related disability is not always a downward decline. People have ups and downs, and conditions can change depending on the cause of the disability. For example, many people recover from a stroke and can regain most if not full function (Guralnik & Simonsick, 1993).

Physical function in this group is primarily assessed with the ADL–IADL inventories, completed as self-reports but more often with assistance from a caregiver or from professional observation. For patients of very limited physical and cognitive functioning,

Table 11.6 Potential Predictors of Physical Disability

Chronic diseases
- Hypertension
- Arthritis
- Angina pectoris
- Coronary heart disease with angina
- Stroke
- Congestive heart failure
- Cancer
- Bone injury
- Obesity
- Diabetes

Lifestyle behaviors and conditions
- Smoking
- Physical inactivity
- Alcohol use
- High fat mass

Cognitive dysfunction
- Depression

Schnelle and colleagues (1995) developed a Mobility Test. The Mobility Test provides categorical data on standing, walking, transferring, and allows for using equipment, such as wheelchairs (see figure 11.4) and continuous data on endurance and speed that, when combined, provide an assessment of mobility

independence. The endurance and speed measures are not susceptible to floor and ceiling effects; thus, they are useful to test various intervention strategies in this severely limited population. Subjects are ranked by the level of assistance needed to perform each item. Speed scores are recorded in seconds, endurance scores by the number of times some tests can be completed within 30 s. The strengths of this test are that it provides scores in time and some other variable, and the assessor also ranks the performance according to quality of movement.

The Physical Disability Index (PDI; Gerety et al., 1993) was developed to provide a comprehensive measure of the physical impairments and disabilities of frail elderly residents of nursing homes. It provides test items for residents whose abilities range from ambulatory and functional to those who are wheelchair bound. The PDI items include observation and timing of bed mobility (such as rolling to the right side, rolling to the left side, bridging, moving up in bed, and moving from a supine position to sitting up in bed), transferring to a chair from the edge of a bed, sitting unassisted, moving from a sitting to a standing position, standing balanced with feet apart and then together, standing with feet in tandem (one forward and one backward) with or without the assistance of a chair, ambulation through a 180° turn, and ambulation for 50 ft (15 m). Finally, the PDI also provides items for wheelchair-bound residents: wheelchair turn through 180° and wheelchair propulsion for 50 ft.

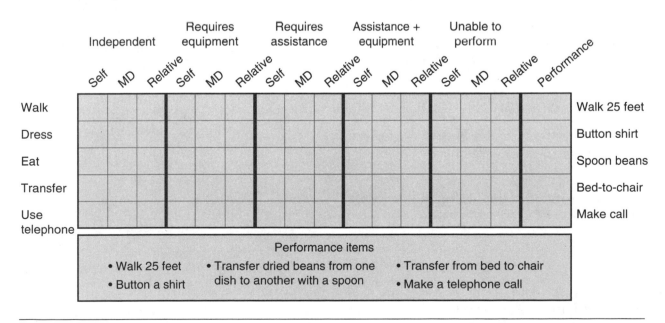

Figure 11.4 Sample self-report and performance test form.

Reprinted, by permission, from J.F. Schnelle et al., 1995, "Functional incidental training, mobility, performance, and incontinence care with nursing home residents," *Journal of American Geriatric Society* 43: 1356-1362.

The Physical Performance and Mobility Examination (PPME) was designed by Lemsky and colleagues (1991) to be a brief performance test appropriate for measuring the physical function of frail, hospitalized elderly adults. In this test, the patient performs the following items: sit up in bed, transfer to a chair, stand up from a chair once and then five times in succession, stand in a tandem and semitandem position, walk 6 m, and step up and down a 9.5-in. (24-cm) step. The test was validated on a sample of 169 patients (average age, 71.5 years) and on another of 98 patients whose average age was 79.63. Three trained raters assessed the patients' abilities on each item. The PPME's reliability was acceptably high, and it correlated moderately with self-reported activities of daily living ($r = .47$-$.66$).

The Medical Outcomes Study Short Form (MOS SF-36) was developed for use with general populations of older adults from the Medical Outcomes Study questionnaire. It has 10 items on physical functioning.

Predicting Disability and Predictive Models

Because physical disability has such a negative impact on quality of life, a substantial amount of attention has been focused on identifying predictors of disability so that interventions can be designed to prevent or postpone dysfunction. Physical function has proven to be a powerful predictor of independent living. Low physical activity level and muscular weakness are predictors of disability later in life. In several longitudinal studies in which physical function was measured at baseline and then dependency was predicted 3 to 5 years later, the amount of physical activity in which the subjects participated was also a strong predictor of dependent living (Guralnik et al., 1994; Hirvensalo et al., 2000; LaCroix et al., 1993; Vita et al., 1998).

> Low physical activity leads to low strength, which leads to low physical function (Rantanen et al., 1999).

When measures of physical performance are combined with self-reported physical activity level, the odds ratio for loss of independence is dramatic (figure 11.5). Older men who did not function well physically and who were sedentary were five times more likely to lose their independence than those who were active and functioned well (Hirvensalo et al., 2000). This was also true for women, but the differences were not as great.

Finally, the likelihood of being admitted into a nursing home is substantially higher for those

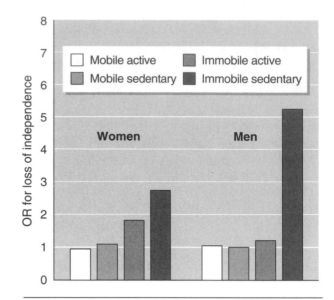

Figure 11.5 Odds ratios (OR) for older adults (age 65-84) categorized by amount of mobility and sedentariness. M = mobile, persons who scored high on a physical performance test of mobility; I = immobile, persons who made low scores on the mobility test; S = sedentary; A = active, based on a self-report of their weekly physical activities.

Adapted from Hirvensalo, Rantanen, and Heikkinen (2000).

who have poor physical function. One of the best examples of this was the study by Guralnik and colleagues (1994), in which they showed a strong relationship to the score on the Physical Performance Test to the number of admissions to nursing homes (figure 11.6). Adults who live independently in the community have higher physical function scores than those who live in assisted living facilities, and they in turn function better physically than those who live in nursing homes (Cunningham et al., 1993; Schroeder et al., 1998). Another example is shown in table 11.7, where the relative risk of being admitted to a nursing home, calculated on the basis of stair climbing scores and physical performance in general, was considerably higher than the relative risk calculated by age alone. Later, Guralnik (1999) argued that measures of lower body function alone are effective predictors of dependency.

An early predictive model, proposed by Nagi (1991), proposed three stages leading to disability:

Pathology → impairment →
functional limitations → disability

Others have since expanded this model to include risk factors, extraindividual factors (medical, professional, and social support), intraindividual factors (lifestyle, psychosocial, and coping skills; Verbrugge & Jette, 1994), and functional limitations (Lawrence &

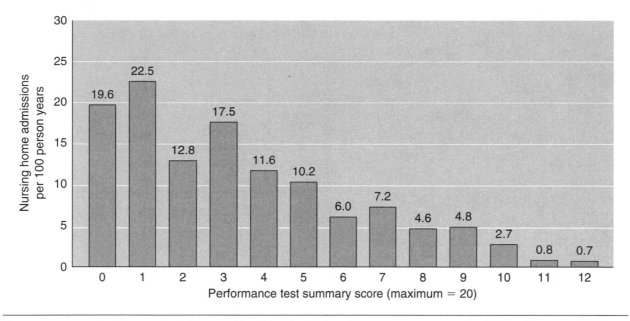

Figure 11.6 Nursing home admissions predicted by Physical Performance Test scores. The higher the score, the better the physical function.

Journals of Gerontology. Series A, Biological Sciences and Medical Sciences by J.M. Guralnik. Copyright 1994 by Gerontological Society of America. Reproduced with permission of Gerontological Society of America in the format textbook via Copyright Clearance Center.

Table 11.7 **Relative Risk of Nursing Home Admission**

	Men	Women
Age	1.8	1.9
ADL	1.1	1.2
Walk 1/2 mile (0.8 kg)	1.2	1.4
Stair climb	1.9	1.2
Performance	2.7	2.2

Note: ADL = activity of daily living. From the Established Populations for the Epidemiologic Study of the Elderly (EPESE). *N* = 5,174 men and women living in nursing homes or community living.

From Guralnik and colleagues (1994).

Jette, 1996). Morey and colleagues (1998) proposed a more comprehensive model that included most of these factors and in addition emphasized the contribution of fitness (cardiorespiratory, muscular performance, and morphologic factors) to the model. A model by Rantanen and colleagues (1999) also found strength and physical activity to be potent predictors of motor disability. In figure 11.7, a conceptual model is shown that combines all of the factors that have been proposed by the several models. Although the relationships shown in the figure are compatible across the different models, no one has actually tested a model such as this. Each previous model included slightly different latent variables and different measurements to represent the latent variables.

Figure 11.7 demonstrates the pathway to disability in old age. Confounding factors such as age, race, gender, education, depression, and cognitive dysfunction can have strong effects on fitness factors. Fitness factors are directly related to functional limitations; that is, even in the absence of pathology, fitness factors affect physical function. Cardiorespiratory fitness is related to pathology, which in turn leads to functional limitations. Many times pathology first produces impairments that then lead to functional limitations. These limitations eventually progress to disability.

Determining Physical Function in the Elderly

Testing the physical function of adults over 60 years of age is challenging. As was emphasized in chapter 2, populations of older adults are extremely heterogeneous. The characteristics of the individuals, the purposes of the evaluation, and the ease with which the test can be administered are all important considerations. As we have seen, three basic methods have been used to test physical function in the old and oldest-old: physical performance and capacity

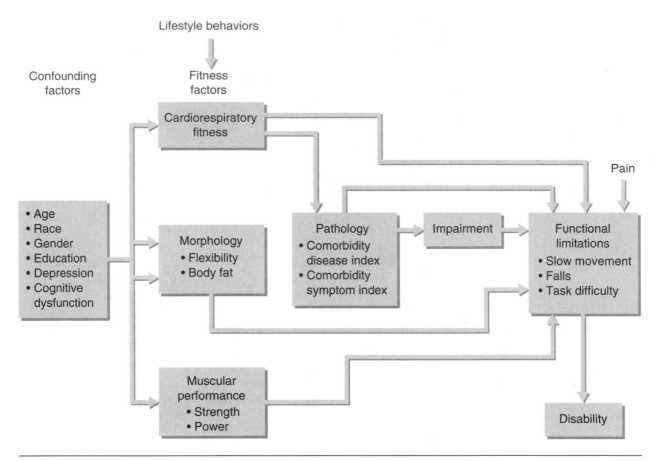

Figure 11.7 Conceptual model of the path toward disability (based on models and research from Lawrence & Jette, 1996; Morey et al., 1998; Nagi et al., 1991; and Verbrugge & Jette, 1994).

tests, observation and functional skill testing, and self-report or caregiver report instruments, such as surveys and interviews. Assessment is a pivotal part of the professional services provided to older adults, but it is a complex and difficult process. It also has some attendant risks of injury or mortality. Several of these issues are discussed in the next session.

Special Issues in Testing the Elderly

Several factors make it more difficult to test older adults:

- Fluctuations in fatigue or pain level
- Temporary distractions or lack of concentration
- Impaired cognitive ability
- Reduced information processing speed
- Changing medical conditions or medications
- Fluctuations in mood, anxiety, and level of depression

As in any testing situation, when one is determining the physical ability of the very old, an important variable to consider is test anxiety and motivation. How nervous and anxious are the subjects about being tested, and how much do they really care about giving their very best effort for the test? When we are determining physical capacities of this age group, we need to know whether the performance observed during testing is representative of daily performance. Older individuals are more likely to be excessively and deleteriously anxious about being tested on their physical abilities if they believe that the test outcomes will have implications for their living independently or participating in other activities that they enjoy. Conversely, if they think the test outcomes have little implication, they may have less motivation to provide their best performance. In either case, the test administrator does not obtain a true picture of the individual's physical abilities.

Finally, it is of interest to compare scores of older adults with younger adults, either to estimate how much function has been lost or for research purposes, other problems surface. Many tests of physical function were first developed on younger subjects, and performance norms were based primarily on those subjects. Consequently, many norms are provided in younger age categories in 10-year intervals, but because of the wide heterogeneity of old adult performance, 10-year intervals are not as instructive as 5-year intervals. The physical performance of a 40-year-old may not be that much different from that of a 30-year-old, but the difference between a 90-year-old and an 80-year-old is usually very large. Five-year norm intervals make much more sense for adults over age 70. Also, some tests that older adults can barely complete are so easy for young adults that the tests do not discriminate among the younger adults. Thus, age comparisons are not possible.

Value of Assessment of Older Adults

Although physical functioning of the elderly is of vital concern to individuals and has substantial implications for national health care costs, the assessment of physical function is not yet a routine clinical procedure for adults over 70, unless they become dysfunctional and require care. Yet routine annual assessments of function have great value in determining physiological reserve, extending active life expectancy, and thus enhancing the quality of life.

Need for Periodic Functional Assessment

Functional or screening assessments usually are conducted when there is evidence that instrumental or basic activities may be compromised. But physical health and function are so important in the elderly that several gerontologists have recommended that a baseline of physical capacity of all individuals over age 65 be established (Rikli & Jones, 1997). Only by establishing a baseline of performance can the degree and rate of change of physical function in these individuals be assessed accurately, and only through periodic assessment can an individual's "reserve" be quantified in various systems. Baseline assessments are valuable for determining whether deterioration in function is age related or potentially treatable. The findings can be applied to questions about driving automobiles, housing accommodations, travel, and participation in specific types of activities, such as exercise programs. Systematic assessments can provide longitudinally based norms of function within the population, so that the effectiveness of prevention or treatment programs can be assessed. Periodic assessments also provide norms of age-related changes in function.

Periodic functional assessment provides a way to determine the extent of functional decline.

For some old and oldest-old adults, a comprehensive geriatric assessment (CGA), which includes much more than just health and physical function, can help determine their capabilities for independent living. Like health and physical function, domains such as cognitive function, affective function, social support, economic status, environmental stressors, and well-being are also important determinants of independent living. The National Institutes of Health (1988) have recommended one CGA that includes all dimensions of life, as shown in table 11.8. Note that a substantial portion of this CGA involves physical health and functioning. The CGA is primarily a diagnostic process that must be linked to the ongoing

Table 11.8 Comprehensive Geriatric Assessment

Physical health
Traditional problem list:
 Disease severity indicators
 Self-ratings of health and disability
 Quantifications of need for, and use of, medical services
 Disease-specific rating scales

Overall functional ability
 Activities of daily living scales (bathing, dressing, eating, toileting, transferring, and walking)
 Instrumental activities of daily living scales (household and money management, use of telephone)

Psychological health
 Cognitive function
 Affective function

Socioeconomic variables
 Social interactions network
 Social support needs and resources
 Quality of life assessment
 Economic resources and access

Environmental characteristics
 Environmental adequacy and safety
 Access to services (shopping, pharmacy, transportation, and recreation)

Adapted, by permission, from D.H. Soloman et al., 1988, "New issues in geriatric care," *Annals of Internal Medicine* 108: 725.

Benefits of Annual Physical Function Assessments

Annual physical function assessments offer many benefits for the elderly. Among them are the following:

- Evaluation of an individual's functional status
- Basis for planning exercise programming
- Way to assess effects of exercise programming
- Basis for motivation to continue exercise program
- Basis for referral to physicians
- Prediction of elderly who are at risk of becoming functionally dependent
- If a person is at risk, determination of type of institutional care needed
- Identification of the distribution and type of services required by the elderly
- Determination of future health and long-term care needs for communities
- Basis for better understanding of physical function in the elderly (research)

care of the clients, and it is more appropriate for the midranges of functional capacity, that is, those who are neither "too well nor too irreversibly disabled" (Reuben & Solomon, 1989, p. 570).

Extension of Active Life Expectancy

Although most individuals hope that they have a quantitatively long life, they may not want a long life if the quality of that life is poor (refer to chapter 1). Being physically independent and having the capacity to be active plays a large role in defining quality of life for all older individuals. In fact, the fear of becoming dependent because of physical disabilities is one of the greatest fears of the old. These fears, in addition to the high social costs of dependency, have led gerontologists and public health policy researchers to distinguish between life expectancy and **active life expectancy (ALE)** for older cohorts. Understanding, through health and physical function assessments, the physical capacities that might reasonably be expected at various advanced ages will enable health professionals and gerontologists to develop preven-

tive and intervention programs that will extend the ALE for thousands of adults.

Active life expectancy, defined by Katz and colleagues (1983), is that period of life that is free of disability in ADLs. It is an important indicator of the quality of life. Figure 11.8 shows the percentage of remaining life in which 65- to 90-year-old individuals in one study were independent (Branch et al., 1991). Several important observations can be made about this figure. First, the ALE declined steadily in all three geographical areas, except for men aged 75 to 85 years in New Haven. Second, the ALE is different for men and women, with the differences increasing in those old subjects over age 85. The percent of remaining independent life is higher in men than in women who live to these older ages. Third, geographical differences are striking. The men in New Haven have a much higher percentage of ALE than do men in the other two geographical locations.

The concept of ALE is an extension of the index of health expectancy (the life expectancy of an individual in several different states of health) proposed earlier by Wilkins and Adams (1983). By calculating the number of years that Canadians spent in different conditions (short-term disabilities, restricted or impossible instrumental or daily activities, or long-term institutionalization), these authors described the age-specific rates of various forms of activity restriction in the total population (figure 11.9). They then calculated the health expectancy at birth for a given cohort. The quality-adjusted life expectancy was 3.2 years greater for Canadians living in cities than for those in rural areas and small towns and 7.7 years greater for persons from high-income families than for persons from low-income families. Non-institutionalized individuals could expect to have some restrictions on their activities—10.8 years for men and 14.0 years for women. Furthermore, men could expect 3 years and women 1.3 years in the most restricted category, that of inability to do work for employment or housework.

Physical disabilities do not always lead to dependent living, because some individuals have transitions in and out of dependency during their later years (Branch et al., 1991). In fact, a significant number of disabled old persons regain independence; thus, the occurrence of disability should not be assumed to lead inevitably to a decline in health and functional status. The story of Eula Weaver in chapter 4 is a good example of a person who, after changing her health and exercise habits, moved from dependent to independent status. One way that ALE might be extended is by making periodic assessments of the physical function of older

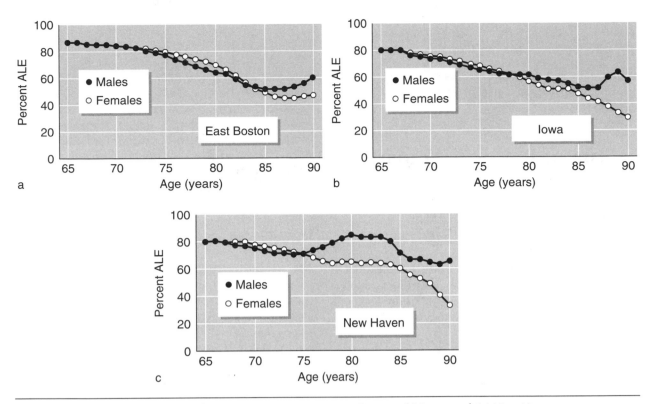

Figure 11.8 Percentage of active life expectancy (ALE) in *(a)* east Boston, *(b)* Iowa, and *(c)* New Haven.

Reprinted, by permission, from L.G. Branch et al., 1991, "Active life expectancy for 10,000 Caucasian men and women in three communities," *Journal of Gerontology: Medical Science* 46: M148.

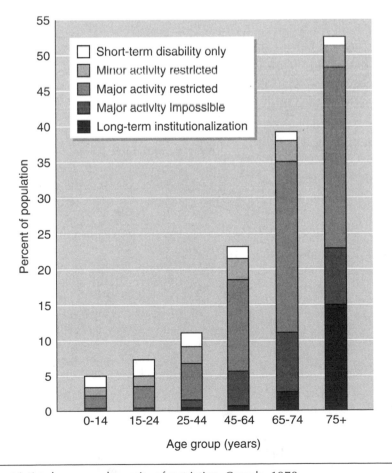

Figure 11.9 Activity restriction by age and severity of restriction, Canada, 1978.

Reprinted, by permission, from R. Wilkins and O.B. Adams, 1983, "Health expectancy in Canada, late 1970s: Demographic, regional and social dimensions," *American Journal of Public Health* 73: 1075. Copyright APHA.

individuals and using the results to prescribe and monitor physical exercise programs and dietary adjustments.

Role of Physical Activity in Postponing Disability and Facilitating Independent Living

There are many causes of disability and reasons other than loss of physical function why some older adults live in nursing homes. The main reasons are loss of cognitive function, uncontrollable depression, economic difficulties, and psychosocial reasons. Evidence is accumulating that social interaction is related to maintenance of health and function in the elderly. Those who experience loneliness also report more fatigue, visit their physicians more, and take more medications than elderly adults who are not lonely (Svanborg, 1993). Certainly the onset of multiple chronic diseases and comorbidities presents a formidable challenge to independent living. Osteoarthritis, vertigo, and diabetes were the strongest predictors of poor ADL and poor physical performance in a study by Kivinen, P., Sulkava, Halonen, & Nissinen (1998).

> *"The mere presence of cardiovascular disease, diabetes, stroke, osteoporosis, depression, dementia, chronic pulmonary disease, chronic renal failure, peripheral vascular disease, or arthritis (which may all be present within a single individual) is not by itself a contraindication to exercise"* (ACSM, 1998).

However, losses of physical function play such a dominant role in the loss of independence that they merit additional discussion. First, the powerful relationship between fitness attributes such as strength, power, and endurance with physical function is discussed. Second, the relationship between physical activity levels and physical function is discussed, and third, the effect of exercise programs on the physical function of the old and oldest-old is considered.

Fitness Components and Physical Function

Virtually all investigators find that aerobic capacity, strength, power, flexibility, and balance are related to physical function in older adults (e.g., Brown, Sina-

core, Ehsani, et al., 2000 ; Seeman et al., 1995). Leg power has accounted for 86% of variance in walking speed in elderly women (Bassey et al., 1992). Strength and balance are strong predictors of severe walking disability (Rantanen et al., 1999). Individuals with poorer strength report more difficulties in motor activities (figure 11.10). It is clear that strength is a limiting factor in old adults, and the older they get, the more it becomes a limiting factor.

Physical Activity Levels

The evidence is overwhelming that the level of physical activity in which adults engage is significant in postponing frailty and disability (Simonsick et al., 1993; Voorrips et al., 1993; Young et al., 1995). Physical activity daily energy expenditure is linearly related to optimal physical function. Moderate to high physical activity groups are 1.5 to 2.0 times more likely than low physical activity groups to receive an optimal score on physical performance, ADLs, home management skills, physical endurance-type tasks, and strength-related tasks. The amount of disability in 75-year-old men and women who had been physically active for the previous 5 years was dramatically less (figure 11.11).

> The frail elderly who never walk at least 1 mile (1.6 km) per week are 1.56 times more likely to decline in function and become unable to perform ADLs and IADLs (Morey et al., 1998).

Physical activity also improves the physical function of patients with chronic diseases. In 1,758 patients with one or more of the following diseases—diabetes, hypertension, congestive heart failure, recent myocardial infarction, depressive symptoms, or current depressive disorder—physical function was better 2 years later in those who maintained higher levels of physical activity throughout the 2 years (Stewart et al., 1994) and 5 years later, in a subset of Japanese American men who had chronic diseases (Young et al. 1995).

Moderate or strenuous physical activity is associated with improvements in balance, gait, and chair-stand (Seeman et al., 1995). Strawbridge and colleagues (1998) reported that the probability for physically inactive people becoming frail was two times greater than that of active people. Rantanen and colleagues (1999) reported that low physical activity levels lead to low strength, and this leads to low physical function. Most dramatically, at the end of a 5-year follow-up study, men and women who were physically active were much more likely to have no

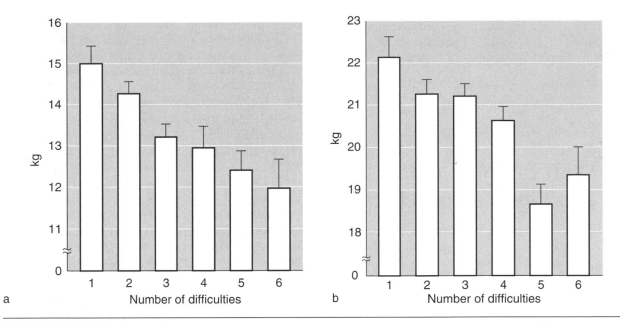

Figure 11.10 Relationship of lower leg *(a)* and grip strength *(b)* to the number of physical function difficulties reported by older adults.

Reprinted, by permission, from T. Rantanen et al., 1999, "Disability, physical activity and muscle strength in older women: The Women's Health and Aging Study," *Archives of Physical Medicine and Rehabilitation* 80: 130-135.

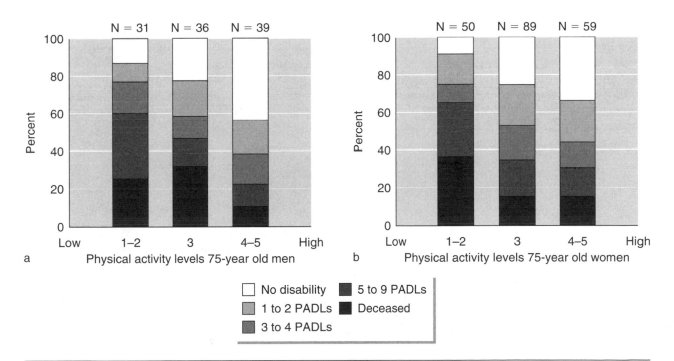

Figure 11.11 The physical activity levels of 75-year-old men *(a)* and women *(b)* were assessed, and 5 years later the number of disabilities that they had were recorded. Almost half of those who were in the high categories of physical activity were free of disabilities, compared with only 12% of those in the lower categories. In stark contrast, 60% of those in the low categories were either deceased or had difficulty with five to nine physical activities of daily living (PADL). The results were similar in the sample of women.

Reprinted, by permission, from P. Laukkanen, M. Kauppinen, and E. Heikkinen, 1998, "Physical activity as a predictor of health and disability in 75- and 80-year-old men and women: A five-year longitudinal study," *Journal of Aging and Physical Activity* 6:141-156.

or one physical disability, whereas those who were sedentary at the baseline of measurement 5 years earlier had a high percentage of disabilities.

Sedentariness appears a far more dangerous condition than physical activity in the very old (ACSM, 1998).

Exercise Interventions and Physical Function

The goals of an exercise program are different for elderly adults. For many young adults, exercise goals are to reach maximum or near-maximum capacity in many or all of their systems. Exercises are planned to produce maximum or competitive endurance, muscular strength and power, flexibility, and agility. The goals for old adults, as recommended by the ACSM Position Stand on Exercise and Physical Activity (ACSM, 1998), are focused on health and maintenance of function.

Even though the evidence is compelling that appropriate physical activity is beneficial for adults over 75, the vast majority of them report no leisure-time physical activity (figure 11.12). For many years, exercise in general was not recommended for very old adults. It was thought to be too hazardous and too likely to lead to falls and debilitating injuries that would shorten life. Most medical and health professionals now realize that physical activity is

beneficial for all ages, but several issues continue to be discussed and some yet remain to be resolved. These issues are (a) the effects of exercise on adults at different levels of base function, (b) the intensity, duration, rest intervals, and type of exercise that are most appropriate for older adults at the various levels of physical function, (c) the role of pain in exercise and recovery, and (d) the appropriateness of exercise for the very frail and disabled. Although there is still much to learn about the principles of effective exercise for the elderly, some basic principles have emerged.

Small increases in physical activity (beginning an exercise program) may have a large positive effect on individuals who have been almost completely sedentary but very little effect on those who were moderately active before the program. That is, a small change in baseline activity makes a big difference in very sedentary adults but almost no perceivable difference in highly active adults. This is shown diagrammatically in figure 11.13 (Haskell, 1994).

Although high-intensity resistance exercise has proven to be an effective and feasible way to increase strength in very old adults (Fiatarone et al., 1994), most experts conclude that frequent low-intensity exercise is more effective in maintaining and improving physical function (Topp & Stevenson, 1994). Low-intensity exercise has produced good results in people older than 78, if all the components of frailty are assessed: flexibility, balance, body handling skills, speed of reaction, coordination, and strength (Brown, Sinacore, Ehsani et al., 2000).

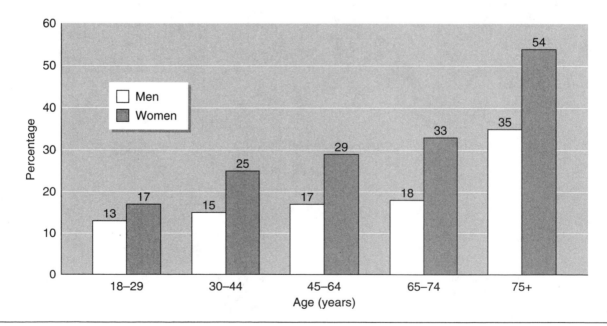

Figure 11.12 Percentage of adults reporting no leisure-time physical activity.
From NHANES III.

Goals of Exercise Are Different for Young and Old Adults

Young adults and old adults differ in their exercise goals. The young should exercise for the following reasons:

- Prevent cardiovascular disease, cancer, and diabetes
- Increase life expectancy
- Reach and maintain optimal weight

The old should exercise for these reasons:
- Combat frailty caused by inactivity
- Minimize biological changes of aging
- Reverse disuse syndromes
- Control chronic diseases
- Maximize psychological health
- Increase mobility and function
- Assist with rehabilitation from acute and chronic illnesses

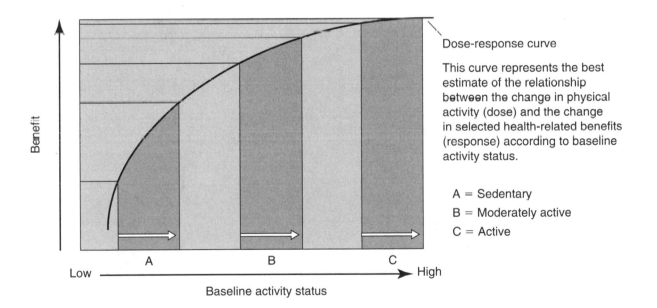

Dose-response curve

This curve represents the best estimate of the relationship between the change in physical activity (dose) and the change in selected health-related benefits (response) according to baseline activity status.

A = Sedentary
B = Moderately active
C = Active

Benefit

Low ——————————————————→ High

Baseline activity status

Figure 11.13 Theoretical dose–response curve demonstrating that the magnitude of the benefit for any given increase in activity is greater for less active persons. That is, the same increase in physical activity level in a sedentary group of individuals (A) produces greater benefits in function than it does in a highly active group (C).

Adapted, by permission, from W.L. Haskell, 1994, "Health consequences of physical activity: Understanding and challenges regarding dose-response," *Medicine and Science in Sports and Exercise.* 26(6): 649-660.

Repetitions of movements, use of Thera-Bands, and use of 1- to 2-lb (0.45- to 0.9-kg) hand-held weights were useful. However, Brown, Sinacore, Ehsani, et al. (2000) also indicated that even though strength was increased through resistance training and balance was increased, many older adults still had difficulty recovering quickly enough from a loss of balance to prevent falling. A potential cause that needs to be studied is whether increased power would enable older adults to prevent a fall. It has been suggested that men could recover from a loss of balance better than women because they could generate leg movement velocity faster and more quickly than women. Moving quickly requires power, and age-related losses lose power more quickly than strength. Evans (2000) suggested that exercise training to prevent disability and frailty should include power exercises.

Almost no study has been made of the role that pain plays in discouraging physical activity, but it most certainly has some impact. (see Vogt et al., 2002).

A final issue that continues to be discussed is whether physical activity and exercise are appropriate for the frail and the disabled. However, evidence is accumulating that with a systematic exercise program, frailty can be modified in many adults (e.g., Brown, Sinacore, Ehsani, et al., 2000; Shumway-Cook et al., 1997; Simonsick et al., 1993)

Following are chronic diseases that are positively affected by exercise.

- Arthritis
- Diabetes
- Coronary artery disease
- Congestive heart failure
- Chronic obstructive pulmonary disease
- Depression
- Disorders of gait and balance
- Falls
- Insomnia

(American College of Sports Medicine, 1998)

Expectations for Physical Performance of the Old and Oldest-Old

It is clear that physical exercise can make significant improvements in the physical functioning of individuals at any age. Even among the oldest participants, aerobic capacity, muscular strength, muscular endurance, flexibility, speed of responses, and coordination all improve following an exercise program. Improvements in some or all of these factors lead to significant improvements in physical functioning. Why, then, do not all of the oldest-old remain more physically active?

Many reasons have been suggested throughout this text, but the most senseless contributor to physical inactivity is the expectation for decreased physical performance, on the part of both the individual and her or his support group. Too many people are con-

tent to believe that when people grow older than 75 years, their physically active life is almost over. Ageism pressures the oldest-old to become inactive.

We expect too little function of older adults, and that is what we get.

A vicious cycle develops. As people age, they become less active. The less active they are, the less physical ability and endurance they have. The less physical ability they have, the less inclined they are to be physically active. And the less active they are, the more physical capacity they lose. The less they move, the less they can move. They begin to feel old and act old, which includes not being physically active. When a child or a teenager takes a bad fall and breaks an arm, people tell him or her to "get back on the horse" as quickly as possible. When an old person has an accident and breaks an arm, people say, "better slow down." The result of this vicious cycle is a steady deterioration of function, depicted by the straight line running from left to right through the circle in figure 11.14. This line represents the classic average decline that occurs in many functions and abilities. Another interpretation of this line may be seen in the familiar logo meaning "do not..." or "not allowed." So why not this line: DO NOT fall into this vicious cycle, or sedentary lifestyle NOT allowed!

Colleagues, friends, health professionals, and, finally, old people themselves begin to expect very little in the way of physical function, and these lowered expectations become a self-fulfilling prophecy. Yet, the amount of physical activity that individuals can accomplish and the contribution that it can make to their own quality of life are as different for

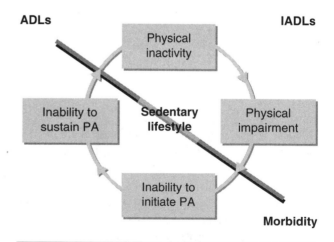

Figure 11.14 The vicious cycle of physical inactivity (PA). ADLs = activities of daily living; IADLs = instrumental activities of daily living.

Adapted from Berger and Hecht (1989).

each individual as is every other aspect of the aging process. The goals for physical functioning among the oldest-old should be maximum goals, set as high as possible for each individual. Health care professionals and family members should be aware of the entire hierarchy of physical function and that many individuals in the lower levels of the hierarchy are not there because of fate but because of inactivity, inadequate information, and low expectations. When everyone around an old individual views disable-

ment and dependency as the inevitable outcomes of advanced age, then it is easier to give up and become dependent. The two highest levels of the hierarchy of physical function in the old and oldest-old bear testimony to the wide range of function possible in these age groups. The individuals in these groups should provide the basis for much optimism among professionals who, when working with their clients, should share with them expectations for their physical function that are as high as possible.

SUMMARY

Adults display a wide range of physical capabilities at all ages, but the differences are very great in the age groups 75 to 85 and from 86 on. Adults differ in their functional independence, functional fitness, and functional performance. The physical function of the oldest adults can be categorized into a hierarchy of five levels: the physically elite, physically fit, physically independent, physically frail, and physically dependent. An important target for those who are physically independent but frail is to maintain reserve in functional fitness, so that they are not operating at minimum levels.

Several performance field tests have been devised that are appropriate for the categories of physically elite, physically fit, and independent. Testing the frail elderly is a challenge, but a number of survey instruments (paper and pencil tests) are effective, in addition to several performance tests that were designed for the frail elderly and for the physically dependent.

Assessing the physical function of the elderly is challenging because many factors make these people difficult to test. Factors such as pain, impaired cognition, and changes in medical conditions and medications increase the within-subject and error variance in measurement. However, the assessment of physical function is extremely important in older adults so that baselines of function can be established. Without baselines of performance, it is difficult for health professionals and caregivers to know whether fluctuations in competency are related to aging, disuse, or pathology.

Physical activity and exercise make a dramatic difference in maintaining physical function throughout the last years of life. The goals of physical activity programs for older adults, as outlined by the American College of Sports Medicine, are different from those recommended for young adults, but the research evidence supporting an activity–function relationship is overwhelming. Physical activity is a crucial requirement for maintaining function and staying mobile.

REVIEW QUESTIONS

1. Describe someone you know or have read about who is over 70 years old and whom you would classify as being in the physically elite category for physical function. Name all of the factors that you think have contributed to his or her physical status at this age.

2. Why is the concept of physical or physiological reserve so important for older persons?

   Think of a way that you could quantify the "reserve" in 60- to 70-year-old women for strength, aerobic endurance, and power.

3. If you were planning to measure the aerobic fitness of men and women over the age of 70, what kinds of precautions should you take, both to ensure safety but also to obtain accurate and reliable scores?

4. What types of exercise programs are appropriate for adults over 70? Should they include resistance training, aerobic training, functional training, or all? What factors should you consider in making this decision?

SUGGESTED READINGS

American College of Sports Medicine. (1998). Exercise and physical activity for older adults: Position stand. *Medicine and Science in Sport and Exercise, 30*(6), 992-1008.

National Institute on Aging. (2000). *Exercise: A guide from the National Institute on Aging.* NIA Information Center, P.O. Box 807, Gaithersburg, MD 20890-8057.

Rantanen, T., Guralnik, J.M., Sakari-Rantala, R., Leveille, S., Simonsick, E.M., Ling, S., & Fried, L.P. (1999). Disability, physical activity, and muscle strength in older women: The Women's Health and Aging Study. *Archives of Physical Medicine & Rehabilitation, 80,* 130-135.

Rikli, R.E., & Jones, C.J. (2001) *Senior fitness test manual.* Champaign, IL: Human Kinetics.

Physically Elite Older Adults

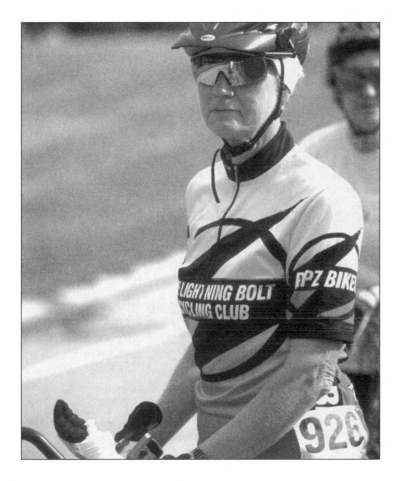

The objectives of this chapter are

- to introduce the reader to the upper limit of older adult physical performance,

- to show how competitive physical performance can be used to enrich scientists' understanding of the effects of aging on physiological systems,

- to point out nonphysiological factors that limit physical performances of masters athletes, and

- to raise health professionals' expectations of the capabilities of older adults.

12

*E*lite is a strong word, because it literally means the very best. Yet, no other word seems potent enough to describe the small percentage of elderly adults who manage to maintain outstanding physical abilities well into their 80s and 90s. Their physical abilities, although not as powerful as those of 20-year-olds, continue to be far superior to the physical abilities of most younger people. When people read the story of Johnny Kelley, who at 83 years of age finished his 60th Boston Marathon 5 hr 42 min 54 s behind the much younger winner (Kardong, 1991), their first thought may be that aging takes a considerable toll on running performance. On further consideration, however, most people remember that a marathon is approximately 26 miles (42 km). How many 20-year-olds can run 26 miles? Kept in perspective, the ability of 80-year-olds to run 26 miles is phenomenal and a testament to the remarkable resilience of the human body when it is properly maintained.

Who Are the "Physically Elite" Older Adults?

The physically elite elderly are older athletes who keep training and competing in tournaments well into their 60s, 70s, and 80s. They physically push themselves daily, competing in masters tournaments, the Senior Sports Classics, and local tournaments. They are those older individuals who do not quit working in occupations that require strength and endurance and who maintain their abilities through physical training so that they outperform most of their colleagues who are many years younger. They are frontline field-working firefighters, police, military personnel, dock workers, scuba divers, forest rangers, Emergency Medical Services workers, and a host of older individuals in occupations that require physical strength and stamina. They are also those individuals like Emil Biener, who has climbed Switzerland's Matterhorn more than 200 times and continues, in his 60s, to guide other climbers (Barnard, 1992). The physical performances of these noncompetitive individuals are not as easy to describe as those of masters athletes because the types of physical activity they do are more difficult to quantify. There are no scores for mountain climbing or scuba diving to make it easy to compare their performances with those of younger persons. But every community has these active seniors, and people who know them admire them.

Athletic competitions, conversely, provide an easy way for researchers to compare the physical abilities of one age group with another. In athletics, physical ability is rank ordered, and one of the purposes of tournaments and competitions is to identify the best physical performance. Elaborate rules and strict monitoring ensure that, inasmuch as possible, the comparisons are fair. Athletics, therefore, is a natural arena to determine how successfully humans can defy the physical effects of aging.

This chapter focuses on the physical accomplishments of older masters athletes, not because they are the only older adults who perform remarkable physical achievements but because their achievements are often accurately quantified, recorded, and publicized. First, this chapter describes the groups of athletes and discusses what can be learned from a study of aged athletes. Then, it describes some of the achievements of masters athletes in track and field, swimming, cycling, rowing, weightlifting, baseball hitting, bowling, and golf and discusses several issues related to the analysis of athletic performance records. Finally, there are the nonphysiological factors that limit the athletic performance of older adults. The chapter closes by considering the question, "How do they do it?"

Masters Athletes

Masters athletes are competitors who exceed a minimum age specific to each sport and who participate in competitive events designed for masters athletes (e.g., the Senior Sports Classics, the World Veterans Games, or local masters competitions). In track and field, masters athletes are older than 35 years old; in race walking, they must exceed 40. The minimum age varies according to the extent to which youth is a requisite for success. In swimming, for example, where many of the world records are held by teenagers, the minimum masters age is 25.

Masters competitions are relatively new in the athletic world. The First World Masters Track-and-Field Championship was held in Toronto in 1975. The National Senior Olympics, which began in 1987, offers competitions every odd year for adults older than age 50 who qualify on the basis of their state Senior Games performance. Since 1999, the participation in these games has ranged from more than 9,000 to 12,000 competitors, making it the largest recurring multisport event in the United States. The events include archery, badminton, basketball, bowling, cycling, golf, horseshoes, racquetball, road races, shuffleboard, softball, swimming, table tennis, tennis, track and field, triathlon, volleyball, 2-mile (3.2-km) racewalk, and washer pitching. Each year

Muscle Mass Declines, But Determination Does Not

In the VIIIth World Veterans Championships, excitement was high for all 4,950 athletes from 58 nations, but the most electrifying moment occurred in the 200-m dash. "Among the men were 94-year-old Wang Chingchang of Taiwan and 90-year-old Herbert Kirk of Bozeman, Montana. Wang bolted to a 5-m lead off the turn. But Kirk charged with 80 meters to go and passed Wang with 40 left, as the crowd stood roaring. Wang, amazingly, dug down and repassed Kirk, winning by a foot, 52.21 to 52.33 sec. But this race wasn't over. Kirk, who had given up tennis at 86 because he could no longer see the ball, didn't see the finish line either. He kept right on sprinting. Wang, fiercely competitive, went with him, and they dueled for another 70 meters before they were stopped. As they trotted back, it was in front of a delirious, tearful throng" (Moore, 1992, p. 44).

the Senior Games has many heartwarming stories of successful performances by the participants, such as that of Peter Laurino, who won the 85+ division of the 5,000-m racewalk four times.

> The World Veterans Games, which is a biennial track-and-field championship for men over age 40 and women over age 35, was first held in 1975.

Masters athletes are also local sports heroes. Every sport and every community have a few legendary elder athletes. Johnny Kelley, at age 83, ran his 60th Boston Marathon in 1991. The race officials set up a special finish line for him and gave him a hat and shirt with the Boston Marathon logo emblazoned on it. Wally Hayward, at 79 years, stunned everyone with his 9 hr, 44 min, 15 s finish in the Charity Challenge 80-km (48-mile) race in South Africa. He finished 5,482nd out of 11,234 starters of all ages. Peter Laurino, a racewalking champion, at 98 years of age won the Charter Hospital's Senior 2-mile (3.2-km) Strut. Ruth Rothfarb and Ida Mintz, both over 80 years old, ran the marathon in just a little over 5 hr.

Studying the Elite Physical Performance of Masters Athletes

One might ask, Why study and discuss these highly exceptional physically elite older adults? After all, they represent an extremely small number of their cohort. There are several reasons for observing and studying these persons, who truly optimize their physical well-being throughout their lives. An obvious reason is that they represent the extreme end of a distribution that ranges from physical disability and dysfunction at one end to elite athletic accom-

plishments at the other. Because they represent one extreme of this distribution, they should be described and understood. But other reasons are more important. These athletes provide official and controlled physical performance data, they offer a barometer of what is possible in physical aging, and their performances are of scientific value in understanding both physical and physiological changes with aging.

Highly Controlled and Motivated Performance

Athletic events have always offered well-documented, quantified evaluations of physical ability. The conditions under which official state, national, and world athletic records are made are highly controlled. Trained officials monitor the performances during events so that no athlete has an unfair advantage. The rules of competition, which take into account weather conditions, facilities, and equipment, are designed to ensure fairness and objectivity of measurement. In fact, considering how highly monitored athletic competitions are, by officials, observers, and media coverage, the quantification and reliability of physical performance during these events must be considered to be as controlled as during field research experiments. Also, the athletes performing in these competitions are doing so willingly and are extremely motivated. Most subjects in laboratory experiments never reach the high level of motivation to produce strength or speed scores that they would reach if they were measured under competitive conditions. This is particularly true for high-level athletes. Hagerman (1994) and Foster and colleagues (1993) indicated that the peak $\dot{V}O_2$ values that they obtained from elite athletes during competition were always higher than the $\dot{V}O_2$ values they obtained from them during a standard incremental exercise protocol.

Barometer of the Possible

Those who break records raise the ceiling for everyone. It is well known in athletics that all events have barriers, performances that seem impossible for anyone to surpass. Yet, when someone does break the barrier, then often a flood of people do, and the new record becomes the next barrier. One of the most famous of these barriers was the 4-min mile, a time that everyone thought no human being could accomplish. But after Roger Bannister broke this barrier, the times tumbled. The same metamorphosis is occurring with physical performances of older adults. Previous ideas about the physical limitations of older adults are being reformulated almost monthly with every masters competition.

More and more older adults are competing in local and state tournaments, and more and more events are being modified to include older individuals. Many masters athletes are training in the atmosphere of a sports club, with other athletes of various ages, and under the aegis of a coach who provides them with knowledge about innovative training techniques and new technologies designed to improve performance. In fact, it is not uncommon to find cases where, because of improved training techniques and technological advances in equipment, masters athletes surpass their own collegiate performances.

Describing, recording, analyzing, and publicizing the physical performance of masters athletes can remind all adults and gerontological professionals that physical ability can be maintained at remarkable levels for a very long time. The training and performance of thousands of older adults in these tournaments show that disability is not inevitable. The athletic performances of all the competitors, not just the winners, show what the aging human can do physically in the absence of disease and physical inactivity. Above all, masters athletes' performances reveal what the aging human can accomplish when talent and ability are optimized.

Masters athletes raise both physical and psychological ceilings and shatter the barriers of expectations that society has for the aged.

Scientific Importance of Analyzing Masters Sports

Outstanding achievements in physical performance can partially answer many questions, such as, Are age-related losses greater in aerobic, anaerobic, strength, or power systems? Is the loss of physical ability linear or curvilinear? Do men and women lose physical ability at the same rate? Is there a breakpoint in performance, an age at which the effects of age accelerate? Different energy mobilization and structural systems are necessary for optimum performance in different sports and even across different distances within a sport. **Athletic power** is the production of a large amount of work within a short amount of time, such as occurs in the 100-m sprint race or the clean-and-jerk weightlifting event (see also chapter 5). These types of performance challenge the peak muscle force generating potential and neuromuscular coordination. In intermediate duration events, ranging from the 400-m dash on the track (or those of about 60 s duration) to the 1,000-m single sculling event on the water (about 4 min), the physiological challenge is to sustain work outputs far in excess of aerobic capacity in the face of an increasing metabolic load. Longer events, such as a marathon race, challenge the capacity of the aging system to supply continued resources to the muscle (aerobic capacity). High jumping requires exquisite multilimb coordination, whereas running a marathon does not. The marathon, on the other hand, challenges the aerobic system, whereas high jumping does not. By studying the rate of decline of performances that rely exclusively or heavily on specific energy systems and structural integrity, scientists can obtain information about aging effects on these physiological systems. They do this by developing mathematical models, the components of which provide the basis for hypotheses about the mechanisms that control human physical performance. With these models, and other statistical comparisons, athletic competitive performances can supplement laboratory physiological measurements and contribute new hypotheses about how physiological mechanisms interrelate in aging.

Finally, yet another reason to study elite masters athletes is that athletic performance represents the functional significance of physiological theory. If systems such as the aerobic capacity system are found to decrease an average of 1% a year and athletic performance, which depends highly on aerobic capacity, parallels this decline, this finding provides a functional congruency to theory. Additionally, laboratory researchers, in order to gain high quantitative validity, can measure only a limited number of components of whole-body performance such as strength, aerobic capacity, or balance. Maximum sport performance, however, is more than the sum of many parts. It is that one brilliant moment for each individual when all the body systems, functioning at their peak, are coordinated with the precise timing required to perform better than any other human ever has. Such a finding is different from laboratory research, but it is valid, relevant, and instructive.

Masters Athletes' Record Performances

Before we address more theoretical issues of age effects on maximal physical performance, it is instructive to describe the performance of older athletes in a few sports. Although most sport associations now provide and encourage masters competition, only a few are discussed in detail in this chapter: track and field, swimming, cycling, rowing, and weightlifting. The track-and-field, swimming, and cycling events are included because more senior adults participate in these competitions than in other sports. Rowing is included because it is a whole-body sport and both field competition and laboratory-rowing ergometer data are available for comparison. Weightlifting is discussed, not because many older adults participate, but because it is a sport that requires extremes of power and strength. The section concludes with a limited discussion of baseball hitting, bowling, and golf, because baseball hitting represents eye–hand, whole-body neuromuscular coordination and reactive capacity, and bowling and golf require flexibility, coordination, and accuracy. Together, the task demands of these sports challenge the full range of physical capacities.

Track and Field

The track-and-field events included in this section are the 100-m, 800-m, 10,000-m, 1-mile (1.6-km), and marathon running events and two throwing events: the discus throw and the shot put.

Running

The percentage decline in running velocity in men's and women's U.S. Masters National records for the 100-m sprint, the 800-m distance, and an endurance event, the 10,000-m (10K) run, are shown in figure 12.1. The percent of loss is approximately 1% each year, which is about the same as the loss in maximum oxygen consumption ($\dot{V}O_2$max) over the same period. The first impression is that a striking decline occurs in running speed over the life span. But even though this decline is apparent, a closer inspection reveals that the male masters runners maintain more than 50% of their ability until approximately 80 years of age. Even more remarkable, the 80- to 84-year-old masters runners' record in the sprint (100-m) race is only 42% slower than the national record. These figures were based on **cross-sectional research** data, which means that the decline in performance is exaggerated. If **longitudinal research** data of highly trained competitors were analyzed, the proportion of world performance

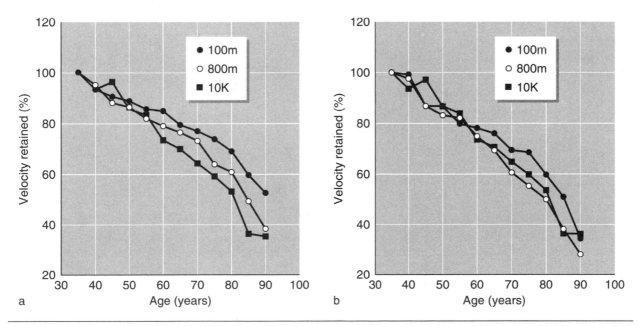

Figure 12.1   Comparison of velocity of male *(a)* and female *(b)* record holders in the U.S. Masters National Championships, 2002, at different ages. Records for males are 100 m = 9.97 sec; 800 m = 1:43 min; 10K = 27.25 min. Records for females are 100 m = 10.85 sec; 800 m = 1:57 min; 10K = 31:20 min.

Data from *Masters Age Records for 1990* (1991).

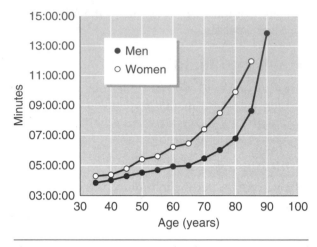

Figure 12.2 Time in minutes taken by U.S. masters record holders to run 1 mile.

Data from *Masters Age Records* (2002).

maintained might be even greater (Hartley & Hartley, 1984; Stones & Kozma, 1982a).

The times of the top 10 competitors at each age level are remarkably similar, and it is notable that the increases in time with age in these highly trained men and women are very gradual, not slowing at an acutely rapid pace until after the age of 70. Past the age of 70, age differences are larger and are more variable, especially in the women's records. Some of the great variability in the older adults records can be attributed to the extremely small number of competitors in these age groups. Nevertheless, it is astonishing that even at the age of 80 some men can run 10K, or roughly 6 miles, in a little over 40 min. A few 80-year-old women can run 6 miles in 58 min. Compare this with the general public. Most people under the age of 60 cannot even jog 10K without stopping, much less finish the distance in 45 to 60 min.

Other incredible performances of these masters are the age group records in the mile run, shown in figure 12.2. It is not until after the age of 80 that the records for the men's mile run increase

dramatically. In women, the times lengthen considerably at about 70 years. But even at that age, these times of 6:43 (80-year-old men) and 7:26 (70-year-old women) are much better than the time that many sedentary 30- and 40-year-olds need to run a mile!

The average running speed (velocity in meters per second) of male runners over age 40 is compared in figure 12.3 with that of world-class men and women. On the abscissa of the graph, the distances over which these average speeds are run are shown on a logarithmic scale. One of the most striking features of this analysis is that the decline in speed with increasing distance is almost parallel for men of four increasingly older age groups. Although men over age 70 slow a little more in the extremely long distances, the 40-, 50-, and 60-year-old men have essentially the same declines with distance as the world-class men. Another striking result is the difference in slopes between the world-class men and women and the other runners. The average running speed of world-class men and women, unlike that of men at all ages shown in the figure, declines more precipitously with increasing distances.

Although large geographical, climatic, altitude, and time differences occur among and within marathons, making them unreliable to use for statistical

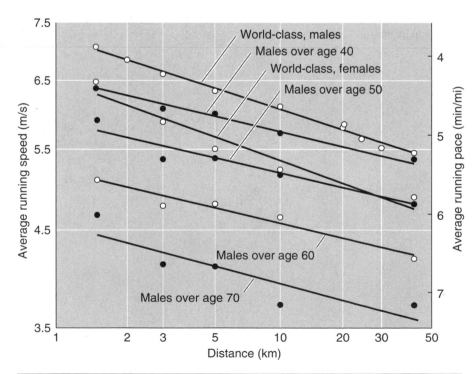

Figure 12.3 Age and gender differences in the average running speed during world record performances.

Reprinted, by permission, from P.S. Riegel, 1981, "Athletic records and human endurance," *American Scientist* 69: 288. Copyright 1981 by Sigma XI, The Scientific Research Society.

age group comparisons, it is clear from national records that with training, high-level competitive men can run a marathon very close to the overall record time until they reach their 70s, and women can stay close until their 60s (figure 12.4). Perhaps because the marathon is so long and dramatic, hundreds of stories are published annually all over the world featuring men and women over 70 years of age who complete marathons (see sidebar on page 294). Not only do many of these older adults run one marathon, but many of them run several a year. In figure 12.5 the exponential decline in aerobic and neuromuscular endurance that begins in the late 60s for women can clearly be seen in both the longitudinal marathon

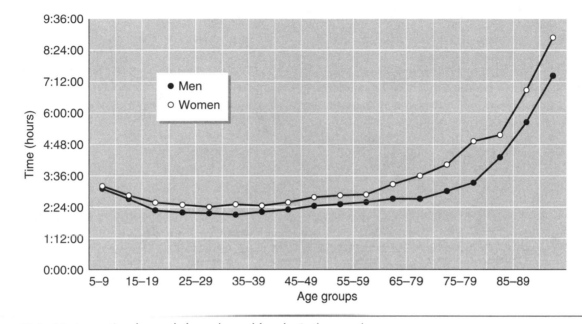

Figure 12.4 Masters national records for males and females in the marathon.

Data from *Masters Age Records* (2002).

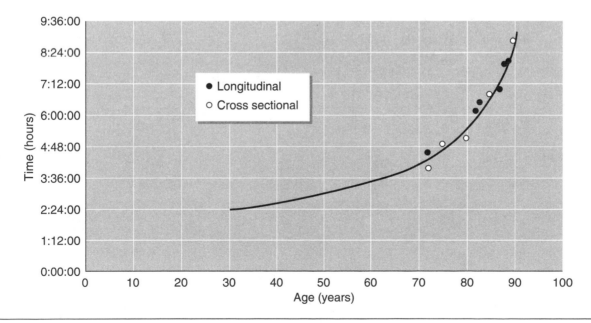

Figure 12.5 The marathon times of Mavis Lindgren in the United States: single age road racing records from 1983 to 2002, compared with the same cross-sectional records for each half decade. The increases in time, for both longitudinal and cross-sectional data, are steep and similar.

Data from *U.S.A. Single Age Road Racing Records* (2002).

times of Mavis Lindgren and the cross-sectional age-group records over a 12-year period. Nevertheless, it is a testament to the potential durability of the human body that if an individual physically trains consistently and tenaciously, aerobic endurance can be maintained into the 10th decade.

Throwing

The world masters records for the discus throw and the shot put for both men and women are shown in figure 12.6. In these throwing events, the records decline approximately 2% each year, which is a greater decline than in the running events. Performance decline is greater in whole-body, neuromuscular coordination–limited events that require substantial outlays of power than in cardiovascular-limited events. However, it must be remembered that each point on these graphs is the record of different individuals, not the record of one person from year to year. These year-to-year differences could be attributable either to a true decline in the performance of a single record holder who nevertheless wins two or more consecutive years or to the individual differences that exist between different people who hold consecutive records. These limitations of records analyses must be considered when interpreting performance graphs and are discussed in more detail later in the chapter.

Running Marathons at 80+

Jenny Wood Allen, 89, of Dundee, Scotland, completed the 2002 London Marathon, making her the oldest woman ever to complete a marathon. She had previously set the record in 1999, finishing in 17 hr, 14 min, and 46 s, to earn a place in the *Guinness Book of World Records*, 2002. She began running marathons when she was 69 and completed 30 marathons before 1999. An American, Abraham Weintraub, 91, was the oldest man to complete the marathon (*U.S.A. Single Age Road Racing Records*, 2002). The fastest marathon time, however, is held by Helen Klein of Rancho Cordova, California, 80, who finished the California International Marathon in 4:31.32, setting the world record by almost 40 min for the 80+ age group. A former emergency room nurse, she has completed 59 marathons and 136 ultramarathons. She completed her first marathon at age 57 (*Faces in the Crowd*, 2002).

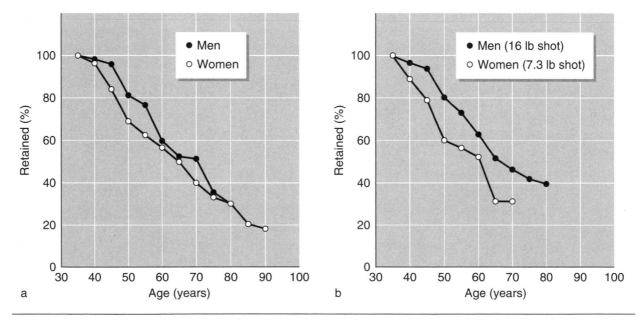

Figure 12.6 Masters world records for males and females in the *(a)* discus throw and *(b)* shot put. *(a)* Percent of the world record retained by men and women of different ages throwing the discus. Records are men = 232 ft 8 in. (70.9 m) (2 kg discus); women = 228 ft 4 in. (69.5 m) (1 kg discus). *(b)* Percent of the world record retained by men and women of different ages putting the shot. Records are men (16-lb [7.2-kg] shot) = 72 ft 9 3/4 in.; women (7.3-lb [3.3-kg] shot) = 70 ft 5 1/4 in. U.S. Masters National Championships.

Data from *Masters Age Records* (2002).

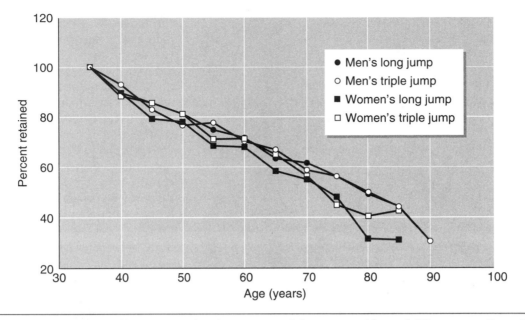

Figure 12.7 Percent retained of long jump and triple jump records by masters athletes of different ages. Records are men's long jump = 27 ft 10 3/4 in. (8.5 m); men's triple jump = 58 ft 9 1/2 in. (17.9 m); women's long jump = 22 ft 11 1/4 in. (7 m); women's triple jump = 46 ft 0 in. (14 m).

Data from *Masters Age Records* (2002).

Women use a lighter discus than do men. Nevertheless, the amount of performance retained in women's records is somewhat poorer between ages 45 and 55. It is difficult to make gender comparisons in the shot put event because women use a 7.3-lb (3.3 kg) shot put and men use a 16-lb (7.2 kg) shot. However, it is clear in these comparisons that the percent of the record accomplished by women is approximately 15% to 20% less than that achieved by men (figure 12.6b).

Jumping

Jumping data for masters men and women are shown in figure 12.7. Both men and women decline in jumping distance, but women decline somewhat more, especially in the oldest decades. In the long jump, the gender difference is 18% at age 35, but it increases linearly to 42% by the age of 85. In the triple jump, the difference ranges between 17 and 37%, but with no linear trend. Women fall below the 50% level about age 75 and men at about age 85.

Swimming

Just as was true of the running records, the swimming speed of masters swimmers slows with age. Swimming is an important sport to study in this context, because it differs in significant ways from most other sports. Performance depends much more on upper body strength and endurance, and it is performed in water and in a supine position rather than an upright position. Thus, buoyancy, gravity, and balance play different roles in swimming than in running. Swimming also differs from most other sports in that the ratio of men to women competitors is more equal. Finally, the injury rate is lower in swimming than it is in land events, allowing more older adults to compete at older ages.

The swimming performance times of the 10 fastest masters swimmers from the United States Masters Swimming Championships were longitudinally tracked over a 12-year period (Donato et al., 2003). All swimmers analyzed had placed in the top 10 at least 3 years, with the average being 5 years. The swimming times for both the 50-m and the 1,500-m freestyle, compared with the 2003 world record times, slowed very gradually until approximately age 70, whereupon they dramatically increased (figure 12.8). As was true for running events, both men and women maintained their performances closer to the world record in the shorter 50-m race than in the longer 1,500-m race, suggesting that anaerobic performance is maintained with aging better than aerobic performance. The decline in the women's times after 70 years was much steeper than that of the men's in the 50-m race but not in the 1,500-m race.

Cycling

At present, older adults maintain their performance capabilities better in cycling than in most other

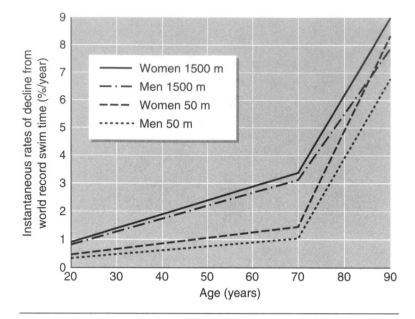

Figure 12.8 The instantaneous (relative) rate of changes in swimming performance times in relation to the present fastest world record time.

Reprinted, by permission, from A.J. Donato et al., 2003, "Declines in physiological functional capacity with age: A longitudinal study in peak swimming performance," *Journal of Applied Physiology* 94: 764-769.

the percent losses are so similar for men and women up to the 60- to 69-year age group, which is the oldest age group for which U.S. records are kept, that the precipitous loss in the oldest age group is probably attributable primarily to the fact that few women over the age of 60 compete in cycling races. For example, in the 10K race, an event that attracts many more older women competitors than cycling events do, the women's losses in running are only 30%, which is the same as those of men. (This sampling problem is discussed in more detail later in this chapter.) It is surprising that more older women do not compete in cycling, because it seems to be a very popular endurance sport for older men. Competitive cycling, however, also presents a fairly high risk for falling, accidents, and injury, and it may be those characteristics of the event that discourage women.

vigorous sports. Shown in figure 12.9a, the velocity of 65-year-old male cyclists is only 9% slower than the record of the 35-year-old cyclists, whereas the velocity of 10K runners at 65 is 30% slower (figure 12.10). It is impressive that highly conditioned men 60 to 69 years old can propel themselves 24.8 miles 39.9 km) in less than 1 hr on a bicycle. Women's cycling records are also impressive (figure 12.9b). The percent losses are very similar for men and women until ages 65 to 69, at which time the women's record is 23% slower than the national women's record. However,

Cycling records must be considered within the context of the sport as well. As a competitive sport, cycling, other than the 40-km time-trials event, is somewhat different from other racing sports. In swimming and running races, the competitors more or less swim or run as fast as they can throughout the race, perhaps saving something at the end for a sprinting finish. In cycling, however, wind resistance plays such an important role that the experienced cyclists ride slightly behind one or more of the competitors, making the leaders bear the brunt of the wind and work harder during the first part of the race. Those trailing the leaders can then

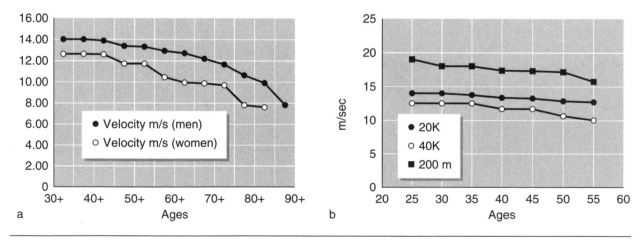

Figure 12.9 *(a)* Records from the 2002 United States Cycling Federation 20K Road Race Trials: absolute time in minutes. *(b)* Comparison of the velocities of male cyclists at 200-m, 20-km, and 40-km distances.

Data from the United States Cycling Federation (1990).

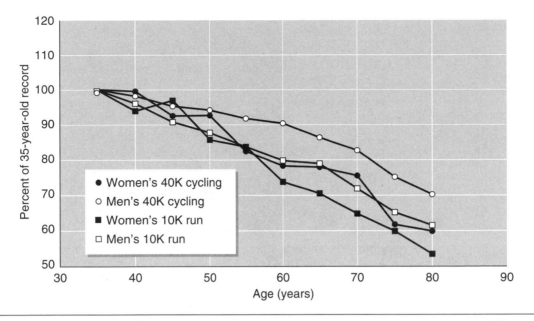

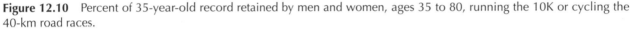

Figure 12.10 Percent of 35-year-old record retained by men and women, ages 35 to 80, running the 10K or cycling the 40-km road races.

Data from the United States Cycling Federation (2002) and the U.S. Masters Track and Field Age Records, *Masters Age Records* (2002).

burst out in front at the moment when they think that the combination of more reserve capacity and the element of surprise will leave their competitors unable to catch them. Thus, road-racing times do not reflect the absolute fastest times that the racers could ride but rather the nature of the race strategy. For the sport of cycling, therefore, only **cycling time trials** in which competitors race singly against the clock are legitimate races from which to judge the effects of aging on cycling.

Rowing

In this sport, one-, two-, four-, or eight-person crews with or without a **coxswain** propel a **shell** (boat) in as straight a line as possible for speed. Rowing requires coordination of almost all of the large muscles of the body (leg, trunk, back, and arms) for relatively long time periods. Most of the events are endurance events and tax the aerobic system. This sport is also somewhat unique in that a rowing ergometer has been developed and performance times on this ergometer have been recorded as world records for the 2,000-m individual race. The results from the ergometer world records provide an interesting comparison to world records in competitive events on the water.

Competitive Events

The results of the 2000 United States Masters Championship in rowing for the heavyweight men's singles competitions are shown in figure 12.11. In this partic-

ular year, the environmental conditions for all three days of the competition were reasonably consistent and good for rowing, so these competitive times are relatively reliable. As shown in the figure, the racing times of the first- through the third-place finishers gradually increase in each older age group. The fastest times were produced by the competitors between ages 28 and 44. The times among the first- through third-place finishers for these age groups were almost identical. These times may be underestimates of this age group, because some of the fastest rowers who would be in the age 27 to 34 category of this tournament rarely enter masters competitions. Rather, these relatively young competitors continue to enter the United States Open Championships. In the masters competitions, both men and women heavyweights row considerably faster than their lightweight counterparts, and men of all ages can move the racing shell much faster than their female cohorts. The age group at which the times slow more acutely is the 50- to 54-year-old-group, which is a decade younger than is seen in running and cycling and still younger than swimming. This age difference may be attributed to the fact that competitive rowing has fewer participants in these older categories than do running and swimming events.

Rowing Ergometer Performance

A **rowing ergometer** is a device that measures physical work output, and as discussed in chapter 4, bicycle ergometers have been used for many years to measure

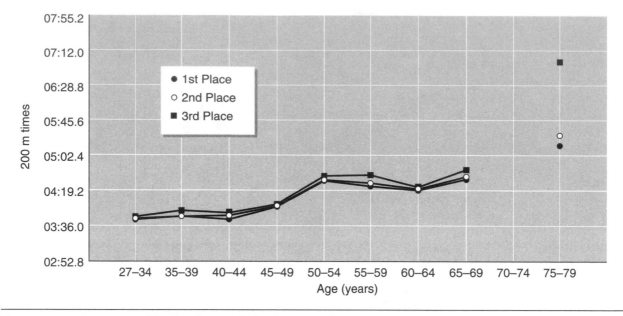

Figure 12.11 Times (min) of the first three male finishers in each age category at the Masters National Rowing Regatta at Lake Merritt, Oakland, CA, 2000. Lake Merritt Rowing Club: http://www.rowlakemerritt.org/ (accessed 6-8-04).

physiological work parameters such as maximum oxygen consumption. The rowing ergometer, however, is calibrated so that the rowing time achieved by an individual on the ergometer is a good estimate of that individual's potential time to row on water. Thus, individuals can test themselves to determine how fast they can row the specified race distance without ever getting on the water. The technical mastery necessary to balance the body in the shell and keep it on line with respect to the finish line limits the on-water performance, so that the velocity that can be developed in the rowing ergometer is about 15% higher than the velocity that can be generated on the water. Nevertheless, the ergometer provides a good estimate of rowing potential. Concept II, Inc., developed the ergometer and has established world rankings based on thousands of entrants from many countries (Concept II World Rankings, 1991). These data, which are updated each year, are particularly useful for analyzing age differences in rowing performances, because they are free of the influences of the weather (rain, wind, choppy water) and equipment differences that usually prevail in an outdoor race.

Good male rowers who compete in ergometer competitions lose about 3 s per year (0.54%), and good female rowers lose about 4 s per year (0.57%). In these rowers, age alone only accounts for about 33% of the variance for men and 21% for women. Thus, many other factors, discussed later, contribute to the time (Seiler, Spirduso, & Martin, 1998). However, when only the top 5% of men and women rowers are analyzed, age accounts for about 90% of the variance (figure 12.12). Several insights can be gained from figure 12.12, where the relative declines in time and performance power are shown for the top 5% of men and women. First, the relative decline in time for women is quite linear, whereas the decline in men's times is curvilinear. Second, the relative decline in men and women is almost the same until about age 35, and then the women's rate of decline accelerates more than that of the men. Third, an increase in the rate of decline occurs in men at about age 55. Fourth, decline in power performance is linear for both men and women, but women lose power at a slightly faster rate than men.

One additional point about figure 12.12: Even though the sample size is very large ($N = 5,000$), the distribution of ages is extremely unequal, as shown in figure 12.13. In this figure almost one fifth of the entire sample were 20-year-olds, and the samples were very small beginning at about age 55. At this particular age, the performance decrement also becomes noticeably greater. Therefore, part of the explanation for slower performances by those over age 55 may be the smaller number of people who compete at that age in the ergometer competitions.

Weightlifting

Competitive **weightlifting** does not attract the large numbers of older athletes that sports such as running, swimming, and cycling do. Weightlifting is a sport in which the muscular, powerful, and anaerobically talented individual may excel. It requires a tremen-

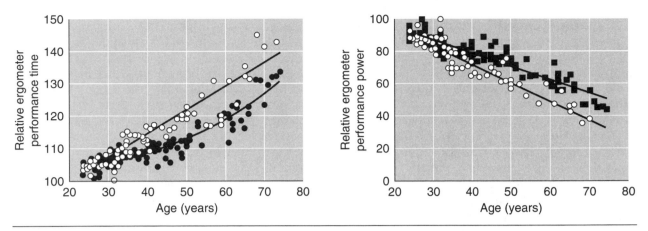

Figure 12.12 Performance of the best male (filled symbols) and female (open symbols) age groups relative to the best overall young individual rowers. Each age group mean is divided by the fastest young male or female result to determine performance across age relative to the best absolute performance. Y-axis values on the left graph are minutes, and on the right graph are percent of maximum power (watts).

Reprinted, by permission, from K.S. Seiler, W.W. Spirduso, and J.D. Martin, 1998, "Gender differences in rowing performance and power with aging," *Medicine and Science in Sports and Exercise* 30: 121-127.

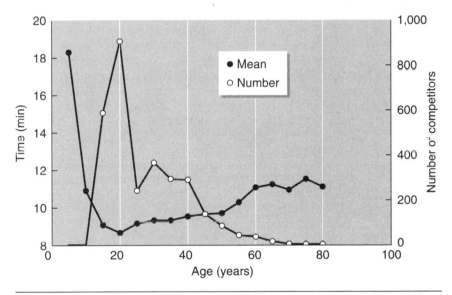

Figure 12.13 Rowing ergometer times and frequencies for data in figure 12.12. The left axis depicts ergometer times (minutes) and the right axis depicts the number of competitors contributing to that mean time.

dous recruitment of energy over a very short period of time and develops extremely high internal pressures during the exertion. Despite the toll that aging takes on muscle mass (and explosive power), many competitive lifters continue to enter contests into their 70s and 80s. Their lifting records provide substantial insight into the decline of muscular strength and power with aging. It is unlikely that elderly subjects in a strength laboratory ever reach the truly maximum effort that is produced by masters-level lifters in competition. Noncompetitive subjects have rarely experienced the sensation of producing a maximum neuromuscular effort. Not only are competitive lift-

ers highly motivated in a contest setting, but as a group they also physically train their muscles far more intensively than do any subjects in experimentally designed strength training programs. From that perspective, the masters-level competitive lifters provide the best data to indicate how much strength can be maintained over the years if a person systematically and scientifically undergoes resistive strength training.

Weightlifting, sometimes called *Olympic lifting*, is a term by which the general public loosely describes all events and activities in which persons lift barbells competitively. From the public's perspective, weightlifting can mean resistance strength training, any competition where the athletes lift heavy weights, or even bodybuilding. Technically, however, there are only two major sports in which the participants compete to determine who can lift the most weight. Weightlifting officially includes two events, the clean and jerk and the snatch. In the clean and jerk, the lifter reaches down to the bar, which is loaded with barbell plates to the necessary weight, and in one quick motion "cleans" the loaded bar to the chest, pauses momentarily, and then explosively "jerks" the bar above the head and holds it with both arms extended until the referee gives the signal that the lift is complete. In the snatch, the lifter must pull the bar all the way from the floor to the fully extended arm position above the head in one motion while at the same time lowering the body by doing a fore and aft split or a deep knee bend. Both the snatch and the clean and jerk require not only tremendous power production during the pulling phase but also inordinate agility and flexibility to lower the body under the bar quickly when it reaches its highest point from the first exertion. These events also require exquisite neuromuscular coordination to time the transfer of weight across the different body muscles that absorb and "catch" the load and then lift it upward until the legs and arms are completely straight. Excellent balance throughout the lift is also required to maintain the weight over the center of gravity throughout the lift. Losing one's balance under a 300-lb (136-kg) bar can be disastrous. Both the snatch and the clean and jerk are sanctioned by the International Olympic Committee and are Olympic events. They are the lifts used in the Olympic Games.

The other major type of competitive lifting is **power lifting.** Power lifting consists of three events: the squat, the bench press, and the deadlift. The squat requires the lifter to begin with the bar placed on the shoulders, squat until the crease between the torso and thigh is below the top of the bent knee, and then return to a full erect position. To perform the bench press, the lifter lies on a bench on his or her back, holds the weight at arms-length above the chest, lowers the bar to the chest, and

returns it to the original position. In the deadlift, the lifter reaches down to the bar and must lift the weight only as high as is necessary to get the arms, legs, and back fully extended. Thus, in all three of the power lifts, absolute force production is at a premium. The term *power lifting* is rather a misnomer for these three events, because speed is not a factor in the lifts. The snatch and the clean and jerk, however, are true power movements, because they require a fast movement to hoist the bar from the floor to a position above the head. Nevertheless, these events acquired their names long before the technical distinctions between strength and power were commonly understood, and it is not likely that they will change.

Age Effects on Weightlifting

Figure 12.14a, which is based on the International Federation of Weightlifting Masters 2002 data, provides a graphic description of the toll that aging takes on weightlifting. Only the clean-and-jerk records are shown in this figure, because the pattern of difference over time is virtually identical for the snatch event. In each successively older decade, lifters in these three weight classes (representing heavy-, middle-, and lightweight) are able to lift less and less weight. The percent difference over the decades is shown in figure 12.14b as percentages of the world record for that weight class for each age group. The record holders, whatever their

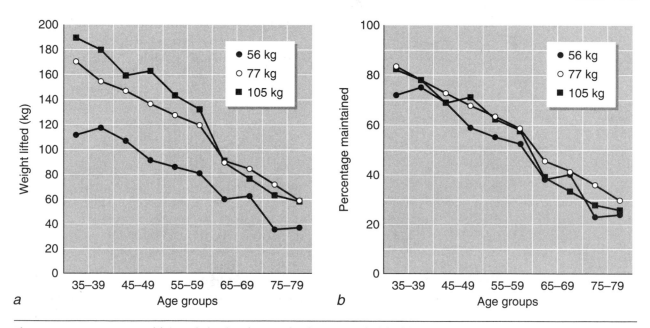

Figure 12.14 Masters world records for the clean and jerk. (a) Weight lifted for lightweights (56-kg class), middle-weights (77-kg class), and heavyweights (105-kg class); (b) percent of the 35-year-old record for each weight class at each age group.

Data from the World Weightlifting Federation (2000).

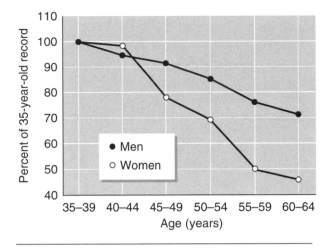

Figure 12.15 Comparison of percent differences across age for men's and women's clean and jerk weightlifting records. Data are averages of the records from 58- to ≥75-kg weight categories in women, and 77- and 105-kg weight categories in men.

Data from the World Weightlifting Federation (2000).

weight class, can only lift about 43% of the world record for their weight by age 79. In all weight classes, the decline from age 65 to 79 (15 years) is much steeper than that from age 35 to 64 (30 years). The smaller, lighter lifters lift substantially less absolute weight than that those in heavier weight classes (figure 12.14a), but when their lifts are expressed as a percentage of their weight records, the decline over age is about the same for all weight classes (figure 12.14b). Large gender differences in the percent

of strength retained occur after age 45 in women's records, compared with men's (figure 12.15). This was also confirmed by Anton and colleagues (2004). However, a large part of these large discrepancies are attributable to the sampling problem that is discussed in more detail later.

Age Effects on Power Lifting

The records of the masters in power lifting, specifically the deadlift event from the U.S.A. Powerlifting national records, 2003, are shown in figure 12.16. All weight-class records decrease with each increasingly older age group, at about the same rate. These record holders at ages 65 to 69 are lifting almost 60% of the world record, which is remarkable. Generally, the deadlift records decline linearly up until age 70 and then decrease at a faster rate (Meltzer, 1994). The decrease from 40 to 69 (~30 years) is 18%, but 20% more is lost in the next 10 years. Differences between men and women power lifters are shown in figure 12.17.

The squat and the bench press events in power lifting provide a way to compare age effects on lower body and upper body strength. Many researchers, therapists, and trainers believe that upper body strength declines at a faster rate than lower body strength. Earlier in this chapter we discussed this as a mechanism to explain the faster age-related declines in swimming performances that rely more heavily on upper body strength. However, in the U.S.A. Powerlifting com-

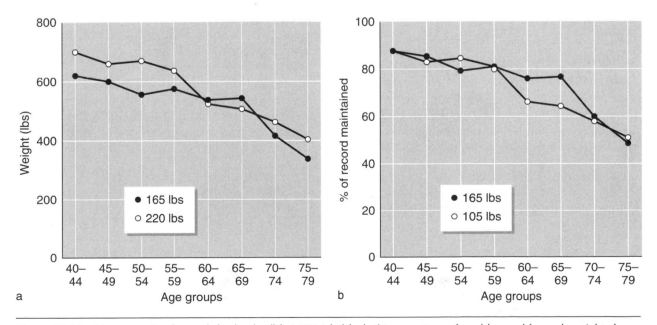

Figure 12.16 Masters national records for the deadlift. *(a)* Weight lifted; *(b)* percentage of world record for each weight class.

Data from the U.S.A. Powerlifting Federation (1991).

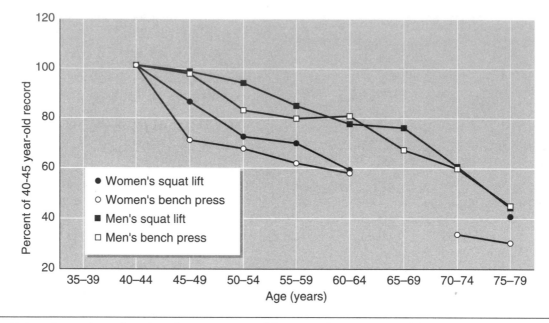

Figure 12.17 Comparison of men's and women's power lifting records as a percent of the 40- to 45-year-old record. From men's and women's records, U.S.A. Powerlifting. Men's data are averages of the 165- (74.8-), 181- (82.1-), and 198-lb (89.8-kg) weight categories, and women's data are averages of the 132- (59.8-), 148.75- (67.4-), and 165.25-lb (74.9-kg) weight categories.

Data from the United States Powerlifting Federation (1991).

petitions, the bench press and squat declined at a similar rate (Anton et al., 2004). Most investigators reporting age-related differences in upper and lower body strength have used isometric strength measures, but the dynamic power lifts seen in competition do not support these differences. Also, arm and leg muscle quality derived from isokinetic dynamometer measures declined at a similar rate in men (Lynch et al., 1999).

Comparison of Power Lifting and Weightlifting

Comparing power lifting and competitive lifting provides a way to compare the effects of age on pure strength (power lifting) versus strength in combination with power, coordination, agility, flexibility, and

balance (weightlifting). The brute strength required for power lifting can be maintained better over the years than the combined attributes of power production, coordination, and balance (weightlifting). This is shown in figure 12.18, in which the percent of performance lost is compared for the two events. Beginning at age 55, the power lifters maintain a higher percentage of the world record in the deadlift than do the weightlifters in the clean and jerk. This difference is greatest in the 65- to 69-year-old age group, where the power lifting record is 70% of the world record and the clean and jerk record is 50% of the record. The cumulative effects of aging on strength production, coordination, flexibility, agility, and balance result in older lifters achieving a lower percentage of the world record in weightlifting events than

Losses of strength and power in the weight-lifting events, which also require considerable coordination and balance to raise the weight above the head, are greater than losses in power lifting, such as the deadlift, squat, and bench press.

	Loss from age 40 to age 69 (30 yrs)	Loss from age 70 to 79 (10 yrs)	Total loss from ~40 to 79 (45 yrs)
Weightlifting	50%	15%	65%
Power lifting	30%	20%	50%

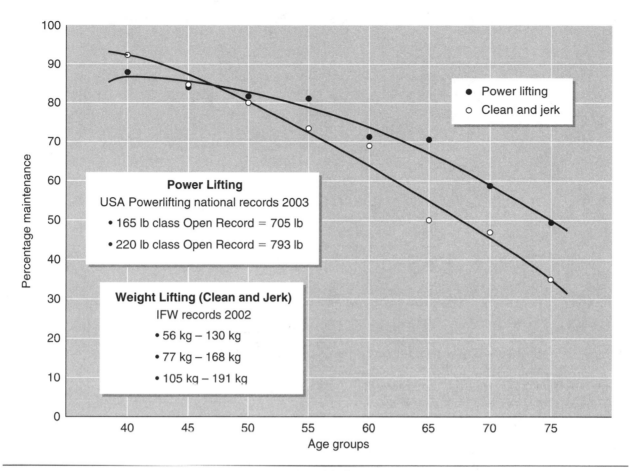

Figure 12.18 Comparison of masters national records for a lift that is purely strength (deadlift) and a lift that requires power, coordination, flexibility, and balance (clean and jerk). Deadlift data are the averages of the 165-lb (74.8-kg) and 220-lb (99.7-kg) cases in the Open Record category. Clean-and-jerk data are the averages of the 56-kg, 77-kg, and 105- to 191-kg classes in the International Federation of Weightlifting records for 2002.

Data from the International Federation of Weightlifting (2002) and the United States Powerlifting Federation (2003).

they achieve in power lifting events, which require primarily maintenance of strength. In fact, the highest peak movement velocity occurs in the snatch and the clean and jerk, the two events in which the difference between old and young competitors is the greatest, and the lowest movement velocity is required in the deadlift and squat, the two events in which the older performers come closest to the world records. Thus, it appears that as the peak power requirement increases in these events, the ability to maintain performance decreases.

Implications of Weightlifting Performances of Masters Competitors

The competitive lifting performances of older competitors are remarkable. When we consider the physical abilities of the vast majority of older people, it is inspiring to observe that some 70-year-old men can lift more than 500 lb (226.7 kg) of steel and iron

from the floor. The world records show that the men who placed in the 70- to 79-year-old category could deadlift two times their own weight. The men in the 80- to 84-year-old category could lift their own body weight. Just as impressive, P. Larsen set the record for 75- to-79-year-old women in the deadlift by lifting 236.75 lb (107.4 kg), and Effie Nielson, in the 90- to 94-year age category, lifted 135 lb (61.2 kg)! These performances by strength-trained individuals suggest that if most men and women were to follow good health habits and to weight train even a moderate amount throughout their lives, they could continue to lift 50 to 75 lb (22-34 kg) well into their 60s and 70s. Thus, it is not unreasonable to suggest that the 16% of adults over age 55 who report having difficulty lifting even 25 lb (11.3 kg) (Kovar & LaCroix, 1987) are experiencing the outcomes of disuse and chronic disease, not the early onset of an inevitable wasting of muscle tissue.

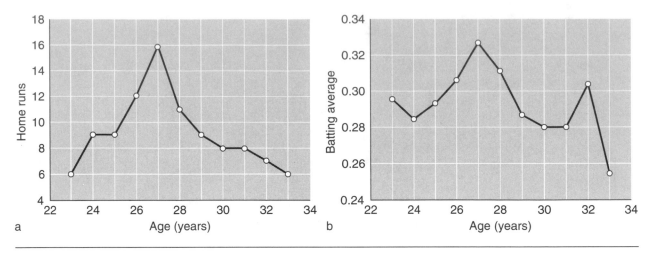

Figure 12.19 *(a)* Home run and *(b)* batting average records for five baseball players listed in the Baseball Hall of Fame.
Data from Langford (1987).

Baseball Hitting

Part of the folklore of baseball is that hitting a fastball is one of the hardest sport skills. Hitting a fastball involves the incredible ability to track a relatively small object (i.e., a baseball) that is moving at a velocity of more than 90 mph and coordinate almost all of the large muscles of the body so that the bat can arrive at the exact point in space at the precise moment in time to contact the ball. Because visual tracking speed, information processing, coordination, and power are required for this skill, the maximum age for effectiveness in baseball hitting is very young. Figure 12.19 presents the annual number of home runs and the batting averages of five members of the Baseball Hall of Fame recorded for a 10-year period of their careers. Both hitting power and accuracy peaked at age 27 for these players and then declined. Their careers were essentially over by age 33. Baseball, like football and basketball, requires power and whole-body coordination, a combination that does not fare well with aging.

Bowling

Unlike the power, endurance, and reactive sports, bowling is a sport that people can perform successfully for many years. Table 12.1 shows the bowling averages of the top 10 bowlers in the Professional Bowling Association compared with those of the top 10 in the Senior Professional Bowling Association. These scores show that older bowlers who continue to bowl can post scores into their 70s that are almost as high as touring pros. This information does not include the age of the senior bowlers, but it does show that high scores can be maintained for a very

Table 12.1 Top 10 Bowlers' Averages on the PBA Tour and Senior Tour

Top 10 Averages	PBA Seniors	PBA Tour
1	226.5	222.7
2	217.2	222.7
3	216.7	222.4
4	216.1	222.0
5	214.9	221.0
6	214.6	221.0
7	214.3	220.6
8	214.3	220.4
9	214.1	220.1
10	213.7	219.5
Average	216.2	221.2
Standard Deviation	3.79	1.14

Note: PBA = Professional Bowling Association.
Data from PBA Tour 2004. www.pba.com/ytdstats.asp?Tour=1&Stype=Average (accessed 9/27/2004).

long time. Ed Easter, who maintained a 193 average during his 16-year career in bowling, did not begin bowling until he was 60 years old. He bowled two of his 300 games when he was more than 70 years old (Hickok, 1971). Thus, bowling can be started late in life and maintained relatively successfully for a great many years.

Improving With Age

Myra Smith, age 95, improved her bowling average in 1992 from 100 to 114. She received her 30-year pin from the Women's International Bowling Congress in 1991, and she is still bowling in 2003. "She has been bowling at least once a week since 1961," her daughter said, "except when she broke her wrist, and even then she was back as soon as the doctor said she could move around." The accident did not affect her form, although she had to switch from a 13-lb (5.8-kg) ball to a 10-lb (4.5-kg) one. "Of course I'm very grateful it wasn't my bowling hand," she said. (Dreckman, 1993)

Golf

Golf is very popular among older adults, because although the game requires many different abilities, the most important of them are primarily abilities of skill and finesse. Power with the driving and fairway woods helps to make approach shots shorter, but in golf accuracy is much more important than power. More than half of the strokes in an average golfer's score are chipping and putting scores, which require almost no strength at all. Older adults can compensate very effectively for a loss of distance when using the long woods and irons by increased precision in approach shots, chipping, and putting. A good example of this is a comparison of the 2002 Professional Golf Association (PGA) tour players' records with those of the PGA Senior tour players (figure 12.20). Excellent golfers drive the ball far, arrive at the green in "regulation" (one stroke for par 3s, two for par 4s, and three for par 5s), get a high percentage of their shots that go in sand bunkers out and in the hole for par (sand saves), have a very low putting average per green (less than two strokes per green), and have a low scoring average. The only one of these in which the top senior players are significantly worse than the top younger PGA players is driving distance. The most important statistic in golf is scoring average, and the difference between the two age groups on this statistic is negligible. In professional tournaments, the seniors do not play as long a course as the PGA players; thus, the age-related difference in driving distance is negated in these statistics. If the seniors were to play the same length of course as the PGA players, their scoring average would be slightly higher (worse) than those of the PGA players. That

is why it is rare for players in their late 40s to win PGA tournaments. Raymond Floyd and Hale Irwin are good examples, however, of the individual differences in older people. Both of them, in their late 40s, won four PGA events. In 1992 Floyd won the Doral Ryder Open tournament at the age of 50. Jack Nicholas won one of the most prestigious PGA tour events, the Masters Tournament, at the age of 46.

Among amateurs, the effect of aging is even less apparent, because people differ so much in their amount of practice, their skill level, and their psychological approach to the game. It is common to find 60- and 70-year-old amateurs who can soundly trounce 20-year-olds in a round of golf, and in any given round, it is not at all unlikely that even an 80-year-old golfer will chip at least one ball as close to the hole as any professional can or sink a putt as long as that of any 20-year-old. Patience, experience, and wisdom are great compensatory mechanisms for older golfers, and these abilities, in addition to practice, enable people to continue to play golf even into their 90s. That may be why golf is one of the most popular participant sports throughout the world. One of the goals of many avid amateur golfers is to be able to "shoot their age," but because par is 72 and almost no amateurs can shoot par, this goal usually is not even possible until a golfer reaches the age of 72. Nevertheless, many people do finally shoot their age, usually in their late 70s and early 80s, and lists of these accomplishments are regularly published in golf magazines throughout the world. The record was made in 1972 when Arthur Thompson, of Victoria, British Columbia, Canada, at 103 years of age, shot 97 on a 6,215-yd (5,683-m) golf course (Hains, 1989).

> Golf is a sport in which dogged determination, constant practice, a positive attitude, and focusing on strengths rather than weaknesses can postpone the negative effects of physical aging on the ultimate goal for a very long time.

Estimating Age-Related Changes in Physiological Functional Capacity

Analyses of aging effects on athletic performance, besides being inherently interesting and serving as a barometer of what is possible at older ages, also supplement scientific knowledge about the effects of aging and other factors on the physiological mechanisms that underpin efficient, powerful physical

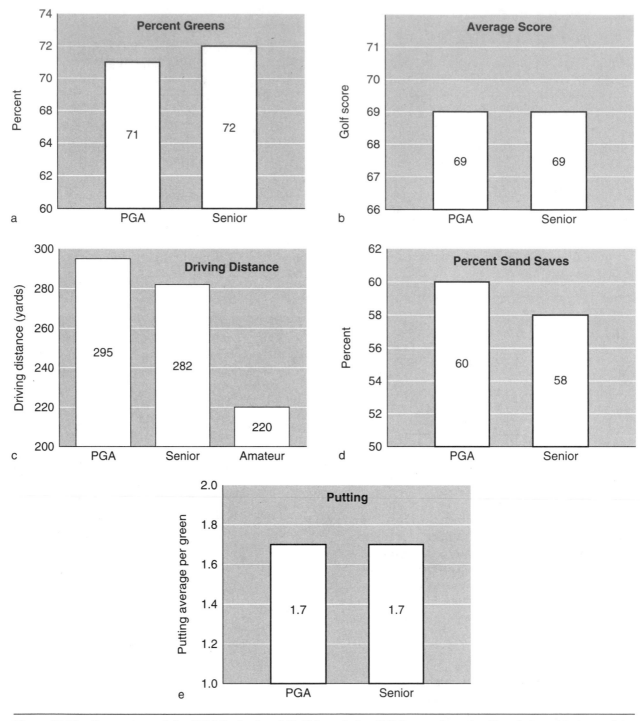

Figure 12.20 Comparison of the 1990 Professional Golf Association (PGA) tour players' golf statistics with those of the Senior PGA players, top 10 players in each tour. *(a)* Percentage of greens in regulation; *(b)* scoring averages (top three players in each tour only); *(c)* driving distance; *(d)* percentage of sand saves; *(e)* putting averages.

performance. One question that has always been of interest is whether aerobic endurance or anaerobic power production is more affected by aging. Another question is whether aging affects one gender more than the other, and if so, in what types of performances. These questions were answered many years ago by exercise physiologists who obtained direct measurements of aerobic and anaerobic capacity, but it has also been of interest to see how those physiological differences are revealed in actual physical performance. In this section, age effects on aerobic and anaerobic systems are considered, followed by a discussion on gender differences, and finally, variability of performance.

The simplest but least accurate way to predict which systems are most affected by aging is to observe the extent and rate of decline in the records held by adults of different ages in specific sports, and then consider which physiological systems are crucial to success in that sport. Running performances over distances that take less than 1 min to run depend primarily on the anaerobic system, whereas races over distances long enough to require several minutes (or more) rely heavily on the aerobic system. In table 12.2, selected sports were ranked on the basis of the percent difference between the 35- or 40-yr-old record and the masters athlete records at increasingly older ages. Two observations from this table are clear. First, swimming and running short distances are the least affected by aging. Both require anaerobic energy in what are basically simple locomotor skills over a very short time period. Swimming is additionally aided by a buoyancy factor, which could account for it having the smallest difference between 35- and 60-yr-olds. The comparisons of the 100-m run with longer races are shown in figure 12.21. The midlevel endurance performances (running 10K, cycling 20K, and swimming 1.5K) also are re-tained almost as well as the sprint

performance. Masters athletes lost the most in the sports requiring complex, whole-body coordination in addition to huge expenditures of power from large muscle mass. The discus and shot put and jumping events also require high levels of coordination, exquisite timing, spatial perception, flexibility, balance, and, in the case of jumping, the ability to withstand jarring force contacts with the ground.

A second observation that is clear from table 12.2 is that for many reasons, discussed later in more detail ("Age and Gender Interactions in Sports Performance"), the performances of women decline more with aging than do those of men. In the last three columns of the table, the percent differences between men and women at ages 35, 60, and 80 are shown. In all but one sport, the differences increase with increasing age. The lack of difference in swimming 1.5 km is probably a fluke that can be attributed to the small samples in all sports in the 80+ age categories.

Predicting Performance From Age and Event Distance

A more accurate way to assess aging effects on different physiological systems is to use regression

Table 12.2 Age and Gender Percent Differences Across Selected Sports

| Approximate rank order of age effects | Unit of measure | Percent difference between 35 and 60 within gender | | Percent difference between 35 and 80 within gender | | Percent difference between men and women at age | | |
		Men	Women	Men	Women	35 or 40	at 60	at 80
Sprint								
Running	100 m	15[a]	22	31	40	8	16	20
Swimming	50 m	10	18	30	36	7	16	17
Endurance								
Running	10K	20	35	40	87.5	14	23	31
Cycling	20K	10	22	30	40	11	28	31
Swimming	1.5K	16	27	43	37	10	22	0
Power								
Discus	2 kg[b], 1 kg[c]	41	44	70	No Cs	wd	wd	wd
Shot put	7.3 kg[b], 4 kg[c]	38	48	61	No Cs	wd	wd	wd
Long jump		29	32	51	68	18	22	46
Triple jump		31	28	50	60	22	20	37
Power lifting		30		50				

Note: No Cs = no competitors in this age range 80+); Wd (weights differ) = men use a heavier discus and shotput than women.
[a]All numbers are percent differences: 15 in this cell means that the difference between 25-yr-old men and 60-yr-old men is 15%.
[b]Weight for men.
[c]Weight for women.

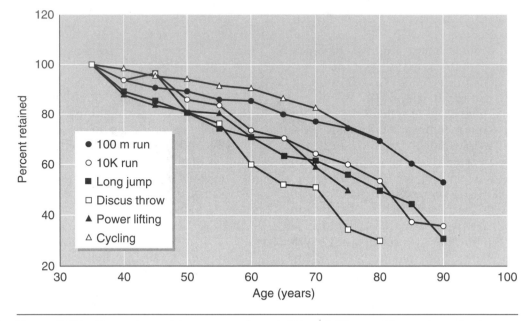

Figure 12.21 Comparison of the percent of men's 35- and 40-year-old records retained across six different sports events.

Data from *Masters Age Records* (2002), United States Cycling Federation (2002), and United States Powerlifting Federation (2003).

statistics to predict sport performance from age, allowing for gender differences. In longitudinal analyses, the regression techniques predict changes that occur within individuals. Both types of analyses provide information about the magnitude and rate of decline of performance. To answer questions about which type of performance declines faster, sprinting (anaerobic) or distance running (aerobic), or whether males decline more slowly in performance than females, regression models have been developed that include age as one predictor and a measure of the type of physiological system primarily used (aerobic or anaerobic) as a second predictor of performance times. Race distances therefore are used as a proxy for the type of physiological system that is being taxed. If running times (or average velocities) can be predicted accurately by including both age and distance traveled, then an analysis of some of the components of the equation should shed some light on the effects of aging on these physiological systems

By far, the most comprehensive study of age effects on maximal physical performance and performance-limiting physiological mechanisms has been made by Stones and Kozma (1980, 1981, 1982a, 1982b, 1984a, 1984b, 1985, 1986a, 1986b). Drawing on their many analyses, they proposed that performance time in running can best be expressed as a product of power function of distance and an exponential function of age (Stones & Kozma, 1980). This exponential function can be simpli-

fied, however, to a general linear model in which performance time is related to both age and event distance:

$$Ln \ (perf) = \ Ln \ (0.049 \ \cdot \ distance^{1.089}) + b \ \cdot \ age$$

where Ln = log to the base n (natural logarithm), perf = the runner's time, distance = distance of event, and b = coefficient specific to the type of race (i.e., anaerobic or aerobic).

This equation implies that perf, expressed as a natural logarithm, is a linear function of age; the intercept is the log function of distance. From their comparison of the b coefficients, which averaged 0.009 for anaerobic events (those <400 m) and 0.011 for aerobic events (those >400 m), these authors concluded that the age effect is greater for middle- and long-distance events than for sprints (figure 12.1, p. 291).

The rate of decline in the middle- and long-distance events is almost the same as the age-related 1% per year rate of decline in aerobics power ($\dot{V}O_2$) when measured by laboratory testing (see chapter 4).

From these results, Stones and Kozma (1985) formulated an energy output–supply ratio hypothesis and later tested its validity against other hypotheses (Stones & Kozma, 1986b). They called their model the power output relative to power available (POrPA) model. The model is based on two assumptions: that age-related decline is greater on tasks in which the maximal output of power taxes the available power more severely, and that more power is available for short-duration performances than for prolonged ones. How does this work?

In short-distance events, the anaerobic system provides a large supply of energy for a brief time. Physiological evidence indicates that the power available from anaerobic sources is three to four times greater than that available from aerobic sources (Bouchard et al., 1981), and that peak muscular power declines at a less rapid rate than maximal aerobic capacity (Larsson et al., 1979). This principle is also observed in tests of absolute muscle strength, where the greater the mass of muscle tested, the greater the age-related decline. Thus, as was discussed in chapter 5, the decline with age is greater in leg and trunk muscles than in the arm muscles (Åstrand & Rodahl, 1977). This principle may be seen in the comparisons of the deadlift, which uses primarily lower limb and back muscles, to the clean and jerk, in which extensor muscles of the upper arms and back must be incorporated into the lift. In long-distance events, the aerobic system provides lower energy supplies but over a longer time period. Because the energy expenditure over a long period is greater than the energy available, age effects are more pronounced in distance events than in short, power events.

Adding Drag to the Equation

Swimming, rowing, and cycling differ from running in that competitors have to contend with overcoming "drag." Locomoting through the medium of water, in the case of swimming and rowing, and against wind, in the case of cycling and rowing, presents a slightly different challenge. Although runners occasionally have to deal with wind, their main challenge is resisting gravity. Does aging affect these performances differently?

Performance records from swimming share many similarities with running. Donato and colleagues (2003) provided the best evidence by analyzing the 12-year longitudinal performances of 321 women and 319 men competing in the United States Masters Swimming Championships. As in running records, these swimming performances deteriorated modestly but inexorably with aging until approximately age 70, after which point they deteriorated more rapidly. This age-related pattern of decline was also observed in a cross-sectional study of the same competitors (Tanaka & Seals, 1997). Performance was maintained better in the short event, the 50-m freestyle, than in

the long events, supporting the laboratory findings that anaerobic power (on which short races depend) declines at a slower rate than aerobic endurance (Larsson et al., 1979).

Although swimmers, like runners, cyclists, and rowers, are confronted with drag, other differences such as buoyancy and emphasis on upper body musculature override these effects. The overall amount of performance loss is smaller in swimming than in running, and the age at which exponential declines begin is older in swimmers than in runners (Tanaka & Seals, 1997). One explanation may be that upper limb muscles of the body deteriorate more slowly than lower limb muscles (McDonagh et al., 1984). In addition, Donato and colleagues (2003) proposed that performances in swimming may decline less rapidly because fast competitive swimming times depend more on biomechanical technique than running times do. Craig and Pendergast (1979) made this suggestion when they found that freestyle swimming performance and distance per stroke are highly correlated. The more efficient each stroke is, the faster the total time.

> In both running and swimming, long-distance endurance events are highly correlated with maximal oxygen uptake and lactate threshold.

In summary, age-related changes in many types of sport performance appear to be linear and gradual until approximately 70 years of age, at which time performance deteriorates more rapidly. Donato and colleagues (2003), noting that this type of deterioration pattern also occurs in preferred walking speed of older adults and in field observations of insects and rodents, suggested that fundamental changes in biological aging processes may occur at about age 70.

Nonphysiological Factors That Influence Maximum Sport Performance

It is clear that aging has a potent negative effect on structural and physiological mechanisms, ensuring that athletic performance must inevitably decline with advancing age. However, several factors other than physical ones also contribute to diminishing performance among most masters athletes. The type of performance analysis that is used, the interaction of gender with aging, and the increase in individual differences with aging influence physical performance. Also, most masters athletes train less intensely, compete with somewhat less verve and in fewer numbers, and have less psychosocial support for their participation.

Cross-Sectional Versus Longitudinal Analyses

The interpretations that are made of physiological functional capacity from sport performance are sometimes influenced by whether the research design is cross-sectional or longitudinal. In chapter 2, we pointed out that usually each age group of a cross-sectional design consists of different people, so that genetic differences, cohort differences, behavior differences, and dropouts of these people at different ages may be as responsible for the regression outcome as age. Conversely, longitudinal designs have other problems. The competitors in a study may change their behavior as the study progresses. Some may practice more, others may reduce their training volume, some may experience injuries, or some may lose large amounts of weight. These can all influence the interpretation of results, and thus all possibilities should be considered when one is evaluating the study findings.

A good example of this is the change in interpretation that Donato and colleagues (2003) made of comparative declines in the swimming performance of men and women over a 50-year period. From cross-sectional data it appeared that the rate and magnitude of declines in swimming performance with age were greater in women than in men (Tanaka & Seals, 1997). However, in their longitudinal follow-up of the same swimmers 12 years later, Donato and colleagues discovered that this gender difference could be observed only in the 50-m sprint and not in the longer distances.

Age and Gender Interactions in Sport Performance

As shown in table 12.2, the performances of women in sport decline at a greater rate than those of men. The greater the aging effect on a sport performance, the bigger the difference is between the men's and women's scores. Several physical and physiological gender differences contribute to this. Although the rate of decline in maximal oxygen consumption is the same in men and women (Holloszy & Kohrt, 1995), the decline in muscular strength and power, particularly in the upper extremities, is greater in women than in men (Skelton et al., 1994). This gender difference in strength and power is even seen as a greater reduction in maximal voluntary strength per cross-sectional area (Phillips et al., 1993). The greater loss of upper body strength is reflected in the greater losses in women's swimming sprints. Within any one swimming event, both men and women endurance swimmers declined linearly from a peak at 35 to 40 years to about 70 years, and then the decline increased exponentially (Tanaka & Seals, 1997). But the rate and magnitude of decline were greater in women only in the shortest distance event, the one that depends the most on upper body strength (Donato et al., 2003).

The relative decline in swimming records of men was not affected by event distance. In a cross-sectional analysis, the percent difference between men and women became smaller from the shortest race to the longest race (figure 12.22; Tanaka & Seals, 1997). This was not true in running events, as no pattern of gender differences emerged across the running events from 100 m to 10 km. In a later longitudinal study of the same subjects, the women declined at a greater rate than men only on the shortest distance race (50 m). A plausible explanation for this gender difference is that the energy cost of swimming is lower in women, perhaps because of their smaller body size (less drag in the water), lower body density, higher percent body fat, and shorter legs (facilitating a more horizontal and streamlined position). The longer the swimming race, the more a high work economy is an advantage, and the closer the performance of women is to men. In contrast, the energy cost of running is similar (Pate et al., 1987), and so gender differences were not linearly related to race distance.

It is also highly probable that several of the nonphysiological factors discussed subsequently that influence physical performance interact with age and gender differences. It is likely that decreases in training, decreased zeal for competition, lower numbers of women competitors in older age groups, and a more negative societal attitude toward old sports competitors play a more predominant role in the decline of women's performances.

Individual Differences

In both genders, individual differences (group standard deviations) increase substantially in increasingly older age groups, even in the top 10 swimmers, who would seem to be a very homogeneous group. Increased variability (individual differences) has been found both cross-sectionally and longitudinally (Donato et al., 2003; Tanaka & Seals, 1997). The greater the individual differences, the more likely that the sampled scores are less representative of the capabilities of individuals of that age group.

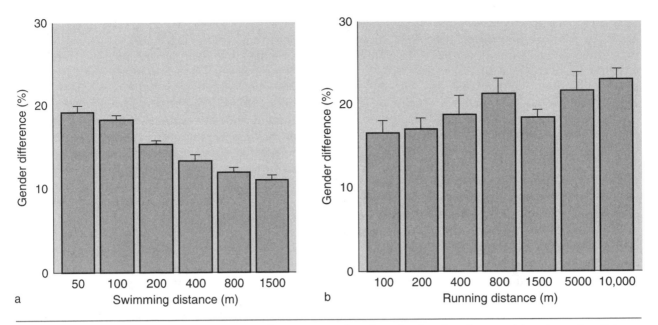

Figure 12.22 Percent gender differences in performance as a function of swimming distance *(a)* and running distance *(b)*. There were significant differences *(p < .05)* between any paired swimming distances except for two distances. Gender differences were not significantly different between 50 and 100 m and between 800 and 1,500 m.

Reprinted, by permission, from H. Tanaka and D.R. Seals, 1997, "Age and gender interactions in physiological functional capacity: Insight from swimming performance," *Journal of Applied Physiology* 82: 846-851.

Decreases in Training

Although empirical data are scarce, most analysts of older adults' athletic performance believe that with increasing age, masters competitors reduce both the frequency and intensity with which they train. Older people train less strenuously for several reasons. First, many older adults maintain full-time managerial, supervisory, or administrative jobs that carry multiple responsibilities. They simply do not have the time to train that they once did. Second, older adults also have a lifetime of experiences that enable them to place training time and sport competition within a broader perspective than 20-year-olds can. Most can only win so many trophies before additional ones begin to lose their luster. Third, the best that older competitors can achieve is a relative victory, that of their age group, whereas 20- to 30-year-olds are striving for an absolute victory—the winner over all ages. For many people, it is harder to maintain an aggressive training program to gain a relative victory than it is to maintain discipline for a collegiate, state, national, or world record. Fourth, old lifters are less likely to adopt performance-enhancing behaviors, such as tight body suits, face slapping, and ammonia inhalation, that are commonly used by young lifters. This could influence the rate of change in lifting performances independent of age effects, although the effects of these enhancers on performance have

not been proved. Fifth, the ravages of time are hard on the body; not only is it difficult psychologically to maintain a heavy training schedule, but it is also difficult physically. Older competitors are plagued much more by muscular and orthopedic training injuries than are the young, and it takes them longer to rehabilitate from injuries. Consequently, they enter competitions without the extensive training base that young competitors have.

Because of these training differences, sports events that require more training to remain in top form reveal greater age declines. It is hard to distinguish whether the greater declines seen in training-dependent events such as distance running, hurdles, and weightlifting are the result of age-related declines in physiological resources, disinclination to train hard, incidence or fear of injury, or a combination of these.

Competitive Fervor Decreases

For some of the same reasons that limit training practices, most masters athletes do not approach competitive events with as much passion as young people do. Besides winning relative rather than absolute victories, and in the life perspective with which older adults view athletic victories, masters athletes are not likely to view athletics as a potential source of revenue or as a way out of an undesirable lifestyle.

The different ways that young and old power lifters approach a competition is a good example. Younger men and women in the power lifting events (not weightlifting events) wear body suits and use other types of lift-enhancing training equipment and techniques, some of which are relatively painful. These external suits and training apparatus enable the competitors to lift significantly more weight than they can lift without them. But these external performance aids also substantially raise the blood pressure during the lift, and they create other physical problems. Older lifters may not use these as enthusiastically; consequently, they do not lift as much as they might be capable of lifting. Also, young competitors do things in competition to evoke the fight-or-flight response just before attempting a lift. Face slapping, ammonia inhalation, and yelling are all part of the game for the younger athlete. For the most part, these types of efforts are absent during masters competitions, suggesting that these age groups also differ psychologically from young competitors.

Another age difference in training techniques is that young athletes are also much more likely to use steroids, growth hormones, or untested supplements to enhance their performance, whereas older athletes probably began their careers before drugs were commonly used and are much less likely to begin drug use at an older age. Older athletes, from experience, have discovered that they are neither invincible nor immortal. Young athletes intellectually know that they will not live in good health forever, but they do not believe it. Consequently, young athletes are willing to take more risks with their health.

Sampling Problem

Perhaps because the motivation to train and to compete decreases with age, many athletes eventually quit competitive sports. Also, many champion athletes do not choose to compete at the masters level when they become less competitive at the national or world level. They would rather not compete at all than compete at what they regard as a lower level. But in other sports, it is considered unseemly for champions to move from world competition to masters competition because they are so much better than amateurs who have not been world-class athletes. This point cannot be made strongly enough: Masters records do not always contain the best performances that adults of each age group can produce.

Because many champions do not compete, and others drop out, the numbers of athletes dwindle with each advancing decade. This is clearly shown in figure 12.13 (p. 299), where the number of rowers at each decade is shown on the right y-axis and their times are shown on the left y-axis. To acquire performance data that are truly representative of each age cohort, however, it is important to have a large pool of competitors, so that the natural screening process of competition can produce the very highest performances that humans can achieve. Generally speaking, if an event has 500 competitors from 50 countries, the winner of that event will probably have a higher score than the winner of an event with 25 competitors from a single city. In all the states but the one in which the champion resides, state records are not as high as the national records, because the state competitions do not sample as wide an array of human resources. In a marathon event, there may be 750 runners between the ages of 20 and 30, 40 runners between the ages of 50 and 60, but only three competitors older than age 80. This contestant-by-age compression phenomenon is even greater in women's events, so performance records and the models that are based on women may be increasingly less representative of actual performance capabilities that could be attained by older age groups. Smaller samples mean less likelihood of high-caliber performances.

The sampling issue is more problematic in some events than in others. Tanaka and Seals (1997) suggested that some of the gender differences observed in age-related swimming and running events may be attributed not just to physiological differences but to the differences that exist in the female-to-male ratio of competitors at each age in the two sports. The number of 80-and-older contestants is much higher in the 10K race than in the shot put, and in the 50-km racewalk than in the high jump. Inequity of sampling is extreme in weightlifting, where the number of weightlifting records dramatically decreases for both men and women, even as early as middle age. Because the competitions at these older ages have fewer and fewer competitors in them, they serve less effectively as a sample of their age group. In sports that have weight classes, such as weightlifting, boxing, wrestling, and rowing, the sample of competitors is divided into even smaller subunits, so that some weight classes in the older masters categories have only one or two competitors.

Psychosocial Influences

Many psychosocial factors influence the participation of older adults in sports, but two are especially pertinent: (a) societal attitudes toward older participants in sports events (ageism), and (b) societal gender bias with regard to sport. The concept of vigorously active, competitive septuagenarians and octogenarians is a relatively new phenomenon in American society. In the first two thirds of the 20th century, at least, societal expectations were that older adults should rest, take it easy, and be relatively inactive, especially after retirement. Indeed, the dictionary definition of retirement includes such phrases as "to withdraw to a secluded place, to go to bed, to retreat, to give up work because of age, to withdraw from use." Societal expectations are a very powerful influence, so when older adults indicated that they were interested in competing in a tournament, it is likely that they were told, either directly in conversation or indirectly by actions, that they should "act their age," meaning they should not compete. Only those few older athletes who were willing to face societal disapproval entered competitions. A large proportion of older adults view masters athletes as "different" from average adults. These societal attitudes still contribute to the sampling problem discussed previously.

Societies also have strong views about what is appropriate behavior for women and men, and although attitudes are changing, gender bias persists in sport. People who harbor these biases believe that tennis and golf are appropriate for women, whereas power lifting and shot putting are not. Similarly, pole vaulting is acceptable for men, but ice skating is not. Gender bias therefore influences the size of the pool of competitive athletes. It also limits the opportunities for training and coaching of athletes in those sports that are considered inappropriate for a specific gender.

Consider weightlifting or power lifting. Comparatively few young women compete in these events, and even fewer continue to lift into their senior years. Very few U.S. records are available for women, and in some weight classes, no records are available. A plausible explanation for why almost no women compete in these sports beyond age 50 is that weightlifting places a premium on power production, and social attitudes toward women, especially older women, as power producers are generally negative. Given the performances of the few women who do compete in their middle-age years, it might be deduced that women cannot maintain strength and power as well as men can. Figure 12.15 (p. 301) compares the percentages of world records achieved by men and women for the clean-and-jerk weightlifting event. The men 60 to 64 years old lift a little more than 70% of the 40-year-old record, whereas the women lift only about 45% of their world record. Much of this is attributable to gender-related strength and power differences, but a substantial amount of differences might also be attributed to the extremely small number of women competing compared with men and to their training

techniques. This is probably also the explanation for the illogical "upturn in capacity" seen in the jumping records of the women's 80-and-older age groups, whereas the men's 80+ records continue their downward trend (figure 12.7, page 295).

Fifty years ago it was socially unacceptable for women to participate in even moderately demanding sports. Within this context, weightlifting not only was unacceptable, it was unthinkable. Consequently, 70-year-old women today have no youthful experiences of weightlifting on which to build. Those few women over 50 who lift weights are usually beginning to lift for the first time in their lives, a pattern of performance that is hardly comparable to that of male masters competitors, many of whom lifted weights in their youth. Even today, when more and more young women are lifting weights, their coaches many times do not require the same demanding training schedules that they demand from their male athletes. These attitude and training differences may also explain in part the findings from laboratory studies, which are generally that the percent loss in women's power and absolute upper body strength is greater than that of men's.

Probably because the baby boomers are aging, and the proportion of the population that is old is increasing, attitudes toward old athletes and women in sport are changing rapidly. The Senior Tour in golf, only 20 years old, has a substantial following and solid financial backing. Both the National Basketball Association and Major League Baseball have initiated shortened Old-Timers All-Star games which precede the All-Star game. Women's professional golf and basketball teams and women's intercollegiate sports are beginning to attract larger followings. The social support system for older athletes, therefore, is improving.

Social Support Systems and the Positive Secular Trend

The performances of all masters athletes are improving with each passing decade. This positive secular trend in athletic performance is illustrated in table 12.3 (modified from Ericsson, 1990). In all categories except the 200-m run, the recent records of master athletes from age 50 to 59 were faster or almost the same as the best times in the Olympic Games of 1896. It is impressive that not only were the 1979 masters times faster than the times of those who won Olympic medals in 1896, but in the longer distances, the

Table 12.3 **Olympic and World Running Records in 1896 compared to Masters Athletes' Records in 1979, 1990, and 2002**

Event	Best time in Olympic games of 1896[a]	Unofficial World record in 1896[b]	Age category for masters athletes in 1979 and 1990											
			50-54			55-59			60-64			65-69		
			1979	1990	2002	1979	1990	2002	1979	1990	2002	1979	1990	2002
100 m (in s)	12.0	10.8	11.4	11.2	11.2	11.6		11.6	12.0		11.7	13.2	12.5	12.5
200 m (in s)	22.2	21.8	23.6	22.9	22.9	23.6		23.4	24.9		24.0	27.9	25.6	25.6
400 m (in s)	54.2	48.2	52.9	52.2	51.39	54.6	53.8	52.6	59.1	55.2	53.9	65.1	61.1	57.5
800 m (in min:s)	2:11.0	1:53.4	2:01.1	2:00.4	1:59.45	2:11.4	2:05.1	2:05.7	2:19.9	2:12.9	2:10.42	2:27.2	2:20.5	2:14.33
1,500 m (in min:s)	4:33.2	4:10.4	4:14.0	4:05.0	4:05.2	4:20.4	4:14.4	4:12.5	4:53.2	4:30.0	4:27.65	4:59.2	4:41.8	4:39.87
Marathon	2:58:5		2:25:17		2:29:11	2:26:3		2:33:49	2:53:03		2:42:44	2:53:03		2:42:49

Adapted from K.A. Ericcson (1990).

1990 and 2002 United States masters records were progressively faster than those established in 1979. The secular trend of masters performances in longer distances, therefore, is toward better and better performances.

Why are athletes performing at older and older ages at the highest levels of sport? The answer may lie not so much in changing physiology but rather in a changing sport society. For example, career longevity in competitive sport seems to be positively correlated with financial incentive. Athletes in professional sports such as baseball, basketball, and football perform at the highest levels of their sport into at least their early 30s (Nolan Ryan at age 44 pitched a no-hitter). Obviously, in these sports high salaries promote career longevity. Conversely, until recently, the track-and-field athlete performed within a very different athletic time frame. Runners generally began running in elementary school, trained and competed in high school and college, and after losing the financial and social support for their passion, retired from competition soon after college and when they were still in their early 20s. It should not be surprising, then, that the age at peak performance in many track-and-field events was approximately 21 years. Today, with elite track-and-field performers negotiating for lucrative appearance fees and endorsements, the age at peak performance is increasing significantly.

Athletes over age 50 may be positively influenced by the impressive increase in popularity of masters competitive events and the intensity of media attention that has been focused on masters participants as well as winners in the past two decades. More masters athletes are training harder and more often. More and more older adults are postponing their retirement from competition, and many older adults are beginning to compete in tournaments. As the baby boomers turn 60 years old, their sheer numbers will increase the number of older athletic competitors. Younger cohorts who have grown up in a social environment that promotes good health habits will be increasingly reluctant to give up physical competition. As more athletes continue competing into their older years, these age categories will be sampled better, and their performances will more accurately reflect human capability. Given their different approaches to competition, it may very well be that the athletic performances of young and old competitors in some sports would be more similar if young competitors performed without performance-enhancing drugs and equipment and the old competitors trained as intensely as the young.

How Do They Do It?

Anyone who studies the physical performances of very old masters athletes, or of those who climb mountains, water ski, or hang glide, must be in awe of their successful physical aging. How do they do it? Many factors contribute to the physical accomplishments of these older adults, not the least of which is a superb genetic makeup that has provided them with talent and physical stamina. With all the discussion of special behaviors of these individuals, it should be remembered that they have inherited relevant abilities and resistance to injury, which enable them to optimize their physical performance. They also have been lucky: They have not been in a fatal or debilitating automobile accident or contracted a disabling disease, such as Parkinson's disease, multiple sclerosis, or muscular dystrophy. But given good inheritance and luck, they have maximized their potential by continuing to train physically and by maintaining good health habits, such as good diet, abstinence from smoking and drug use, and low alcohol consumption. They have a psychological makeup in which the body and its functioning are a very important component of their self-awareness and esteem. The combination of these factors produces an individual who physically ages extremely well.

SUMMARY

One of the best ways to determine human physical potential throughout the life span is to study athletic performances of individuals at different ages. Record performances from events such as the World Masters Track-and-Field Championships, the World Veterans Games, the United States Amateur Union Masters Swimming Championships, and the United States Weightlifting Federation's competition provide measures of maximum human performance throughout aging. These national and world records contribute to an understanding of aging physical abilities, because in masters competitions, the physical efforts are very highly motivated and the performances occur under highly controlled circumstances. These records provide information about the physical abilities of the small percentage of elderly who maintain the maximum amount of strength and fitness possible throughout a lifetime. The records provide a marker of what is physically possible for human beings. In addition, information about the shape of the curve that describes these losses assists scientists in understanding the physiological, psychological, and sociological mechanisms that curtail physical performance.

This chapter described and compared the masters records for selected track-and-field events (running, jumping, and throwing), swimming, cycling, rowing, and weightlifting. The most important conclusion to be drawn from these analyses is that masters athletes produce remarkable physical performances. In a world in which far too many elderly are disabled and physically dysfunctional, the masters athletes stand as a symbol of human strength and resilience. The most striking example is that for men aged 60 to 69 years, the United States record in the 40-km (24.8-mile) cycling road race event is only 14% lower than the U.S. record set by young men. This phenomenal maintenance of function occurs in events such as cycling, running, swimming, and rowing, sports in which the systems most resistant to aging—aerobic endurance and strategy—are predominant.

Although national and world records are an important source of information with regard to understanding aged human physical potential, several caveats must be considered when interpreting the records. The older the age group, the fewer the competitors. Also, most researchers believe that even the most zealous of elderly competitors usually do not train as intensely as young athletes do. Both of these caveats are particularly true for women. Thus, individual differences, even in these homogeneous and highly select groups, become greater and greater with increasing age, and because of this sampling problem, it is likely that observed age decrements in the oldest groups, as well as gender differences, are overestimated. Age records have been improving every year as the popularity of masters competitions increases and more and more people compete.

That many adults over age 70 participate in noncompetitive, physically demanding activities or occupations bears repeating. This chapter has focused on competitors because their performances are quantified, yet those who remain physically active in other ways are equally admirable. Although those elderly who participate intensely in physical activity, like masters athletes, represent a very small percentage of the old and oldest-old population, they are an important group to study and to emulate. They reveal the limits of human physical potential in all adult age categories. Because they are remarkable and an inspiration, and because they epitomize optimal physical aging, their story is a most appropriate last chapter. They inspire an upward look, provide a standard, and give hope, and that is the note on which any book about the physical dimensions of aging should conclude.

REVIEW QUESTIONS

1. What are three main contributions that the study of masters sports record performances add to the scientific information that we have about physiological capabilities of older adults?

2. Discuss three psychosocial outcomes of the study of physically elite older adults.

3. In which sports are the records most negatively affected by increased aging? Rank order these six sports in terms of how resistant they are to the aging process, with the first on the list being the most resistant and the last on the list being very vulnerable to the aging process: marathon running, triple jump, 50-m swimming, power lifting, hitting a baseball, and golf. Justify your ranking on the basis of information provided in chapters 4 through 8.

4. Name three competitive sports other than the ones discussed in this chapter. Where would you place them in your rank ordering of the sports in question number 3? Why?

5. Why does the variability of performance records get increasingly larger in increasingly older age groups?

SUGGESTED READINGS

Clark, E. (1986). *Growing old is not for sissies. Portraits of senior athletes.* Petaluma, CA: Pomegranate Calendars and Books.

Ford, D. (1993, January). The golden years. *Skiing,* pp. 56-64, 147.

Glossary

abductor muscle groups—Muscles that are used to move a limb in a lateral direction away from the body.

acceleration—Rate of change of velocity.

active life expectancy (ALE)—Period of life that is free of disability in activities of daily living (ch. 1; Katz et al., 1983).

adductor muscle groups—Muscles that are used to move a limb in a lateral direction toward the body.

affect—The way a person, situation, or an event makes one feel; described as positive or negative.

ageism—Expecting certain behaviors or abilities based solely on someone's chronological age.

allostatic load—A cumulative, multisystem view of the physiologic toll that may be exacted on the body through attempts at adaptation.

anemia—Condition in which there are too few red blood cells in the bloodstream, resulting in insufficient oxygen to tissues and organs.

angiogenesis—Formation of new capillaries from existing capillaries.

ankle strategy—Strategy used to maintain standing balance. The body sways as a single entity about the ankle joints as force is exerted against the surface.

anthropometry—Branch of science dealing with the measurement of the human body.

anticipatory postural control—Process whereby a movement is planned before it actually begins.

arteriovenous oxygen difference, or $(a-\bar{v})O_2$ **difference**—Difference between the amount of oxygen transported in the arterial blood and the amount transported in the mixed venous blood.

arthritis—Condition or disease that involves inflammation of a joint.

atherosclerosis—A form of heart disease in which the inner layers of artery walls become thick and irregular because of deposits of fat, cholesterol, and other substances (plaque). This narrowing of the arteries reduces the flow of blood through the arteries.

athletic power—Production of a large amount of work within a short amount of time, such as occurs in the 100-m sprint race or the clean-and-jerk weight-lifting event. Technically, power is the physical work accomplished per unit time, or $(F \times D)/T$, where F is force, D is the distance through which the force is moved, and T is the duration of the work period (ch. 12; McArdle et al., 2001).

autoimmunity theory—Theory that during aging the immune system, which normally attacks foreign substances such as viruses or cancerous cells in the body, loses the capacity to distinguish foreign antigens from normal body materials. Antibodies are formed that react with normal cells and destroy them or that fail to recognize and destroy the small detrimental mutations that occur in cells.

average life span—The average age by which all but a very small percentage of the members of a species are deceased.

balance—Process by which we control the body's center of mass (COM) with respect to the base of support, whether it is stationary or moving.

base of support (BOS)—Area of an object that is in contact with the support surface (e.g., feet, hands).

best practice approaches—Approaches that are based on accumulated research evidence.

between-group variability—Spread of scores of group means around the group mean of means.

bimanual—Movement that is made by using both arms or both hands.

biological aging—Process or group of processes that causes the eventual breakdown of mammalian homeostasis with the passage of time.

biomarker(s) of aging—Measure or group of biological measures that quantify the status of basic biological processes, separating biological status from disease status and chronological age. Such markers are highly sought, because they would enable a quantification of the organism's biological rate of aging. At present, no biomarkers have been found that fulfill all of the requirements for a true biomarker.

blood pressure—Force or pressure that the circulating blood exerts on the walls of the arteries.

body competence—Subjective evaluation of the body's ability to accomplish the physical goals that individuals create for themselves.

body consciousness—A concept that has three aspects: body image, perception of body function, and body competence.

body image—Subjective feelings that people have about their physical appearance, the private perception of body function, and body competence.

body mass index—Rough estimate of fatness derived by dividing body weight by height. It is calculated in kilograms and meters as kg/m^2.

brain plasticity—Conduciveness of the brain to change physiologically and morphologically to changes in task and environmental demands. Young brains are very malleable, or "plastic" in that physiological changes occur very quickly. As brains age, their ability to respond to change and to adapt lessens.

caloric restriction—A diet in which the major nutrients, minerals, and vitamins that are necessary for health are supplied, but the total amount of food is reduced to about two thirds of normal consumption. This is the only known way to change the rate of aging, and it has only been shown in nonhuman species.

capillarity—Number of capillaries per muscle fiber, or the number of capillaries surrounding muscle fibers.

cardiac output (Q)—Total amount of blood ejected from each ventricle of the heart in one minute.

center of gravity (COG)—Vertical projection of the center of mass.

center of mass (COM)—Point at the center of the total body mass being measured.

central component—Component of an intrinsic system that includes all central nervous system structures such as afferent pathways.

central pattern generators—Hypothesized circuits of neurons in the spinal cord that are believed to produce certain rhythmic movements such as locomotion and breathing

change score—Measure of the amount of change that occurs within one individual over a period of time. It is measured by subtracting the second observed score from the first observed score.

choice reaction time (CRT)—Time interval between stimulus and response when a specific response is paired with a specific stimulus, and the reactor has to observe the stimulus and then choose the correct response that is paired with it.

cholesterol—One of several types of fats that play an important role in the body. High concentrations of high-density lipoprotein cholesterol or "good" cholesterol in the blood are associated with a lower risk of heart disease, whereas high concentrations of low-density lipoprotein cholesterol or "bad" cholesterol in the blood are associated with a higher risk for heart disease.

chronometric measures—Measures such as simple and choice reaction time, movement time, and response time.

coefficient of variation—Measure of the spread of scores around a mean. It is calculated by relating the standard deviation of a group to its mean, that is, by dividing the standard deviation by the mean. Coefficient of variation can only be used with ratio scale scores, but because it is a calculated score that provides a ratio of the variability to the magnitude of the mean, it is very useful for comparing within-group variability (individual differences) across variables with different units of measure.

compression of morbidity—Reducing the period of time at the end of life in which older individuals live in a state of morbidity.

concentric muscle contraction—Muscle shortening during contraction.

control—Process by which the temporal and spatial patterns of movement are constrained.

controlled processes—Cognitive processes that require control to complete the task.

coordination—"The patterning of body and limb motions relative to the patterning of environmental objects and events" (ch. 8; Magill, 2001, p. 37).

coronary arteries—Arteries that supply the heart with oxygenated blood.

coxswain—Person who sits in the stern of the boat, facing the crew (who row backward) and guiding the boat so that it goes in a straight line.

cross-sectional research—Research design in which the data are obtained from different people of different ages, and differences among the age groups are inferred to be related to the aging process. Described in detail in chapter 1.

cumulative disadvantage—Accumulated effect of multiple negative social factors, such as unemployment, low social class, low education level, and long-term caregiver status, which disadvantage individuals in the labor market, depress their financial incomes, and negatively influence health status.

cycling time trials—Events in which cyclists race singly against the clock for 40 yd (36.5 m).

dermis—Underlying connective tissue layer beneath the epidermis of the skin.

diastolic blood pressure—Highest pressure generated by the heart during ventricular relaxation.

disability—A physical or mental limitation that interferes with a person's performance of socially defined life tasks expected of an individual within a typical sociocultural and physical environment (ch. 11; Jette et al., 2002).

discrimination reaction time—Time interval between stimulus and response when the reactor is not sure whether a "go" stimulus will follow the "ready" signal.

dispersion—Rate of decline is not the same across multiple tasks; people age more in some tasks than in others.

displacement—Act of the body moving through space and time.

diversity—Individual differences; individuals decline at different rates.

double-support time—Amount of time in which both feet are in contact with the floor surface.

dynamic (isotonic) strength—Strength production in which muscle fibers shorten or lengthen so that movement of the skeleton occurs.

dynamic systems theory—Research perspective that views motor control as subject to self-organization; that "regularities of movement patterns . . . emerge naturally (that is, physically) as the result of complex interactions among numerous connected elements" (ch. 8; Schmidt & Wrisberg, 2004, p. 143).

dynamometer—Instrument that quantifies forces; generally a hand dynamometer, in which a handle is squeezed as hard as possible to measure grip strength.

eccentric muscle contraction—Muscle lengthening during contraction.

effortful processing—Tasks that require multiple allocations of resources and focus of attention to different aspects of the task at different times and thus require considerable mental effort to perform.

epidermis—Outer layer of the skin composed of epithelium.

executive control/executive function—Planning, scheduling, coordination, inhibition, and working memory functions of the brain.

exercise—Subset of physical activity; physical activity that is planned, structured, repetitive, and purposive in the sense that improvement or maintenance of one or more components of physical fitness is an objective.

exercise ceiling effect—Level of exercise above which no addition benefit accrues to a given variable.

exercise dose—Level of exercise used as an independent variable in an experimental study of the effects of exercise on some variable. The "dosage" might be four levels: none, 40%, 60%, or 75% of maximum effort; or it might be three levels: sedentary, moderate, or high physical activity levels.

exercise threshold effect—Level of exercise that is the minimum amount necessary to produce an effect on a given variable.

fat free mass—Total body mass minus fat mass; water, protein, and bone mineral.

fat mass—Estimate of the amount of fat in the body. It is estimated most commonly in clinics by skinfold measures and underwater weighing and in research laboratories by air plethysmography, bioimpedance, DEXA, computed tomography, and magnetic resonance imaging.

feedforward—Process in which vision is used to prepare the motor system before the movement begins.

flexibility—Range of motion around a joint or multiple joints.

force plate—Systems that are designed to measure the changing pressures under the feet as the body maintains a static posture or moves through space.

frailty—"Condition or syndrome that results from a multi system reduction in reserve capacity to the extent that a number of physiological systems are close to, or past, the threshold of symptomatic clinical failure" (ch. 11; Campbell & Buchner, 1997, p. 315).

free-radical theory—Theory that free radicals oxidize and attack other cellular components, causing alterations and malfunctions that accumulate throughout life. Eventually, so much cellular damage has occurred that the cell dies.

functional fitness—Maintenance of fitness components (strength, power, flexibility, balance, and endurance) necessary to perform normal everyday activities safely and independently without undue fatigue.

functional health—The way individuals function within the constraints of their objective health.

functional health status—Degree to which physical conditions and diseases limit activity.

functional independence—Ability to maintain activities of daily living without undue difficulty; operating at least at the minimal levels of physical, cognitive, and mental health.

functional performance—Observable ability to perform tasks of daily living.

gait cycle—Arbitrarily defined as the time between the first contact the heel of one foot makes with the ground to the next heel–floor contact made with the same foot.

genotypes—Genetic constitution of an organism or cell: the internally coded, inheritable information that is used as a blueprint or set of instructions for building and maintaining a living creature. The genotype provides the codes that result in the expressed features or physical manifestations of the organism (phenotype).

Hayflick limit—Theory that cells will divide and reproduce themselves only a genetically programmed, limited number of times.

health—Attribute of people that is related to many factors such as genetics, nutrition, sleep, psychological stress, and abstinence from smoking and drugs.

health-related quality of life—Health and physical function contributions to a psychological feeling of well-being (does not include environment, economic status, availability of resources, or climate).

hip strategy—Movement strategy used to control sway in a standing position that requires the activation of hip muscles. The upper and lower body move in opposite directions when this strategy is used.

hypertension—Persistent high blood pressure.

inconsistency—Older individuals are more inconsistent than young, and their inconsistence across tasks is greater than in young individuals.

individual differences—Differences that exist among individuals on a given variable. The extent of these differences within a group is represented by the coefficient of variation ([group standard deviation]/ group mean).

information processing theory—a model that considers the individual a "black-box," taking in environmental information through the senses and processing it in various ways through several stages until it results in motor output that fulfills a goal.

isometric (static) strength—Muscle activation in which no observable change occurs in muscle length.

kilojoule (kJ)—An international standard for expressing energy. $4.2 \cdot 1$ kcal = 1 kJ; a kilocalorie is the amount of energy necessary to raise the temperature of 1 kg of water $1°$ C.

kinematic—Qualities of motion without regard to force.

kinematics—Scientific description of movement without regard to force or mass; it includes displacement, velocity, and acceleration.

kinetic—Internal and external forces that contribute to the quality of motion.

kinetics—Scientific description of the cause of motion.

kyphotic posture—Increased posterior curve of the spine.

life expectancy—The average number of years of life remaining for a population of individuals, all of the same age, usually expressed from birth as the average number of years of life that newborns might expect to live.

life satisfaction—Degree to which feelings of well-being pertain to one's entire life.

longitudinal research—Research design in which the same individuals are observed over several years and the changes that occur in their performance times are recorded.

masters athletes—Individuals who compete in any sport in age categories. Each sport has a different minimum age at which the age groups begin. In some sports, the age at which competitors become masters is 27; in other sports in may be 30, 35, or 40.

maximal aerobic capacity ($\dot{V}O_2$max)—Maximal rate at which oxygen can be taken up, distributed, and used by the body in the performance of exercise that engages a large muscle mass.

maximum life span—Survival potential of members of a species, defined by the oldest living member of that species.

mobility—Ability to move oneself independently and safely from one place to another.

mood—Concepts of depression, anxiety, anger, vigor, fatigue, confusion, pleasantness, and euphoria.

morbidity—Condition in which an individual is so physically or mentally disabled by chronic disease or condition that he or she becomes immobile and dependent on the care of others.

morphological changes—Structural changes in neural components, such as neurons, axons, and dendrites.

motor control—Study of movements and postures and the processes that underlie them.

motor learning—"A change in the capability of a person to perform a skill that must be inferred from a relatively permanent improvement in performance as a result of practice or experience" (ch. 8; Magill, 2001, p. 129).

motor preparation period—Period preceding a movement to be made in response to an executive control task.

motor unit—Motor neuron and all the muscle fibers that it innervates.

muscle atrophy—Wasting away of muscle; loss of protein in muscle cells and loss of muscle cells (fibers).

muscle hypertrophy—Enlargement of a muscle by the increase in size of muscle cells (fibers).

muscle power—Generation of force over a short period of time; work/time; measured in watts.

muscle quality—Specific force; newtons of force per fiber cross-sectional area.

muscle response synergies—Groups of muscles that are constrained to act together.

muscle strength—Amount of force (or torque) that a muscle or group of muscles can produce with a single maximum contraction; measured in newtons or newton-meters.

myocardial infarction—Irreversible injury to the heart muscle; heart attack.

neurotrophins—Proteins that maintain, protect, and promote growth in neuronal populations.

newton (N)—Force applied to a mass of 1 kg that gives it an acceleration of $1 \text{ m} \cdot \text{s}^{-2}$.

osteopenia—Loss of bone tissue; defined as having bone mineral density values between 1.0 and 2.5 standard deviations below the mean for young women.

osteoporosis—Degenerative bone disease; deterioration or breakdown of bone tissue.

oxygen transport—Transport of oxygen in the blood primarily through its attachment to hemoglobin to cells where it is used.

perception–action cycle—Interplay that occurs between the sensory and motor systems and creates a cyclical feedback loop between perception and action. Perception drives action while the feedback derived from action alters or confirms the original perception.

perception of body function—Awareness that people have of internal body sensations that are not visible to others.

performance outcome—Result of performance.

performance production—Provides information about the behavior that produced the outcome.

peripheral component—Component of an intrinsic system that includes all peripheral nervous system structures (e.g., sensory receptors and nerve pathways leading to and from the spinal cord).

peripheral neuropathy—A partial or complete loss of sensation beginning in the hands or feet and moving proximally toward the arms or legs.

physical activity—Any bodily movement produced by skeletal muscles that results in energy expenditure.

physical condition—Professionally diagnosed presence or absence of disease.

physical fitness—Set of attributes that people have or achieve that relates to the ability to perform physical activity.

physical reserve—Distance from frailty; that is, maintaining a reserve of functional fitness components that provide a margin of safety.

plantar surface—Surface of the feet in contact with the ground.

postural hypotension—Also known as orthostatic hypotension, a condition in which blood pressure regulation is somewhat compromised, leading to a sudden decrease in blood pressure following a rapid change in body position. The decrease in blood pressure can cause light-headedness or fainting. It happens most frequently when older adults rise quickly from sitting in a chair or lying in bed, sometimes after illnesses, and when they are fatigued.

posture—Biomechanical alignment of each body part and the orientation of the whole body with respect to the environment.

power—Work rate or the product of force produced and movement velocity.

power lifting—Type of weightlifting competition consisting of three events: the deadlift, squat, and bench press.

premotor time—Component that best represents the beginning of a response.

processing speed—Amount of time it takes to go through the sequential or parallel stages of mental function and movement initiation necessary to complete a task. In Colcombe and Kramer's (2003) definition (ch. 9 in this text), it refers primarily to relatively low level functions such as stimulus perception, encoding, and storage retrieval.

proprioceptors—Sensory receptors within the body that provide uninterrupted knowledge about the position of the body in space before and during movements.

reaction time response—Response that is made to a stimulus. The response may be a large skeletal muscle response, or a smaller one, such as an oral response, or that of a very small movement of an eyelid. Reaction times have even been recorded by EMG for single motor units, in which case no visible movement is seen.

reaction time—Time interval from the onset of a stimulus to the initiation of a volitional response.

reaction time stimulus—Onset of a signal, which may be visual, auditory, or tactiles, to which the subject is to initiate a response as quickly as possible.

reactive postural control—Movements that cannot be planned in advance of the action.

relative phase—Measure that has been commonly used as a reflection of coordination at the behavioral level. This measure reflects the difference in phase between the limbs. The relative phase of an in-phase pattern is 0°, whereas the relative phase of an antiphase pattern is 180°.

response–response compatibility—Ease with which responses are performed simultaneously or individually when paired with another alternative response.

rheumatism—General term that indicates pain and stiffness affecting the skeletal and muscular systems.

risk factors—Personal habits or characteristics that medical research has shown to be associated with an increased risk of a particular disease or condition.

rowing ergometer—Indoor rowing machine that has a calibrated flywheel to provide resistance and a monitoring device that provides distance rowed, rate of rowing, power output, real-time, calories expended, and several various combinations of these.

saccadic fixation—Ballistic movement of the eyeball that directs the eye to a target of interest. The saccade is a movement of the fovea of the eye to the target that is so fast that it is almost impossible to correct once in motion. The fovea is a small spot in the retina that is the central area of highest visual acuity.

sarcopenia—Age-related decline in muscle mass; muscle wasting.

secular effects—Environmental effects that influence all people who live within an identified period.

selective mortality—Loss of individuals in a research study or program because of nonrandom factors. Older age groups ordinarily lose more subjects throughout the course of a study through death than do younger age groups. Experimentally, selective mortality can refer to the nonrandom

loss of subjects attributable to their reactions to the research project, the researchers, the tests being taken, or the subject's characteristics and biases.

self-concept—Conscious awareness and perception of self.

self-efficacy—An individual's perception of his or her capability to execute a certain behavior successfully.

self-esteem—Regard with which people view themselves in all dimensions of their lives.

shell—Small boat that single rowers use to row. It holds one person and has two oars.

simple reaction time (SRT)—Time interval from the onset of a simple stimulus to make a simple response.

specific force—Newtons of force per fiber cross-sectional area.

stability limits—Maximum distance a person is willing or able to lean in any direction without changing the base of support.

step strategy—Postural control strategy.

stochastic processes—Processes that appear to be random rather than being explained by a theory.

stroke volume—Amount of blood that is pumped from the heart with each beat.

subcutaneous layer—Tissue that separates the skin from the deep fascia around other organs, such as muscles and bones, and contains a large number of adipose (fat) cells.

subjective health—Perception of individuals of their own health.

systems theory—A contemporary theoretical approach to the study of posture, balance, and locomotion that assumes that multiple systems within the body collaborate to control bodily orientation and locomotion. The goal of the action being performed and the properties of the environment are also believed to play an important contributing role in this theory.

systolic blood pressure—Highest pressure generated by the heart during ventricular contraction.

tandem stance—Stance where a person stands with one foot front directly lined up and behind the other foot, with the toe of one foot immediately behind and touching the heel of the other foot.

telomere—Region of DNA at the end of each chromosome in dividing cells that contains no genetic information, grows shorter with each replication of the chromosome, and has been proposed as the clock that times the cell's death (telomere hypothesis).

torque—Degree to which a force tends to rotate an object about a specified fulcrum: the magnitude of a force times the length of its moment arm (ch. 5; Baechle & Earle, 2000).

total peripheral resistance—Total resistance to blood flow in the arteries involved in systemic circulation.

transfer—Ability to adapt a movement pattern learned in one context to a similar but related skill or context.

unimanual—Movement that is made by using one arm or one hand.

variability—Spread of scores around a mean value for a group of scores.

velocity—Rate of change in position over the change in time.

vestibular system—Proprioceptive structure that forms part of the membranous labyrinth of the inner ear. It is comprised of three semi-circular canals, an utricle, and a scale that provide information about the position and movement of the head in space.

vestibulo-ocular reflex (VOR)—Reflex that generates eye movements to ensure clear vision while the head is moving.

visuospatial processing—Transformation or recall of visual and spatial information.

watt (W)—Power that in 1 s generates the energy of 1 J ($1 \text{ W} = 1 \text{ J} \cdot \text{s}^{-1}$).

weight lifting—Type of weightlifting competition consisting of two events: the clean and jerk and the snatch.

within-group variability—Also called individual differences; the spread of scores of all individuals in a group around the group mean. It is usually measured with the standard deviation. Groups that have small standard deviations are homogeneous, and those in which the individuals are vastly different from each other are heterogeneous.

within-individual variability—Also known as within-subject variability; the spread of scores provided by one person about that person's own mean. The scores within the distribution could be several trials by the same person or the same person's scores on different levels of some test.

References

Chapter 1

Arbuckle, T.Y., Sissons, M.E., & Harsany, M. (1986/1987). Development of a measure of intellectual, social, and physical activity for use with young and older adults. *Research Bulletins of the Centre for Research in Human Development, Concordia University, 5*(4).

Arking, R. (1998). *Biology of aging: Observations and principals* (2nd ed.). Sunderland, Massachusetts. Sinauer Associates, Inc.

Bjorksten, J. (1989). The role of aluminum and age-dependent decline. *Environmental Health Perspectives, 81*, 241-242.

Blair, S., Kampert, J.B., Kohl, H.W., III, Barlow, C.E., Macera, C.A. Paffenbarger, R.S., Jr., & Gibbons, L.W. (1996). Influences of cardiorespiratory fitness and other precursors on cardiovascular disease and all-cause mortality in men and women. *Journal of the American Medical Association, 276*, 205-210.

Busse, E.W. (1969). Theories of aging. In E.W. Busse & E. Pfeiffer (Eds.), *Behavior and adaptation in later life* (pp. 11-32). Boston: Little Brown.

Casey, A.E., & Casey, J.G. (1971). Long-lived male population with high cholesterol intake in Slieve Loughner, Ireland. *Alabama Journal of Medical Science, 7*, 21.

Chlebowski, R.T., Hendrix, S.L., Langer, R.D., Stefanick, M.S., Gass, M., Lane, D., Rodabough, R.J., Gilligan, M.A., Cyr, M.G., Thomson, C.A., Khandekar, J., Petrovitch, H., & McTierman (2003). Risks and benefits of estrogen plus progestin in healthy postmenopausal women. *Journal of the American Medical Association, 289*, 3243-3257.

Crandall, R.C. (1991). *Gerontology: A behavioral science approach* (2nd ed.). New York: McGraw-Hill.

Department of Family and Community Services. (2001). Australia's fertility rate: Trends and issues. [Online]. 9:4. Available: via e-mail *Research.Sheet @facs.gov.au* [February 2001].

Drori, D., & Folman, Y. (1976). Environmental effects on longevity in the male rat: Exercise, mating, castration, and restricted feeding. *Experimental Gerontology, 11*, 25-32.

Edington, D., Cosmas, A.C., & McCafferty, W.B. (1972). Exercise and longevity: Evidence for a threshold age. *Journal of Gerontology, 27*, 341-343.

Ekonomov, A.L., Rudd, C.L., & Lomakin, A.J. (1989). Actuarial aging rate is not constant within the human life span. *Gerontology, 35*, 113-120.

Enstrom, J.E. (1984). Smoking and longevity studies. *Science, 225*, 878.

Finch, C.E. (1976). The regulation of physiological changes during mammalian aging. *Quarterly Review of Biology, 51*, 49-83.

Friedman, G.D., Dalles, L.G., & Ury, N. (1979). Mortality in middle-aged smokers and nonsmokers. *New England Journal of Medicine, 300*, 213-217.

Fries, J.F. (1980). Aging, natural death, and the compression of morbidity. *New England Journal of Medicine, 303*, 130-135.

Fries, J.F. (2002). Successful aging—An emerging paradigm of gerontology. *Clinical Geriatric Medicine, 18*, 371-382.

Fries, J.F., & Crapo, L.M. (1981). *Vitality and aging*. New York: Freeman.

Fries, J.F., Green, L.W., & Levine, S. (1989). Health promotion and the compression of morbidity. *Lancet, 8636*, 481-483.

Frolkis, V.V. (1968). Regulatory process in the mechanisms of aging. *Experimental Gerontology, 3*, 113-123.

Ganrot, P.O. (1986). Metabolism and possible health effects of aluminum. *Environmental Health Perspectives, 56*, 363-441.

Gill, T. (2002). Geriatric medicine: It's more than caring for old people. *American Journal of Medicine, 113*, 85-89.

Goodrick, C.L. (1980). Effects of long-term voluntary wheel exercise on male and female Wistar rats. *Gerontology, 26*, 22-33.

Goodrick, C.L., Ingram, D.K., Reynolds, M.A., Freeman, J.R., & Cider, N.L. (1983). Differential effects of intermittent feeding and voluntary exercise on body weight and life span in adult rats. *Journal of Gerontology, 38*, 36-45.

Guralnik, J.M., LaCroix, A.Z., Everett, D.F., & Kovar, M.G. (1989). Aging in the eighties: The prevalence of comorbidity and its association with disability. *Advance Data, National Center for Health Statistics, 170*, 1-8.

Hayflick, L. (1977). The cellular basis for biological aging. In C.E. Firch & L. Hayflick (Eds.), *Handbook of the biology of aging* (pp. 159-186). New York: Van Nostrand Reinhold.

Hayflick, L. (1994). *How and why we age.* New York: Ballantine Books.

Hershey, D. (1984). *Must we grow old?* Cincinnati: Basal Books.

Hogstel, M.O., & Kashka, M. (1989, January/February). Staying healthy after 85. *Geriatric Nursing*, pp. 16-18.

Holden, C. (1987). Why do women live longer than men? *Science, 238*, 158-160.

Holden, C. (1996). New populations of old add to poor nations' burdens. *Science, 273*, 46-48.

Holloszy, J. (1993). Exercise increases average longevity of female rats despite increased food intake and no growth retardation. *Journal of Gerontology: Biological Sciences, 48*, B97-B100.

Hubert, H.B., Bloch, D.A., Ochlert, J.W., & Fries, J.F. (2002). Lifestyle habits and compression of morbidity. *Journal of Gerontology: Medical Sciences, 57*, M347-M351.

Jazwinski, S.M. (1996). Longevity, genes, and aging. *Science, 273*, 54-59.

Johnson, H.A. (1985). Is aging physiological or pathological? In H.A. Johnson (Ed.), *Relations between normal aging and disease* (pp. 239-247). New York: Raven Press.

Johnson, T.E. (1990). Increased life span of age-1 mutants in *Caenorhabditis elegans* and lower Gompertz rate of aging. *Science, 249*, 908-912.

Katz, S., Branch, L.G., Branson, M.H., Papsidero, J.A., Beck, J.C., & Greek, D.S. (1983). Active life expectancy. *New England Journal of Medicine, 309*, 1218-1224.

Kemnitz, J.W., Weindruch, R., Roecker, E.B., Crawford, K., Kaufmann, P.L., & Ershler, W.B. (1993). Dietary restriction of adult male rhesus monkeys: Findings from the first year of study. *Journal of Gerontology: Biological Sciences, 48*, B17-B26.

Krach, C.A., & Velkoff, V.A. (1999). Centenarians in the United States. National Institute of Aging, U.S. Department of Commerce, Economic & Statistics Administration, U.S. Census Bureau. [Online]. Available: http://www.census.gov/prod/99pubs/p23-199.pdf [05.29.04].

Lee, D.J., & Markides, K.S. (1990). Activity and mortality among aged persons over an eight-year period. *Journal of Gerontology: Social Sciences, 45*, S39-S42.

Lee, I.M., Hsieh, C.C., & Paffenbarger, R.S. (1995). Exercise intensity and longevity in men. *Journal of the American Medical Association, 273*, 1179-1184.

Ljungquist, B., Berg, S., Lanke, J., McClearn, G., & Pedersen, N.L. (1998). The effect of genetic factors for longevity: A comparison of identical and fraternal twins in the Swedish twin registry. *Journal of Gerontology: Medical Sciences, 53A*, M441-M446.

Ly, D.H., Lockhart, D.J., Lerner, R.A., & Schultz, P.G. (2000). Mitotic misregulation and human aging. *Science, 287*, 2486-2492.

McEwen, B.S. (1998). Protective and damaging effects of stress mediators. *New England Journal of Medicine, 338*, 171-179.

Miguel, J. (1991). An integrated theory of aging as the result of mitochondrial-DNA mutation in differentiated cells. *Archives of Gerontology and Geriatrics, 12*, 99-117.

Miller, G.H. (1986). Is the longevity gender gap decreasing? *New York State Journal of Medicine, 86*, 59-60.

Miller, G.H., & Gerstein, D.R. (1983). The life expectancy of nonsmoking men and women. *Public Health Report, 98*, 343-349.

Miller, R.A. (1999). Kleemeier award lecture: Are there genes for aging? *Journal of Gerontology: Biological Sciences, 54A*, B297-B307.

Montague, A. (1953). *The natural superiority of women.* New York: Macmillan.

Nabarra, B., & Andrianarison, I. (1996). Ultrastructural study of thymic microenvironment involution in aging mice. *Experimental Gerontology, 31*, 489-506.

Nascher, J.L. (1979). *Geriatrics: The diseases of old age and their treatment.* New York: Arno Press. (Original work published 1914)

Older Americans 2000. (2000). Administration on Aging. [Online]. Available: www.aoa.gov/agingstats/chartbook2000 [05.29.04].

Olshansky, S.J., Carnes, B.A., & Cassel, C. (1990). In search of Methuselah: Estimating the upper limits to human longevity. *Science, 250*, 634-640.

Olshansky, S.J., Carnes, B.A., & Desesquelles, A. (2001). Demography. Prospects for human longevity. *Science, 291*, 1491-1492.

Olshansky, S.J., Hayflick, L., & Carnes, B.A. (2002). No truth to the fountain of youth. *Scientific American, 286*, 92-95.

Paffenbarger, R.S., Jr., Hyde, R.T., Wing, A.L., & Steinmetz, C.H. (1984). A natural history of athleticism and cardiovascular health. *Journal of the American Medical Association, 252,* 491-495.

Pennisi, E. (1996). Premature aging gene discovered. *Science, 272,* 193-194.

Rakowski, W., & Mor, V. (1992). The association of physical activity with mortality among older adults in the longitudinal study of aging (1984-1988). *Journal of Gerontology: Medical Sciences, 47,* M122-M129.

Retzlaff, E., Fontaine, J., & Futura, W. (1966). Effect of daily exercise on life span of albino rats. *Geriatrics, 21,* 171-177.

Rothenberg, R., Lentzner, H.R., & Parker, R.A. (1991). Population aging patterns: The expansion of mortality. *Journal of Gerontology: Social Sciences, 46,* S66-S70.

Rowe, J.W. (1997). The new gerontology. *Science, 278,* 367.

Rowe, J.W., & Kahn, R.L. (1998). *Successful aging.* New York: Pantheon Books.

Sarna, S., Sahi, T., Koskenvuo, M., & Kaprio, J. (1993). Increased life expectancy of world class male athletes. *Medicine and Science in Sports and Exercise, 25,* 237-244.

Schneider, E.L., & Guralnik, J. (1990). The aging of America: Impact on health care costs. *Journal of the American Medical Association, 263,* 2335-2340.

Seeman, T.E., Singer, B.H., Rowe, J.W., Horwitz, R.I., & McEwen, B.S. (1997). Price of adaptation—Allostatic load and its health consequences. *Archives of Internal Medicine, 157,* 2259-2268k.

Sperling, G.A., Loosli, J.K., Lupien, P., & McCay, C.M. (1978). Effect of sulfamerazine and exercise on life span of rats and hamsters. *Gerontology, 24,* 220-224.

Stones, M.J., Dornan, B., & Kozma, A. (1989). The prediction of mortality in elderly institution residents. *Journal of Gerontology: Psychological Sciences, 44,* P72-P79.

Stones, M.J., & Kozma, A. (1986). "Happy are they who are happy . . ." A test between two causal models of relationships between happiness and its correlates. *Experimental Aging Research, 12,* 23-29.

Topp, B., Windsor, L.A., Sans, L.P., Gorman, K.M., Bleiman, M., Cherkas, L., & Posner, J.D. (1989). The effect of exercise on morbidity patterns of healthy older adults. *Gerontologist, 29,* 192A.

U.S. Census Bureau. (2000). Population projections of the United States by age, sex, race, Hispanic origin, and nativity: 1999-2100. [Online]. Available: www.census.gov/population/www/projections/natproj.html [05.29.04].

U.S. Department of Health and Human Services. (1996). *Physical activity and health: A report of the Surgeon General.* Atlanta, GA: U.S. Department of Health and Human Services, Public Health Service, CDC, National Center for Chronic Disease Prevention and Health Promotion.

van Saase, J.L.C.M., Noteboom, W.M.P., & Vandenbroucke, J.P. (1990). Longevity of men capable of prolonged vigorous physical exercise: A 32-year follow-up of 2,259 participants in the Dutch Eleven Cities Ice Skating Tour. *British Medical Journal, 301,* 1409-1411.

Vita, A.J., Terry, R.B., Hubert, H.B., & Fries, J.F. (1998). Aging, health risks, and cumulative disability. *New England Journal of Medicine, 338,* 1035-1041.

Walford, R. (1983). *Maximum life span.* New York: Norton.

Walford, R.L., & Crew, M. (1989, Winter). How dietary restriction retards aging: An integrative hypothesis. *Growth, Development, and Aging,* pp. 139-140.

Weindruch, R. (1995). Diet restriction. In G. Maddox (Ed.), *The encyclopedia of aging* (2nd ed., pp. 276-279). New York: Springer.

Wilkins, R., & Adams, O. (1983). Health expectancy in Canada, late 1970s: Demographic, regional, and social dimensions. *American Journal of Public Health, 73,* 1073-1080.

World Health Organization, Global Population Profile, International Populations Reports, U.S. Department of Commerce, Economics and Statistics Administration, U.S. Census Bureau, 2002.

Chapter 2

Baker, G.T.I., & Sprott, R. L. (1988). Biomarkers of aging. *Experimental Gerontology, 23,* 223-239.

Bandura, A. (1977). Self-efficacy: Toward a unifying theory of behavior change. *Psychological Review, 84,* 191-215.

Borkan, G.A., & Norris, A.H. (1980). Assessment of biological age using a profile of physical parameters. *Journal of Gerontology, 35,* 177-184.

Botwinick, J. (1973). *Aging and behavior.* New York: Springer.

Botwinick, J. (1984). Research methods. In J. Botwinick (Ed.), *Aging behavior* (pp. 381-403). New York: Springer.

Botwinick, J., West, R., & Storandt, M. (1978). Predicting death from behavioral test performance. *Journal of Gerontology, 33,* 755-762.

Buss, A.H., & Plomin, R. (1984). *A temperament theory of personality development.* Hillsdale, NJ: Erlbaum.

Chodzko-Zajko, W., & Ringle, R.L. (1989). Evaluating the influence of physiological health on sensory and motor performance changes in the elderly. In A.C. Ostrow (Ed.), *Aging and work behavior* (pp. 307-323). Indianapolis: Benchmark Press.

Clarkson-Smith, L., & Hartley, A.A. (1990). The game of bridge as an exercise in working memory and reasoning. *Psychology and Aging: Psychological Sciences, 45,* P233-P238.

Collier, T.J., & Coleman, P.D. (1991). Divergence of biological and chronological aging: Evidence from rodent studies. *Neurobiology of Aging, 12,* 685-693.

Costa, P.T., Jr., & McCrae, R.R. (1980). Functional age: A conceptual and empirical critique. In S.G. Haynes & M. Feinlab (Eds.), *Proceedings of the second conference on the epidemiology of aging* (p. 23; NIH Publication No. 80-969). Washington, DC: U.S. Government Printing Office.

Costa, P.T., Jr., & McCrae, R.R. (1985). Concepts of functional and biological age: A critical view. In R. Andres (Ed.), *Principles of geriatric medicine* (pp. 30-37). New York: McGraw-Hill.

Fozard, J.L., Metter, E.J., & Brant, L.J. (1990). Next steps in describing aging and disease in longtitudinal studies. *Journal of Gerontology: Psychological Sciences, 45,* P119.

Fozard, J.L., Thomas, J.C., & Waugh, N.C. (1976). Effects of age and frequency of stimulus repetitions on two-choice reaction time. *Journal of Gerontology, 31,* 556-563.

Hertzog, C. (1985). An individual differences perspective: Implications for cognitve research in gerontology. *Research on Aging, 7,* 7-45.

Holmes, P. (In press). Current findings in neurobiological systems response to exercise. In L.W. Poon, W Chozko-Zajko, & P. Tomporowski (Eds.), Active living, cognitive functioning, and aging. Champaign, IL: Human Kinetics.

Jackson, J.S., Antonucci, T.C., & Gibson, R.C. (1990). Cultural, racial, and ethnic minority influences on aging. In J.E. Birren & K.W. Schaie (Eds.), *Handbook of the psychology of aging* (3rd ed., pp. 103-123). New York: Academic Press.

Johnson, H.A. (1985). Is aging physiological or pathological? In H.A. Johnson (Ed.), *Relations between normal aging and disease* (pp. 239-247). New York: Raven Press.

Kausler, D.H. (1990). Motivation, human aging, and cognitive performance. In J.E. Birren & K.W. Schaie (Eds.), *Handbook of the psychology of aging* (3rd ed., pp. 172-182). New York: Academic Press.

Lachman, M.E., & McArthur, L.Z. (1986). Adult age differences in casual attributions for cognitive, physical, and social performance. *Psychology and Aging, 1,* 127-132.

Levine, S. (1962). Plasma-free corticosteroid response to electric shock in rats stimulated in infancy. *Science, 135,* 795-796.

Light, K.E., Reilly, M.A., Behrman, A.L., & Spirduso, W.W. (1996). Reaction times and movement times: Benefits of practice to younger and older adults. *Journal of Aging and Physical Activity, 4,* 27-41.

Ludwig, F.C., & Smoke, M.E. (1980). The measurement of biological age. *Experimental Aging Research, 6,* 497-522.

Maddox, G.L., & Douglass, E.B. (1974). Aging and individual differences: A longitudinal analysis of social, psychological, and physiological indicators. *Journal of Gerontology, 29,* 555-563.

Nagi, S.Z. (1991). Disability concepts revisited: Implication for prevention. In A.M. Pope & A.R. Tarlov (Eds.), *Disability in America: Toward a national agenda for prevention* (pp. 309-327). Washington, DC: National Academy Press.

Older Americans 2000. (2000). Administration on Aging. [Online]. Available: www.aoa.gov/ agingstats/chartbook2000 [05.29.04].

O'Rand, A. (1996). The precious and the precocious: Understanding cumulative disadvantage and cumulative advantage over the life course. *Gerontologist, 36,* 230-238.

Palmore, E. (1981). *Social patterns in normal aging* . Durham, NC: Duke University Press.

Pescosolido, B. (1992) Beyond rational choice: The social dynamics of how people seek help. *American Journal of Sociology, 97,* 1096-1138.

Plomin, R., Pedersen, N.L., McClearn, G.E., Nesselroade, J.R., & Bergeman, C.S. (1988). EAS temperaments during the last half of the life span: Twins reared apart and twins reared together. *Psychology of Aging, 4,* 43-49.

Powell, D.A., Furchtgott, E., Henderson, M., Prescott, L., Mitchell, A., Harris, P., Valentine, J. D., & Milligan, W.L. (1990). Some determinants of attrition in prospective studies on aging. *Experimental Aging Research, 16,* 17-24.

Rikli, R.E., & Jones, C.J. (1997). Assessing physical performance in independent older adults: Issues and guidelines. *Journal of Aging and Physical Activity, 5,* 244-261.

Salthouse, T.A. (1988). Cognitive aspects of motor functioning. In J.A. Joseph (Ed.), *Central determi-*

nants of age-related declines in motor function. New York: New York Academy of Sciences.

Schaie, K.W. (1990). Intellectual development in adulthood. In J.E. Birren & K.W. Schaie (Eds.), *Handbook of the psychology of aging* (3rd ed., pp. 291-309). New York: Academic Press.

Shock, N.W. (1962). The science of gerontology. In E.C. Jeffers (Ed.), *Proceedings seminars, 1951-69* (pp. 123-140). Durham, NC: Council on Gerontology & Duke University Press.

Shock, N.W. (1967). Physical activity and the rate of aging. *Canadian Medical Association Journal, 96,* 836-840.

Shock, N.W., Greulich, R.C., Andres, R., Arenberg, D., Costa, P.T., Jr., Lakatta, E.G., & Tobin, J. D. (1984). *Normal human aging: The Baltimore Longitudinal Study of Aging.* Washington, DC: U.S. Department of Health and Services.

Sprott, R.L. (1999). Biomarkers of aging. *Journal of Gerontology: Biological Sciences, 54A,* B464-B465.

Stones, M.J., Dornan, B., & Kozma, A. (1989). The prediction of mortality in elderly institution residents. *Journal of Gerentology: Psychological Sciences, 44,* P72-P79.

Stones, M.J., & Kozma, A. (1986). Happiness and activities as propensities. *Journal of Gerontology, 41,* 85-90.

Stones, M.J., & Kozma, A. (1988). Physical activity, age, and cognitive/motor performance. In M.L. Howe & C.J. Brainerd (Eds.), *Cognitive development in adulthood: Progress in cognitive development research* (pp. 273-321). New York: Springer-Verlag.

Verhoff, J., Reuman, D., & Feld, S. (1984). Motives in American men and women across the adult life span. *Developmental Psychology, 20,* 1142-1158.

Webster, I.W., & Logie, A.R. (1976). A relationship between functional age and health status in female subjects. *Journal of Gerontology, 31,* 546-550.

Chapter 3

ACSM Position Stand. (1998). Exercise and physical activity for older adults. *Medicine, Science, in Sports and Exercise, 30,* 992-1008.

American Geriatrics Society Panel on Exercise and Osteoarthritis. (2001). Exercise prescription for older adults with osteoarthritis pain: Consensus practice recommendations. *Journal of the American Geriatrics Society, 49,* 808-823.

Arthritis Fact Sheet. [Online]. Available: www.arthritis.org [9.17.02].

Badley, E.M., Wagstaff, S., & Wood, P.H.N. (1984). Measures of functional ability (disability) in arthritis in relation to impairment of range of joint movement. *Annals of Rheumatic Disease, 43,* 563-569

Baumgartner, R.N. (2000). Body composition in healthy aging. *Annals of New York Academy of Science, 904,* 437-448.

Baumgartner, R.N., Roche, A.F., Gleo, S., Lohman, T., Baileall, R.A., & Slaughter, M.H. (1986). Adipose tissue distribution: The stability of principal components by sex, ethnicity, and maturation stage. *Human Biology, 58,* 719-735.

Beck, B., & Marcus, R. (1999). Impact of physical activity on age-related bone loss. In C.J. Rosen, J. Glowacki, & J.P. Bilezikian (Eds.), *The aging skeleton* (pp. 467-478). New York: Academic Press.

Beck, B.R., & Snow, C.M. (2003). Bone health across the lifespan—Exercising our options. *Exercise and Sport Sciences Review, 31,* 117-122.

Bell, R.D., & Hoshizaki, T.B. (1981). Relationships of age and sex with range of motion of seventeen joint actions in human. *Canadian Journal of Applied Sports Science, 6,* 202-206.

Bevier, W.C., Wiswell, R.A., Pyka, C., Kozak, K.C., Newhall, K.M., & Marcus, R. (1989). Relationship of body composition, muscle strength, and aerobic capacity to bone mineral density in older men and women. *Journal of Bone and Mineral Research, 4,* 421-432.

Blackman, M.R., Sorkin, J.D., Munzer, T., Bellantoni, M.F., Busby-Whitehead, J., Stevens, T.E., Jayme, J., O'Connor, K.G., Christmas, C., Tobin, J.D., Stewart, K.J., Cottrell, E., St. Clair, C., Pabst, K.M., & Harman, S.M. (2002). Growth hormone and sex steroid administration in healthy aged women and men: A randomized controlled trial. *Journal of American Medical Association, 288,* 2282-2292.

Bray, G.A. (1985). Obesity: Definition, diagnosis, and disadvantages. *Medical Journal of Australia, 142,* 52-58.

Calle, E.E., Thun, M.J., Petrelli, J.M., Rodriguez, C., & Heath, C.W. (1999). Body-mass index and mortality in a prospective cohort of U.S. adults. *The New England Journal of Medicine, 341,* 1097-1105.

Chandler, P.J., & Bock, R.D. (1991). Age changes in adult stature: Trend estimation from mixed longitudinal data. *Annals of Human Biology, 18,* 433-440.

Despres, J.P. (1997). Visceral obesity, insulin resistance, and dyslipidemia: Contribution of endurance exercise training to the treatment of the plurimetabolic syndrome. *Exercise and Sports Science Reviews, 25,* 271.

Drinkwater, B. (1986). Osteoporosis and the female masters athlete. In J.R. Sutton & R.M. Brock (Eds.), *Sports medicine for the mature athlete* (pp. 353-359). Indianapolis: Benchmark Press.

Dunn, L.B., Damesyn, M., Moore, A.A., Reuben, D.B., Greendale, G.A. (1997). Does estrogen prevent skin aging? *Archives of Dermatology, 133,* 339-342.

Durnin, J.V.G.A., & Womersley, J. (1974). Body fat assessed from total body density and its estimation from skinfold thickness: Measurements of 481 men and women aged from 16 to 72 years. *British Journal of Nutrition, 32,* 77-97.

Einkauf, D.K., Gohdes, M.L., Jensen, G.M., & Jewell, M.J. (1987). Changes in spinal mobility with increasing age in women. *Physical Therapy, 67,* 370-375.

Ettinger, W.H., Burns, R., Messier, S.P., Applegate, W., Rejeski, W.J., Morgan, T., Shumaker, S., Berry, M.J., O'Toole, M., Monu, J., & Craven, T. (1997). A randomized trial comparing aerobic exercise and resistance exercise with a health education program in older adults and seniors trial (FAST). *Journal of the American Medical Association, 277,* 25-31.

Evans, W.J., & Campbell, W.W. (1993). Sarcopenia and age-related changes in body composition and functional capacity. *Journal of Nutrition, 123,* 465-468.

Felson, D.T., Lawrence, R.C., Dieppe, P.A., Hirsch, R., Helmick, C.G., Jordan, J.M., Kington, R.S., Lane, N.E., Nevitt, M.C., Zhang, Y., Sowers, M., McAlindon, T., Spector, T.D., Poole, A.R., Yanovski, S.Z., Ateshian, G., Sharma, L., Buckwalter, J.A. Brandt, K.D., Fries, J.F. (2000). Osteoarthritis: New insights. Part 1: The disease and its risk factors. *Annals of Internal Medicine, 133,* 635-646.

Felson, D.T., Zhang, Y., Hannan, M.T., Naimark, A., Weissman, B., Aliabadi, P., & Levy, D. (1997). Risk factors for incident radiographic knee osteoarthritis in the elderly: The Framingham Study. *Arthritis and Rheumatism, 40,* 728-733.

Feskanich, D., Willett, W., & Colditz, G. (2002). Walking and leisure-time activity and risk of hip fracture in postmenopausal women. *Journal of the American Medical Association, 288,* 2300-2306.

Fiatarone Singh, M.A. (1998). Combined exercise and dietary intervention to optimize body composition in aging. *Annals of New York Academy of Science, 854,* 378-393.

Fields, D.A., Goran, J.I., & McCrory, M.A. (2002). Body-composition assessment via air-displacement plethysmography in adults and children: A review. *American Journal of Clinical Nutrition, 75,* 453-467.

Fields, K.A. (2000). Skin breakthroughs in the year 2000. *International Journal of Fertility, 45,* 175-181.

Finch, S., Doyle, W., Lowe, C., Bates, C.J., Prentice, A., Smithers, G., & Clarke, P.C. (1998). *National diet and nutrition survey of people aged 65 years and over.* London: H.M. Stationery Office.

Finkelstein, J.S., Lee, M.L., Sowers, M., Ettinger, B., Neer, R.M., Kelsey, J.L., Cauley, J.A., Huang, M.H., & Greendale, G.A. (2002). Ethnic variation in bone density in premenopausal and early perimenopausal women: Effects of anthropometric and lifestyle factors. *Journal of Clinical Endocrinology and Metabolism, 87,* 3057-67.

Flegal, K.M., Carroll, M.D., Kuczmarski, R.J., & Johnson, C.L. (1998). Overweight and obesity in the United States: Prevalence and trends, 1960-1994. *International Journal of Obesity Related Metabolic Disorders, 22,* 39-47.

Franck, H., Beuker, F., & Gurk, S. (1991). The effect of physical activity on bone turnover in young adults. *Experimental and Clinical Endocrinology, 98,* 42-46.

Frisancho, A.R. (1990). *Anthropometric standards for the assessment of growth and nutritional status.* Ann Arbor: University of Michigan Press.

Frost, H.M. (1989). Mechanical usage, bone mass, bone fragility: A brief overview. In M. Kleerekoper & S.M. Krane (Eds.), *Clinical disorders of bone and mineral metabolism: Proceedings of the Laurence and Dorothy Fallis International Symposium* (pp. 15-40). New York: Mary Ann Liebert.

Frost, H.M. (2000). Growth hormone and osteoporosis: an overview of endocrinological and pharmacological insights from the Utah paradigm of skeletal physiology. *Hormone Research, 54, Suppl 1,* 36-43.

Fusco, F.J. (2001). The aging face and skin: Common signs and treatment. *Clinics in Plastic Surgery, 28,* 1-12.

Gallagher, D., Heymsfield, S.B., Moonseong, H., Jebb, S.A., Murgatroyd, P.R., & Sakamoto, Y. (2000). Healthy percentage body fat ranges: An approach for developing guidelines based on body mass index. *American Journal of Clinical Nutrition, 72,* 694-701.

Gardsell, P., Johnell, O., & Nilsson, B.E. (1991). The predictive value of bone loss for fragility fractures in women: A longitudinal study over 15 years. *Calcified Tissue International, 49,* 90-94.

Gillum, R.F. (1987). The association of body fat distribution with hypertension, hypertensive heart disease, coronary heart disease, diabetes, and cardiovascular risk factors in men and women aged 18-79 years. *Journal of Chronic Diseases, 40,* 421-428.

Golding, L.A., & Lindsay, A. (1989). Flexibility and age. *Perspective, 15,* 28-30.

Greendale, G.A., Edelstein, S., & Barrett-Connor, E. (1997). Endogenous sex steriods and bone mineral density in older women and men: The Rancho Bernardo Study. *Journal of Bone Mineral Research, 12,* 1833-1843.

Gregg, E.W., Pereira, M.A., Caspersen, C.J. (2000). Physical activity, falls, and fractures among older adults: A review of the epidemiologic evidence. *Journal of the American Geriatric Society, 48,* 883-93.

Hagino, H., Yamamoto, K., Teshima, R., Kishimoto, H., & Kagawa, T. (1992). Radial bone mineral changes in pre- and postmenopausal healthy Japanese women: Cross-sectional and longitudinal studies. *Journal of Bone and Mineral Research, 7,* 147-152.

Halle, J.S., Smidt, G.L., O'Dwyer, K., & Lin, S. (1990). Relationship between trunk muscle torque and bone mineral content of the lumbar spine and hip in healthy postmenopausal women. *Physical Therapy, 70,* 690-699.

Harris, S., Dallal, G.E., & Dawson-Hughes, B. (1992). Influence of body weight on rates of change in bone density of the spine, hip, and radius in postmenopausal women. *Calcified Tissue International, 50,* 19-23.

Heaney, R.P. (1986). Calcium, bone health, and osteoporosis. *Journal of Bone and Mineral Research, 4,* 255-301.

Heaney, R.P. (1992). Calcium in the prevention and treatment of osteoporosis. *Journal of Internal Medicine, 231,* 169-180.

Heikkinen, J., Kurttila-Matero, E., Kyllonen, E., Vuori, J., Takala, T., & Vuaananen, H.K. (1991). Moderate exercise does not enhance the positive effect of estrogen on bone mineral density in postmenopausal women. *Calcified Tissue International, 49,* (Suppl.), 583-584.

Heinonen, A., Kannus, P., Sievanen, H., Oja, P., Pasanen, M., Rinne, M., Uusi-Rasi, K., Vuori, I. (1996). Randomized controlled trial of effect of high-impact exercise on selected risk factors for osteoporotic fractures. *Lancet, 348,* 1343-1347.

Heymsfield, S.B., Nunez, C., Testolin, C. & Gallagher, D. (2000). Anthropometry and methods of body composition measurement for research and field application in the elderly. *European Journal of Clinical Nutrition, 54,* S26-S32.

Holland, G.J., Tanaka, K., Shigematsu, S., & Nakagaichi, M. (2002). Flexibility and physical functions of older adults: A review. *Journal of Aging and Physical Activity, 10,* 169-206.

Huddleston, A.L, Rockewell, D., Kulund, D.N., & Harrison, R.B. (1980). Bone mass in lifetime tennis athletes. *Journal of the American Medical Association, 244,* 1107-1109.

Hughes, V.A., Frontera, W.R., Roubenoff, R., Evans, W.J., & Fiatarone Singh, M.A. (2002). Longitudinal changes in body composition in older men and women: Role of body weight change and physical activity. *American Journal of Clinical Nutrition, 76,* 473-481.

Hui, S.L., Slemenda, C.W., & Johnston, C.C. (1988). Age and bone mass as predictors of fracture in a prospective study. *Journal of Clinical Investigation, 81,* 1804-1809.

Hulley, S., Grady, D., Bush, T., Furberg, C., Herrington, D, Riggs, B., Vittinghoff, E. (1998). Randomized trial of estrogen plus progestin for secondary prevention of coronary heart disease in postmenopausal women: Heart and Estrogen/progestin Replacement Study (HERS) Research Group. *Journal of the American Medical Association, 280,* 605-613.

Hunter, G.R., Kekes-Szabo, T., Snyder, S.W., Nicholson, C., Nyikos, I., Berland, L. (1997). Fat distribution, physical activity, and cardiovascular risk factors. *Medicine and Science in Sports and Exercise, 29,* 362-369.

Hunter, G.R., Kekes-Szabo, T., Treuth, M.S., Williams, M.J., Goran, M., Pichon, C. (1996). Intra-abdominal adipose tissue, physical activity and cardiovascular risk in pre- and post-menopausal women. *International Journal of Obesity and Related Metabolic Disorders, 20,* 860-865.

Hurley, B.F., & Hagberg, J.M. (1998). Optimizing health in older persons: Aerobic or strength training. *Exercise and Sports Science Reviews, 26,* 61-90.

Joisten, U., & Albrecht, H.J. (1992). Physical activity and spondylarthritis. In H.-W. Baenkler (Ed.), Rheumatic diseases and sport. *Rheumatology* (Vol. 16, pp. 153-159). Basel: Karger.

Jones, H.H., Priest, J.D., Hayes, W.C., Tichenor, C.C., & Nagel, D.A. (1977). Humeral hypertrophy in response to exercise. *Journal of Bone and Joint Surgery, 59A,* 204-208.

Karlsson, M. (2004). Has exercise an antifracture efficacy in women? *Scandinavian Journal of Medicine and Science in Sport, 14,* 2-15.

Karlsson, M.K., Linden, C., Karlsson, C., Johnell, O., Obrant, K., & Seeman, E. (2000). Exercise during growth and BMD and fractures in old age. *Lancet, 355*, 469-470.

Kavanaugh, T., & Shephard, R.J. (1990). Can regular sports participation slow the aging process? *Physician and Sportsmedicine, 18*, 94-104.

Kemmler, W., Lauber, D., Weineck, J., Hensen, J., Kalender, W., & Engelke, K. (2004). Benefits of 2 years of intense exercise on bone density, physical fitness, and blood lipids in early postmenopausal osteopenic women: Results of the Erlangen Fitness Osteoporosis Prevention Study (EFOPS). *Archives of Internal Medicine, 164*, 1084-1091.

Kiebzak, G.M. (1991). Age-related bone changes. *Experimental Gerontology, 26*, 171-187.

Kirk, S., Sharp, C.F., Elbaum, N., Endres, K., Simons, S.M., Mohler, J.G., & Rude, R.K. (1989). Effect of long-distance running on bone mass in women. *Journal of Bone and Mineral Research, 4*, 515-522.

Kissebah, A.H., Freedman, D.S., & Prinis, A.N. (1989). Health risks of obesity. *Medical Clinics of North America, 73*, 111-138.

Kohrt, W.M., Ehsani, A.A., & Birge, S.J., Jr. (1998). HRT preserves increases in bone mineral density and reductions in body fat after a supervised exercise program. *Journal of Applied Physiology, 84*, 1506-1512.

Konczak, J., Meeuwsen, H.J., & Cress, M.E. (1992). Changing affordances in stair climbing: The perception of maximum climbability in young and old adults. *Journal of Experimental Psychology: Human Perception and Performance, 18*, 691-697.

Kotz, C.M., Billington, C.J., & Levine, A.S. (1999). Obesity and aging. *Clinics in Geriatric Medicine, 15*, 391-412.

Krølner, B., & Toft, B. (1983). Vertebral bone loss: An unheeded side effect of therapeutic bed rest. *Clinical Science, 64*, 537-540.

Lan, C., Lai, J.S., Chen, S.U., & Wong, M.K. (1998). 12 month Tai Chi training in the elderly, its effects on health fitness. *Medicine and Science in Sports and Exercise, 30*, 345-351.

Lane, N., Bloch, D.A., Jones, H.H., Marshall, W.H., Jr., Wood, D.D., & Fries, J.F. (1986). Long-distance running, bone density, and osteoarthritis. *Journal of the American Medical Association, 255*, 1147-1151.

Lane, N., Michel, B., Bjorkengren, A., Oehlert, J., Shi, H., Bloch, D.A., & Fries, J. F. (1993). The risk of osteoarthritis with running and aging: A 5-year longitudinal study. *Journal of Rheumatology, 20*, 461-469.

Launer, L.J., & Harris, T. (1996). Weight, height, and body mass index distributions in geographically and ethnically diverse samples of older persons. *Age and Aging, 25*, 300-306.

LeBlanc, A., & Schneider, V. (1991). Can the adult skeleton recover lost bone? *Experimental Gerontology, 26*, 189-201.

Looker, A.C., Orwoll, E.S., Johnston, C.C., Lindsay, R.L., Wahner, H.W., Dunn, W.L., Calvo, M.S., Harris, T.B. & Heyse, S.P. (1997). Prevalence of low femoral bone density in older US adults from NHANES III. *Journal of Bone Mineral Research, 12*, 1761-1768.

Malina, R.M., & Bouchard, C. (1991). *Growth, maturation, and physical activity.* Champaign, IL: Human Kinetics.

McArdle, W.D., Katch, F.I., & Katch,V.L. (2001). *Exercise physiology: Energy, Nutrition and Human Performance.* New York: Lippincott, Williams, & Wilkins.

Messier, S.P., Royer, T.D. Gaven, T.E., O'Toole, M.L., Burns, R., Ettinger, W.H. Jr. (2000). Long term exercise and its effect on balance in older, osteoarthritic adults: Results from the Fitness, Arthritis, and Senior Trial (FAST). *Journal of the American Geriatric Society, 48*, 131-138.

Morley, J.E. (1996). Anorexia in older persons: Epidemiology and optimal treatment. *Drugs and Aging, 8*, 134-155.

Mosekilde, L. (2000). Age-related changes in bone mass, structure, and strength—Effects of loading. *Zeitschrift für Rheumatologie, 59*, 1-9.

Muller, D.C., Elahi, D., Tobin, J. & Andres, R. (1996). The effect of age on insulin resistance and secretion: A review. *Seminars in Nephrology, 16*, 289-298.

National Academy of Sciences. (1997). Dietary reference intakes for calcium, phosphorus, magnesium, vitamin D, and fluoride. [Online]. Available: lab.nap.edu/nap-cgi/discover.cgi?term=calcium+recommendations+1997 [9.15.03].

National Institutes of Health. (2001a). Osteoporosis and Related Bone Diseases National Resource Center. Available: www.osteo.org [8.28.03].

National Institutes of Health. Consensus Development Panel on Osteoporosis Prevention, Diagnosis, and Therapy. (2001b). Osteoporosis prevention, diagnosis, and therapy. *Journal of the American Medical Association, 285*, 785-795.

Nelson, H.D. (Jan, 2003). Harvard Women's Health Watch. Postmenopausal hormones: Where do we go from here? www.health.harvard.edu.

Nelson, H.D., Humphrey, L.L., Nygren, P., Teutsch, S.M., & Allan, J.D. (2002). Postmenopausal hormone replacement therapy. *Journal of the American Medical Association, 288,* 872-881.

Nelson, M.E., Fiatarone, M.A., Morganti, C.M., Trice, I., Greenberg, R.A., & Evans, W.J. (1994). Effects of high-intensity strength training on multiple risk factors for osteoporotic fractures. *Journal of the American Medical Association, 272,* 1909-1914.

Nevitt, M.C., Ross, P.D., Palermo, L., Musliner, T., Genant, H.K. & Thompson, D.E. (1999). Association of prevalent vertebral fractures, bone density, and alendronate treatment with incident vertebral fractures: Effect of number and spinal location of fractures. The Fracture Intervention Trial Research Group. *Bone, 25,* 613-619.

Nevitt, M.C., Xu, L., Zhang,Y., Lui, L., Yu, W., Lane, N.E., Qin, M., Hochberg, M.C., Cummings, S.R., & Felson, D.T. (2002). Very low prevalence of hip osteoarthritis among Chinese elderly in Beijing, China, compared with whites in the United States. *Arthritis and Rheumatism, 46,* 1773-1779.

Nieman, D.C. (2003). *Exercise testing and prescription.* Boston: McGraw Hill.

Nillsson, B.E., & Westlin, N.E. (1971). Bone density in athletes. *Clinical Orthopaedics, 77,* 179-182.

Panush, R.S., Schmidt, C., Caldwell, J.R., Edwards, N.L., Longley, S., Yonker, R., Webster, E., Stork, J., & Pettersson, H. (1986). Is running associated with degenerative joint disease? *Journal of the American Medical Association, 255,* 1152-1154.

Partridge, S.M. (1970). Biological role of cutaneous elastin. In W. Montagna, J.P. Bentley, & R.L. Dobson (Eds.), *Advances in biology of skin* (Vol. 10, pp. 69-87). New York: Meredith Corporation.

Pocock, N.A., Eisman, J.A., Gwinn, T.H., Sambrook, P.N., Yeates, M.G., & Freund, J. (1988). Regional muscle strength, physical fitness, and weight but not age predict femur bone mass. *Journal of Bone and Mineral Research, 3,* 584.

Pollock, M.L., Foster, C., Knapp, D., Rod, J.L., & Schmidt, D.H. (1987). Effect of age and training on aerobic capacity and body composition of master athletes. *Journal of Applied Physiology, 62,* 725-731.

Pollock, M.L., Mengelkoch, L.J., Graves, J.E., Lowenthal, D.T., Limacher, M.C., Foster, C., & Wilmore, J.H. (1997). Twenty-year follow-up of aerobic power and body composition of older track athletes. *Journal Applied Physiology, 82,* 1508-1516.

Popkin, B.M., & Dorak, C.M. (1998). The obesity epidemic is a worldwide phenomenon. *Nutritional Review, 56,* 106-114.

Puhl, W., Maier, P., & Gunther, K.P. (1992). Effects of physical activity on degenerative joint disease. In H.-W. Baenkler (Ed.), Rheumatic diseases and sport. *Rheumatology* (Vol. 16, pp. 129-141). Basel: Karger.

Rebuffé-Scrive, M., Anderson, B., Olbe, L., Bjorntorp, P. (1990). Metabolism of adipose tissue in intraabdominal depots in severely obese men and women. *Metabolism, 39,* 1021-1025.

Rider, R.A., & Daly, J. (1991). Effects of flexibility training on enhancing spinal mobility in older women. *Journal of Sports Medicine and Physical Fitness, 31,* 213-217.

Rikli, R.E., & Jones, C.J. (1999). Functional fitness normative scores for community residing older adults, ages 60-94. *Journal of Aging and Physical Activity, 7,* 162-181.

Rikli, R.E., & Jones, C.J. (2001). *Senior fitness test manual.* Champaign, IL: Human Kinetics.

Rosen, C.J. (2003). Restoring aging bones. *Scientific American, 288,* 71-77.

Rudman, D., Feller, A.G., Cohn, L., Shetty, K.R., Rudman, I.W., & Draper, M.W. (1991). Effects of human growth hormone on body composition in elderly men. *Hormone Research, 36 (Suppl. 1),* 73-81.

Schneider, V.S., & McDonald, J. (1984). Skeletal calcium homeostasis and countermeasures to prevent disuse osteoporosis. *Calcified Tissue International, 36,* S151-S154.

Schultheis, L. (1991). The mechanical control system of bone in weightless spaceflight and in aging. *Experimental Gerontology, 26,* 203-214.

Schwartz, R., Shuman, W.P., Bradbury, V.L., Cain, K.C., Fellingham, G.W., Beard, J.C., Kahn, S.E., Stratton, J.R., Cerqueira, M.D., & Abrass, I.B. (1990). Body fat distribution in healthy young and older men. *Journal of Gerontology: Medical Sciences, 45,* M181-M185.

Seeman, E. (2002). Pathogenesis of bone fragility in women and men. *Lancet, 359,* 1841-50.

Seidell, J.C., & Visscher, T.L.S. (2000). Body weight and weight change and their health implications for the elderly. *European Journal of Clinical Nutrition, 54,* S33-S39.

Slemenda, C.W., Brandt, K.D., Heliman, D.K., Mazzuca, S., Braunstein, E.M., Katz, B.P., & Wolinsky, F.D. (1997). Quadriceps weakness and osteoarthritis of the knees. *Annals of Internal Medicine, 127,* 97-104.

Snow, C.M., Shaw, J.M., Winters, K.M., & Witzke, K.A. (2000). Long-term exercise using weighted vests prevents hip bone loss in postmenopausal women. *Journal of Gerontology Series A: Biological and Medical Sciences, 55,* M489-491.

Sorkin, J.D., Muller, D.C., & Andres, R. (1999). Longitudinal change in the heights of men and women: Consequential effects on body mass index. *Epidemiologic Reviews, 21,* 247-260.

Specker, B.L. (1996). Evidence for an interaction between calcium intake and physical activity on change sin bone mineral density. *Journal of Bone Mineral Research, 11,* 1539-1544.

Thompson, M.P., & Morris, L.K. (1991). Unexplained weight loss in the ambulatory elderly. *Journal of the American Geriatrics Society, 39,* 497-500.

Toda, Y., Toda, T., Takemura, S., Wada, T., Morimoto, T., Ogawa, R. (1998). Change in body fat, but not body weight or metabolic correlates of obesity, is related to symptomatic relief of obese patients with knee osteoarthritis after a weight control program. *Journal of Rheumatology, 25,* 2181-2186.

Torpy, J.M., Lynm, C., Glass, R.M. (2002). Hormone replacement therapy patient page. *Journal of the American Medical Association, 288,* 3230.

Toth, J.J., Beckett, T., & Poehlman, E.T. (1999). Physical activity and the progressive change in body composition with aging: Current evidence and research issues. *Medicine, Science, in Sports and Exercise, 31,* S590-596.

Trappe, S.W., Costill, D.L., Vukovich, M.D., Jones, J., & Melham, T. (1996). Aging among elite distance runners: A 22-yr longitudinal study. *Journal of Applied Physiology, 80,* 285-290.

U.S. Department of Agriculture, Agricultural Research Service, Dietary Guidelines Advisory Committee. (1995). Report of the Dietary Guidelines Advisory Committee on the Dietary Guidelines for Americans, 1995, to the Secretary of Health and Human Services and the Secretary of Agriculture. Washington, DC: U.S. Government Printing Office.

U.S. Department of Health and Human Services. (1998). *Clinical guidelines on the identification, evaluation, and treatment of overweight and obesity in adults* (Vol. 98-4083). Washington, DC: U.S. Department of Health and Human Services. [Online]. Available: www.nhlbi.nih.gov. [5.23.03].

U.S. Department of Health and Human Services. (2000). *Tracking Healthy People 2010.* Washington, DC: U.S. Government Printing Office.

Vandervoort, A.A., Chesworth, B.M., Cunningham, D.A., Paterson, D.H., Rechnitzer, P.A., & Koval, J.J. (1992). Age and sex effects on mobility of the human ankle. *Journal of Gerontology: Medical Sciences, 47,* M17-M21.

Warren, R., Gartstein, V., Kligman, A.M., Montagna, W., Allendorg, R.A., & Ridder, G.M. (1991). Age, sunlight, and facial skin: A histologic and quantitative study. *Journal of the American Academy of Dermatology, 25,* 751-760.

Watson, R.C. (1973). Bone growth and physical activity in young males. In R.B. Mazess (Ed.), *International Conference on Bone Mineral Measurement* (NIH #75-683; pp. 380-386). Chicago, IL: Department of Health, Education, & Welfare.

Weinreb, M., Rodan, G.A., & Thompson, D.D. (1989). Osteopenia in the immobilized rat hind limb is associated with increased bone resorption and decreased bone formation. *Bone, 10,* 187-194.

Williams, J.A., Wagner, J., Wasnich, R., & Heilbrun, L. (1984). The effect of long-distance running upon appendicular bone mineral content. *Medicine and Science in Sport and Exercise, 16,* 223-227.

World Health Organization. (1998a). *Obesity: Preventing and managing the global epidemic. Report of a WHO consultation on obesity.* Geneva: World Health Organization.

World Health Organization. Report by The Expert Subcommittee on the Use and Interpretation of Anthropometry in the Elderly (1998b). Uses and interpretation of anthropometry in the elderly for the assessment of physical status report to the nutrition unit of the world health organization. *Journal of Nutrition, Health, and Aging, 2,* 15-17.

Writing Group for the Women's Health Initiative Investigators (2002). Risks and benefits of estrogen plus progestin in healthy postmenopausal women. *Journal of the American Medical Association, 288,* 321-333.

Chapter 4

American College of Sports Medicine. (1993). Position stand: Physical activity, physical fitness, and hypertensions. *Medicine and Science in Sports and Exercise, 25,* i-x.

American College of Sports Medicine. (1998a). Position stand: Exercise and physical activity for older adults. *Medicine and Science in Sports and Exercise, 30,* 992-1008.

American College of Sports Medicine. (1998b). *ACSM's resource manual for guidelines for exercise testing and prescription* (3rd ed). Philadelphia: Lippincott Williams & Wilkins.

American Heart Association. (2001). *2001 heart and stroke statistical update. Heart and stroke facts.* Dallas: American Heart Association.

Bacon, C.G., Mittleman, M.A., Kawachi, I., Giovannucci, E., Glasser, D.B., & Rimm, E.B. (2003). Sexual function of men older than 50 years of age: Results from the Health Professions Follow-up Study. *Annals of Internal Medicine, 139,* 161-168.

Biegel, L. (1984). *Physical fitness and the older person.* Rockville, MD: Aspen.

Binder, E.F., Schechtman, K.B., Ehsani, A.A., Sinacore, D.R., Brown, M., Yarasheski, K.E., Steger-May, K., & Holloszy, J. (2002). Effects of exercise training on frailty in community-dwelling elderly adults: Results of a randomized, controlled trial. *Journal of the American Geriatrics Society, 50,* 1921-1932.

Blair, S.N., Kampert, J.B., Kohl, H.W., III, Barlow, C.E., Macera, C.A., Paffenbarger, R.S., & Gibbons, L.W. (1996). Influences of cardiorespiratory fitness and other precursors on cardiovascular disease and all-cause mortality in men and women. *Journal of the American Medical Association, 276,* 205-210.

Booth, F.W. (1982). Effect of limb immobilization on skeletal muscle. *Journal of Applied Physiology: Respiration, Environment, and Exercise Physiology, 52,* 1113-1118.

Bortz, W.M., II. (1983). On disease . . . aging . . . and disuse. *Executive Health, 20*(3), 1-6.

Bouchard, C., & Malina, R.M. (1983). Genetics of physical fitness and motor performance. *Exercise and Sport Sciences Reviews, 11,* 306-339.

Brooks, S.V., & Faulkner, J.A. (1995). Effects of aging on the structure and function of skeletal muscle. In C. Roussos (Ed.), *The thorax* (pp. 295-312). New York: Academic Press.

Clark, D.O. (1996). The effects of walking on lower body disability among older blacks and whites. *American Journal of Public Health, 86,* 57-61.

Convertino, V.A., Montgomery, L.D., & Greenleaf, J.E. (1984). Cardiovascular responses during orthostasis: Effect of an increase in VO_2. *Aviation, Space, and Environmental Medicine, 55,* 702-708.

Davidson, W.R., Jr., & Fee, E.C. (1990). Influence of aging on pulmonary hemodynamics in a population free of coronary artery disease. *American Journal of Cardiology, 65,* 1454-1458.

DiPetro, L. (1996). The epidemiology of physical activity and physical function in older people. *Medicine and Science in Sports and Exercise, 28,* 596-600.

Docherty, J.R. (1990). Cardiovascular responses in aging: A review. *Pharmacological Review, 42,* 103-125.

Fleg, J.L. (1986). Alterations in cardiovascular structure and function with advancing age. *American Journal of Cardiology, 57,* 33C-44C.

Fleg, J.L., Tzankoff, S.P., & Lakatta, E.G. (1985). Age-related augmentation of plasma catecholamines during dynamic exercise in healthy males. *Journal of Applied Physiology, 59,* 1033-1039.

Gerstenblith, G., Renlund, D.G., & Lakatta, E.G. (1987). Cardiovascular response to exercise in younger and older men. *Federation Proceedings, 46,* 1834-1839.

Greenleaf, J.E. (1984). Physiological responses to prolonged bed rest and fluid immersion in humans. *Journal of Applied Physiology: Respiration, Environment, and Exercise Physiology, 57,* 619-633.

Hagberg, J.M., Allen, W.K., Seals, D.R., Hurley, B.F., Ehsani, A.A., & Holloszy, J.O. (1985). A hemodynamic comparison of young and older endurance athletes during exercise. *Journal of Applied Physiology, 58,* 2041-2046.

Hagberg, J.M., Graves, J.E., Limacher, M., Woods, D.R., Leggett, S.H., Cononie, C., Gruber, J.J., & Pollock, M.L. (1989). Cardiovascular responses of 70- to 79-year-old men and women to exercise training. *Journal of Applied Physiology, 66,* 2589-2594.

Harris, T., Lipsitz, L.A., Kleinman, J.C., & Cornoni-Huntley, J. (1991). Postural change in blood pressure associated with age and systolic blood pressure. *Journal of Gerontology: Medical Sciences, 46,* M159-M163.

Haskell, W.L., Sims, C., Myll, J., Bortz, W.M., Goar, F.G., & Alderman, E.L. (1993). Coronary artery size and dilating capacity in ultradistance runners. *Circulation, 87,* 1076-1082.

Hawkins, S.A., Marcell, T.J., Jaque, S.V., & Wiswell, R.A. (2001). A longitudinal assessment of change in VO_2max and maximal heart rate in master athletes. *Medicine and Science in Sports and Exercise, 33*(10), 1744-1750.

Joint National Committee on Prevention, Detection, Evaluation and Treatment of High Blood Pressure. (2004). Available: www.nhlbi.nih.gov/guidelines/hypertension/express.pdf. [Accessed May 15, 2004.]

Kasch, F.W., Boyer, J.L., Schmidt, P.K., Wells, R.H., Wallace, J.P., Verity, L.S., Guy, H., & Schneider, D. (1999). Ageing of the cardiovascular system during 33 years of aerobic exercise. *Age and Ageing, 28,* 531-536.

Katzel, L.I., Sorkin, J.D., & Fleg, J.L. (2001). A comparison of longitudinal changes in aerobic fitness in older endurance athletes and sedentary men. *Journal of the American Geriatrics Society, 49*, 1657-1664.

Klag, M.J., Whelton, P.K., & Appel, L.J. (1990). Effect of age on the efficacy of blood pressure treatment strategies. *Hypertension, 26*, 700-705.

Lakatta, E.G. (1986). Diminished beta-adrenergic modulation of cardiovascular function in advanced age. *Cardiac Clinics, 4*, 185-200.

Lakatta, E.G. (1990). Heart and circulation. In E.L. Schneider & S.W. Rowe (Eds.), *Handbook of the biology of aging*, 181-216.

Lakatta, E.G. (2002). Age-associated cardiovascular changes in health: Impact on cardiovascular disease in older persons. *Heart Failure Reviews, 7*, 29-49.

Lipsitz, L.A. (1989). Altered blood pressure homeostasis in advanced age: Clinical and research implications. *Journal of Gerontology: Medical Sciences, 44*, M179-M183.

Manson, J.E., Tosteson, H., Ridker, P.M., Satterfield, S., Hebert, P., O'Connor, G.T., Buring, J.E., & Hennekens, C.H. (1992). The primary prevention of myocardial infarction. *New England Journal of Medicine, 326*, 1406-1413.

Marti, B., & Howald, H. (1990). Long-term effects of physical training on aerobic capacity: Controlled study of former elite athletes. *Journal of Applied Physiology, 69*, 1451-1459.

Martin, W.H., Kohrt, W.M., Malley, M.T., Korte, E., & Stoltz, S. (1990). Exercise training enhances leg vasodilatory capacity of 65-year-old men and women. *Journal of Applied Physiology, 69*, 1804-1809.

Martin, W.H., III, Ogawa, T., Kohrt, M., Malley, M.T., Korte, E., Kieffer, P.S., & Schechtman, K.B. (1991). Effects of aging, gender, and physical training on peripheral vascular function. *Circulation, 84*, 654-664.

Mazzeo, R.S., Cavanagh, P., Evans, W.J., Fiatarone, M., Hagberg, J., McAuley, E., & Startzell, J. (1998). Position stand from the American College of Sports Medicine. Exercise and physical activity for older adults. *Medicine and Science in Sports and Exercise, 30*, 992-1008.

Mazzeo, R.S. & Tanaka, H. (2001). Exercise prescription for the elderly. *Sports Medicine, 31*, 809-818.

McArdle, W.D., Katch, F.I., & Katch, V.L. (1991). *Exercise physiology.* Philadelphia: Lea & Febiger.

McArdle, W.D., Katch, F.I., & Katch, V.L. (2001). *Exercise physiology: Energy, nutrition and human performance.* New York: Academic Press.

McGuire, D.K., Levine, B.D., Williamson, J.W., Snell, P.G., Blomquist, C.G., Saltin, B., & Mitchell, J.H. (2001). 30 year follow-up of the Dallas bed rest and training study. *Circulation, 104*, 1358-1366.

National Center for Health Statistics. (2001). Available: www.nlm.nih.gov/medlineplus/highblood pressure.html#generaloverviews. [Accessed June 5, 2003.]

Nieman, D.C. (2003). *Exercise testing and prescription.* New York: McGraw-Hill.

NIH Consensus Development Panel on Physical Activity and Cardiovascular Health. (1996). Physical activity and cardiovascular health. *Journal of the American Medical Association, 276*, 241-246.

O'Leary, D.H., Polak, J.F., Kronmal, R.A., Manolio, T.A., Burke, G.L., & Wolfson, S.K., Jr., for the Cardiovascular Health Study Collaborative Research Group. (1999). Carotid-artery intima and medial thickness as a risk factor for myocardial infarction and stroke in older adult. *New England Journal of Medicine, 340*, 14-22.

Paffenbarger, R.S., & Lee, I.M. (1996). Physical activity and fitness for health and longevity. *Research Quarterly in Exercise and Sport, 62*(Suppl.), S11-S28

Pickering, G.P., Fellmann, N., Morio, B., Ritz, P., Amonchot, A., Vermorel, M., & Coudert, J. (1997). Effects of endurance training on the cardiovascular system and water compartments in elderly subjects. *Journal of Applied Physiology, 83*, 1300-1306.

Pollock, M.L., Mengelkoch, L.J., Graves, J.E., Lowenthal, D.T., Limacher, M.C., Foster, C., & Wilmore, J.H. (1997). Twenty-year follow-up of aerobic power and body composition of older track athletes. *Journal Applied Physiology, 82*, 1508-1516.

Powell, K.E., Thompson, P.D., Caspersen, C.J., & Kendrick, J.S. (1987). Physical activity and the incidence of coronary heart disease. *Annual Reviews of Public Health, 8*, 253-287.

Rossi, A., Ganassini, A., Tantucci, C., & Grassi, V. (1996). Aging and the respiratory system. *Aging (Milano), 8*, 143-161.

Safar, M. (1990). Aging and its effects on the cardiovascular system. *Drugs, 39*(Suppl. 1), 1-18.

Sahyoun, N.R., Lentzner, H., Hoyert, D., & Robinson, K.N. (2001). Trends *in causes of death among the elderly. Aging trends, 1.* Hyattsville, MD: National Center for Health Statistics.

Saltin, B., & Grimby, G. (1968). Physiological analysis of middle-aged and old former athletes. Comparison of still-active athletes of the same age. *Circulation, 38*, 1104-1115.

Seals, D.R. (2003). Habitual exercise and the age-associated decline in large artery compliance. *Exercise and Sport Sciences Reviews, 31*, 68-72.

Seals, D.R., Taylor, J.A., Ng, A.V., & Esler, M.D. (1994). Exercise and aging: Autonomic control of the circulation. *Medicine and Science in Sports and Exercise, 26*, 568-576.

Shepherd, R.J. (1987). *Physical activity and aging.* Rockville, MD: Aspen.

Shepherd, R.J., Kavanagh, T., Mertens, D.J., Qureshi, S., & Clark, M. (1995). Personal health benefits of masters athletics competition. *British Journal of Sports Medicine, 29*, 35-40.

Shiraki, K., Sagawa, S., & Yousef, M.K. (2001). *Physical fitness and health promotion in active aging.* Leiden: Backhuys.

Spina, R.J. (1999). Cardiovascular adaptations to endurance exercise training in older men and women. *Exercise and Sport Sciences Reviews, 27*, 317-332.

Tanaka, H., Dinenno, F.A., Monahan, K.D., Clevenger, C.M., DeSouza, C.A., & Seals, D.R. (2000). Aging, habitual exercise, and dynamic arterial compliance. *Circulation, 102*, 1270-1275.

Tanaka, H., Monahan, K.D., & Seals, D.R. (2001). Age-predicted maximal heart rate revisited. *Journal of the American College of Cardiology, 37*, 153-156.

Timiras, M.L., & Brownstein, H. (1987). Prevalence of anemia and correlation of hemoglobin with age in a geriatric screening clinic population. *Journal of the American Geriatrics Society, 35*, 639-643.

U.S. Department of Health and Human Services. (1996). *Physical activity and health: A report of the Surgeon General.* Atlanta, Georgia: U.S. Department of Health and Human Services, Public Health Service, CDC, National Center for Chronic Disease Prevention and Health Promotion.

U.S. Department of Health and Human Services. (2000). *Healthy People 2010.* [Online]. www.health.gov/healthypeople. [Accessed December 10, 2002].

Vaitkevicius, P.V., Ebersold, C., Shah, M.S., Gill, N.S., Katz, R.L., Narrett, M.J., Applebaum, G.E., Parrish, S.M., O'Conner, F.C., & Fleg, J.L. (2002). Effects of aerobic training in community-based subjects aged 80 and older: A pilot study. *Journal of the American Geriatrics Society, 50*, 2009-2013.

Wang, B.W., Ramey, D.R., Schettler, J.D., Hubert, H.B., & Fries, J.F. (2002). Postponed development of disability in elderly runners: A 13-year longitudinal study. *Archives of Internal Medicine, 162*, 2285-2294.

Williams, P.T. (2001). Health effects resulting from exercise versus those from body fat loss. *Medicine and Science in Sports and Exercise, 33*, S611-S621.

Wilson, T.M., & Tanaka, H. (2000). Meta-analysis of the age-associated decline in maximal aerobic capacity in men: Relation to training status. *American Journal of Physiology and Heart Circulatory Physiology, 278*, H829-H834.

Zaugg, M., & Lucchinetti, E. (2000). Respiratory function in the elderly. *Anesthesiology Clinics of North America, 18*, 47-58.

Chapter 5

Ades, P.A., Waldmann, M.L., Meyer, W.L., Brown, K.A., Poehlman, E.T., Pendlebury, W.W., Leslie, K.O., Gray, P.R., Lew, R.R., & LeWinter, M.M. (1996). Skeletal muscle and cardiovascular adaptations to exercise conditioning in older coronary patients. *Circulation, 94*, 323-330.

American College of Sports Medicine. (1998). Position stand. Exercise and physical activity for older adults. *Medicine and Science in Sports and Exercise, 30*, 992-1008.

Andersen, J.L., Terzis, G., & Kryger, A. (1999). Increase in the degree of coexpression of myosin heavy chain isoforms in skeletal muscle fibers of the very old. *Muscle and Nerve, 22*, 449-454.

Aniansson, A., Grimby, G., & Hedberg, M. (1992). Compensatory muscle fiber hypertrophy in elderly men. *Journal of Applied Physiology, 73*, 812-816.

Aniansson, A., Sperling, L., Rundgren, A., & Lehnberg, E. (1983). Muscle function in 75-year-old men and women: A longitudinal study. *Scandinavian Journal of Rehabilitation Medicine, 193*(Suppl.), 92-102.

Bassey, E.J., Fiatarone, M.A., O'Neill, E.F., Kelly, M., Evans, W.J., & Lipsitz, L.A. (1992). Leg extensor power and functional performance in very old men. *Clinical Science, 82*, 321-327.

Baechle T., & Earle, R.W. (2000). *Essentials of strength training and conditioning.* Champaign, Ill: Human Kinetics. Chapter 2, p. 15-24 and Ch 9, p. 169-186.

Bean, J.F., Leveille, S.G., Kiely, D.K., Bandinelli, S., Guralnik, J.M., & Ferrucci, L. (2003). A comparison of leg power and leg strength within the InCHIANTI study: Which influences mobility more? *Journal of Gerontology: Medical Sciences, 58A*, 728-733.

Brooks, G.A., Fahey, T.D., White, T.P., & Baldwin, K.M. (2000). *Exercise physiology* (3rd ed.). Mountain View, CA: Mayfield.

Brooks, S.V., & Faulkner, J.A. (1988). Contractile properties of skeletal muscles from young, adult and aged mice. *Journal of Physiology, 404,* 71-82.

Brooks, S.V., & Faulkner, J.A. (1994). Skeletal muscle weakness in old age: Underlying mechanisms. *Medicine and Science in Sport and Exercise, 26,* 432-439.

Brose, A., Parise, G., & Tarnopolsky, M.A. (2003). Creatine supplementation enhances isometric strength and body composition improvements following strength exercise training in older adults. *Journal of Gerontology: Biological Sciences, 58,* 11-19.

Brown, M. (2000). Strength training and aging. *Topics in Geriatric Rehabilitation, 15,* 1-5.

Cartee, G.D. (1994). Aging skeletal muscle: Response to exercise. *Exercise and Sport Sciences Reviews, 22,* 91-120.

Charette, S.L., McEvoy, L., Pyka, G., Snow-Harter, C., Guido, D., Wiswell, R.A., & Marcus, R. (1991). Muscle hypertrophy response to resistance training in older women. *Journal of Applied Physiology, 70,* 1912-1916.

Clarence Bass's testing at the Cooper Clinic: Personification of lifetime body building and balanced training. (1993). *Master Trainer, 3,* 1-4.

Connelly, D.M., & Vandervoort, A.A. (2000). Effects of isokinetic strength training on concentric and eccentric torque development in the ankle dorsiflexors of older adults. *Journal of Gerontology, 55A*(9), B1-B8.

Doherty, T.J., & Brown, W.F. (1997). Age-related changes in the twitch contractile properties of human ulnar motor units. *Journal of Applied Physiology, 82,* 93-101.

Earles, D.R., Judge, J.O., & Gunnarsson, O.T. (2001). Velocity training induces power-specific adaptations in highly functioning older adults. *Archives of Physical Medical Rehabilitation, 82,* 872-878.

Essen-Gustavsson, B., & Borges, O. (1986). Histochemical and metabolic characteristics of human skeletal muscle in relation to age. *Acta Physiologica Scandinavica, 126,* 107-114.

Esmarck, B., Andersen, J.L., Olsen, S., Richter, A., Mizuno, M., & Kjaer, M. (2001). Timing of postexercise protein intake is important for muscle hypertrophy with resistance training in elderly humans. *Journal of Physiology, 535,* 301-311.

Faulkner, J.A., Claflin, D.R., & McCulley, K.K. (1986). Power output of fast and slow fibers from human skeletal muscles. In N.L. Jones, N.M. McCartney, & A.J. McComas (Eds.), *Human muscle power* (pp. 81-94). Champaign, IL: Human Kinetics.

Fiatarone, M.A., Marks, E.C., Ryan, N.D., Meredith, C., Lipsitz, L.A., & Evans, W.J. (1990). High intensity strength training in nonagenerians. *Journal of the American Medical Association, 263,* 3029-3034.

Fiatarone, M.A., O'Neill, E.F., Ryan, N.D., Clements, K.M., Solares, G.R., Nelson, M.E., Roberts, S.B., Kehayias, J.J., Lipsitz, L.A., & Evans, W.J. (1994). Exercise training and nutritional supplementation for physical frailty in very elderly people. *New England Journal of Medicine, 330*(25), 1769-1775.

Fiatarone Singh, M.A. (2002). Exercise comes of age: Rationale and recommendations for a geriatric exercise prescription. *Journal of Gerontology: Medical Sciences, 57A,* M262-M282.

Fiatarone Singh, M.A., Ding, W., Manfredi, T.J., Solares, G.S., O'Neill, E.F., Clements, K.M., Ryan, N.D., Kehayias, J.J., Fielding, R.A., & Evans, W.J. (1999). Insulin-like growth factor I in skeletal muscle after weight-lifting exercise in frail elders. *American Journal of Physiology, 277,* E135-e143.

Fielding, R.A., LeBrasseur, N.K., Cuoco, A., Bean, J., Mizer, K., & Fiatarone-Singh, M.A. (2002). High-velocity resistance training increases skeletal muscle peak in older women. *Journal of the American Geriatrics Society, 50,* 655-662.

Foldvari, M., Clark, M., Laviolette, L.D., Bernstein, M.A., Kaliton, D., Castaneda, C., Pu, C.T., Hausdorff, J.M., Fielding, R.A., & Singh, M.A.F. (2000). Association of muscle power with functional status in community-dwelling elderly women. *Journal of Gerontology: Medical Sciences, 55A,* M192-M199.

Frontera, W.R., Hughes, V.A., Fielding, R.A., Fiatarone, M.A., Evans, W.J., & Roubenoff, R. (2000). Aging of skeletal muscle: A 12-yr longitudinal study. *Journal of Applied Physiology, 88,* 1321-1326.

Frontera, W.R., Meredith, C.N., O'Reilly, K.P., Knuttgen, H.G., & Evans, W.J. (1988). Strength conditioning in older men: Skeletal muscle hypertrophy and improved function. *Journal of Applied Physiology, 64,* 1038-1044.

Hagerman, F.C., Walsh, S.J., Staron, R.S., Hikida, R.S., Gilders, R.M., Murray, T.F., Toma, K., & Ragg, K.E. (2000). Effects of high-intensity resistance training on untrained older men. I. Strength, cardiovascular, and metabolic responses. *Journal of Gerontology, 55A*(7), B336-B346.

Hakkinen, K., Kallinen, M., Izquierdo, M., Jokelainen, K., Lassila, H., Malkia, E., Kraemer, W.J., Newton, R.U., & Alen, M. (1998). Changes in agonist-antagonist EMG, muscle CSA, and force during strength training in middle-aged and older people. *Journal of Applied Physiology, 84*, 1341-1349.

Hakkinen, K., Newton, R.U., Gordon, S.E., McCormick, M., Volek, J.S., Nindl, B.C., Gotshalk, L.A., Campbell, W.W., Evans, W.J., Hakkinnen, A., Humphries, B.J., & Kraemer, W.J. (1998). Changes in muscle morphology, electromyographic activity, and force production characteristics during progressive strength training in young and older men. *Journal of Gerontology: Biological Sciences, 53*, B415-B423.

Hall, C.D., & Jensen, J.L. (2002). Age related differences in lower extremity power after support surface perturbations. *Journal of American Geriatrics Society, 50*, 1782-1788.

Hicks, A.L., Cupido, C.M., Martin, J., & Dent, J. (1991). Twitch potentiation during fatigue exercise in the elderly: The effects of training. *European Journal of Applied Physiology, 63*, 278-281.

Hikida, R.S., Staron, R.S., Hagerman, F.C., Walsh, S., Kaiser, E., Shell, S., & Hervey, S. (2000). Effects of high-intensity resistance training on untrained older men. II. Muscle fiber characteristics and nucleo-cyoplasmic relationships. *Journal of Gerontology: Biological Sciences, 55*, B347-B354.

Hortobagyi, T., Tunnel, D., Moody, J., Beam, S., & DeVita, P. (2001). Low- or high-intensity strength training partially restores impaired quadriceps force accuracy and steadiness in aged adults. *Journal of Gerontology: Biological Sciences, 56*, B38-b47.

Hughes, V.A., Frontera, W.R., Wood, M., Evans, W.J., Dallal, G.E., Roubenoff, R., & Fiatarone Singh, M.A. (2001). Longitudinal muscle strength changes in older adults: Influence of muscle mass, physical activity, and health. *Journal of Gerontology: Biological Sciences, 56A*, B209-B217.

Hunter, S.K., Thompson, M.W., Ruell, P.A., Harmer, A.R., Thom, J.M., Gwinn, T.H., & Adams, R.D. (1999). Human skeletal sarcoplasmic reticular Ca^{2+} uptake and muscle function with ageing and strength training. *Journal of Applied Physiology, 86*, 1858-1865.

Jozsi, A.C., Campbell, W.W., Joseph, L., Davey, S.L., & Evans, W.J. (1999). Changes in power with resistance training in older and younger men and women. *Journal of Gerontology, 54A*(11), M591-M596.

Kallman, D.A., Plato, C.C., & Tobin, J.D. (1990). The role of muscle loss in the age-related decline of grip strength: Cross-sectional and longitudinal perspectives. *Journal of Gerontology: Medical Sciences, 45*, M82-M88.

Kent-Braun, J.A., Ng, A.V., & Young, K. (2000). Skeletal muscle contractile and non-contractile components in young and elderly women and men. *Journal of Applied Physiology, 88*, 662-668.

Kirkendall, D.T., & Garrett, W.E. (1998). The effects of aging and training on skeletal muscle. *American Journal of Sports Medicine, 26*, 598-602.

Laforest, S., St-Pierre, D.M.M., Cyr, J., & Gayton, D. (1990). Effects of age and regular exercise on muscle strength and endurance. *European Journal of Applied Physiology, 60*, 104-111.

Larsson, L., Grimby, G., & Karlsson, J. (1979). Muscle strength and speed of movement in relation to age and muscle morphology. *Journal of Applied Physiology, 46*, 451-456.

Larsson, L., Sjodin, B., & Karlsson, J. (1978). Histochemical and biochemical changes in human skeletal muscle with age in sedentary males, age 22-65 years. *Acta Physiologica Scandinavica, 103*, 31-39.

Lewis, S.F., Taylor, W.F., Bastian, B.C., Graham, R.M., Pettinger, W.A., & Blomqvist, C.G. (1983). Haemodynamic responses to static and dynamic handgrip before and after autonomic blockage. *Clinical Science, 64*, 593-599.

Lexell, J. (2000). Strength training and muscle hypertrophy in older men and women. *Topics in Geriatric Rehabilitation, 15*, 41-46.

Lexell, J., Downham, D.Y., Larsson, Y., Bruhn, E., & Morsing, B. (1995). Heavy-resistance training for Scandinavian men and women over seventy: Short- and long-term effects on arm and leg muscles. *Scandinavian Journal of Medicine and Science in Sports, 5*, 329-341.

Lexell, J., Taylor, C., & Sjostrom, M. (1988). What is the cause of ageing atrophy? Total number, size, and proportion of different fiber types studied in whole vastus lateralis muscle from 15- to 83-year-old men. *Journal of Neurological Sciences, 84*, 275-294.

Lord, S.R., Menz, H.M., & Tiedemann, A. (2003). A physiological profile approach to falls risk assessment and prevention. *Physical Therapy, 83*, 237-252.

Lynch, N.A., Metter, E.J., Lindle, R.S., Fozard, J.L., Tobin, J.D., Roy, T.A., Fleg, J.L., & Hurley, B.F. (1999). Muscle quality. I. Age associated differences between arm and leg muscle groups. *Journal of Applied Physiology, 86*, 188-194.

Maki, B.E., & McIlroy, W.E. (1996). Postural control in the older adult. *Clinics in Geriatric Medicine, 12*, 635-658.

Martin, J.C., Farrar, R.P., Wagner, B.M., & Spirduso, W.W. (2000). Maximal power across the lifespan. *Journal of Gerontology, 55A*(6), M311-M316.

McArdle, W.D., Katch, F.I., & Katch, V.L. (2001). *Exercise physiology: Energy, nutrition and human performance.* New York: Lippincott Williams & Wilkins.

McCarter, R., & McGee, J. (1987). Influence of nutrition and aging on the composition and function of rat skeletal muscle. *Journal of Gerontology, 42,* 432-441.

McCartney, N., Hicks, A.L., Martin, J., & Webber, C.E. (1996). A longitudinal trial of weight training in the elderly: Continued improvements in year 2. *Journal of Gerontology: Biological Sciences, 51A*(6), B425-B433.

McIlroy, W., & Maki, B. (1993). Do anticipatory adjustments precede compensatory stepping reactions evoked by perturbation? *Neuroscience Letters, 164,* 199-202.

Metter, E.J., Conwitt, R., Tobin, J., & Fozard, J.L. (1997). Age-associated loss of power and strength in the upper extremities in women and men. *Journal of Gerontology: Biological Sciences, 52A*(5), B267-B276.

Miszko, T.A., Cress, M.E., Slade, J.M., Covey, C.J., Agrawal, S.K., & Doerr, C.E. (2003). Effect of strength and power training on physical function in community-dwelling older adults. *Journal of Gerontology: Medical Sciences, 58A,* 171-175.

Nashner, L.M. (1990). Dynamic posturography in the diagnosis and management of dizziness and balance disorders. *Neurologic Clinics, 8*(2), 331-349.

Newman, A.B., Haggerty, C.L., Goodpaster, B., Harris, T., Kritchevsky, S., Nevitt, M., Miles, T.P., & Visser, M. (2003). Strength and muscle quality in a zwell-functioning cohort of older adults: The Health, Aging, and Body Composition Study. *Journal of the American Geriatric Society, 51,* 323-330.

Newton, R.U., Hakkinen, K., Hakkinen, A., McCormick, M., Volek, J., & Kraemer, W.J. (2002). Mixed-methods resistance training increases power and strength of young and older men. *Medicine and Science in Sports, 34,* 1367-1375.

Nieman, D.C. (2003). *Exercise testing and prescription.* Boston: McGraw-Hill.

Petrofsky, J.S., & Lind, A.R. (1975). Aging, isometric strength and endurance, and cardiovascular responses to static effort. *Journal of Applied Physiology, 38,* 91-95.

Porter, M.M., Vandervoort, A.A., & Kramer, J.F. (1997). Eccentric peak torque of the plantar and dorsiflexors is maintained in older women. *Journal of Gerontology: Biological Sciences, 52,* B125-B131.

Prior, B.M., Lloyd, P.G., Yang, H.T., & Terjung, R.L. (2003). Exercise-induced vascular remodeling. *Exercise and Sport Sciences Reviews, 31,* 26-33.

Rantanen, T. (2003). Muscle strength, disability, and mortality. *Scandinavian Journal of Medicine and Science in Sports, 13,* 3-8.

Rice, C.L. (2000). Muscle function at the motor unit level: Consequences of aging. *Topics in Geriatric Rehabiliation, 15,* 70-82.

Rikli, R., & Busch, S. (1986). Motor performance of women as a function of age and physical activity level. *Journal of Gerontology, 41,* 645-649.

Skelton, D.A., Greig, C.A., Davies, J.M., & Young, A. (1994). Strength, power and related functional ability of health people aged 65-89 years. *Age and Ageing, 23,* 371-377.

Skelton, D.A., Young, A., Greig, C.A., & Malbut, K.E. (1995). Effects of resistance training on strength, power, and selected functional abilities of women aged 75 and older. *Journal of American Geriatrics Society, 43,* 1081-1087.

Stanley, S.N., & Taylor, N.A.S. (1993). Isokinematic muscle mechanics in 4 groups of women of increasing age. *European Journal of Applied Physiology, 66,* 178-184.

Stump, T., Clark, D.O., Johnson, R.J., & Wolinsky, F.D. (1997). The structure of health status among Hispanic, African American, and White older adults. *Journal of Gerontology: Psychological Sciences and Social Sciences, 52,* Spec No:49-60.

Taaffe, D.R., Duret, C., Wheller, S., & Marcus, R. (1999). Once-weekly resistance exercise improves muscle strength and neuromuscular performance in older adults. *Journal of the American Geriatrics Society, 47,* 1208-1214.

Terjung, R.L., Zarzeczny, R., & Yang, H.T. (2002). Muscle blood flow and mitochondrial function: Influence of aging. *International Journal of Sport Nutrition and Exercise Metabolism, 12,* 368-378.

Tinetti, M.E., & Speechley, M. (1989). Prevention of falls among the elderly. *New England Journal of Medicine, 320,* 1055-1059.

Tracy, B.L., Ivey, F.M., Hurlbut, D., Martel, G.F., Lemmer, J.T., Siegel, E.L., Metter, E.J., Fozard, J.L., Fleg, J.L., & Hurley, B.F. (1999). Muscle quality. II. Effects of strength training in 65- to 75-yr-old men and women. *Journal of Applied Physiology, 86,* 195-201.

Trappe, S., Williamson, D., Godard, M., Porter, D., Rowden, G., & Costill, D. (2000). Effect of resistance training on single muscle fiber contractile function in older men. *Journal of Applied Physiology, 89,* 143-152.

Vandervoort, A.A. (2002). Aging of the human neuromuscular system. *Muscle and Nerve, 25,* 17-25.

Whipple, R.H., Wolfson, L.I., & Amerman, P.M. (1987). The relationship of knee and ankle weakness to falls in nursing home residents: An isokinetic study. *Journal of the American Geriatrics Society, 35,* 13-20.

Yarasheski, K.E., Pak-Loduca, J., Hasten, D.L., Obert, K.A., Brown, M.B., & Sinacore, D.R. (1999). Resistance exercise training increases mixed muscle protein synthesis rate in frail women and men >76 yr old. *American Journal of Physiology, 277,* E118-E125.

Young, A., & Skelton, D.A. (1994). Applied physiology of strength and power in old age. *International Journal of Sports Medicine, 15,* 149-151.

Young, A., Stokes, M., & Crowe, M. (1985). The size and strength of the quadriceps muscles of old and young men. *Clinical Physiology, 5,* 145-154.

Chapter 6

Alexander, N.B. (1994). Postural control in older adults. *Journal of the American Geriatrics Society, 42,* 93-108.

American Academy of Orthopedic Surgeons (1998). *Don't let a fall be your last trip.* Brochure, available at www.aaos.org [accessed 6.10.04].

American Geriatrics Society, British Geriatrics Society, and American Academy of Orthopaedic Surgeons Panel on Falls Prevention. (2001). Guideline for the prevention of falls in older persons. *Journal of the American Geriatrics Society, 49,* 664-672.

Basmajian, J.V., & De Luca, C.J. (1985). *Muscles alive: Their functions revealed by electromyography* (5th ed.). Baltimore: Williams & Wilkins.

Berg, K., Wood-Dauphinee, S., Williams, J., & Maki, B.E. (1992). Measuring balance in the elderly: Validation of an instrument. *Canadian Journal of Public Health, 83,* S7-S11.

Berthoz, A., & Pozzo, T. (1994). Head and body coordination during locomotion and complex movements. In S.P. Swinnen, H. Heuer, J. Massion, & P. Casaer (Eds.), *Interlimb coordination: Neural, dynamical, and cognitive constraints* (pp. 147-165). San Diego: Academic Press.

Bohannon, R.W. (1997). Comfortable and maximum walking speed of adults aged 20-79 years: Reference values and determinants. *Age and Ageing, 26,* 15-19.

Brauer, S., Woollacott, M., & Shumway-Cook, A. (2001). The interacting effects of cognitive demand and recovery of postural stability in balance-impaired elderly. *Journal of Gerontology: Medical Sciences, 56A,* M489-M496.

Braun, B.L. (1998). Knowledge and perception of fall-related risk factors and fall-reduction techniques among community-dwelling elderly individuals. *Physical Therapy, 78,* 1262-1276.

Brill, P.A., Matthews, M., Mason, J., Davis, D., Mustafa, T., & Macera, C. (1998). Improving functional performance through a group-based free weight strength training program in residents of two assisted living communities. *Physical and Occupational Therapy in Geriatrics, 15(3),* 57-69.

Brown, L.A., Shumway-Cook, A., & Woollacott, M.H. (1999). Attentional demands and postural recovery: The effects of aging. *Journal of Gerontology: Medical Sciences, 54A,* M165-M171.

Bruce, M.F. (1980). The relation of tactile thresholds to histology in the fingers of the elderly. *Journal of Neurology, Neurosurgery, and Psychiatry, 43,* 730.

Buchner, D.M., Cress, M., de Lateur, B., Esselman, P., Margherita, A., Price, R., & Wagner, E. (1997). The effect of strength and endurance training on gait, balance, fall risk, and health services use in community-living older adults. *Journal of Gerontology: Medical Sciences, 52A(4),* M218-M224.

Campbell, A., Robertson, M., Gardner, M., Norton, R., & Buchner, D. (1999). Falls prevention over 2 years: A randomised controlled trial in women 80 years and older. *Age and Ageing, 28,* 513-518.

Campbell, A., Robertson, M., Gardner, M., Norton, R., Tilyard, M., & Buchner, D. (1997). Randomised controlled trial of a general practice program of home based exercise to prevent falls in elderly women. *British Medical Journal, 315,* 1065-1069.

Carr, J.H., & Shephard, R.B. (1998). *Neurologic rehabilitation: Optimizing motor performance.* Oxford: Butterworth and Heinemann.

Chen, H., Ashton-Miller, J.A., Alexander, N.B., & Schultz, A.B. (1991). Stepping over obstacles: Gait patterns of healthy young and old adults. *Journal of Gerontology, 46,* M196-M203.

Chen, H.C., Schultz, A.B., Ashton-Miller, J.A., Giordani, B., Alexander, N.B., & Guire, K. (1996). Stepping over obstacles: Dividing attention impairs performance of old more than young adults.

Journal of Gerontology: Medical Sciences, 51A, M116-M122.

Close, J., Ellis, M., Hooper, R., Glucksman, E., Jackson, S., & Swift, C. (1999). Prevention of falls in the elderly trial (PROFET): A randomised controlled trial. *Lancet, 353*, 93-97.

Cordo, P., & Nashner, L. (1982). Properties of postural adjustments associated with rapid arm movements. *Journal of Neurophysiology, 47*, 287-302.

Cumming, R., Thomas, M., Szonyi, G., Salkeld, G., O'Neill, E., Westbury, C., & Frampton, G. (1999). Home visits by an occupational therapist for assessment and modification of environmental hazards: A randomised controlled trial. *Journal of the American Geriatrics Society, 47*, 1397-1402.

Day, L., Fildes, B., Gordon, I., Fitzharris, M., Flamer, H., & Lord, S. (2002). Randomised factorial trial of falls prevention among older people living in their own homes. *British Medical Journal, 325*, 128-133.

Do, M.C., Bussel, B., & Breniere, Y. (1990). Influence of plantar cutaneous afferents on early compensatory reactions to forward fall. *Experimental Brain Research, 79*, 319-324.

Do, M.C., & Roby-Brami, A. (1991). The influence of a reduced plantar support surface area on the compensatory reactions to a forward fall. *Experimental Brain Research, 84*, 439-443.

Duncan, P., Weiner, D.K., Chandler, J., & Studenski, S. (1990). Functional reach: A new clinical measure of balance. *Journal of Gerontology, 45*, 192-195.

Elble, R.J. (1997). Changes in gait with normal aging. In J.C. Masdeu, L. Sudarsky, & L. Wolfson (Eds.), *Gait disorders of aging. Falls and therapeutic strategies* (pp. 93-106). Philadelphia: Lippincott-Raven.

Elble, R.J., Thomas, S.S., Higgins, C., & Colliver, J. (1991). Stride-dependent changes in gait of older people. *Journal of Neurology, 238*, 1-5.

Erim, Z., Beg, M.F., Burke, D.T., & De Luca, C.J. (1999). Effects of aging on motor-unit control properties. *Journal of Neurophysiology, 82*, 2081-2091.

Evans, W.J. (2000). Exercise strategies should be designed to increase muscle power. *Journal of Gerontology: Medical Sciences, 55A*, M309-M310.

Fernie, G.R., Gryfe, C.I., Holliday, P.J., & Llewellyn, A. (1982). The relationship of postural sway in standing: The incidence of falls in geriatric subjects. *Age and Ageing, 11*, 11-16.

Fiatarone, M.A., O'Neill, E., Doyle Ryan, N., Clements, K., Solares, G., Nelson, M., Roberts, S., Kehayias, J., Lipstiz, L., & Evans, W. (1994). Exercise training and nutritional supplementation for physical frailty in the oldest old. *New England Journal of Medicine, 330*, 1769-1775.

Foldvari, M.M., Clark, L.A., Laviolette, M.A., Bernstein, D., Kaliton, C., Castaneda, C.T., Pu, J.M., Hausdorff, R.A., Fielding, R.A., & Fiatarone Singh, M. (2000). Association of muscle power with functional status in community-dwelling elderly women. *Journal of Gerontology, 55A*, M192-M199.

Foy, A. (1993). Withdrawing benzodiazepines. *Australian Practitioner, 16*, 12-14.

Frank, J.S., Patla, A.E., & Brown, J.E. (1987). Characteristics of postural control accompanying voluntary arm movement in the elderly. *Society for Neuroscience Abstracts, 13*, 335.

Gill, T.M., Robison, J.T., Williams, C.S., & Tinetti, M.E. (1999). Mismatches between the home environment and physical capabilities among community-living older persons. *Journal of the American Geriatrics Society, 47*, 88-92.

Gillespie, L.D., Gillespie, W.J., Cumming, R., Lamb, S.E., & Rowe, B.H. (2002). Interventions for preventing falls in elderly people (Cochrane Review). In: *The Cochrane Library, Issue 3*. Oxford: Update Software.

Hill, K., Smith, R., Murray, K., Sims, J., Gough, J., Darzins, P., & Vrantsidis, F. (2000). An analysis of research on preventing falls and falls injury in older people: Community, residential aged-care and acute care settings. Report to the Commonwealth Department of Health and Aged Care, Injury Prevention Section by National Ageing Research Institute, Melbourne, Australia.

Horak, F.B. (1992). Effects of neurological disorders on postural movement strategies in the elderly. In B. Vellas, M. Toupet, L. Rubenstein, J.L. Albarede, & Y. Christen (Eds.), *Falls, balance, and gait disorders in the elderly* (pp. 137-152). Paris: Elsevier.

Horak, F.B., & Diener, H.C. (1994). Cerebellar control of postural scaling and central set in stance. *Journal of Neurophysiology, 72*, 479-493.

Horak, F.B., Diener, H.C., & Nashner, L.M. (1989). Influence of central set on human postural responses. *Journal of Neurophysiology, 62*, 167-177.

Horak, F.B., & Nashner, L. (1986). Central programming of postural movements: Adaptation to altered support surface configurations. *Journal of Neurophysiology, 55*, 1368-1381.

Hornbrook, M.C., Stevens, V.J., Wingfield, D.J., Hollis, J., Greenlick, M.R., & Ory, M.G. (1994). Preventing falls among community-dwelling older persons: Results from a randomized trial. *Gerontologist, 34,* 16-23.

Howland, J., Lachman, M.E., Peterson, E.W., Cote, J., Kasten, L., & Jette, A. (1998). Covariates of fear of falling and associated activity curtailment. *Gerontologist, 38(5),* 549-555.

Howland, J., Peterson, E.W., Levin, W., Fried, L., Pordon, D., & Bak, S. (1993). Fear of falling among the community-dwelling elderly. *Journal of Aging and Health, 5(2),* 229-243.

Inglin, B., & Woollacott, M.H. (1988). Age-related changes in anticipatory postural adjustments associated with arm movements. *Journal of Gerontology, 43,* M105-M113.

Inglis, J.T., Horak, F.B., Shupert, C.L., & Rycewicz, C. (1994). The importance of somatosensory information in triggering and scaling automatic postural responses in humans. *Experimental Brain Research, 101,* 159-164.

Jensen, J.L., Bothner, K.E., & Woollacott, M.H. (1996). Balance control: The scaling of the kinetic response to accommodate increasing perturbation magnitudes. *Journal of Sport and Exercise Psychology, 18,* S45.

Kannus, P., Parkkari, J., Niemi, S., Pasanen, M., Palvanen, M., Jarvinen, M., & Vuori, I. (2000). Prevention of hip fracture in elderly people with use of a hip protector. *New England Journal of Medicine, 343(21),* 1506-1513.

Lauritzen, J., Peterson, M., & Lund, B. (1993). Effect of external hip protectors on hip fractures. *Lancet, 341,* 11-13.

Leipzig, R., Cumming, R., & Tinetti, M. (1999a). Drugs and falls in older people: A systematic review and meta-analysis: II Cardiac and analgesic drugs. *Journal of the American Geriatrics Society, 47,* 40-50.

Leipzig, R., Cumming, R., & Tinetti, M. (1999b). Drugs and falls in older people: A systematic review and meta-analysis: I. Psychotropic drugs. *Journal of the American Geriatrics Society, 47,* 30-9.

Lin, S.I. (1998). *Adapting to dynamically changing balance threats: Differentiating young, healthy older adults and unstable older adults.* Unpublished doctoral dissertation, University of Oregon.

Lindle, R.S., Metter, E.J., Lynch, N.A., Fleg, J.L., Fozard, J.L., Tobin, J., Roy, T.A., & Hurley, B.F. (1997). Age and gender comparisons of muscle strength in 654 women and men aged 20-93 yr. *Journal of Applied Physiology, 83,* 1581-1587.

Lord, S.E., Halligan, P.W., & Wade, D.T. (1998). Visual gait analysis: The development of a clinical assessment and scale. *Clinics in Rehabilitation, 12,* 107-119.

Lord, S.R., Ward, J.A., Williams, P., & Strudwick, M. (1995). The effect of a 12-month exercise trial on balance, strength, and falls in older women: A randomized controlled trial. *Journal of the American Geriatrics Society, 43,* 1198-1206.

MacRae, P.G., Feltner, M.E., & Reinsch, S.A. (1994). A one-year exercise program for older women: Effects on falls, injuries, and physical performance. *Journal of Aging and Physical Activity, 2,* 127-142.

Maki, B.E., & McIlroy, W.E. (1996). Postural control in the older adult. *Clinics in Geriatric Medicine, 12,* 635-658.

Maki, B.E., & McIlroy, W.E. (1998). Control of compensatory stepping reactions: Age-related impairment and the potential for remedial intervention. *Physiotherapy Theory and Practice. 15,* 69-90.

McIlroy, W., & Maki, B. (1996). Age-related changes in compensatory stepping in response to unpredictable perturbations. *Journal of Gerontology, 51A,* M289-M296.

Means, K.M., Rodell, D.E., O'Sullivan, P.S., & Cranford, L.A. (1996). Rehabilitation of elderly fallers: Pilot study of a low to moderate intensity exercise program. *Archives of Physical Medicine and Rehabilitation, 77,* 1030-1036.

Meuleman, J.R., Brechue, W.M., Kubilis, P.S., & Lowenthal, D.T. (2000). Exercise training in the debilitated aged: Strength and functional outcomes. *Archives of Physical Medicine and Rehabilitation, 81,* 312-318.

Mulrow, C.D., Gerety, M.B., Kanten, D., Comeil, J.E., DeNino, L.A., Chiodo, L., Aguilar, C., O'Neil, M.B., Rosenberg, J., & Solis, R.M. (1994). A randomized trial of physical rehabilitation for very frail nursing home residents. *Journal of the American Medical Association, 271,* 519-524.

Nashner, L.M. (1990). Dynamic posturography in the diagnosis and management of dizziness and balance disorders. *Neurologic Clinics 8(2),* 331-349.

Nashner, L.M. (1997). Physiology of balance, with special reference to the healthy elderly. In J.C. Masdeu, L. Sudarsky, & L. Wolfson, L. (Eds.), *Gait disorders of aging. Falls and therapeutic strategies* (pp. 37-54). Philadelphia: Lippincott-Raven.

Nevitt, M.C., Cummings, S.R., Kidd, S., & Black, D. (1989). Risk factors for recurrent nonsyncopal falls. *Journal of the American Medical Association, 261,* 2663-2668.

Newton, R.A. (1997). Balance screening of an inner city older adult population. *Archives of Physical Medicine and Rehabilitation, 78,* 587-591.

Newton, R.A. (2001). Validity of the multi-directional reach test: A practical measure for limits of stability in older adults. *Journal of Gerontology: Medical Sciences, 56A(4)*, M248-M252.

Nowalk, M.P., Prendergast, J.M., Bayles, C.M., D'Amico, F.J., & Colvin, G.C. (2001). A randomized trial of exercise programs among older individuals living in two long-term care facilities: The FallsFREE Program. Journal of the *American Geriatrics Society, 49*, 859-865.

Paige, G.D. (1991). The aging vestibule-ocular reflex (VOR) and adaptive plasticity. *Acta Otolaryngolica, 481(Suppl.)*, 297.

Patla, A.E. (1997). Understanding the roles of vision in the control of human locomotion. *Gait and Posture, 5*, 54-69.

Patla, A.E., Winter, D.A., Frank, J.S., Walt, S.E., & Prasad, S. (1990). Identification of age-related changes in the balance-control system. In P.W. Duncan (Ed.), *Balance* (pp. 43-56). Alexandria, VA: American Physical Therapy Association.

Perret, E., & Reglis, F. (1970). Age and the perceptual threshold for vibratory stimuli. *European Journal of Neurology, 4*, 65-76.

Plautz, B., Beck, D., Selmer, C., & Radetsky, M. (1996). Modifying the environment: A community-based injury-reduction program for elderly residents. *American Journal of Preventative Medicine 12(Suppl.)*, 33-38.

Province, M., Hadley, E., Hornbrook, M., Lipsitz, L., Miller, J., Mulrow, C., Ory, M., Sattin, R., Tinetti, M., & Wolf, S. (1995). The effects of exercise on falls in elderly patients: A preplanned m-analysis of the FICSIT trials. *Journal of the American Medical Association, 273*, 1341-1347.

Pynoos, J., Sabata, D., Abernethy, G., Alley, D., Nishita, C., & Overton, J. (2003). Prevention of falls at home: Home and environmental modification. In: Preventing falls in older Californians. A California blueprint for fall prevention. *Proceedings of the California Blueprint Fall Prevention Conference*, February 5-6, Sacramento, CA.

Ray, W., Taylor, J., Meador, K., Thapa, P., Brown, A., Kalihara, H., Davis, C., Gideon, P., & Griffin, M. (1997). A randomised trial of a consultation service to reduce falls in nursing homes. *Journal of the American Medical Association, 278*, 557-562.

Reinsch, S., MacRae, P., Lachenbruch, P., & Tobias, J. (1992). Attempts to prevent falls and injury: A prospective community study. *Gerontologist, 32*, 114-122.

Ring, C., Nayak, U.S.L., & Isaacs, B. (1988). Balance function in elderly people who have and who have not fallen. *Archives of Physical Medicine and Rehabilitation, 69*, 261-264.

Rose, D.J. (1997). *A multilevel approach to the study of motor control and learning.* Boston: Allyn & Bacon.

Rose, D.J. (2003). *FallProof. A comprehensive balance and mobility program.* Champaign, IL: Human Kinetics.

Rosenhall, U., & Rubin, W. (1975). Degenerative changes in the human vestibular sensory epithelia. *Acta Otolaryngolica, 79*, 67-81.

Rubenstein, L.Z. (1999). The importance of including the home environment in assessment of frail older persons. *Journal of the American Geriatrics Society, 47*, 111-112.

Rubenstein, L.Z., & Josephson, K.R. (2002). The epidemiology of falls and syncope. In R.A. Kenny & D. O'Shea (Eds), *Falls and syncope in elderly patients. Clinics in geriatric medicine* (pp. 141-158). Philadelphia: Saunders.

Rubenstein, L.Z., Josephson, K.R., Trueblood, P.R., Loy, S., Harker, J.O., Pietruszka, F.M., & Robbins, A.S. (2000). Effects of a group exercise program on strength, mobility, and falls among fall-prone elderly men. *Journal of Gerontology: Medical Sciences, 55A*, M317-M321.

Rubenstein, L.Z., & Powers, C. (1999). *Falls and mobility problems: Potential quality indicators and literature review (the ACOVE Project).* Santa Monica, CA: RAND Corporation.

Runge, C.F., Shupert, C.L., Horak, F.B., & Zajac, F.E. (1999). Postural strategies defined by joint torques. *Gait and Posture, 10*, 161-170.

Scott, V.J., Dukeshire, S., Gallagher, E.M., & Scanlan, A. (2001). *A best practices guide for the prevention of falls among seniors living in the community.* A report prepared on behalf of the Federal/Provincial/Territorial Committee of Officials (Seniors) for the Ministers Responsible for Seniors. Minister of Public Works and Government Services, Ottawa, Ontario, Canada.

Shumway-Cook, A., & Horak, F.B. (1986). Assessing the influence of sensory interaction on balance. *Physical Therapy, 66*, 1548-1550.

Shumway-Cook, A., & Woollacott, M.H. (2001). *Motor control. Theory and practical applications.* Philadelphia: Lippincott Williams & Wilkins.

Shumway-Cook, A., Woollacott, M., Baldwin, M., & Kerns, K. (1997). The effects of cognitive demands on postural sway in elderly fallers and nonfallers. *Journal of Gerontology: Medical Sciences, 52A*, M232-M240.

Sloane, P.D. (1989). Dizziness in primary care: Results from national ambulatory medical care survey. *Journal of Family Practice, 29(1)*, 33-38.

Spirduso, W.W. (1995). *Physical dimensions of aging.* Champaign, IL: Human Kinetics.

Stelmach, G.E., Phillips, J., DiFabio, R.P., & Teasdale, N. (1989). Age, functional postural reflexes, and voluntary sway. *Journal of Gerontology: Biological Sciences, 44*, B100-B106.

Studenski, S., Duncan, P.W., & Chandler, J. (1991). Postural responses and effector factors in persons with unexplained falls: Results and methodologic issues. *Journal of the American Geriatrics Society, 39*, 229-234.

Sullivan, D.H., Wall, P.T., Bariola, J.R., Bopp, M.M., & Frost, Y.M. (2001). Progressive resistance muscle strength training of hospitalized frail elderly. *American Journal of Physical Medicine and Rehabilitation, 80*, 503-509.

Sundermeier, L., Woollacott, M., Jensen, J., & Moore, S. (1996). Postural sensitivity to visual flow in aging adults with and without balance problems. *Journal of Gerontology: Medical Sciences, 51A*, M45-M52.

Tennstedt, S.L. (Guest Ed.) (2003). Falls and fall-related injuries. *Generations, 26 (4)*, 1-100.

Thelen, D.G., Muriuki, M., James, J., Schultz, A.B., Ashton-Miller, J.A., & Alexander, N.B. (2000). Muscle activities used by young and old adults when stepping to regain balance during a forward fall. *Journal of Electromyography and Kinesiology, 10*, 93-101.

Thelen, D.G., Wojcik, L.A., Schultz, A.B., Ashton-Miller, J.A., & Alexander, N.B. (1997). Age differences in using a rapid forward step to regain balance during a forward fall. *Journal of Gerontology: Medical Sciences, 52A*, M8-M13.

Thompson, P.G. (1996). Preventing falls in the elderly at home: A community-based program. *Medical Journal of Australia, 164*, 530-532.

Tinetti, M.E. (1986). Performance oriented assessment of mobility problems in elderly patients. *Journal of the American Geriatrics Society, 34*, 119-126.

Tinetti, M.E., Baker, D.I., McAvay, G., Clans, E.B., Garrett, P., Gottschalk, M., Koch, M.L., Trainor, K., & Horwitz, R.I. (1994). A multifactorial intervention to reduce the risk of falling among elderly people living in the community. *New England Journal of Medicine, 331*, 821-827.

Tinetti, M.E., Speechley, M., & Ginter, S.F. (1988). Risk factors for falls among elderly people living in the community. *New England Journal of Medicine, 319*, 1701-1707.

Van Swearingen, J.M., Paschal, K.A., Bonino, P., & Yang, J-F. (1996). The modified gait abnormality rating scale for recognizing the risk of recurrent falls in community-dwelling elderly adults. *Physical Therapy, 76*, 994-1001.

Wade, M.G., Lindquist, R., Taylor, J.R., & Treat-Jacobsen, D. (1995). Optical flow, spatial orientation, and the control of posture in the elderly. *Journal of Gerontology: Psychological Sciences, 50B*, P51-P58.

Whipple, R., & Wolfson, L.I. (1990). Abnormalities of balance, gait, and sensorimotor function in the elderly population. In P.W. Duncan (Ed.), *Balance* (pp. 61-68) Alexandria, VA: American Physical Therapy Association.

Winter, D.A., Patla, A.E., Frank, J.S., & Walt, S.E. (1990). Biomechanical walking pattern changes in the fit and healthy elderly. *Physical Therapy, 70(6)*, 340-347.

Wojcik, L.A., Thelen, D.G., Schultz, A.B., Ashton-Miller, J.A., & Alexander, N.B. (1999). Age and gender differences in single-step recovery from a forward fall. *Journal of Gerontology: Medical Sciences, 54A*, M38-M43.

Wolf, S.L., Barnhart, H.X., Kutner, N.G., McNeely, E., Coogler, C., & Xu, T. (1996). Reducing frailty and falls in older persons: An investigation of tai chi and computerized balance training. Atlanta FICSIT Group. Frailty and injuries: Cooperative studies of intervention techniques. *Journal of the American Geriatrics Society, 44*, 489-497.

Wolfson, L. (1997). Balance decrements in older persons: Effects of age and disease. In J.C. Masdeu, L. Sudarsky, & L. Wolfson (Eds.), *Gait disorders of aging. Falls and therapeutic strategies* (pp. 79-92). Philadelphia: Lippincott-Raven.

Wolfson, L., Judge, J., Whipple, R., & King, M. (1995). Strength is a major factor in balance, gait, and the occurrence of falls. *Journal of Gerontology: Biological Sciences and Medical Sciences, 50*, Spec No: 64-67.

Wolfson, L.I., Whipple, R.H., Amerman, P., & Tobin, J.N. (1990). Gait assessment in the elderly: A gait abnormality rating scale and its relation to falls. *Journal of Gerontology, 45*, M12-M19.

Woollacott, M.H., Shumway-Cook, A., & Nashner, L.M. (1986). Aging and posture control: Changes in sensory organization and muscular coordination. *International Journal of Aging and Human Development, 23*, 97-114.

Yaffe, K., Barnes, D., Nevitt, M., Lui, L-Y., & Covinski, K. (2001). A prospective study of physical activity and cognitive decline in elderly women: Women who walk. *Archives of Internal Medicine, 161*, 1703-1708.

Chapter 7

Amrhein, P.C., Goggin, N.L., & Stelmach, G.E. (1991). Age differences in the maintenance and restructuring of movement preparation. *Psychology and Aging, 6(3)*, 451-466.

Bashore, T.R., Osman, A., & Heffley, E.F. (1989). Mental slowing in elderly persons: A cognitive psychophysiological analysis. *Psychology and Aging, 4*, 235-244.

Bashore, T.R., Ridderinkhof, K.R., & van der Molen, M.W. (1997). The decline of cognitive processing speed in old age. *Current Directions in Psychological Science, 6(6)*, 163-169.

Brogmus, G.E. (1991). Effects of age and sex on speed and accuracy of hand movements and the refinements they suggest for Fitts' law. *Proceedings of the Human Factors Society, 35th Annual Meeting* (pp. 208-212). Santa Monica, CA: Human Factors and Ergonomics Society.

Cabeza, R., Anderson, N.D., Locantroe, J.K., & McIntosh, A.R. (2002). Aging gracefully: Compensatory brain activity in high-performing older adults. *Neuroimage, 17*, 1394-1402.

Cerella, J., Poon, L.W., & Williams, D. (1980). Age and the complexity hypothesis. In L.W. Poon (Ed.), *Aging in the 1980s* (pp. 332-340). Washington, DC: American Psychological Association.

Christiansen, H., Korten, A.E., Jorm, A.F., Henderson, A.S., Jacomb, P., Rogers, B., & Mackinnon, A.J. (1999). An analysis of diversity in the cognitive performance of elderly community dwellers: Individual differences in change scores as a function of age. *Psychology and Aging, 14(3)*, 365-379.

Dixon, R.A., & Backman, L. (1999). Principles of compensation in cognitive neurorehabilitation. In D.T. Stuss, G. Winocur, & I.H. Robertson (Eds.), *Cognitive neurorehabilitation* (pp. 59-72). Cambridge, UK: Cambridge University Press.

Elbert, T., Pantev, C., Wienbruch, C., Rockstroh, B., Taub, E. (1995). Increased cortical representation of the fingers of the left hand in string players. *Science, 270*, 305-307.

Elbert, T., Sterr, A., & Rockstroh, B. (1996). Untersuchungen zu corticaler Plastizität beim erwachsenen Menschen: was lernt das Gehirn beim Geige spielen? [Studies of cortical plasticity in adults: What does the brain learn from playing the violin?]. *Musikphysiol Musikmedizin, 3*, 57-65.

Ferris, S., Crook, T., Sathananthan, G., & Gershon, S. (1976). Reaction time as a diagnostic measure in senility. *Journal of the American Geriatrics Society, 24*, 529-533.

Fitts, P.M. (1954). The information capacity of the human motor system in controlling the amplitude of movement. *Journal of Experimental Psychology, 47*, 381-391.

Fozard, J.L., Vercruyssen, M., Reynolds, S.L., Hancock, P.A., & Quilter, R.E. (1994). Age differences and changes in reaction time: The Baltimore longitudinal study. Journal of Gerontology: *Psychological Sciences, 49*, P179-P189.

Galton, F. (1899). Exhibition of instruments (1) for testing perception of differences of tint and (2) for determining reaction-time. *Journal of the Anthropological Institute, 19*, 27-29.

Gottsdanker, R. (1982). Age and simple reaction time. *Journal of Gerontology, 37*, 342-348.

Hale, S., Meyerson, J., & Wagstaff, D. (1987). General slowing of nonverbal information processing: Evidence for a power law. *Journal of Gerontology, 42*, 131-136.

Henderson, L., Harrison, J., & Kennard, C. (2001). Selectively impaired reaction time in Parkinson's disease: Persistent absence of simple reaction time advantage in a patient with frontal complications. *Neurocase, 7*, 319-330.

Hultsch, D.F., MacDonald, S.W.S., & Dixon, R.A. (2002). Variability in reaction time performance of younger and older adults. *Journal of Gerontology: Psychological Sciences, 57B(2)*, P101-P115.

Jahanshahi, M., Brown, R.G., & Marsden, C.D. (1993). Motor slowness in Parkinson's disease. In G.E. Stelmach & V. Homberg (Eds.), *Sensorimotor impairments of the elderly* (pp. 269-261). Dortdrecht: Kluver.

Johnson, R.C., McClearn, G.E., Yuen, S., Nagoshi, C.T., Ahern, F.M., & Cole, R.E. (1985). Galton's data a century later. *American Psychologist, 40*, 875-892.

Karni, A., Meyer, G., Jezzard, P. Adams, M., Turner, R., & Ungerleider, L. (1995). Functional MRI evidence for adult motor cortex plasticity during motor skill learning. *Nature, 377(6545)*, 155-158.

Koga, Y., & Morant, G.M. (1923). On the degree of association between reaction times in the case of different senses. *Biometrika, 15*, 346-372.

Kraiuhin, C., Yiannikis, C., Coyle, S., Gordon, E., Rennie, C.J., Howson, A., & Meares, R.A. (1989). The relationship between reaction time and latency of the P300 event-related potential in normal subjects and Alzheimer's disease. *Clinical and Experimental Neurology, 26,* 81-88.

Krampe, R.T. (2002). Aging, expertise and fine motor movement. *Neuroscience and Biobehavioral Reviews, 26,* 769-776.

Krampe, R.T., & Ericsson, K.A. (1996). Maintaining excellence: Deliberate practice and elite performance in younger and older pianists. *Journal of Experimental Psychology: General, 125,* 331-359.

Li, S.C., & Lindenberger, U. (1999). Cross-level unification: A computational exploration of the link between deterioration of neurotransmitter systems and dedifferentiation of cognitive abilities in old age. In L.G. Nilsson & H. Markowitsch (Eds.), *Cognitive neuroscience and memory* (pp. 103-146). Toronto: Hogrefe & Huber.

Light, K., & Spirduso, W. (1990). Effects of adult aging on the movement complexity factor response programming. *Journal of Gerontology: Psychological Sciences, 45,* P107-P109.

Light, K.E., & Spirduso, W.W. (1996). Age factors influencing response-response compatability in reaction time tasks. *Journal of Aging and Physical Activity, 4,* 179-193.

Lima, S.D., Hale, S., & Myerson, J. (1991). How general is general slowing? Evidence from the lexical domain. *Psychology and Aging, 6,* 416-425.

Madden, D.J. (2001). Speed and timing of behavioral processes. In J.E. Birren & K.W. Schaie (Eds.), *Handbook of the psychology of aging* (pp. 313-348). New York: Academic Press.

Madden, D.J., Welsh-Bohmer, K.A., & Tupler, L.A. (1999). Task complexity and signal detectional analyses of lexical decision performance in Alzheimer's disease. *Developmental Neuropsychology, 16,* 1-18.

Melis, A., Soetens, E., & van der Molen, M.W. (2002). Process-specific slowing with advancing age: Evidence derived from the analysis of sequential effects. *Brain and Cognition, 49,* 420-435.

Myerson, J., Hale, S., Hirschman, R., Hansen, C., & Christiansen, B. (1989). Global increase in response latencies by early middle age: Complexity effects in individual performances. *Journal of the Experimental Analysis of Behavior, 52,* 353-362.

Nebes, R.D., & Madden, D.J. (1988). Different patterns of cognitive slowing produced by Alzheimer's disease and normal aging. *Psychology and Aging, 3,* 102-104.

Pirozzolo, F.J., & Hansch, E.C. (1981). Oculomotor reaction time in dementia reflects degree of cerebral dysfunction. *Science, 214,* 349-351.

Raz, N. (2000). Aging of the brain and its impact on cognitive performance: Integration of structural and functional findings. In F.I.M. Craik & T.A. Salthouse (Eds.), *The handbook of aging and cognition* (2nd ed., pp. 1-90). Mahwah, NJ: Erlbaum.

Salthouse, T.A. (2000). Aging and measure of processing speed. *Biological Psychology, 54,* 35-54.

Smulders, F.T.Y., Kenemans J.L., Schmidt, W.F., & Kok, A. (1999). Effects of task complexity in young and old adults: Reaction time and P300 latency are not always associated. *Psychophysiology, 36,* 118-125.

Vercruyssen, M. (1991). Age-related slowing of behavior. *Proceedings of the Human Factors Society 35th Annual Meeting* (pp. 188-192). Santa Monica, CA: Human Factors and Ergonomics Society.

Walker, N., Philbin, D.A., & Fisk, A. D. (1997). Age-related differences in movement control: Adjusting submovement structure to optimize performance. *Journal of Gerontology, 52B(1),* P40-P52.

Wilkinson, R.T., & Allison, S. (1989). Age and simple reaction time: Decade differences for 5,325 subjects. *Journal of Gerontology: Psychological Sciences, 44,* P29-P35.

Chapter 8

Backman, L., & Molander, B. (1991). On the generalizability of the age-related decline in coping with high-arousal conditions in a precision sport: Replication and extension. *Journal of Gerontology: Psychological Sciences, 46,* P79-P81.

Ball, K., Beard, B., Roenker, D., Miller, R., & Griggs, D. (1988). Age and visual search: Expanding the useful field of view. *Journal of the Optical Society of America, 5,* 2210-2219.

Ball, K., Owsley, C., Sloane, M.E., Roenker, D.L., & Bruni, J.R. (1993). Visual attention problems as a predictor of vehicle crashes in older drivers. *Investigative Ophthalmology and Visual Science, 34,* 3110-3123.

Barrett, G.V., Alexander, R.A., & Forbes, B.J. (1977). Analysis of performance measurement and training requirements for decision making in emergency situations. *JSAS Catalog of Selected Documents in Psychology, 7,* 126.

Bennett, K.M.B., & Castiello, U. (1994). Reach to grasp: Changes with age. *Journal of Gerontology, 49B(1),* 1-7.

Birren, J.E. (1974). Translations in gerontology—From lab to life. *American Psychologist, 29,* 808-815.

Birren, J.E., & Botwinick, J. (1951). The relation of writing speed to age and to the senile psychoses. *Journal of Consulting Psychology, 15*, 243-249.

Bolton, C.F., Winkelman, M.D., & Dyck, P.J. (1996). A quantitative study of Meissner's corpuscles in man. *Neurology, 16*, 1-9.

Brocklehurst, J.C., Robertson, D., & James-Groom, P. (1982). Clinical correlates of sway in old age—Sensory modalities. *Age and Ageing, 11(1)*, 1-10.

Brouwer, W.H., Waternink, W., van Wolffelaar, P.C., & Rothengatter, T. (1991). Divided attention in experienced young and older drivers: Lane tracking and visual analysis in a dynamic driving simulator. *Human Factors, 33(5)*, 573-582.

Cerella, J. (1990). Aging and information-processing rate. In J.E. Birrin & K.W. Schaie (Eds.), *Handbook of the psychology of aging* (3rd ed., pp. 201-221). New York: Academic Press.

Clark, J.E. (1994). Motor development. In V.S. Ramachadran (Ed.), *Encyclopedia of human behavior* (pp. 245-255). San Diego: Academic Press.

Cole, K.J. (1991). Grasp force control in older adults. *Journal of Motor Behavior, 23(4)*, 251-258.

Cole, K.J., & Beck, C.L. (1994). The stability of precision grip force in older adults. *Journal of Motor Behavior, 26(2)*, 171-177.

Cole, K.J., & Rotella, D.L. (2002). Old age impairs the use of arbitrary visual cues for predictive control of fingertip forces during grasp. *Experimental Brain Research, 143*, 35-41.

Cole, K.J., Rotella, D.L., & Harper, J.G. (1998). Tactile impairments cannot explain the effect of age on a grasp and lift task. *Experimental Brain Research, 121*, 263-269.

Cole, K.J., Rotella, D.L., & Harper, J.G. (1999). Mechanisms for age-related changes of fingertip forces during precision gripping and lifting in adults. *Journal of Neuroscience, 19(8)*, 3238-3247.

Contreras-Vidal, J.L., Teulings, H.L., & Stelmach, G.E. (1998). Elderly subjects are impaired in spatial coordination in fine motor control. *Acta Psychologica, 100*, 25-35.

Cremer, R., Snel, J., & Brouwer, W.H. (1990). Age-related differences in timing position and velocity identification. *Accident Annals Preview, 22*, 467-474.

Dixon, R.A., Kurzman, D., & Friesen, I. C. (1993). Handwriting performance in younger and older adults: Age, familiarity, and practice effects. *Psychology and Aging, 8(3)*, 360-370.

Donatelle, R.J., Davis, L.G., Hoover, C.F., & Harding, A. (1991). *Access to aging.* Englewood Cliffs, NJ: Prentice Hall.

Evans, L. (1988). Older driver involvement in fatal and severe traffic crashes. *Journal of Gerontology: Social Sciences, 43*, S186-S193.

Floeter, M., & Greenough, W.T. (1979). Cerebellar plasticity: Modification of Purkinje cell structure by differential rearing in monkeys. *Science, 206*, 227-229.

Gentile, A., Behesti, Z., & Held, J.M. (1987). Environment vs. exercise effects on motor impairments following cortical lesions in rats. *Behavior and Neural Biology, 47*, 321-332.

Gilhorta, J.G., Mitchell, P., Ivers, R., & Cumming, R.G. (2001). Impaired vision and other factors associated with driving cessation in the elderly: The Blue Mountains Eye Study. *Clinical and Experimental Ophthalmology, 29*, 104-107.

Goggin, N.L., & Meeuwsen, H.J. (1992). Age-related differences in the control of spatial aiming movements. *Research Quarterly for Exercise and Sport, 63(4)*, 366-372.

Grant, E., Storandt, M., & Botwinick, J. (1978). Incentive and practice in the psychomotor performance of the elderly. *Journal of Gerontology, 33*, 413-415.

Greene, L.S., & Williams, H.G. (1996). Aging and coordination from a dynamic pattern perspective. In A. Ferrandez & N. Teasdale (Eds.), *Changes in sensory motor behavior in aging* (pp. 89-132). New York: Elsevier Science.

Greenwood, M., Meeuwsen, H., & French, R. (1993). Effects of cognitive learning strategies, verbal reinforcement, and gender on the performance of closed motor skills in older adults. *Activities, Adaptation & Aging, 17(3)*, 39-53.

Hakamies-Blomqvist, L., Mynttinen, S., Backman, M., & Mikkonen, V. (1999). Age-related differences in driving: Are older drivers more serial? *International Journal of Behavioral Development, 23(3)*, 575-589.

Harrington, D.L., & Haaland, K.Y. (1992). Skill learning in the elderly: Diminished implicit and explicit memory for a motor sequence. *Psychology and Aging, 7(3)*, 425-434.

Held, J., Gordon, J., & Gentile, A.M. (1985). Environmental influences on locomotor recovery following cortical lesions in rats. *Journal of Behavioral Neuroscience, 99*, 678-690.

Henderson, R.L., & Burg, A. (1974). *Vision and audition in driving* (Report No. NTIS PB-238-278). Washington, DC: U.S. Department of Transportation.

Hertzog, C.K., Williams, M.V., & Walsh, D.A. (1976). The effect of practice on age differences in central perceptual processing. *Journal of Gerontology, 31*, 428-433.

Johansson, B.B., & Ohlsson, A.L. (1996). Environment, social interaction, and physical activity as determinants of functional outcome after cerebral infarction in the rat. *Experimental Neurology, 139(2)*, 322-327.

Kausler, D.H. (1990). Motivation, human aging, and cognitive performance. In J.E. Birren & K.W. Schaie (Eds.), *Handbook of the psychology of aging* (3rd ed., pp. 171-182). New York: Academic Press.

Ketcham, C.J., Seidler, R.D., Van Gemmert, A.W.A., & Stelmach, G.E. (2002). Age-related kinematic differences as influenced by task difficulty, target size, and movement amplitude. *Journal of Gerontology: Psychological Sciences, 57B*, 54-64.

Kinoshita, H., & Francis, P.R. (1996). A comparison of prehension force control in young and elderly individuals. *European Journal of Applied Physiology, 74*, 450-460.

Klavora, P., & Heslegrave, R.J. (2002). Senior drivers: An overview of problems and intervention strategies. *Journal of Aging and Physical Activity, 10*, 322-335.

Kline, D.W., Kline, T.J.B., Fozard, J.L., Kosnik, W., Schieber, F., & Sekuler, R. (1992). Vision, aging, and driving: The problems of older drivers. *Journal of Gerontology: Psychological Sciences, 47*, P27-P34.

Kokmen, E., Bossemeyer, R.W.J., & Williams, W. J. (1978). Quantitative evaluation of joint motion sensation in an aging population. *Journal of Gerontology, 33*, 62-67.

Korteling, J.E. (1994). Effects of aging, skill modification, and demand alternation on multiple-task performance. *Human Factors, 36(1)*, 27-43.

LaRiviere, J.E., & Simonson, E. (1965). The effect of age and occupation on speed of writing. *Journal of Gerontology, 20*, 415-416.

Lazarus, J.C., & Haynes, J.M. (1997). Isometric pinch force control and learning in older adults. *Experimental Aging Research, 23*, 179-200.

Li, K.Z.H., Lindenberger, U., Freund, A.M., & Baltes, P.B. (2001). Walking while memorizing: Age-related differences in compensatory behavior. *Psychological Science, 12(3)*, 230-237.

Lovelace, E.A., & Aikens, J.E. (1990). Vision, kinesthesis, and control of hand movement by young and old adults. *Perceptual and Motor Skills, 70*, 1131-1137.

Lovelace, E.A., Vella, B.A., & Anderson, D.M. (1993). Judging age from handwritting done with and without visual feedback. *Bulletin of the Psychonomic Society, 31(2)*, 111-113.

Lowe, B. D. (2001). Precision grip force control of older and younger adults, revisited. *Journal of Occupational Rehabilitation, 11(4)*, 267-279.

Magill, R.A. (2001). *Motor learning: Concepts and applications* (6th ed.). New York: McGraw-Hill.

Manchester, D., Woollacott, M., Zederbauer-Hylton, N., & Marin, O. (1989). Visual, vestibular, and somatosensory contributions to balance control in the older adult. *Journal of Gerontology: Medical Sciences, 44*, M118-M127.

Margolis, K.L., Kerani, R.P., McGovern, P., Songer, T., Cauley, J.A., & Ensrun, K.E. (2002). Risk factors for motor vehicle crashes in older women. *Journal of Gerontology: Medical Sciences, 57A(3)*, M186-M191.

McDowd, J.M., & Craik, I.M.(1988). Effects of aging and task difficulty on divided attention performance. *Journal of Experimental Psychology: Human Perception and Performance, 14*, 267-280.

McDowd, J.M., Vercruyssesn, M., & Birren, J.E. (1991). Aging, divided attention, and dual task performance. In D.L. Damos (Ed.), *Multiple-task performance* (pp. 386-414). Washington, DC: Taylor & Francis.

McFarland, R.A., Tune, G.S., & Welford, A.T. (1964). On the driving of automobiles by older people. *Journal of Gerontology, 19*, 190-197.

Meyer, D.E., Kornblum, S., Abrams, R.A., Wright, C.E., & Smith, J.E.K. (1988). Optimality in human motor performance: Ideal control of rapid aimed movements. *Psychological Review, 95(3)*, 340-370.

Molander, B., & Backman, L. (1990). Age differences in the effects of background noise on motor and memory performance in a precision sport. *Experimental Aging Research, 16*, 55-60.

Molander, B., & Backman, L. (1994). Attention and performance in miniature golf across the lifespan. *Journal of Gerontology, 49(2)*, 35-41.

Morgan, M., Phillips, J.G., Bradshaw, J.L., Mattingley, J., Iansek, R., & Bradshaw, J.A. (1994). Age-related motor slowness: Simply strategic? *Journal of Gerontology: Medical Sciences, 49(3)*, M133-M139.

National Highway Traffic Safety Administration. (2001). Traffic safety facts 2000: Older population. U.S. Department of Transportation: National Highway Traffic Safety Administration. [Online]. Available: www.nhtsa.dot.gov. [May 15, 2004].

Nedbor, R.G. (2003, July 14). Those hand gestures didn't mean "hello." *Newsweek*, Feature: My Turn.

Nelson, D.E., Sacks, J.J., & Chorba, T.L. (1992). Required vision testing for older drivers [letter to the editor]. *New England Journal of Medicine, 326*, 1784-1785.

Owlsey, C., Ball, K., McGwin, G., Jr., Sloane, M.E., Roenker, D.L., White, M.F., & Overley, T. (1998). Visual processing impairment and risk of motor vehicle crash among older adults. *Journal of the American Medical Association, 279(14)*, 1083-1088.

Panek, P.E., Barrett, G.V., Sterns, H.L., & Alexander, R.A. (1978). Age differences in perceptual style, selective attention, and perceptual-motor reaction time. *Experimental Aging Research, 4*, 377-387.

Persson, D. (1993). The elderly driver: Deciding when to stop. *Gerontologist, 33*, 88-91.

Philips, J.G., Mueller, F., & Stelmach, G.E. (1989). Movement disorders and the neural basis of motor control. In S.A. Wallace (Ed.), *Perspectives on the coordination of movement* (pp. 367-417). Amsterdam: North-Holland.

Plude, D.J., & Hoyer, W.J. (1985). Attention and performance: Identifying and localizing age deficits. In N. Charness (Ed.), *Aging and human performance* (pp. 47-99). Chichester, UK: Wiley.

Ponds, R.W.H.M., Brouwer, W.H., & van Wolffelaar, P.C. (1988). Age differences in divided attention in a simulated driving task. *Journal of Gerontology: Psychological Sciences, 43*, P151-P156.

Potvin, A.R., Syndulko, K., Tourtellotte, W.W., Lemmon, J.A., & Potvin, J.H. (1980). Human neurologic function and the aging process. *Journal of the American Geriatrics Society, 28*, 1-9.

Pratt, J., Chasteen, A.L., & Abrams, R.A. (1994). Rapid aimed limb movements: Age differences and practice effects in component submovements. *Psychology and Aging, 9(2)*, 325-334.

Prinz, P.N., Dustman, R.E., & Emmerson, R. (1990). Electrophysiology and aging. In J.E. Birren & K.W. Schaie (Eds.), *Handbook of the psychology of aging* (3rd ed., pp. 135-149). New York: Academic Press.

Pysh, J.J., & Weiss, G.M. (1979). Exercise during development induces an increase in Purkinje cell dendritic tree size. *Science, 206*, 230-231.

Rabbitt, P.M.A., & Rogers, M. (1965). Age and choice between responses in a self-paced repetitive task. *Ergonomics, 8*, 435-444.

Ranganathan, V.K., Siemionow, V., Vinod, S., Liu, J.Z., & Yue, G.H. (2001). Skilled finger movement exercise improves hand function. *Journal of Gerontology: Medical Sciences, 56A(8)*, M518-M522.

Retchin, S.M., & Anapolle, J. (1993). An overview of the older driver. *Clinics in Geriatric Medicine, 9(2)*, 297-310.

Roberton, M.A. (1977). Stability of stage categorizations across trials: Implications for the "stage-theory" of overarm throw development. *Journal of Human Movement Studies, 3*, 49-59.

Rose, D.J. (1997). *Motor control and learning*. Boston: Allyn & Bacon.

Rothstein, D., Larish, D., Petruzzello, S., Crews, D., & Naham, A. (1989). Bimanual coordination in the healthy old. *Gerontologist, 29*, 258-259A.

Salthouse, T.A. (1984). Effects of age and skill on typing. *Journal of Experimental Psychology: General, 113*, 345-371.

Schmidt, R.A. (1988). *Motor control and learning*. Champaign, IL: Human Kinetics.

Schmidt, R.A., & Wristberg, C.A. (2004). *Motor learning and performance* (3rd ed.). Champaign, IL: Human Kinetics.

Scialfa, C.T., Guzy, L.T., Leibowitz, H.W., Garvey, P.M., & Tyrrell, R.A. (1991). Age differences in estimating vehicle velocity. *Psychology and Aging, 6*, 60-66.

Seidler, R.D., Alberts, J.L., & Stelmach, G.E. (2002). Changes in multi-joint performance with age. *Motor Control, 6*, 19-31.

Seidler-Dobrin, R.D., & Stelmach, G.E. (1998). Persistence in visual feedback control by the elderly. *Experimental Brain Research, 119*, 467-474.

Sekuler, A.B., & Bennett, P.J. (2000). Effects of aging on the useful field of view. *Experimental Aging Research, 26*, 103-120.

Sekuler, R., & Hutman, L.P. (1980). Spatial vision and aging. I: Contrast sensitivity. *Journal of Gerontology, 35*, 692-699.

Sekuler, R., Hutman, L., & Owlsey, C. (1980). Human aging and spatial vision. *Science, 209*, 1255-1256.

Sheldrick, M.G. (1992). Technology for the elderly. *Electronic News, 38*, 22.

Skinner, H.B., Barrack, R.L., & Cook, S.D. (1988). Age-related declines in proprioception. *Clinical Orthopaedics, 184*, 208-211.

Slavin, M.J., Phillips, J.G., & Bradshaw, J.L. (1996). Visual cues and the handwriting of older adults: A kinematic analysis. *Psychology and Aging, 11(3)*, 524.

Smith, K., & Greene, D. (1962). Scientific motion study and aging process in performance. *Ergonomics, 5*, 155-164.

Spirduso, W.W., & Choi, J.H. (1993). Age and practice effects on force control of the thumb and index fingers in precision pinching and bilateral coordination. In G.E. Stelmach & V. Hömberg (Eds.), *Sensorimotor impairments in the elderly: Are they reversible?* (pp. 393-412). Dordrecht, The Netherlands: Kluwer Academic.

Staplin, L., & Fisk, A.D. (1991). A cognitive engineering approach to improving signalized left turn intersections. *Human Factors, 33(5)*, 559-571.

Stelmach, G.E., Amrhein, P.C., & Goggin, N.L. (1988a). Age differences in bimanual coordination. Journal of Gerontology: *Psychological Sciences, 43*, P18-P23.

Stelmach, G.E., Goggin, N.L., & Amrhein, P.C. (1988b). Aging and the restructuring of precued movements. *Psychology and Aging, 3*, 152.

Surburg, P.R. (1976). Aging and the effect of physical-mental practice upon acquisition and retention of motor skill. *Journal of Gerontology, 31*, 64-67.

Swinnen, S.P., Verschueren, S.M.P., Bogaerts, H., Dounskaia, N., Lee, T.D., Stelmach, G.E., & Serrien, D.J. (1998). Age-related deficits in motor learning and the differences in feedback processing during the production of a bimanual coordination pattern. *Cognitive Neuropsychology, 15(5)*, 439-466.

Tasca, L. (1992). *Review of the literature on senior driving performance* (Rep. No. RUSO-92-107). Toronto: Ontario Ministry of Transportation.

Transportation Research Board. (1988). *Transportation in an aging society: Improving mobility and safety for older people* (Special Rep. 218, No. 1). Washington, DC: National Research Council.

Underwood, M. (1992). The older driver: Clinical assessment and injury prevention. Archives of *Internal Medicine, 152*, 735-740.

Von Donkelaar, P.V., & Franks, I.M. (1991). Preprogramming vs. on-line control in simple movement sequences. *Acta Psychologia, 77*, 1-19.

Walser, N. (1991). When to hang up the keys. *Harvard Health Letter, 17*, 1-4.

Weir, P.L., MacDonald, J.R., Mallat, B.J., Leavitt, J.L., & Roy, E.A. (1998). Age-related differences in prehension: The influence of task goals. *Journal of Motor Behavior, 30(1)*, 79-89.

Welford, A.T. (1958). *Ageing and human skill*. Oxford, UK: Oxford University Press.

Welford, A.T. (1977). Motor performance. In J.E. Birren & K.W. Schaie (Eds.), *Handbook of the psychology of aging* (pp. 450-496). New York: Van Nostrand Reinhold.

Whanger, A.D., & Wang, H.S. (1974). Clinical correlates of the vibratory sense in elderly psychiatric patients. *Journal of Gerontology, 29(1)*, 39-45.

Williams, H. (1983). *Perceptual and motor development*. Englewood Cliffs, NJ: Prentice-Hall.

Winstein, C.J., & Schmidt, R.A. (1990). Reduced frequency of knowledge of results enhances motor skill learning. *Journal of Experimental Psychology: Learning, Memory, and Cognition, 16*, 677-691.

Wishart, L.R., Lee, T.D., Cunningham, S.J., & Murdoch, J.E. (2002). Age-related differences and the role of augmented visual feedback in learning a bimanual coordination pattern. *Acta Psychologica, 110*, 247-263.

Wyke, B. (1979). Conference on the ageing brain. Cervical articular contributions to posture and gait: Their relation to senile disequilibrium. *Age and Ageing, 8*, 251-257.

Yan, J.H., Thomas, J.R., Stelmach, G.E., & Thomas, K.T. (2000). Developmental features of rapid aiming arm movements across the lifespan. *Journal of Motor Behavior, 32*, 126.

Chapter 9

Abourezk, T., & Toole, T. (1995). Effect of task complexity on the relationship between physical fitness and reaction time in older women. *Journal of Aging and Physical Activity, 3*, 251-260.

Anch, A.M., Browman, C.P., & Mitler, J.K. (1988). *Sleep: A scientific perspective*. Englewood Cliffs, NJ: Prentice Hall.

Anstey, K.J., & Smith, G.A. (1999). Interrelationships among biological markers of aging, health, activity, acculturation, and cognitive performance in late adulthood. *Psychology and Aging, 14*, 605-618.

Barry, A.J., Steinmetz, J.R., Page, H.F., & Rodahl, K. (1966). The effects of physical conditioning on older individuals. II. Motor performance and cognitive function. *Journal of Gerontology, 21*, 182-191.

Baylor, A.M., & Spirduso, W.W. (1988). Systematic aerobic exercise and components of reaction time in older women. *Journal of Gerontology: Psychological Sciences, 43*, P121-P126.

Black, J.E., Greenough, W.T., Anderson, B.J., & Isaacs, K.R. (1987). Environment and the aging brain. *Canadian Journal of Psychology, 41*, 111-130.

Black, J.E., Isaacs, K.R., Anderson, B.J., Alcontara, A.A., & Greenough, W.T. (1990). Learning causes synaptogenesis, while motor activity causes angiogenesis, in cerebellar cortex of adult rats. *Proceedings of the National Academy of Science USA, 87*, 5568-5572.

Black, J.E., Isaacs, K.R., & Greenough, W.T. (1991). Usual vs. successful aging: Some notes on experiential factors. *Neurobiology of Aging, 12,* 325-328.

Black, J.E., Polinsky, M., & Greenough, W.T. (1989). Progressive failure of cerebral angiogenesis supporting neural plasticity in aging rats. *Neurobiology of Aging, 10,* 353-358.

Blumenthal, J.A., Emery, C.F., Madden, D.J., George, L.K., Coleman, E., Riddle, M.W., McKee, D.C. Reasoner, J., & Williams, R.S. (1989). Cardiovascular and behavioral effects of aerobic exercise training in healthy older men and women. *Journal of Gerontology: Medical Sciences, 44,* M147-M157.

Blumenthal, J.A., & Madden, D.J. (1988). Effects of aerobic exercise training, age, and physical fitness on memory search performance. *Psychology and Aging, 3,* 280-285.

Botwinick, J., & Birren, J.E. (1963). Cognitive processes: Mental abilities and psychomotor responses in aged men. In J.E. Birren, R.N. Butler, S.W. Greenhouse, L. Sokoloff, & M.R. Yarrow (Eds.), *Human aging: A biological and behavioral study* (pp. 143-156). Washington, DC: U.S. Government Printing Office.

Botwinick, J.E., & Storandt, M. (1974). Cardiovascular status, depressive effect, and other factors in reaction time. *Journal of Gerontology, 29,* 543-548.

Boutcher, S.H. (2000). Cognitive performance, fitness, and ageing. In S.J.H. Biddle, K.R. Fox, & S.H. Boutcher (Eds.), *Physical activity and psychological well-being* (pp. 118-129). New York: Routledge.

Boutcher, S.H., Nugent, F.W., McLaren, P.F., & Weltman, A.L. (1998). Heart period variability of trained and untrained men at rest and during mental challenge. *Psychophysiology, 35,* 16-22.

Brown, B.S., Payne, T., Kim, C., Moore, G., Krebs, P., & Martin, W. (1979). Chronic response of rat brain norepinephrine and serotonin levels to endurance training. *Journal of Applied Physiology, 46,* 12-23.

Carlow, T.J., Appenzeller, O., & Rodriguez, M. (1978). Neurology of training: VEPs before and after a run. *Neurology, 2,* 390.

Casperson, C.J., Powell, K.E., & Christenson, G.M. (1985). Physical activity, exercise, and physical fitness: Definitions and distinctions for health-related research. *Public Health Reports, 100,* 126-131.

Chen, Y.C., Chen, Q.S., Lei, J.L., & Wang, S.L. (1998). Physical training modifies the age-related decrease of GAP-43 and synaptophysin in the hippocampal formation in C57BL/6J mouse. *Brain Research, 806,* 238-245.

Chodzko-Zajko, W.J. (1991). Physical fitness, cognitive performance, and aging. *Medicine and Science in Sports and Exercise, 23,* 868-872.

Chodzko-Zajko, W.J., & Moore, K.A. (1994). Physical fitness and cognitive functioning in aging. *Exercise and Sport Sciences Reviews, 22,* 195-220.

Chodzko-Zajko, W.J., & Ringel, R.L. (1987). Physiological fitness measures and sensory and motor performance in aging. *Experimental Gerontology, 22,* 317-328.

Chodzko-Zajko, W.J., Schuler, P.B., Solomon, J.S., Heinl, B., & Ellis, N. (1992). The influence of physical fitness on automatic and effortful memory changes in aging. *International Journal of Aging & Human Development, 35,* 265-285.

Clarkson, P.M. (1978). The effect of age and activity level in simple and choice fractionated response time. *European Journal of Applied Physiology, 40,* 17-25.

Clarkson-Smith, L., & Hartley, A.A. (1989). Relationships between physical exercise and cognitive abilities in older adults. *Psychology and Aging, 4,* 183-189.

Colcombe, S.J., Erickson, B.S., Raz, N., Webb, A.G., Cohen, N.J., McAuley, F., & Kramer, A.F. (2003). Aerobic fitness reduces brain tissue loss in aging humans. *Journal of Gerontology: Medical Sciences, 58A,* 176-180.

Colcombe, S., & Kramer, A.F. (2003). Fitness effects on the cognitive function of older adults: A meta-analytic study. *Psychological Science, 2,* 125-130.

Diamond, M.C., & Connor, J.R., Jr. (1982). Plasticity of the aging cerebral cortex. In S. Hoyer (Ed.), *Experimental brain research* (Suppl. 5, pp. 36-44). Berlin: Springer-Verlag.

Diamond, M.C., Johnson, R.E., Protti, A.M., Ott, C., & Kajisa, L. (1985). Plasticity in the 904-day-old male cerebral cortex. *Experimental Neurology, 87,* 309-317.

Dustman, R.E., Emmerson, R.Y., Ruhling, R.O., Shearer, D.E., Steinhaus, L.A., Johnson, S.C., Bonekat, H.W., & Shigeoka, J.W. (1990). Age and fitness effects on EEG, ERPs, visual sensitivity, and cognition. *Neurobiology of Aging, 11,* 193-200.

Dustman, R.E., Ruhling, R.O., Russell, E.M., Shearer, D.E., Bonekat, H.W., Shigeoka, J.W., Wood, J.S., & Bradford, D.C. (1984). Aerobic exercise training and improved neuropsychological function of older individuals. *Neurobiology of Aging, 5,* 35-42.

Earles, J.L., & Salthouse, T.A. (1995). Interrelations of age, health, and speed. *Journal of Gerontology: Psychological Sciences, 50B,* P33-P41.

Elias, M.F., & Schlager, G. (1974). Discrimination learning in mice genetically selected for high and low blood pressure: Initial findings and methodological implications. *Physiology and Behavior, 13,* 261-267.

Elsayed, M., Ismail, A.H., & Young, R.J. (1980). Intellectual differences of adult men related to age and physical fitness before and after an exercise program. *Journal of Gerontology, 35,* 383-387.

Emery, C.F., & Gatz, M. (1990). Psychological and cognitive effects of an exercise program for community-residing older adults. *Gerontologist, 30,* 184-188.

Emery, C.F., Huppert, F.A., & Schein, R.L. (1995). Relationships among age, exercise, health, and cognitive function in a British sample. *Gerontologist, 35,* 378-385.

Emmerson, R.Y., Dustman, R.E., & Shearer, D.E. (1989). P3 latency and symbol digit performance correlations in aging. *Experimental Aging Research, 15,* 151-159.

Era, P. (1988). Sensory, psychomotor, and motor functions in men of different ages. *Scandinavian Journal of Social Medicine, 39,* (Supplement), 9-77.

Etnier, J.E., Johnston, R., Dagenbach, D., Pollard, R.J., Rejeski, W.J., & Berry, M. (1999). The relationships among pulmonary function, aerobic fitness, and cognitive functioning in older COPD patients. *Chest, 116,* 953-960.

Etnier, J.L., & Landers, D.M. (1997). The influence of age and fitness on performance and learning. *Journal of Aging and Physical Activity, 5,* 175-189.

Floeter, M.K., & Greenough, W.T. (1979). Cerebellar plasticity: Modification of Purkinje cell structure by differential rearing in monkeys. *Science, 206,* 227-229.

Fordyce, D.E., & Farrar, R.P. (1991a). Enhancement of spatial learning in F344 rats by physical activity and related learning-associated alterations in hippocampal and cortical cholinergic functioning. *Behavioural Brain Research, 46,* 123-133.

Fordyce, D.E., & Farrar, R.P. (1991b). Physical activity effects on hippocampal and parietal cortical cholinergic function and spatial learning in F344 rats. *Behavioural Brain Research, 43,* 115-125.

Friedland, R.P. (1990). Brain imaging and cerebral metabolism. In F. Boller & J. Grafman (Eds.), *Handbook of neuropsychology* (pp. 197-211). North Holland: Elsevier Science.

Gentile, A., Behesti, Z., & Held, J.M. (1987). Environment vs. exercise effects on motor impairments following cortical lesions in rats. *Behavior and Neural Biology, 47,* 321-332.

Gibson, D., Karpovich, P.V., & Gollnick, P.D. (1961). *Effect of training upon reflex and reaction time* (Research Report DA-49-007-MD-889). Washington, DC: Office of the Surgeon General.

Gilliam, P.E., Spirduso, W.W., Martin, T.P., Walters, T.J., Wilcox, R.E., & Farrar, R.P. (1984). The effects of exercise training on (3H)-spiperone binding in rat striatum. *Pharmacology, Biochemistry, and Behavior, 20,* 863-867.

Gur, R.C., Gur, R.E., Obrist, W.D., Skolnick, B.E., & Reivich, M. (1987). Age and regional cerebral blood flow at rest and during cognitive activity. *Archives of General Psychiatry, 44,* 617-621.

Guralnik, J.M., Simonsick, E.M., & Ferrucci, L., Glynn, R.J., Berkman, L.F., Blazer, D.G., et al. (1994). A short physical performance battery assessing lower extremity function: Association with self-reported disability and prediction of mortality and nursing home admission. *Journal of Gerontology, Medicine, & Science, 49,* M85-M94.

Hall, C.D., Smith, A.L., & Keele, S.W. (2001). The impact of aerobic activity on cognitive function in older adults: A new synthesis based on the concept of executive control. *European Journal of Cognitive Psychology, 13,* 279-300.

Hall, J.L., Gonder-Frederick, L.A., Chewning, W.W., Silveira, J., & Gold, P.E. (1989). Glucose enhancement of performance on memory tests in young and aged humans. *Neuropsychologia, 27,* 1129-1138.

Hawkins, H.L., Kramer, A.F., & Capaldi, D. (1992). Aging, exercise, and attention. *Psychology and Aging, 7,* 643-653.

Held, J., Gordon, J., & Gentile, A.M. (1985). Environmental influences on locomotor recovery following cortical lesions in rats. *Journal of Behavioral Neuroscience, 99*(4), 678-690.

Hillman, C.H., Weiss, E.P., Hagberg, J.M., & Hatfield, B.D. (2002). The relationship of age and cardiovascular fitness to cognitive and motor processes. *Psychophysiology, 39,* 303-312.

Jacobs, E.A. (1971). Paper presented at the National Institute of Health Conference on Drug and Hyperbaric Oxygenation Therapies and Lucidity in the Aged, San Francisco, July 1971.

Jones, T.A., Hawrylak, N., Klintsova, A.Y., & Greenough, W.T. (1998). Brain damage, behavior rehabilitation recovery, and brain plasticity. *Mental Retardation and Developmental Disabilities Research Reviews, 4,* 231-237.

Kennedy, D.O., & Scholey, A.B. (2000). Glucose administration, heart rate and cognitive performance: Effects of increasing mental effort. *Psychopharmacology, 149*, 63-71.

Kramer, A.F., Colcombe, S., Erickson, K., Belopolsky, A., McAuley, E., Cohen, N.J., et al. (2002). Effects of aerobic fitness training on human cortical function: A proposal. *Journal of Molecular Neuroscience, 19*, 227-231.

Kramer, A.F., Hahn, S., McAuley, E., Cohen, N.J., Banich, M.T., Harrison, C., Chason, J., Boileau, R.A., Bardell, L., Colcombe, A., & Vakil, E. (2001). Exercise, aging and cognition: Healthy body, healthy mind? In A.D. Fisk & W. Rogers (Eds.), *Human factors interventions for the health care of older adults*. Hillsdale, NJ: Erlbaum: 91-120.

Kramer, A.F., Sowon, H., Cohen, N.J., Banich, M.T., McAuley, E., Harrison, C.R., Chason, J., Vakil, E., Bardell, L., Boileau, R.A., & Colcombe, A. (1999). Ageing, fitness, and neurocognitive function. *Nature, 400*, 418-419.

Landfield, P.W., & Lynch, G. (1977, November). Brain aging and plasma steroids: Quantitative correlations. *Society for Neuroscience Abstracts*.

Lehr, U., & Thomae, H. (1973). Determinants of "aging": Findings from a longitudinal study. *Zeitschrift für Alternsforschung, 27*, 369-372.

MacRae, P.G., Lee, C., Crum, C.Y., Giessman, D., Greene, J.S., & Ugolini, J.A. (1995). Fractionated reaction time in women as a function of age and physical activity level. *Journal of Aging and Physical Activity, 4*, 14-26.

MacRae, P.G., Spirduso, W.W., Walters, T.J., Farrar, R.P., & Wilcox, R.E. (1987). Endurance training effects on striated D2 dopamine receptor binding and striatal dopamine metabolites in presenescent older rats. *Psychopharmacology, 92*, 236-241.

Manning, C.A., Stone, W.S., Korol, D.L., & Gold, P.E. (1998). Glucose enhancement of 24-h memory retrieval in healthy elderly humans. *Behavior and Brain Research, 93*, 71-76.

McCloskey, D.P., Adamo, D.S., & Anderson, B.J. (2001). Exercise increases metabolic capacity in the motor cortex and striatum, but not in the hippocampus. *Brain Research, 891*, 168-175.

Meltzer, C.C., Cantwell, M.N., Greer, P.J., Ben-Eliezer, D., Smith, G., Frank, G., et al. (2000). Does cerebral blood flow decline in healthy aging? A PET study with partial-volume correction. *Journal of Nuclear Medicine, 41*, 1842-1848.

Milligan, W.L., Powell, D.A., Harley, C., & Furchtgott, E. (1984). A comparison of physical health and psychosocial variables as predictors of reaction time and serial learning performance in elderly men. *Journal of Gerontology, 39*, 704-710.

Moss, M.C., & Scholey, A.B. (1996). Oxygen administration enhances memory formation in healthy young adults. *Psychopharmacology, 124*, 255-260.

Moss, M.C., Scholey, A.B., & Wesnes, K. (1998). Oxygen administration selectively enhances cognitive performance in healthy young adults: A placebo-controlled double blind crossover study. *Psychopharmacology, 138*, 27-33.

Panton, L.B., Graves, J.E., Pollock, M.L., Hagberg, J.M., & Chen, W. (1990). Effect of aerobic and resistance training on fractionated reaction time and speed of movement. *Journal of Gerontology: Medical Sciences, 45*, M26-M31.

Perlmutter, M., & Nyquist, L. (1990). Relationships between self-reported physical and mental health and intelligence performance across adulthood. *Journal of Gerontology: Psychological Sciences, 45*, P145-P155.

Pysh, J.J., & Weiss, G.M. (1979). Exercise during development induces an increase in Purkinje cell dendritic tree size. *Science, 206*, 230-231.

Rikli, R.E., & Edwards, D.J. (1991). Effects of a three-year exercise program on motor function and cognitive processing speed in older women. *Research Quarterly for Exercise and Sport, 62*, 61-67.

Rogers, R.L., Meyer, J.S., & Mortel, K.F. (1990). After reaching retirement age physical activity sustains cerebral perfusion and cognition. *Journal of the American Geriatrics Society, 38*, 123-128.

Russo-Neustadt, A., Ha, T., Ramirez, R., & Kesslak, J.P. (2001). Physical activity antidepressant treatment combination: Impact on brain-derived neurotrophic factor and behavior in an animal model. *Behavioral Brain Research, 120*, 87-95.

Salthouse, T.A. (1991). *Theoretical perspectives on cognitive aging*. Hillsdale, NJ: Erlbaum.

Sands, L.P., & Meredith, W. (1992). Blood pressure and intellectual functioning in late midlife. *Journal of Gerontology: Psychological Sciences, 47*, P81-P84.

Schneider, W., & Shiffrin, R.M. (1977). Controlled and automatic human information processing I: Detection, search, and attention. *Psychological Review, 84*, 1-66.

Scholey, A.B., Harper, S., & Kennedy, D.O. (2001). Cognitive demand and blood glucose. *Physiology and Behavior, 73*, 585-592.

Scholey, A.B., Moss, M.C., Neave, N., & Wesnes, K. (1999). Cognitive performance, hyperoxia, and heart rate following oxygen administration in healthy young adults. *Physiology and Behavior, 67,* 783-789.

Scholey, A.B., Moss, M.C., & Wesnes, K. (1998). Oxygen and cognitive performance: The temporal relationship between hyperoxia and enhanced memory. *Psychopharmacology, 140,* 123-126.

Shaw, T.G., Mortel, K.F., Meyer, J.S., Rogers, R.L., Hardenberg, J., & Cutaia, M.M. (1984). Cerebral blood flow changes in benign aging and cerebrovascular disease. *Neurology, 34,* 855-862.

Sherwood, D.E., & Selder, D.J. (1979). Cardiorespiratory health, reaction time, and aging. *Medicine and Science in Sports, 11,* 186-189.

Shumway-Cook, A., Woollacott, M., Kerns, K.A., & Baldwin, M. (1997). The effects of two types of cognitive tasks on postural stability in older adults with and without a history of falls. *Journal of Gerontology: Biological and Medical Scences, 52,* M232-M240.

Slosman, D.O., Chicherio, C., Ludwig, C., Genton, L., deRibaupierre, S., Hans, D., et al. (2001). ^{133}Xe SPECT cerebral blood flow study in a healthy population: Determination of T-scores. *Journal of Nuclear Medicine, 42,* 864-870.

Spirduso, W.W. (1975). Reaction and movement time as a function of age and physical activity level. *Journal of Gerontology, 30,* 435-440.

Spirduso, W.W. (1980). Physical fitness, aging, and psychomotor speed: A review. *Journal of Gerontology, 35,* 850-865.

Spirduso, W.W., & Clifford, P. (1978). Neuromuscular speed and consistency of performance as a function of age, physical activity level, and type of activity. *Journal of Gerontology, 33,* 26-30.

Spirduso, W.W., & Farrar, R.P. (1981). Effects of aerobic training on reactive capacity: An animal model. *Journal of Gerontology, 36,* 654-662.

Stacey, C., Kozma, A., & Stones, M.J. (1985). Simple cognitive and behavioral changes resulting from improved physical fitness in persons over 50 years of age. *Canadian Journal on Aging, 4,* 67-73.

Stewart, S.T., Zelinski, E.M., & Wallace, R.B. (2000). Age, medical conditions, and gender as interactive predictors of cognitive performance: The effects of selective survival. *Journal of Gerontology: Psychological Sciences, 55B,* P381-P383.

Stones, M.J., & Kozma, A. (1988). Physical activity, age, and cognitive/motor performance. In M.L. Howe & C.J. Brainerd (Eds.), *Cognitive development in adulthood: Progress in cognitive development research* (pp. 273-321). New York: Springer-Verlag.

Stones, M.J., & Kozma, A. (1989). Age, exercise, and coding performance. *Psychology and Aging, 4,* 190-194.

Suominen, H., Heikkinen, E., Parkatti, T., Forsberg, S., & Kiiskinen, A. (1980). Effects of "lifelong" physical training on functional aging in men. *Scandinavian Journal of Social Medicine, 55,* 225-240.

Thomas, J.R., Landers, D.M., Salazar, W., & Etnier, J. (1994). Exercise and cognitive function. In C. Bouchard, R.J. Shephard, & T. Stephens (Eds.), *Physical activity, fitness, and health* (pp. 521-529). Champaign, IL: Human Kinetics.

Tomporowski, P.D. (2003). Effects of acute bouts of exercise on cognition. *Acta Psychologica,* 112: 297-324.

Tomporowski, P.D., & Ellis, N.R. (1986). Effects of exercise on cognitive processes: A review. *Psychological Bulletin, 99,* 338-346.

Van Boxtel, M.P.J., Buntinx, F., Houx, P.J., Metsemakers, J.F.M., Knottnerus, A., & Jolles, J. (1998). The relation between morbidity and cognitive performance in a normal aging population. *Journal of Gerontology: Medical Sciences, 53:* M147-M154.

Vanfraechem, A., & Vanfraechem, R. (1977). Studies of the effect of a short training period on aged subjects. *Journal of Sports Medicine and Physical Fitness, 17,* 373-380.

Vissing, J., Andersen, M., & Diemer, N.H. (1996). Exercise-induced changes in local cerebral glucose utilization in the rat. *Journal of Cerebral Blood Flow and Metabolism, 16,* 729-736.

Vogt, C., & Vogt, O. (1946). Aging of nerve cells. *Nature, 58,* 304.

Warren, L.R., Butler, R.W., Katholi, C.R., & Halsey, J.H., Jr. (1985). Age differences in cerebral blood flow during rest and during mental activation measurements with and without monetary incentive. *Journal of Gerontology, 40,* 53-59.

Wechsler, D. (1981). *Manual for the Weschler Adult Intelligence Scale–Revised.* New York: Psychological Corporation.

Williams, M., & Hornberger, J.A. (1984). A quantitative method of identifying older persons at risk for increasing long-term care services. *Journal of Chronic Diseases, 37,* 705-711.

Winder, R., & Borrill, J. (1998). Fuels for memory: The role of oxygen and glucose in memory enhancement. *Psychopharmacology, 136,* 349-356.

Woodruff, D. (1985). Arousal, sleep, and aging. In J.E. Birren & K.W. Schaie (Eds.), *Handbook of the psychology of aging* (2nd ed., pp. 261-295). New York: Van Nostrand Reinhold.

Woods, A.M. (1981). *Age differences in the effect of physical activity and postural changes on information processing speed.* Doctoral dissertation, University of Southern California, Los Angeles.

Ylikoski, R., Ylikoski, A., Raininko, R., Keskivaara, P., Sulkava, R., Tilvis, R., & Erkinjuntti, T. (2000). Cardiovascular diseases, health status, brain imaging findings and neurologically healthy elderly individuals. *Archives of Gerontology and Geriatrics, 30,* 115-130.

Chapter 10

Appenzeller, O., & Schade, D.R. (1979). Neurology of endurance training III: Sympathetic activity during a marathon run. *Neurology, 29,* 542.

Arent, S.M., Landers, D.M., & Etnier, J. (2000). The effects of exercise on mood in older adults: A meta-analytic review. *Journal of Aging and Physical Activity, 8,* 407-430.

Bahrke, M.S., & Morgan, W.P. (1978). Anxiety reduction following exercise and meditation. *Cognitive Therapy and Research, 2,* 323-333.

Barchas, J.D., & Freedman, D.X. (1963). Brain amines: Response to physiological stress. *Biochemistry and Pharmacology, 12,* 1232-1235.

Bandura, A. (1986). *Social foundations of thought and action: A social cognitive theory.* Englewood Cliffs, NJ: Prentice Hall.

Bandura, A. (1997). Health promotion from the perspective of social cognitive theory. *Psychology and Health, 13,* 623-649.

Beck, A.T., & Beamesderfer, A. (1974). Assessment of depression: The Depression Inventory. In P.Pichot (Ed.). *Psychological measurements in psychopharmacology* (pp. 1-10). Basel: Karger.

Billig, N. (1987). *To be old and sad.* New York: Lexington Books.

Blumenthal, J.A., Babyak, M.A., Moore, K.A., Craighead, W.E., Herman, S., Khatri, P., Waugh, R., Napolitano, M.A., Forman, L.M., Appelbaum, M., Doraiswamy, P.M., & Krishnan, K.R. (1999). Effects of exercise training on older patients with major depression. *Archives of Internal Medicine, 159,* 2349-2356.

Blumenthal, J.A., Emery, C.F., Madden, D.J., George, L.R., Coleman, R.E., Roddle, M.W., et al. (1989). Cardiovascular and behavioral effects of aerobic exercise training in healthy older men and women.

Journal of Gerontology: Medical Science, 44, M147-M157.

Brown, B.S., Payne, T., Kim, C., Moore, G., Krebs, P., & Martin, W. (1979). Chronic response of rat brain norepinephrine and serotonin levels to endurance training. *Journal of Applied Physiology, 46,* 19-23.

Brown, B.S., & Van Huss, W. (1973). Exercise and rat brain catecholamines. *Journal of Applied Physiology, 34,* 664-669.

Brown, R.S., Ramirez, D.E., & Taub, J.M. (1978). The prescription of exercise for depression. *Physician and Sportsmedicine, 6,* 34-45.

Brown, W.J., Mishra, G., Lee, C., & Bauman, A. (2000). Leisure time physical activity in Australian women: Relationship with well being and symptoms. *Research Quarterly of Exercise and Sport, 71,* 206-218.

Camacho, T.C., Roberts, R.E., Lazarus, N.B., Kaplan, G.A., & Cohen, R.D. (1991). Physical activity and depression: Evidence from the Alameda County Study. *American Journal of Epidemiology, 134,* 220-231.

Cannon, J.G., & Kluger, M.J. (1983). Endogenous pyrogen activity in human plasma after exercise. *Science, 220,* 617-619.

Carr, D., Bullen, B.A., Skrinar, G.S., Arnold, M.A., Rosenblatt, M., Beitins, I.Z., Martin, J.B., & McArthur, J.W. (1981). Physical conditioning facilities for the exercise-induced secretion of beta-endorphins and beta-lipoprotein in women. *New England Journal of Medicine, 305,* 560-563.

Centers for Disease Control. (1996). Suicide among older persons—United States, 1980-1992. *Morbidity and Mortality Weekly Report, 45*(01), 3.

Clark, D.O. (1996). Age, socioeconomic status, and exercise self-efficacy. *Gerontologist, 36,* 157-164.

Clark, D.O. (1999). Physical activity and its correlates among urban primary care patients aged 55 years or older. *Journal of Gerontology, 54B,* S41-S48.

Conn, V.S. (1998). Older adults and exercise: Path analysis of self-efficacy related constructs. *Nursing Research, 47,* 180-189.

Craft, L.L., & Landers, D.M. (1998). The effect of exercise on clinical depression and depression resulting from mental illness: A meta-analysis. *Journal of Sport and Exercise Psychology, 20,* 339-357.

Crandall, R.C. (1991*). Gerontology: A behavioral science approach.* New York: McGraw-Hill.

DeCastro, J.M., & Duncan, G. (1985). Operantly conditioned running: Effects on brain catecholamine concentrations and receptor densities in the rat. *Pharmacology, Biochemistry & Behavior, 23,* 495-500.

deVries, H.A. (1987). Tension reduction with exercise. In W.P. Morgan & S.E. Goldston (Eds.), *Exercise and mental health* (pp. 99-104). Washington, DC: Hemisphere.

deVries, H.A., Wiswell, R.A., Bulbulian, R., & Moritani, T. (1981). Tranquilizer effect of exercise. *American Journal of Physical Medicine, 60,* 57-66.

Diener, E. (1984). Subjective well-being. *Psychological Bulletin, 95,* 542-575.

Diener, E., & Suh, M.E. (1997). Subjective well-being and age: An international analysis. In K.W. Schaie & M.P. Lawton (Eds.), *Annual review of gerontology and geriatrics* (Vol. 8, pp. 304-324). New York: Springer.

Dishman, R.K. (1985). Medical psychology in exercise and sport. *Medical Clinics of North America, 69,* 123-143.

Dishman, R.K. (1997). Brain monoamines, exercise, and behavioral stress: Animal models. *Medicine and Science of Exercise and Sport, 29,* 63-74.

Doyne, E.J., Ossip-Klein, D.J., Bowman, E.D., Osborn, K.M., McDougall-Wilson, I.B., & Neimeyer, R.A. (1987). Running versus weight lifting in the treatment of depression. *Journal of Consulting and Clinical Psychology, 55,* 748-754.

Dulac, S., Brisson, G.R., Proteau, L., Peronnet, F., Ledoux, M., & DeCarufel, D. (1982). Selected hormonal response to repeated short bouts of anaerobic exercise. *Medicine and Science in Sports and Exercise, 14,* 173-174.

Dunn, A.L., Trivedi, M.H., Kampert, J.B., O'Neal, H.A., & Clark, C.G. (2002). Exercise dose-response and the treatment of major depression. *Medicine and Science in Sports and Exercise, 34,* S239.

Ekkekakis, P., & Petruzzello, S.J. (1999). Acute aerobic exercise and affect. *Sports Medicine, 28,* 337-374.

Engels, H. J., Drouin, J., Zhu, W., & Kazmierski, J.F. (1998). Effects of low-impact, moderate-intensity exercise training with and without wrist weights on functional capacities and mood states in older adults. *Gerontology, 44,* 239-244.

Farrell, P.A., Gustafson, A.B., Garthwaite, T.L., Kalkhoff, R.K., Cowley, A.W., Jr., & Morgan, W.P. (1986). Influence of endogenous opioids on the response of selected hormones to exercise in humans. *Journal of Applied Physiology, 61,* 1051-1057.

Folkins, C.H., & Sime, W.E. (1981). Physical fitness training and mental health. *American Psychologist, 36,* 373-389.

Ford, H.T., Puckett, J.R., Reeve, T.G., & Lafavi, R.G. (1991). Effects of selected physical activities on global self-concept and body-cathexis score. *Psychological Reports, 68,* 1339-1343.

Forrester, D.A. (1987). Affective disorders and suicide. In J. Norris, M. Kunes-Connell, S. Stockard, P. Mayer-Ehrhart, & G.R. Renschler-Newton (Eds.), *Mental health psychiatric nursing—A continuum of care* (pp. 761-767). New York: Wiley.

Freudenheim, E. (1996). *Chronic care in America: A 21st century challenge.* Princeton, NJ: Robert Wood Johnson Foundation.

Gauvin, L., & Rejeski, W.J. (1993). The exercise induced feeling inventory: Development and initial validation. *Journal of Sport and Exercise Psychology, 15,* 403-423.

George, L.K. (1979). The happiness syndrome: Methodological and substantive issues in the study of social-psychological well-being in adulthood. *The Gerontologist, 19,* 210-216.

Gergen, K.J. (1971). *The concept of self.* New York: Holt, Rinehart, & Winston.

Gergen, K.J. (1981). The functions and foibles of negotiating self-conceptions. In M.D. Lynch, A.A. Norem-Hebeisen, & K.J. Gergen (Eds.), *Self-concept: Advances in theory and research* (pp. 59-73). Cambridge, MA: Ballingurt.

Gill, T.M. (2002). Geriatric medicine: It's more than caring for old people. *American Journal of Medicine, 113,* 85-89.

Glasser, W. (1976). *Positive addiction.* New York: Harper & Row.

Grembowski, D., Patrick, D., Diehr, P., Durham, M., Beresford, S., Kay, E., & Hecht, J. (1993). Self-efficacy and health behavior among older adults. *Journal of Health and Social Behavior, 34,* 89-104.

Harris, M.B. (1994). Growing old gracefully: Age concealment and gender. *Journal of Gerontology, 49,* 149-158.

Hassmén, P., & Kolvula, N. (1997). Mood, physical working capacity and cognitive performance in the elderly as related to physical activity. *Aging Clinical and Experimental Research, 9,* 136-142.

Hatfield, B.D., & Landers, D.M. (1987). Psychophysiology in exercise and sport research: An overview. *Exercise and Sport Sciences Reviews, 15,* 351-387.

HealthyPlace.com (2004). The suicide of older men and women. [Online http://www.healthyplace.com/communities/depression/related/suicide_3.asp [Accessed 6.14.04]

Hollmann, W., Rost, R., DeMeirleir, K., Liesen, H., Heck, H., & Mader, A. (1986). Cardiovascular effects of extreme physical training. *Acta Medica Scandinavia, Suppl. 711*, 193-203.

Hughes, J.R., Casal, D.C., & Leon, A.S. (1986). Psychological effects of exercise: A randomized cross-over trial. *Journal of Psychosomatic Research, 10*, 355-360.

Jacobs, B.L. (1994). Serotonin, motor activity and depression-related disorders. *American Scientist, 82*, 456-463.

Kennedy, M.M., & Newton, M. (1997). Effect of exercise intensity on mood in step aerobics. *Journal of Sports Medicine and Physical Fitness, 37*, 200-204.

King, A.C., Baumann, K., O'Sullivan, P., Wilcox, S., & Castro, C. (2002). Effects of moderate-intensity exercise on physiological, behavioral, and emotional responses to family caregiving: A randomized controlled trial. *Journal of Gerontology: A Biological and Medical Sciences, 57*, M26-M36.

King, A.C., Taylor, C.B., & Haskell, W.L. (1993). Effects of differing intensities and formats of 12 months of exercise training on psychological outcomes in older adults. *Health Psychology, 12*, 292-300.

King, A.C., Taylor, C.B., Haskell, W.L., & DeBusk, R.F. (1989). Influence of regular aerobic exercise on psychological health: A randomized, controlled trial of healthy middle-aged adults. *Health Psychology, 8*, 305-324.

Kirkcaldy, B.D., & Shephard, R.J. (1990). Therapeutic implications of exercise. *International Journal of Sport Psychology, 21*, 165-184.

Kunzmann, U., Little, T.D., & Smith, J. (2000). Is age-related stability of subjective well-being a paradox? Cross-sectional and longitudinal evidence from the Berlin aging study. *Psychology and Aging, 15*, 511-526.

Laraia, M.T. (1987). Psychopharmacology. In G.W. Stuart & S.J. Sundeen (Eds.), *Principles and practice of psychiatric nursing* (pp. 699-738). St Louis: Mosby.

Larson, R. (1978). Thirty years of research on the subjective well-being of older Americans. *Journal of Gerontology, 33*, 109-125.

Lobstein, D.D., Rasmussen, C.L., Dunphy, G.E., & Dunphy, M.J. (1989). Beta-endorphin and components of depression as powerful discriminators between joggers and sedentary middle-aged men. *Journal of Psychosomatic Research, 33*, 293-305.

Loland, N.W. (2000). The aging body: Attitudes toward bodily appearance among physically active and inactive women and men of different ages. *Journal of Aging and Physical Activity, 8*, 197-213.

Lox, C.L., & Freehill, A.J. (1999). The impact of pulmonary rehabilitation on self-efficacy, quality of life, and exercise tolerance. *Rehabilitative Psychology, 44*, 1-14.

Martinsen, E.W. (1990). Benefits of exercise for the treatment of depression. *Sports Medicine, 9*, 380-389.

Matheny, K.B., Aycock, D.W., Pugh, J.L., Curlette, W.L., & Cannella, K.A.S. (1986). Stress coping : A qualitative and quantitative synthesis with implications for treatment. *Counseling Psychologist, 14*, 499-549.

Mather, A.S., Rodriguez, C., Guthrie, M.F., McHarg, A.M., Reid, I.C., & McMurdo, M.E. (2002). Effects of exercise on depressive symptoms in older adults with poorly responsive depressive disorder: Randomized controlled trial. *British Journal of Psychiatry, 180*, 411-415.

McAuley, E., & Blissmer, B. (2000). Self-efficacy determinants and consequences of physical activity. *Exercise and Sport Sciences Reviews, 28*, 85-88.

McAuley, E., & Courneya, K.S. (1994). The Subjective Exercise Experiences Scale (SEES): Development and preliminary validation. *Journal of Sport and Exercise Psychology, 16*, 163-177.

McAuley, E., Lox, C., & Duncan, T. (1993). Long-term maintenance of exercise, self-efficacy, and physiological change in older adults. *Journal of Gerontology, 48*, 218-224.

McAuley, E., & Rudolph, D. (1995). Physical activity, aging, and psychological well-being. *Journal of Aging and Physical Activity, 3*, 67-96.

McNeil, J.K., LeBlanc, E.M., & Joyner, M. (1991). The effect of exercise on depressive symptoms in the moderately depressed elderly. *Psychology and Aging, 6*, 487-488.

Meeusen, R., Piacentini, M.F., Van den Eynde, S., Magnus, L., & De Meirleir, K. (2001). Exercise performance is not influenced by a 5-HT reuptake inhibitor. *International Journal of Sports Medicine, 22*, 329-336.

Mendes de Leon, C.F., Seeman, T.E., Baker, D.I., Richardson, E.D., & Tinetti, M.E. (1996). Self-efficacy, physical decline, and change in functioning in community-living elders: A prospective study. *Journal of Gerontology: Psychological Science and Social Sciences, 51B*, S183-S190.

Miller, L.C., Murphy, R., & Buss, A.H. (1981). Consciousness of body: Private and public. *Journal of Personality and Social Psychology, 41*, 397-406.

Moore, K.A., Babyak, M.A., Wood, C.E., Napolitano, M.A., Khatri, P., Craighead, W.E., Herman, S., Krishnan, R., & Blumenthal, J.A. (1999). The association between physical activity and depression in older depressed adults. *Journal of Aging and Physical Activity, 7*, 55-61.

Morgan, W.P. (1985). Affective beneficence of vigorous physical activity. *Medicine and Science in Sports and Exercise, 17*, 94-100.

Morgan, W.P., & O'Connor, P.J. (1988). Exercise and mental health. In R.K. Dishman (Ed.), *Exercise adherence: Its impact on public health* (pp. 91-121). Champaign, IL: Human Kinetics.

Moses, J., Steptoe, A., Matthews, A., & Edwards, S. (1989). The effects of exercise on mental well-being in the normal population: A controlled trial. *Journal of Psychonomic Research, 33*, 47-61.

Moss, F.E., & Halamandaris, V.J. (1977). *Too old, too sick, too bad: Nursing homes in America.* Germantown, MD: Aspen Systems.

National Institute of Mental Health (2003). Older Adults: Depression and suicide facts. [Online] http://www.nimh.nih.gov/publicat/elderlydepsuicide.cfm [06.13.04]

Nicoloff, G., & Schwenk, T.L. (1995). Using exercise to ward off depression. *Physician and Sportsmedicine, 23*, 44-58.

North, T.C., McCullagh, P., & Tran, Z.V. (1990). Effect of exercise on depression. In K.B. Pandolph & J.O. Holloszy (Eds.), *Exercise and sport science reviews.* 18, 379-415. Baltimore: Williams & Wilkins.

O'Connor, P.J., Aenchbacher, L.E., & Dishman, R.K. (1993). Physical activity and depression in the elderly. *Journal of Aging and Physical Activity, 1*, 34-58.

Okun, M.A., & Stock, W.A. (1987). Correlates and components of subjective well-being among the elderly. *Journal of Applied Gerontology, 6*, 95-112.

Oleson, J. (1971). Contralateral focal increase of cerebral blood flow in man during arm work. *Brain, 94*, 635-646.

Olson, M.I. (1975). *The effects of physical activity on the body image of nursing home residents.* Unpublished master's thesis, Springfield College, Springfield, MA.

Osterweis, M., Solomon, F., & Green, M. (Eds.) (1984). *Bereavement: Reactions, consequences, and care.* Washington, DC: National Academy Press.

Penninx, B.W.J.H., Rejeski, W.J., Pandya, J., Miller, M.E., Di Bari, M., Applegate, W.B., & Pahor, M. (2002). Exercise and depressive symptoms: A comparison of aerobic and resistance exercise effects on emotional and physical function in older persons with high and low depressive symptomatology. *Journal of Gerontology: Psychological Sciences, 57B*, P124-P132.

Plante, T.G., & Rodin, J. (1990). Physical fitness and enhanced psychological health. *Current Psychology: Research and Reviews, 9*, 3-24.

Raglin, J.S., & Morgan, W.P. (1987). Influence of exercise and quiet rest on state anxiety and blood pressure. *Medicine and Science in Sports and Exercise, 19*, 456-463.

Rahkila, P., Hakala, E., Salminen, K., & Laatkainen, T. (1987). Response of plasma endorphins to running exercises in male and female endurance athletes. *Medicine and Science in Sports and Exercise, 19*, 451-455.

Ransford, C.P. (1982). A role for amines in the antidepressant effect of exercise: A review. *Medicine and Science in Sports and Exercise, 14*, 1-10.

Resnick, B. (2001). Testing a model of overall activity in older adults. *Journal of Aging and Physical Activity, 9*, 142-160.

Risch, S.C. (1982). B-endorphin hypersecretion in depression: Possible cholinergic mechanisms. *Biological Psychiatry, 17*, 1071-1079.

Robbins, J.M., & Joseph, P. (1985). Experiencing exercise withdrawal: Possible consequences of therapeutic and mastery running. *Journal of Sport Psychology, 7*, 23-29.

Ruuskanen, J.M., & Ruoppila, I. (1995). Physical activity and psychological well-being among people aged 65 to 84 years. *Age and Ageing, 24*, 292-296.

Ryff, C.D. (1989). In the eye of the beholder: Views of psychological well-being among middle-aged and older adults. *Psychology and Aging, 4*, 206.

Schaie, K.W., & Geiwitz, J. (1982). *Adult development and aging.* Boston: Little, Brown.

Schieman, S., & Turner, H. (1998). Age, disability, and the sense of mastery. *Journal of Health and Social Behavior, 39*, 169-186.

Seeman, T.E., Berkman, L.F., & Charpentier, P.A. (1995). Behavioral and psychosocial predictors of physical performance: MacArthur Studies of Successful Aging. *Journal of Gerontology: Medical Sciences, 50A*, M177-M183.

Seeman, T.E., Unger, J.B., McAvay, G., & Mendes de Leon, C.F. (1999). Self-efficacy beliefs and perceived declines in functional ability: MacArthur studies of successful aging. *Journal of Gerontology: Psychological Science, 54B*, P214-P222.

Shavelson, R.J., Hubner, J.J., & Stanton, J.C. (1976). Self-concept: Validation of construct interpretations. *Review of Educational Research, 46*, 407-441.

Shephard, R.J. (1987). *Physical activity and aging* (2nd ed.). Rockville, MD: Aspen Publishers.

Siever, L.J., & Davis, K.L. (1985). Overview: Toward a dysregulation hypothesis of depression. *American Journal of Psychiatry, 142*, 1017-1031.

Sime, W.E. (1984). Psychological benefits of exercise training in the healthy individual. In J.D. Matarazzo, S.M. Weiss, J.A. Herd, N.A. Miller, & S.M. Weiss, (Eds.). *Behavioral health: A handbook of health enhancement and disease prevention* (pp. 488-508). New York: Wiley.

Simonsick, E.M., Lafferty, M.E., Phillips, C.L., Mendes de Leon, C.F., Kasl, S.V., Seeman, T.E., et al. (1993). Risk due to inactivity in physically capable older adults. *American Journal of Public Health, 83*, 1443-1450.

Singh, N.A., Clements, K.M., & Fiatarone, M.A. (1997). A randomized controlled trial of the effect of exercise on sleep. *Sleep, 20*, 95-101.

Singh, N.A., Clements, K.M., & Singh, M.A. (2001). The efficacy of exercise as a long-term antidepressant in elderly subjects: A randomized, controlled trial. *Journal of Gerontology: Biological and Medical Sciences, 56*, M497-504.

Sonstroem, R.J. (1984). Exercise and self-esteem. *Exercise and Sport Sciences Reviews, 12*, 123-155.

Sonstroem, R.J., & Morgan, W.P. (1989). Exercise and self-esteem: Rationale and model. *Medicine and Science of Sports and Exercise, 64*, 335-342.

Sonstroem, R.J., Harlow, L.L., & Josephs, L. (1994). Exercise and self-esteem: Validity of model expansion and exercise associations. *Journal of Sport and Exercise Psychology, 16*, 29-42.

Spirduso, W., & Cronin, L. (2001). Exercise dose-response effects on quality of life and independent living in older adults. *Medicine and Science in Sports and Exercise, 33*(Suppl.), S598-S608.

Stathi, A., Fox, K.R., & McKenna, J. (2002). Physical activity and dimensions of subjective well-being in older adults. *Journal of Aging and Physical Activity, 10*, 76-92.

Steptoe, A., & Cox, S. (1988). Acute effects of aerobic exercise on mood. *Health Psychology, 7*, 329-340.

Stewart, A.L., & King, A.C. (1991). Evaluating the efficacy of physical activity for influencing quality-of-life outcomes in older adults. *Annals of Behavioral Medicine, 13*, 111.

Stewart, A.L, King, A.C., & Haskell, W.L. (1993). Endurance exercise and health-related quality of life in 50-65 year old adults. *Gerontology, 33*, 782-789.

Stewart, A.L., Mills, K.M., Sepsis, P.G., King, A.C., McLellan, B.Y., Roitz, K., & Ritter, P.L. (1997). Evaluation of CHAMPS, a physical activity promotion program for older adults. *Annals of Behavioral Medicine, 19*, 353-361.

Stidwell, H.F., & Rimmer, J.H. (1995). Measurement of physical self-efficacy in an elderly population. *Clinical Kinesiology, 49*, 58-63.

Strawbridge, W.J., Cohen, R.D., Shema, S.J., & Kaplan, G.A. (1996). Successful aging: Predictors and associated activities. *American Journal of Epidemiology, 144*, 135-141.

Tafarodi, R.W., & Swann, W.B. (1995). Self-liking and self-competence as dimensions of global self-esteem: Initial validation of a measure. *Journal of Personality Assessment, 65*, 322-342.

Takkinen, S., Suutama, T., & Ruoppila, I. (2001). More meaning by exercising? Physical activity as a predictor of a sense of meaning in life. *Journal of Aging and Physical Activity, 9*, 128-141.

Thoren, P., Floras, J.S., Hoffman, P., & Seals, D.R. (1990). Endorphins and exercise: Physiological mechanisms and clinical implications. *Medicine and Science in Sports and Exercise, 22*, 417-428.

Tsutsumi, T., Don, B.M., Zaichkowsky, L.D., Takenaka, K., Oka, K., & Ohno, T. (1998). Comparison of high and moderate intensity of strength training on mood and anxiety in older adults. *Perceptual and Motor Skills, 87*, 1003-1011.

Veale, D.M.W. (1987). Exercise dependence. *British Journal of Addiction, 82*, 735-740.

Von Euler, C., & Soderberg, U. (1956). The relation between gamma motor activity and electroencephalogram. *Experimentia, 12*, 278-279.

Von Euler, C., & Soderberg, U. (1957). The influence of hypothalamic thermoceptive structures on the electroencephalogram and gamma motor activity. *EEG and Clinical Neurophysiology, 9*, 391-408.

Watson, D., Clark, L.A., & Telegen, A. (1988). Development and validation of brief measures of Positive and Negative affect: The PANAS Scales. *Journal of Personality and Social Psychology, 54*, 1063-1070.

Watson, D., & Tellegen, A. (1985). Toward a consensual structure of mood. *Psychological Bullentin, 98*, 219-235.

Williams, P., & Lord, S.R. (1997). Effects of group exercise on cognitive functioning and mood in older women. *Australian and New Zealand Journal of Public Health, 21,* 45-52.

Wolinsky, F.D., Stump, T.E., & Clark, D.O. (1995). Antecedents and consequences of physical activity and exercise among older adults. *The Gerontologist,* 35, 451-462.

Wolpe, J., Salter, A., & Reyna, L.J. (1964). *The conditioning therapies.* New York: Holt, Rinehart, & Winston.

Wood, R.H., Reyes-Alvarez, R., Maraj, B., Metoyer, K.I., & Welsch, M.A. (1999). Physical fitness, cognitive function, and health-related quality of life in older adults. *Journal of Aging and Physical Activity,* 7, 217-230.

Chapter 11

American college of Sports Medicine. (1991). *Guidelines for exercise testing and prescription.* Philadelphia: Lea and Febiger.

American College of Sports Medicine. (1998). Exercise and physical activity for older adults: Position stand. *Medicine and Science in Sports and Exercise,* 30(6), 992-1008.

Anderson-Ranberg, K., Christensen, K., Jeune, B., Skytthe, A., Vasegaard, L., & Vaupel, J.W. (1999). Declining physical abilities with age: A cross-sectional study of older twins and centenarians in Denmark. *Age and Ageing,* 28, 373-377.

Bassey, E.J., Fiatarone, M.A., O'Neill, E.F., Kelly, M., Evans, W.J., & Lipsitz, L.A. (1992). Leg extensor power and functional performance in very old men and women. *Clinical Science* (London). 82, 321-327.

Berger, B.G., & Hecht, L. (1989). Exercise, aging, and psychological well-being: The mind-body question. In A.C. Ostrow (Ed.), *Aging and motor behavior* (pp. 117-157). Indianapolis, IN: Benchmark Press.

Branch, L.G., Guralnik, J.M., Foley, D.J., Kohout, F.J., Wetle, T.T., Ostfeld, A., & Katz, S. (1991). Active life expectancy for 10,000 caucasian men and women in three communities. *Journal of Gerontology: Medical Sciences,* 46, M148.

Bravo, G., Gauthier, P., Roy, P., Tessier, D., Gaulin, P., Dubois, F., & Peloquin, L. (1994). The Functional Fitness Assessment Battery: Reliability and validity data for elderly women. *Journal of Aging and Physical Activity,* 2, 67-79.

Brown, M., Sinacore, D.R., Binder, E.F., & Kohrt, W.M. (2000). Physical and performance measures for the identification of mild to moderate frailty. *Journal of Gerontology: Medical Sciences,* 55A(6), M350-M355.

Brown, M., Sinacore, D.R., Ehsani, A.A., Binder, E.F., Holloszy, J.O., & Kohrt, W.M. (2000). Low-intensity exercise as a modifier of physical frailty in older adults. *Archives of Physical Medicine and Rehabilitation,* 81, 960-965.

Bruce, R.A. (1973). Exercise testing, for ventricular function. *New England Journal of Medicine,* 296, 671-675.

Campbell, A.J., & Buchner, D.M. (1997). Unstable disability and the fluctuations of frailty. *Age and Ageing,* 26, 315-318.

Cress, M.E., Buchner, D.M., Questad, K.A., Esselman, P.C., deLateur, B.J., & Schwartz, R.S. (1996). Continuous-scale physical functional performance in healthy older adults: A validation study. *Archives of Physical Medicine and Rehabilitation,* 77, 1243-1250.

Cunningham, D.A., Paterson, D.H., Himann, J.E., & Rechnitzer, P.A. (1993). Determinants of independence in the elderly. *Canadian Journal of Applied Physiology,* 18, 243-254.

Evans, W.J. (2000). Exercise strategies should be designed to increase muscle power. *Journal of Gerontology: Medical Sciences,* 55A(6), M309-M310.

Federal Interagency Forum on Aging Related Statistics. (2000). Older Americans 2000: Key indicators of well-being. [Online]. Available: www.aoa.gov/agingstats/chartbook2000 [05.29.04].

Fiatarone, M.A., O'Neill, E.F., Ryan, N.D., Clements, K.M., Solares, G.R., Nelson, M.E., Roberts, S.B., Kehayias, J.J., Lipsitz, L.A., & Evans, W.J. (1994). Exercise training and nutritional supplementation for the physical frailty in very elderly people. *New England Journal of Medicine,* 330(25), 1769-1775.

Fried, L.P., Bandeen-Roche, K., Williamson, J.D., Prasada-Rao, P., Chee, E., Tepper, S., & Rubin, G.S. (1996). Functional decline in older adults: Expanding methods of ascertainment. *Journal of Gerontology: Medical Sciences,* 51A(5), M206-M214.

Fries, J.F., Green, L.W., & Levine, S. (1989). Health promotion and the compression of morbidity. *The Lancet,* 8636, 481-483.

Gerety, M.B., Mulrow, M.R., Tuley, M.R., Huzuda, H., Lichtenstein, J.M., O'Neil, M., Gorton, A., & Bohannon, R. (1993). Development and validation of a physical performance instrument for the functionly impaired elderly: The Physical Disability Index (PDI). *Journal of Gerontology: Medical Sciences,* 48, M33-M38.

Granger, C.V., Mailton, B.B., Ketih, R.A., Zielezny, M., & Sherwin, F.S. (1986). Advances in functional assessment for medical rehabilitation. *Topics in Geriatric Rehabilitation,* 1(3), 59-74.

Guralnik, J.M., Ferrucci, L., Penninx, B.W., Kasper, J.D., Leveille, S.G., Bandeen-Roche, K., Fried, L.P. (1999). New and worsening conditions and change in physical and cognitive performance during weekly evaluations over 6 months: The Women's Health and Aging Study. *Journal of Gerontology: Biological Sciences, 54,* M410-M22.

Guralnik, J.M. & Simonsick, E.M. (1993). Physical disability in older Americans. *Journal of Gerontology, 48,* Special Review, No. 3-10.

Guralnik, J.M., Simonsick, E.M, Ferrucci, L., Glynn, R.J., Berkman, L.F., Blazer, D.G., et al. (1994). A short physical performance battery assessing lower extremity function: Association with self-reported disability and prediction of mortality and nursing home admission. *Journal of Gerontology; Medicine & Science, 49,* M85-M94.

Haskell, W.L. (1994). Health consequences of physical activity: Understanding and challenges regarding dose-response. *Medicine and Science in Sports and Exercise, 26(6),* 649-660.

Hirvensalo, M., Rantanen, T., & Heikkinen, E. (2000). Mobility difficulties and physical activity as predictors of mortality and loss of independence in the community-living older population. *Journal of the American Geriatrics Society, 48,* 1-6.

Hughes, S.L., Edelman, P., Chang, R.W., Singer, R.H., & Schuette, P. (1991). The GERI-AIMS. Reliability and validity of the arthritis impact measurement scales adapted for elderly respondents. *Arthritis and Rheumatism, 34,* 856-865.

Jette, A.M., Branch, L.G., & Berlin, J. (1990). Musculoskeletal impairments and physical disablement among the aged. *Journal of Gerontology: Medical Sciences, 45,* M203-M208.

Jette, A.M., Haley, S.M., Coster, W.J., Kooyoomjian, J.T., Levenson, S., Heeren, T., & Ashba, J. (2002). Late life function and disability instrument: I. Development and evaluation of the disability component. *Journal of Gerontology: Medical Sciences, 57A,* M209-M216.

Katz, G.H., Ford, A.B., Moskowitz, R.W., Jackson, B.A., & Jaffe, M.W. (1963). Studies of illness in the aged. The index of ADL: A standardized measure of biological and psychosocial function. *Journal of the American Medical Association, 185,* 914-919.

Katz, S., Branch, L.G., Branson, M.H., Papsidero, J.A., Beck, J.C., & Greer, D.S. (1983). Active life expectancy. *New England Journal of Medicine, 309,* 1218-1224.

Kempen, G.I.J.M., & Suurmeijer, T.P.B.M. (1990). The development of a hierarchical polychotomous ADL-IADL scale for noninstitutionalized elders. *The Gerontologist, 30,* 497-502.

Kimura, M., Hirakawa, K., & Morimoto, T. (1990). Physical performance survey in 900 aged individuals. In M. Kaneko (Ed.), *Fitness for the aged, disabled, and industrial worker* (pp. 55-60), Champaign, IL: Human Kinetics.

Kivinen, P., Sulkava, R., Halonen, P., & Nissinen, A. (1998). Self-reported and performance-based functional status and associated factors among elderly men: The Finnish cohorts of the Seven Countries Study. *Journal of Clinical Epidemiology, 51,* 1243-1252.

Kuo, G.H. (1990). Physical fitness of the people in Taipei including the aged. In M. Kaneko (Ed.), *Fitness for the aged, disabled, and industrial worker* (p. 22). Champaign, IL: Human Kinetics.

LaCroix, A.Z., Guralnik, J.M., Berkman, L., Wallace, R.B., & Satterfield, S. (1993). Maintaining mobility in late life II. Smoking, alcohol consumption, physical activity, and body mass index. *American Journal of Epidemiology, 137,* 858-869.

Laukkanen, P., Kauppinen, M., & Heikkinen, E. (1998). Physical activity as a predictor of health and disability in 75- and 80-year-old men and women: A five-year longitudinal study. *Journal of Aging and Physical Activity, 6,* 141-156.

Lawrence, R.H., & Jette, A.M. (1996). Disentangling the disablement process. *Journal of Gerontology: Social Sciences, 51B,* S173-S182.

Lawton, M.P., & Brody, E.M. (1969). Assessment of older people: Self-maintaining and instrumental activities of daily living. *The Gerontologist, 9,* 179-186.

Lemsky, C., Miller, C.J., Nevitt, M., & Winograd, C. (1991). Reliability and validity of a physical performance and mobility examination for hospitalized elderly. *Society of Gerontology (Abstracts), 31,* 221.

Manton, K.G., Corder, L.S., & Stallard, E. (1993). Estimates of change in chronic disability and institutional incidence and prevalence rates in the U.S. elderly population from the 1982, 1984, and 1989 National Long Term Care Survey. *Journal of Gerontology, 48,* S153-S166.

McArdle, W.D., Katch, F.I., & Katch, V.L. (2001). *Exercise physiology: Energy, nutrition, and human performance.* Baltimore: Lippincott Williams & Wilkins.

Morey, M.C., Pieper, C.F., & Cornoni-Huntley, J.C. (1998). Physical fitness and functional limitations in community-dwelling older adults. *Medicine and Science in Sports and Exercise, 30(5),* 715-723.

Nagi, S. (1991). Disability concepts revisited: Implication for prevention. In A. Pope & A.J. Tarlov (Eds.), *Disability in America: Toward a national agenda for prevention* (pp. 1309-1327). Washington, DC: National Academy Press.

National Institute on Aging. (2000). *Exercise: A guide from the National Institute on Aging*. NIA Information Center, P.O. Box 807. Gaithersburg, MD 20890-8057.

National Institutes of Health Consensus Development Conference Statement. (1988). Geriatric assessment methods for clinical decision-making. *Journal of the American Geriatrics Society, 36*, 342-347.

NHANES III (The National Health and Nutrition Examination Survey; Center for Disease Control; National Center for Health Statistics, 1996). http://www.cdc.gov/nchs/products/pubs/journal/journal03.htm [Accessed 05.30.04].

Osness, W.H. (1996). *Functional fitness for assessment of adults over 60 years*. Reston, VA: American Association for Health, Physical Education, Recreation and Dance. 36 pp.

Rantanen, T., Guralnik, J.M., Sakari-Rantala, R., Leveille, S., Simonsick, E.M., Ling, S., & Fried, L.P. (1999). Disability, physical activity, and muscle strength in older women: The Women's Health and Aging Study. *Archives of Physical Medicine and Rehabilitation, 80*, 130-135.

Reuben, D.B., Laliberte, L., Hiris, J., & Mor, V. (1990). A hierarchical exercise scale to measure function at the advanced activities of daily living (AADL) level. *Journal of American Geriatric Society, 38*, 855-861.

Reuben, D.B. & Solomon, D.H. (1989). Assessment in geriatrics: Of caveats and names. *Journal of the American Geriatrics Society, 37*, 570-572.

Reuben, D.B., & Sui, A.L. (1990). An objective measure of physical function of elderly outpatients: The physical performance test. *Journal of the American Geriatrics Society, 38*, 1108.

Rikli, R.E., & Jones, C.J. (1997). Assessing physical performance in independent older adults: Issues and guidelines. *Journal of Aging and Physical Activity, 5*, 244-261.

Rikli, R.E., & Jones, C.J. (2001). *Senior fitness test manual*. Champaign, IL: Human Kinetics.

Schnelle, J.F., MacRae, P.G., Ouslander, J.G., Simmons, S., & Nitta, M. (1995). Functional incidental training, mobility performance, and incontinence care with nursing home residents. *Journal of American Geriatric Society, 43*, 1356-1362.

Schroeder, J.M., Nau, K.L., Osness, W.H., & Potteiger, J.A. (1998). A comparison of life satisfaction, functional ability, physical characteristics, and activity level among older adults in various living settings. *Journal of Aging Physical Activity, 6*, 340-349.

Seeman, T.E., Berkman, L.F., Charpentier, P.A., Blazer, D.G., Albert, M.S., & Tinetti, M.E. (1995). Behavioral and psychosocial predictors of physical performance: MacArthur Studies of Successful Aging. *Journal of Gerontology: Medicine & Science, 50A*, M177-M183.

Shaulis, D., Golding, L.A., & Tandy, R.D. (1994). Reliability of the AAHPERD Functional Fitness Assessment across multiple practice sessions in older men and women. *Journal of Aging and Physical Activity, 2*, 273-279.

Shumway-Cook, A., Gruber, W., Baldwin, M., & Liao, S. (1997). The effect of multidimensional exercises on balance, mobility, and fall risk in community-dwelling older adults. *Physical Therapy, 77*, 46-57.

Simonsick, E.M., Lafferty, M.E., Phillips, C.L., Mendes de Leon, C.F., Kasl, S.V., Seeman, T.E., Fillenbaum, G., Hert, P., & Lemke, J.H. (1993). Risk due to inactivity in physically capable older adults. *American Journal of Public Health, 83*, 1443-1450.

Solomon, D.H., Judd, H.L., Sier, H.C., Rubenstein, L.Z., & Morley, J.E. (1988). New issues in geriatric care. *Annals of Internal Medicine, 108*, 725.

Spector, W.D., & Fleishman, J.A. (1998). Combining activities of daily living with instrumental activities of daily living to measure functional disability. *Journal of Gerontology: Social Sciences, 53B(1)*, S46-S57.

Stewart, A.L., Hays, R.D., Wells, K.B., Rogers, W.H., Spritzer, K.L., & Greenfield, S. (1994). Long-term functioning and well-being outcomes associated with physical activity and exercise in patients with chronic conditions in the medical outcomes study. *Journal of Clinical Epidemiology, 47*, 719-730.

Strawbridge, W.J., Shema, S.J., Balfour, J.L., Higby, H.R., & Kaplan, G.A. (1998). Antecedents of frailty over three decades in an older cohort. *Journal of Gerontology: Social Sciences, 53B*, S9-S16.

Svanborg, A. (1993). A medical-social intervention in a 70-year-old Swedish population: Is it possible to postpone functional decline in aging? *Journal of Gerontology, 48*, 84-88.

Tahara, J., Sakimoto, S., Uchino, K., & Matsumoto, F. (1990). *Longitudinal study on motor fitness tests for the aged*. In M. Kaneko (Ed.), Fitness for the aged, disabled, and industrial worker (pp. 15-17). Champaign, IL: Human Kinetics.

Tinetti, M.E. (1986). Performance-oriented assessment of mobility problems in elderly patients. *Journal of the American Geriatrics Society, 34*, 119-126.

Topp, R., & Stevenson, J.S. (1994). The effects of attendance and effort on outcomes among older adults in a long-term exercise program. *Research on Nursing Health, 17*, 15-24.

Verbrugge, L., & Jette, A.M. (1994). The disablement process. *Social Science Medicine, 38*, 1-14.

Vita, A.J., Terry, R.B., Hubert, H.B., & Fries, J.F. (1998). Aging, health risks, and cumulative disability. *New England Journal of Medicine, 338*, 1035-1041.

Vogt, M.T., Lauerman, W.C., Chirumbole, M., & Kuller, L.H. (2002). A community-based study of postmenopausal white women with back and leg pain: Health status and limitation in physical activity. *Journal of Gerontology: Biological Science & Medical Science, 57*, M544-M550.

Voorrips, L.E., Lemmink, K.A.P.M., van Heuvelen, M.J.G., Bult, P., & van Staveren, W.A. (1993). The physical condition of elderly women differing in habitual physical activity. *Medicine and Science in Sports and Exercise, 25*, 1152-1157.

Wilkins, R., & Adams, O.B. (1983). Health expectancy in Canada, late 1970s: Demographic, regional, and social dimensions. *American Journal of Public Health, 73*, 1075.

Williams, J.H., & Greene, L.S. (1990). *Williams-Greene Test of Physical/Motor Function.* Laboratory report from the Motor Development/Motor Control laboratory, Department of Exercise Science, University of South Carolina, Columbia.

Young, D.R., Masaki, K.H., & Curb, J.D. (1995). Associations of physical activity with performance-based and self-reported physical functioning in older men: The Honolulu Heart Program. *Journal of the American Geriatrics Society, 43*, 845-854.

Zedlewski, S.R., Barnes, R.O., Burt, M.R., McBride, T.D., & Meyer, J.A. (1990). *The needs of the elderly in the 21st century.* Washington, DC: Urban Institute Press.

Chapter 12

Anton, M.M., Spirduso, W.W., & Tanaka, H. (2004). Age-associated declines in anaerobic muscular performance: Insight from weightlifting and powerlifting records. *Medicine and Science of Exercise and Sports, 36*, 143-147.

Åstrand, P.O., & Rodahl, K. (1977). *Textbook of work physiology.* New York: McGraw-Hill.

Barnard, C. (1992, February-March). Half a mountain . . . the Matterhorn. *Modern Maturity,* pp. 43-49, 66.

Bouchard, C., Thibault, M.C., & Jobin, J. (1981). Advances in selected areas of work physiology. *Yearbook of Physical Anthropology, 24*, 275-286.

Concept II World Rankings. (1991). *Current world records for 2,500 meters on the Concept II Rowing Ergometer as of April 15, 1991.* Morrisville, VT: Concept II.

Craig, A.B., & Pendergast, D.R. (1979). Relationship of stroke rate, distance per stroke, and variation in competitive swimming. *Medicine and Science in Sports and Exercise, 11*, 278-283.

Donato, A.J., Tench, K., Glueck, D.H., Seals, D.R., Eskurza, I., & Tanaka, H. (2003). Declines in physiological functional capacity with age: A longitudinal study in peak swimming performance. *Journal of Applied Physiology, 94*, 764-769.

Dreckman, M. (1993). Austin woman rocks and rolls on 95th birthday. *Austin American Statesman,* Lifestyle Section, p. 1, December 9.

Ericsson, K.A. (1990). Peak performance and age: An examination of peak performance in sports. In P.B. Baltes & M.M. Baltes (Eds.), *Successful aging: Perspectives from the behavioral sciences.* Cambridge: Cambridge University Press.

Foster, C., Green, M.A., Snyder, A.C., Thompson, N.N. (1993). Physiological responses during simulated competition. *Medicine and Science in Sports and Exercise, 25*, 877-882.

Guinness Book of World Records (2002). http://www.guinnessworldrecords.com/index.asp?id=45714.

Hagerman, F.C. (1994). Applied physiology of rowing. In D.R. Lamb & H.H. Knuttgen (Eds.), *Perspectives in exercise science and sports medicine: Vol. 7. Physiology and nutrition of competitive sport.* Indianapolis: Brown & Benchmark.

Hains, L. (1989, October). Rarities. *Golf Digest,* p. S-105.

Hartley, A.A., & Hartley, J.T. (1984). Performance changes in champion swimmers aged 30-84 years. *Experimental Aging Research, 10*, 141-147.

Hickok, R. (1971). *Who was who in American sports.* New York: Hawthorn Books.

Holloszy, J.O., & Kohrt, W.M. (1995). Exercise. In E.J. Masaro (Ed.), Aging. *Handbook of physiology* (Section 11, Chapter 24, pp.633-666). Bethesda, MD: American Physiological Society.

International Federation of Weight Lifting, 2002 records. Website: www.iat.uni-leipzig.de/scripts/dbneight.exe?site=2&wkid=3000002.

Kardong, D. (1991). Young at heart. *Runner's World, 26*, 29, 73.

Kovar, M.G., & LaCroix, A.Z. (1987). Aging in the eighties, ability to perform work-related activities. *National Center for Health Statistics Advance Data, 136*, 1-12.

Langford, W.M. (1987). *Legends of baseball: An oral history of the game's golden age.* South Bend, IN: Diamond Communications.

Larsson, L., Grimby, G., & Karlsson, J. (1979). Muscle strength and speed of movement in relation to age and muscle morphology. *Journal of Applied Physiology, 46*, 1979.

Lynch, N.A., Metter, E.J., Lindle, R.S., Fozard, J.L., Tobin, J.D., Roy, T.A., Fleg, J.L., & Hurley, B.F. (1999). Muscle quality. I. Age-associated differences between arm and leg muscle groups. *Journal of Applied Physiology, 86*, 188-194.

Masters Age Records 1990 Edition. (1991). Available from National Masters News, P.O. Box 5185, Pasadena, CA 91107.

Masters Age Records 2002 Edition. (2003) Approved by the USA Track & Field (USATF) Masters Track & Field Committee and available from the National Masters News, P.O. Box 50098, Eugene, OR 97405.

Masters National Rowing Regatta at Lake Merrit. (2000). Archived rowing records of the 2000 National Masters Rowing Championships, http://www.rowlakemerritt.org/

McArdle, W.D., Katch, F.I., & Katch, V.L. (2001). *Exercise physiology: Energy, nutrition and human performance.* New York: Lippincott Williams & Wilkins.

McDonagh, M.J.N., White, M.J., & Davies, C.T.M. (1984). Different effects of ageing on the mechanical properties of human arm and leg muscles. *Gerontology, 30*, 49-54.

Meltzer, D.E. (1994). Age dependence of Olympic weightlifting ability. *Medicine and Science in Sports and Exercise, 26*, 1053-1067.

Moore, K. (1992). The times of their lives. *Runner's World, 20*, 44-47.

Pate, R.R., Sparling, P.B., Wilson, G.E., Cureton, K.J., & Miller, B.J. (1987). Cardiorespiratory and metabolic responses to submaximal and maximal exercise in elite women distance runners. *International Journal of Sports Medicine, 8*, 91-95.

Phillips, S.K., Rook, K.M., Siddle, N.C., Bruce, S.A., & Woledge, R.C. (1993). Muscle weakness in women occurs at an earlier age than in men, but strength is preserved by hormone replacement therapy. *Clinical Science (London) 84*, 95-98.

Riegel, P.S. (1981). Athletic records and human endurance. *American Scientist, 69*, 285-290.

Seiler, K.S., Spirduso, W.W., & Martin, J.D. (1998). Gender differences in rowing performance and power with aging. *Medicine and Science in Sports and Exercise, 30*, 121-127.

Skelton, D.A., Greig, C.A., Davies, J.M., & Young, A. (1994). Strength, power and related functional ability of healthy people aged 65-89 years. *Age and Ageing, 23*, 371-377.

Sports Illustrated. (2002-2003). Faces in the crowd. Dec 30, 2002- Jan 6, 2003, Double Issue, Vol 97 (26), 38. Also available on http://sportsillustrated.cnn.com/si_online/faces/2002/1230/.

Stones, M.J., & Kozma, A. (1980). Adult age trends in record running performances. *Experimental Aging Research, 6*, 407-416.

Stones, M.J., & Kozma, A. (1981). Adult trends in athletic performance. *Experimental Aging Research, 7*, 269-280.

Stones, M.J., & Kozma, A. (1982a). Cross-sectional, longitudinal, and secular age trends in athletic performances. *Experimental Aging Research, 8*, 185-188.

Stones, M.J., & Kozma, A. (1982b). Sex differences in changes with age in record running performances. *Canadian Journal on Aging, 1*, 12-16.

Stones, M.J., & Kozma, A. (1984a). In response to Hartley and Hartley. Cross-sectional age trends in swimming records; decline is greater at the longer distances. *Experimental Aging Research, 10*, 159-150.

Stones, M.J., & Kozma, A. (1984b). Longitudinal trends in track and field performances. *Experimental Aging Research, 10*, 107-110.

Stones, M.J., & Kozma, A. (1985). Physical performance. In N. Charness (Ed.), *Aging and human performance* (pp. 261-292). London: Wiley.

Stones, M.J., & Kozma, A. (1986a). Age by distance effects in running and swimming records: A note on methodology. *Experimental Aging Research, 12*, 203-206.

Stones, M.J., & Kozma, A. (1986b). Age trends in maximal physical performance: Comparison and evaluation of models. *Experimental Aging Research, 12*, 207-215.

Tanaka, H., & Seals, D.R. (1997). Age and gender interactions in physiological functional capacity: Insight from swimming performance. *Journal of Applied Physiology, 82*, 846-851.

United States Cycling Federation. (2002). *Masters National Records*, pp. 127-132. Available on line: www.usacycling.org [accessed 07.06.04].

United States Cycling Federation. (1990). *Rule book, United States Cycling Federation.* Colorado Springs: Author.

U.S.A. Powerlifting Federation. (1991). www.usa powerlifting.com

U.S.A. Powerlifting Federation. (2003). www.usa powerlifting.com

U.S.A. Single Age Road Racing Records (2002). Available from www.runningusa.org/index_ rankings.html

World Weightlifting Federation. (2000). www.iwf.net/ wrec/world.html [accessed 10.27.04].

Index

Note: The italicized *f* and *t* following page numbers refer to figures and tables, respectively.

challenges to 236
death of friends and loved ones 236
fears of the elderly 236
fitness, exercise interventions, and
positive affect 238-239
fitness and negative affect 239,
239f, 240-244
health and emotional well-being
237, 238
losses 237
mood 237
risk factors for suicide in elderly 240
using exercise to control depression
242
epidermis 82
Erasmus, Darwin 14
exercise 213
exercise characteristics and well-being
acute or habitual exercise exposure
254, 255f
characteristics of exercise 254
effects of environment 255
negative effects of exercise 255-256
questions regarding 254
type of exercise 254
exercise effects on cardiovascular
function
average maximal oxygen consumption 93, 93f, 94
blood constituents, flow, and pressure, effects on 96
cardiac output and O2 difference
94-95, 96
consistent exercise, importance of
92, 93
exercise reducing resting blood pressure, mechanisms 96
maximal aerobic capacity 93
percent of inactive adults 93, 93f
sexual function and physical activity
95
exercise intervention studies
controlled processing 217
executive control 217-218
exercise interventions affecting categories of cognitive function 218,
218f
processing speed 216
visuospatial processing 216, 217

F
falling, when balance fails
medication and falling 151
prevalence of 150
risk factors contributing to 151
fall risk assessment 151-152
falls, prevention of
environmental modifications 153
exercise 152
health promotion and education
153-154
hip protector garments 154
medication withdrawal 154
multifactorial risk factor assessment
and intervention 153

fitness and cognitive function
composite score of 220, 221, 221f
conceptual frameworks of 217
electrophysiological evidence of fit-
ness-cognition relationship 218,
219, 219f, 220, 220f
exercise intervention studies 216,
217-218
global intelligence 220
meta-analysis of fitness effects on
cognition 219
psychological outcomes and cognitive function 214f, 221
relationships of fitness to cognition
studies 216
research studies 215-216
flexibility
description and measurement of
77-79, 79f, 80
exercise effects on 79-80
Floyd, Raymond 305
force plate 141
frailty
assessment of 270
components of 270
description of 269
performance tests 271, 272t
surveys, inventories, diaries 270,
270t, 271
Williams-Greene classification
schema, upper extremity
function/mobility 271
functional health 212
functional health status 234

G
gait
age-associated changes in 149, 150,
150t
cycle, overview 146, 147-148, 147f
measuring 150
gender differences and age
female survival advantage 11, 12f
gender gap 12
genetics theory 12
hormonal differences 12-13
social explanations 13, 14, 14f
generalized slowing theory, challenges to
physiological evidence of process-
specific slowing 169, 169f, 170
selective slowing in cognitive-motor
experts 171
sequential effects of process-specific
slowing 170, 170f
genetic theories of aging
controversy of 16
death gene 15
gene-programmed aging process 15
Hayflick limit 15
telomere hypothesis 15, 16
*Geriatrics: The Diseases of Old Age and
Their Treatment* (Nascher) 14
global perceptions of well-being and
life satisfaction

health and global well-being 248,
249f
life satisfaction, components of 248
gradual imbalance theories
autoimmunity theory 18
description of 17
genetic and environmental stresses
affecting life maintenance reserve
18, 19f
immunological theories 18
neuroendocrine regulatory systems
17-18
regulatory system 18

H
handwriting
importance of 196, 197
number tracing 198, 198f
performance 198, 199f
speed 197, 198f
Hayflick, Leonard 15
Hayflick limit 15
Hayward, Wally 289
health 212
health, exercise, and cognitive function
cognition relationship for older
adults 231
cognitive function, health and physical activity effects on 213-222
concepts of 212-213
fitness beneficial to cognitive function, process 229-231
physical activity beneficial to cognition 222-229
health-related quality of life
exercise on well-being 250-254
exercise related to well-being, characteristics of 254-256
physical function, physical activity,
fitness, and exercise 248-249, 250
quality of life 234-235
well-being 235-249
heart disease (cardiovascular disease)
cholesterol 97
coronary arteries 97
exercise program for 98, 99
myocardial infarction 97
relative risk of death 98, 98f
risk, achievable reductions 98
risk factors 97, 97t
surgeon general's report on physical
activity and health 99
heart function
blood pressure 92
cardiac output (Q) 91
description of 90
heart rate 91, 91f
National Heart, Lung, and Blood
Institute 2004 blood pressure
guidelines 92
oxygen that is circulated 91-92
stroke volume (SV) 91
Hippocrates 14
hip strategy 133

369